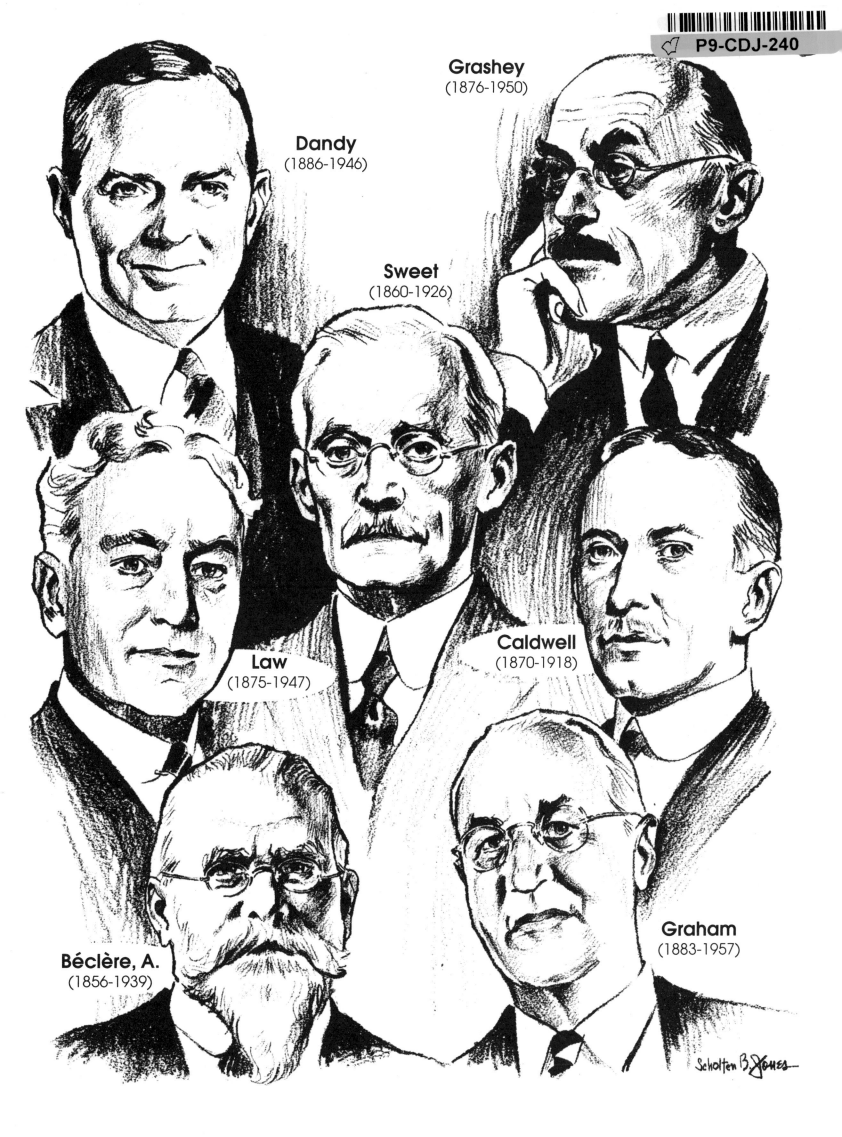

Grashey
(1876-1950)

Dandy
(1886-1946)

Sweet
(1860-1926)

Law
(1875-1947)

Caldwell
(1870-1918)

Béclère, A.
(1856-1939)

Graham
(1883-1957)

Scholten B. Jones

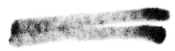

Volume Two

MERRILL'S ATLAS *of*

RADIOGRAPHIC POSITIONING & PROCEDURES

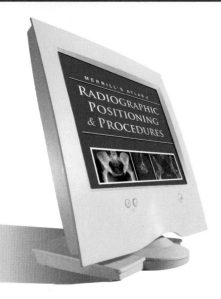
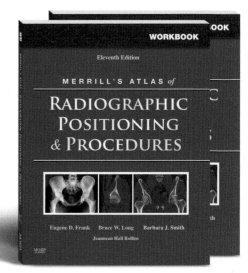
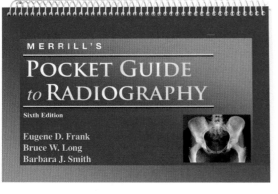

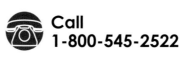
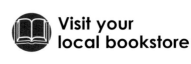
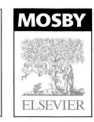

Eleventh Edition
Volume Two

MERRILL'S ATLAS *of*

RADIOGRAPHIC POSITIONING & PROCEDURES

Eugene D. Frank, MA, RT(R), FASRT, FAERS

Director, Radiography Program
Riverland Community College
Austin, Minnesota;
Retired, Assistant Professor of Radiology
Mayo Clinic College of Medicine
Rochester, Minnesota

Bruce W. Long, MS, RT(R)(CV), FASRT

Director and Associate Professor
Radiologic Sciences Programs
Indiana University School of Medicine
Indianapolis, Indiana

Barbara J. Smith, MS, RT(R)(QM), FASRT

Instructor, Radiologic Technology
Medical Imaging Department
Portland Community College
Portland, Oregon

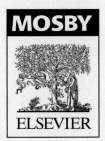

MOSBY

ELSEVIER

11830 Westline Industrial Drive
St. Louis, Missouri 63146

MERRILL'S ATLAS OF RADIOGRAPHIC POSITIONING AND PROCEDURES, EDITION 11
Volume Two

Three-Volume Set

ISBN-13: 978-0-323-04211-6
ISBN-10: 0-323-04211-2
ISBN-13: 978-0-323-03317-6
ISBN-10: 0-323-03317-2

Notice

Knowledge and best practice in this field are constantly changing. As new research and experience broaden our knowledge, changes in practice, treatment, and drug therapy may become necessary or appropriate. Readers are advised to check the most current information provided (i) on procedures featured or (ii) by the manufacturer of each product to be administered, to verify the recommended dose or formula, the method and duration of administration, and contraindications. It is the responsibility of the practitioner, relying on his or her own experience and knowledge of the patient, to make diagnoses, to determine dosages and the best treatment for each individual patient, and to take all appropriate safety precautions. To the fullest extent of the law, neither the Publisher nor the Authors assume any liability for any injury and/or damage to persons or property arising out or related to any use of the material contained in this book.

The Publisher

ISBN-13: 978-0-323-04211-6 (Volume Two)
ISBN-13: 978-0-323-03317-6 (Three-Volume Set)
ISBN-10: 0-323-04211-2 (Volume Two)
ISBN-10: 0-323-03317-2 (Three-Volume Set)

Publisher: Andrew Allen
Executive Editor: Jeanne Wilke
Senior Developmental Editor: Linda Woodard
Publishing Services Manager: Patricia Tannian
Project Manager: Kristine Feeherty
Cover Designer: Paula Ruckenford
Text Designer: Paula Ruckenford
Medical Illustrator: Jeanne Robertson

Printed in the United States of America

Last digit is the print number: 9 8 7 6 5 4 3

PREVIOUS AUTHORS

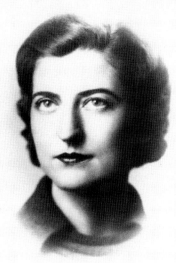

Vinita Merrill

1905-1977

Vinita Merrill had the foresight, talent, and knowledge to write the first
edition of this atlas in 1949. The text she wrote became known
as *Merrill's Atlas* in honor of the significant contribution she made
to the profession of radiography and in acknowledgment of the benefit
of her work to generations of students and practitioners.

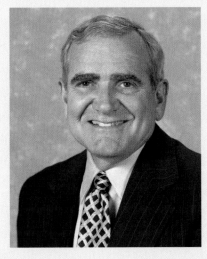

Philip Ballinger became the author of *Merrill's Atlas* in its fifth edition,
which published in 1982. He served as author through the tenth edition, helping to launch successful careers for thousands of students
who have learned radiographic positioning from *Merrill's*. Phil is now
Assistant Professor Emeritus in the Radiologic Technology Division of
the School of Allied Medical Professions at The Ohio State University.
In 1995, he retired after a 25-year career as Radiography Program
Director, and after ably guiding *Merrill's Atlas* through six editions, he
retired as *Merrill's* author. Phil continues to be involved in professional
activities, such as speaking engagements at state, national, and international meetings.

AUTHORS

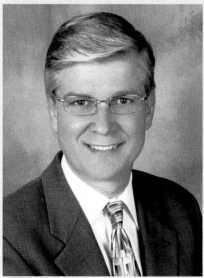

Eugene D. Frank, MA, RT(R), FASRT, FAERS, retired from the Mayo Clinic/Foundation in 2001 after 31 years of employment. He was Assistant Professor of Radiology in the College of Medicine and Director of the Radiography Program. He continues to work in radiography education as Director of the Radiography Program at Riverland Community College, Austin, Minnesota. He frequently presents at professional gatherings throughout the world and has held leadership positions in state, national, and international organizations. He is the coauthor of two radiography textbooks (*Quality Control in Diagnostic Imaging* and *Radiography Essentials for Limited Practice),* two radiography workbooks, and two book chapters, in addition to being coauthor of the atlas. The eleventh edition is Gene's third edition as coauthor.

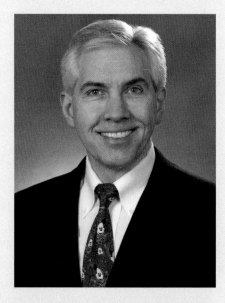

Bruce W. Long, MS, RT(R)(CV), FASRT, is Director and Associate Professor of the Indiana University Radiologic Sciences Programs, where he has taught for 20 years. A life member of the Indiana Society of Radiologic Technologists, he frequently presents at state and national professional meetings. His publication activities include 28 articles in national professional journals and two books, *Orthopaedic Radiography* and *Radiography Essentials for Limited Practice.* The eleventh edition is Bruce's first as coauthor of the atlas.

Barbara J. Smith, MS, RT(R)(QM), FASRT, is an instructor in the Radiologic Technology program at Portland Community College, where she has taught for 22 years. The Oregon Society of Radiologic Technologists inducted her as a life member in 2003. She presents at state, regional, and national meetings and is involved in professional activities at these levels. Her publication activities include articles, book reviews, and chapter contributions. The eleventh edition is Barb's first as coauthor of the atlas.

ADVISORY BOARD

This edition of *Merrill's Atlas* benefits from the expertise of a special advisory board. The following board members have provided professional input and advice and have helped the authors make decisions about atlas content throughout the preparation of the eleventh edition:

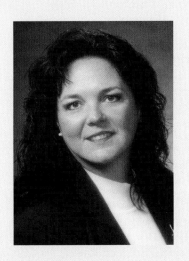

Valerie J. Palm, RT(R), ACR, ID, MEd, FCAMRT

Instructor, Medical Radiography Program
School of Health
British Columbia Institute of Technology
Burnaby, British Columbia

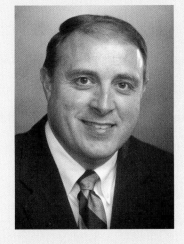

Roger A. Preston, MSRS, RT(R)

Program Director, Reid Hospital & Health Care Services
School of Radiologic Technology
Richmond, Indiana

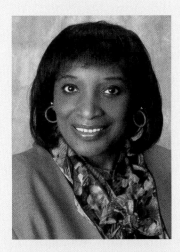

Ms. Johnnie B. Moore, MEd, RT(R)

Chair, Radiography Program
Barnes-Jewish College of Nursing and Allied Health
St. Louis, Missouri

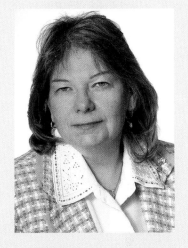

Diedre Costic, MPS, RT(R)(M)

Associate Professor and Department Chair, Diagnostic Imaging Program
Orange County Community College
Middletown, New York

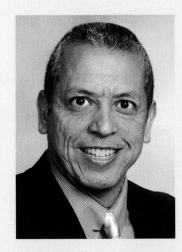

Joe A. Garza, MS, RT(R)

Associate Professor, Radiography Program
Montgomery College
Conroe, Texas

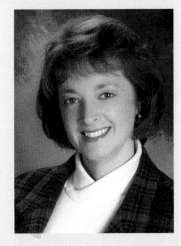

Andrea J. Cornuelle, MS, RT(R)

Associate Professor, Radiologic Technology Program
Northern Kentucky University
Highland Heights, Kentucky

CONTRIBUTORS

Valerie F. Andolina, RT(R)(M)
Imaging Technology Manager
Elizabeth Wende Breast Clinic
Rochester, New York

Albert Aziza, BHA, BSc, MRT(R)
Manager, Imaging Guided Therapy
The Hospital for Sick Children
Toronto, Canada

Peter J. Barger, MS, RT(R)(CT)
Radiography Program Director
College of Nursing and Health Sciences
Cape Girardeau, Missouri

Terri Bruckner, MA, RT(R)(CV)
Clinical Instructor and Clinical
    Coordinator
The Ohio State University
Columbus, Ohio

Thomas H. Burke, RT(R)(CV), FAVIR
Clinical Manager
Microvention, Inc.
Grosse Pointe Woods, Michigan

Leila A. Bussman-Yeakel, BS, RT(R)(T)
Director, Radiation Therapy Program
Mayo School of Health Sciences
Mayo Clinic College of Medicine
Rochester, Minnesota

JoAnn P. Caudill, RT(R)(M)(BD),CDT
Bone Health Program Manager
Erickson Retirement Communities
Catonsville, Maryland

Ellen Charkot, MRT(R)
Chief Technologist, Diagnostic Imaging
    Department
The Hospital for Sick Children
Toronto, Ontario

Sharon A. Coffey, MS, RT(R)
Instructor in Medical Radiography
Houston Community College
Coleman College of Health Sciences
Houston, Texas

**Luann J. Culbreth, MEd,
RT(R)(MR)(QM), CRA, FSMRT**
Director of Imaging Services
Baylor Regional Medical Center at Plano
Plano, Texas

**Sandra L. Hagen-Ansert, MS, RDMS,
RDCS, FSDMS**
Scripps Clinic, Torrey Pines
Cardiac Sonographer
San Diego, California

Nancy L. Hockert, BS, ASCP, CNMT
Program Director, Nuclear Medicine
    Technology
Assistant Professor
Mayo Clinic College of Medicine
Rochester, Minnesota

Steven C. Jensen, PhD, RT(R)
Director, Radiologic Sciences Program
Southern Illinois University
Carbondale, Illinois

Timothy J. Joyce, RT(R)(CV)
Clinical Group Manager
Microvention, Inc.
Dearborn, Michigan

Sara A. Kaderlik, RT(R)
Special Procedures Radiographer
Providence St. Vincent Cardiovascular Lab
Beaverton, Oregon

**Eric P. Matthews, MSEd,
RT(R)(CV)(MR), EMT**
Visiting Assistant Professor, Radiologic
    Sciences Program
Southern Illinois University
Carbondale, Illinois

Elton A. Mosman, MBA, CNMT
Clinical Coordinator, Nuclear Medicine
    Program
Mayo Clinic College of Medicine
Rochester, Minnesota

Sandra J. Nauman, BS, RT(R)(M)
Clinical Coordinator, Radiography
    Program
Riverland Community College
Austin, Minnesota

**Paula Pate-Schloder, MS,
RT(R)(CV)(CT)(VI)**
Associate Professor, Medical Imaging
    Department
College Misericordia
Dallas, Pennsylvania

Joel A. Permar, RT(R)
Surgical Radiographer
University of Alabama Hospital
Birmingham, Alabama

**Jeannean Hall Rollins, MRC,
BSRT(R)(CV)**
Associate Professor, Radiologic Sciences
Arkansas State University
Jonesboro, Arkansas

Kari J. Wetterlin, MA, RT(R)
Unit Supervisor, Surgical Radiology
Mayo Clinic/Foundation
Rochester, Minnesota

Gayle K. Wright, BS, RT(R)(MR)(CT)
Instructor, Radiologic Technology Program
Portland Community College
Portland, Oregon

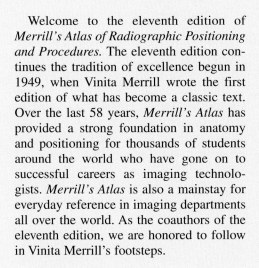

PREFACE

Welcome to the eleventh edition of *Merrill's Atlas of Radiographic Positioning and Procedures*. The eleventh edition continues the tradition of excellence begun in 1949, when Vinita Merrill wrote the first edition of what has become a classic text. Over the last 58 years, *Merrill's Atlas* has provided a strong foundation in anatomy and positioning for thousands of students around the world who have gone on to successful careers as imaging technologists. *Merrill's Atlas* is also a mainstay for everyday reference in imaging departments all over the world. As the coauthors of the eleventh edition, we are honored to follow in Vinita Merrill's footsteps.

Learning and Perfecting Positioning Skills

Merrill's Atlas has an established tradition of helping students learn and perfect their positioning skills. After covering preliminary steps in radiography, radiation protection, and terminology in introductory chapters, *Merrill's* then teaches anatomy and positioning in separate chapters for each bone group or organ system. The student learns to position the patient properly so that the resulting radiograph provides the information the physician needs to correctly diagnose the patient's problem. The atlas presents this information for commonly requested projections, as well as those less commonly requested, making it the most comprehensive text and reference available.

The third volume of the atlas provides basic information about a variety of special imaging modalities, such as mobile, surgical, geriatrics, computed tomography, cardiac catheterization, magnetic resonance imaging, ultrasound, nuclear medicine technology, and radiation therapy.

Merrill's Atlas is not only a sound resource for students to learn from but also an indispensable reference as they move into the clinical environment and ultimately into their practice as imaging professionals.

New to This Edition

Since the first edition of *Merrill's Atlas* in 1949, many changes have occurred. This new edition incorporates many significant changes designed not only to reflect the technologic progress and advancements in the profession but also to meet the needs of today's radiography students. The major changes in this edition are highlighted as follows.

NEW ORTHOPEDIC PROJECTION

One new projection, the Coyle Method for demonstrating the elbow after trauma, has been added to this edition. Also added is a modification of the Judet Method of demonstrating the acetabulum on trauma patients.

NEW ABBREVIATIONS BOXES AND ADDENDUM

Each chapter in this edition contains all the essential abbreviations used in the chapter that have not been introduced in previous chapters. Students become familiar with the common abbreviations, which are then used throughout the chapter. All the abbreviations used in Volumes 1 and 2 are summarized in addendums at the end of the volume.

NEW CHAPTER AND REVISED CHAPTERS

A new chapter on the theory and use of compensating filters is included in this edition. The compensating filters chapter contains high-quality radiographs made with and without filters to demonstrate the positive effect of the filter. In addition, projections that benefit from the use of a filter are identified in the text with the use of a special icon and heading titled "Compensating Filter." The new filter icon is shown here:

◥ COMPENSATING FILTER

The Sectional Anatomy chapter in Volume 3 had been entirely revised with new high-resolution CT and MRI images and correlating art. This chapter will provide instructors and students with information needed for the proposed ASRT curriculum updates.

The Geriatrics chapter has been updated to include patient positioning photographs and radiographs with common pathology.

DIGITAL RADIOGRAPHY UPDATED

Because of the rapid expansion and acceptance of computed radiography (CR) and direct digital radiography (DR), either selected positioning considerations and modifications or special instructions are indicated where necessary. A special icon alerts the reader to digital notes. The icon is shown here:
DIGITAL RADIOGRAPHY

ESSENTIAL PROJECTIONS

Essential projections are identified with the special icon shown here: ✳
One new projection has been designated essential for this edition: the Coyle Method for demonstrating the elbow for trauma. Essential projections are those most frequently performed and determined to be necessary for competency of entry-level practitioners. Of the more than 375 projections described in this atlas, 184 have been identified as essential based on the results of two extensive surveys performed in the United States and Canada.[1]

OBSOLETE PROJECTIONS DELETED

Projections identified as obsolete by the authors and the advisory board have been deleted. A summary is provided at the beginning of any chapter containing deleted projections so that the reader may refer to previous editions for information. Several projections have been deleted in this edition, most of them in the cranial chapters.

CHAPTERS DELETED OR MERGED

The chapters "Radiation Protection" and "Computed Radiography" have been eliminated from this edition of the atlas because these chapters are more closely aligned to physics and exposure and are best studied in comprehensive texts devoted to these topics. The Temporal Bone chapter of the skull has been merged with the general Skull chapter. The Digital Angiography chapter had been merged with the Circulatory System chapter. The Positron Emission Tomography chapter has been merged with the Nuclear Medicine chapter. These merges will enable students to more easily learn the concepts presented in these chapters.

[1]Ballinger PW, Glassner JL: Positioning competencies for radiography graduates, *Radiol Technol* 70:181, 1998.

NEW 3D LINE ART

Many new line illustrations have been added to this edition. Each is designed to clarify anatomy or projections that are difficult to visualize. More than 24 new line art figures appear throughout the three volumes, including the Compensating Filters chapter of Volume 1.

NEW RADIOGRAPHS

Nearly every chapter contains new and additional optimum radiographs, including many that demonstrate pathology. With the addition of more than 30 new radiographic images, the eleventh edition has the most comprehensive collection of high-quality radiographs available to students and practitioners.

NEW MRI AND CT IMAGES INTEGRATED INTO THE TEXT

Nearly every chapter in Volumes 1 and 2 contains new MRI or CT images in the anatomy section to aid the reader in learning radiographic anatomy. These 40 images not only help the student to learn the exact size, shape, and placement of anatomical parts, but also help the reader become familiar with images produced by these commonly used modalities.

NEW PATIENT PHOTOGRAPHY

More than 35 new color anatomy, patient positioning, or procedure-related photographs have been added. These added or replacement photographs aid students in learning radiography positioning concepts.

Learning Aids for the Student

POCKET GUIDE TO RADIOGRAPHY

A new edition of *Merrill's Pocket Guide to Radiography* complements the revision of *Merrill's Atlas*. In addition to instructions for positioning the patient and the body part for all the essential projections, the new pocket guide includes information on digital radiography and automatic exposure control (AEC). kVp information has been added. Tabs have been added to help the user locate the beginning of each section. Space is provided for writing department techniques specific to the user.

RADIOGRAPHIC ANATOMY, POSITIONING, AND PROCEDURES WORKBOOK

The new edition of this two-volume workbook retains most of the features of the previous editions: anatomy labeling exercises, positioning exercises, self-tests, and an answer key. The exercises include labeling of anatomy on drawings and radiographs, crossword puzzles, matching, short answers, and true/false. At the end of each chapter is a multiple-choice test to help students assess their comprehension of the whole chapter. New to this edition are exercises for the Pediatrics, Geriatrics, Mobile, Surgical, and Computed Tomography chapters in Volume 3. Also new to this edition are more image evaluations to give students additional opportunities to evaluate radiographs for proper positioning and more positioning questions to complement the workbook's strong anatomy review. Exercises in these chapters will help students learn the theory and concepts of these special techniques with greater ease.

Teaching Aids for the Instructor

INSTRUCTOR'S ELECTRONIC RESOURCE (IER)

This comprehensive resource provides valuable tools, such as teaching strategies, power point slides, and an electronic test bank, for teaching an anatomy and positioning class. The test bank includes more than 1500 questions, each coded by category and level of difficulty. Four exams are already compiled within the test bank to be used "as is" at the instructor's discretion. The instructor also has the option of building new tests as often as desired by pulling questions from the pool or using a combination of questions from the test bank and questions that the instructor adds.

All the images, photographs, and line illustrations in *Merrill's Atlas* are also available on the Electronic Image Collection on the IER CD-ROM.

More information about the IER is available from an Elsevier sales representative.

MOSBY'S RADIOGRAPHY ONLINE

Mosby's Radiography Online: Anatomy and Positioning is a well-developed online course companion that includes animations with narration and interactive activities and exercises to assist in the understanding of anatomy and positioning. Used in conjunction with the *Merrill's Atlas* textbook, it offers greater learning opportunities while accommodating diverse learning styles and circumstances. This unique program promotes problem-based learning with the goal of developing critical thinking skills that will be needed in the clinical setting.

EVOLVE—ONLINE COURSE MANAGEMENT

Evolve is an interactive learning environment designed to work in coordination with *Merrill's Atlas*. Instructors may use Evolve to provide an Internet-based course component that reinforces and expands on the concepts delivered in class.

Evolve may be used to publish the class syllabus, outlines, and lecture notes; set up "virtual office hours" and e-mail communication; share important dates and information through the online class Calendar; and encourage student participation through Chat Rooms and Discussion Boards. Evolve allows instructors to post exams and manage their grade books online. For more information, visit http://www.evolve.elsevier.com or contact an Elsevier sales representative.

We hope you will find this edition of *Merrill's Atlas of Radiographic Positioning and Procedures* the best ever. Input from generations of readers has helped to keep the atlas strong through ten editions, and we welcome your comments and suggestions. We are constantly striving to build on Vinita Merrill's work, and we trust that she would be proud and pleased to know that the work she began 58 years ago is still so appreciated and valued by the imaging sciences community.

Eugene D. Frank
Bruce W. Long
Barbara J. Smith

ACKNOWLEDGMENTS

In preparing for the eleventh edition, our advisory board continually provided professional expertise and aid in decision making on the revision of this edition. The advisory board members are listed on p. vii. We are most grateful for their input and contributions to this edition of the atlas.

The new Coyle Method for demonstrating the elbow for trauma was written by **Tammy Curtis, MS, RT(R),** from Northwestern State University, Shreveport, Louisiana. Ms. Curtis also performed the research and wrote all of the abbreviations for this edition of the atlas.

Special thanks goes out to a former student and 3D reconstruction specialist, **J. Louis Rankin, BS, RT(R)(MR),** from Indiana University Hospital, Indianapolis, Indiana, for the significant amount of time he spent assisting in acquiring new CT and MRI images used in the non–Sectional Anatomy chapters in the atlas.

Reviewers

The group of radiography professionals listed below reviewed aspects of this edition of the atlas and made many insightful suggestions for strengthening the atlas. We are most appreciative of their willingness to lend their expertise.

Kenneth Bontrager, MA, RT(R)
Radiography Author
Sun City West, Arizona

Kari Buchanan, BS, RT(R)
Mayo Clinic Foundation
Rochester, Minnesota

Barry Burns, MS, RT(R), DABR
University of North Carolina
Chapel Hill, North Carolina

Linda Cox, MS, RT(R)(MR)CT)
Indiana University School of Medicine
Indianapolis, Indiana

Tammy Curtis, MS, RT(R)
Northwestern State University
Shreveport, Louisiana

Timothy Daly, BS, RT(R)
Mayo Clinic Foundation
Rochester, Minnesota

Dan Ferlic, RT(R)
Ferlic Filters
White Bear Lake, Minnesota

Ginger Griffin, RT(R), FASRT
Baptist Medical Center
Jacksonville, Florida

Henrique da Guia Costa, MBA, RT(R)
Radiographer
Radiography Consultant
Lisbon, Portugal

Dimitris Koumoranos, MSc, RT(R)(CT)(MR)
Radiographer, General Hospital Elpis
Athens, Greece

Seiji Nishio, BA, RT(R)
Radiographer, Komazawa University
Tokyo, Japan

Rosanne Paschal, PhD, RT(R)
College of DuPage
Glen Ellyn, Illinois

Susan Robinson, MS, RT(R)
Indiana University School of Medicine
Indianapolis, Indiana

Lavonne Rohn, RT(R)
Mankato Clinic
Mankato, Minnesota

Jeannean Hall Rollins, MRC, BSRT(R)(CV)
Associate Professor, Radiologic Sciences
Arkansas State University
Jonesboro, Arkansas

Carole South-Winter, MEd, RT(R), CNMT
Reclaiming Youth International
Lennox, South Dakota

Richard Terrass, MEd, RT(R)
Massachusetts General Hospital
Boston, Massachusetts

Beth Vealé, MEd, RT(R)(QM)
Midwestern State University
Wichita Falls, Texas

CONTENTS

Volume Two

MERRILL'S ATLAS *of*

RADIOGRAPHIC POSITIONING & PROCEDURES

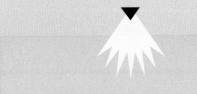

11

LONG BONE MEASUREMENT

Leg measurement showing that the right leg is shorter than the left leg.

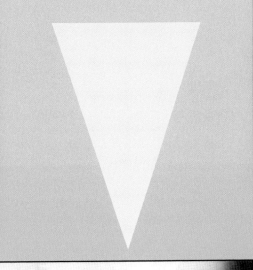

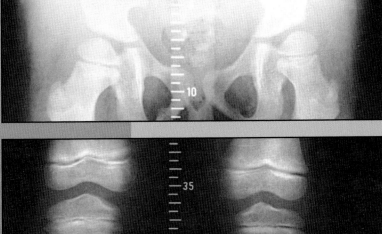

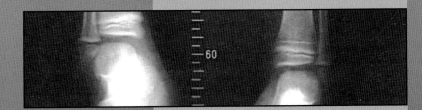

Radiography provides the most reliable means of obtaining accurate measurements of the length of long bones, specifically length differences between the two sides. Although studies are occasionally made of the upper limbs, radiography is most frequently applied to the lower limbs. This chapter considers only a few of the many radiographic methods that have been devised for long bone measurement.

NEW ABBREVIATIONS USED IN CHAPTER 11

AP	Anteroposterior
CT	Computed tomography
IR	Image receptor

See Addendum B for a summary of all abbreviations used in Volume 2.

Radiation Protection

Differences in limb length are not uncommon in children and may occur in association with a variety of disorders. Patients with unequal limb growth may require yearly radiographic evaluations. More frequent examinations may be necessary in patients who have undergone surgical procedures to equalize limb length. One treatment method controls bone growth on the normal side. This is usually accomplished by means of metaphysial-epiphysial fusion at the distal femoral or proximal tibial level. Another treatment technique is to increase the growth of the shorter limb. This is achieved by surgically cutting the femur or tibia-fibula, or both. A frame is then placed around the cut ends and extended to the outside of the body. Gradual pressure on the frame separates the bone, extends the leg, and promotes healing at the same time.

Because patients with limb length differences require checkups at regular intervals over a period of years, gonad shielding is necessary to guard their well-being. In addition, careful patient positioning, secure immobilization, and accurate centering of a closely collimated beam of radiation are important to prevent unnecessary repeat exposures.

Position of Patient

Three exposures are made of each limb, with the accuracy of the examination depending on the patient not moving the limb or limbs even slightly. Small children must be carefully immobilized to prevent motion. If movement of the limb occurs before the examination is completed, all radiographs may need to be repeated.

- Place the patient in the supine position for all techniques, and examine both sides for comparison.
- When a soft tissue abnormality (swelling or atrophy) is causing rotation of the pelvis, elevate the low side on a radiolucent support to overcome the rotation, if necessary.

Position of Part

The limb to be examined should be positioned as follows:

- Adjust and immobilize the limb for an AP projection.
- If the two lower limbs are examined simultaneously, separate the ankles 5 to 6 inches (13 to 15 cm) and place the specialized ruler under the pelvis and extended down between the legs.
- If the limbs are examined separately, position the patient with a special ruler beneath each limb.
- When the knee of the patient's abnormal side cannot be fully extended, flex the normal knee to the same degree and support each knee on one of a pair of supports of *identical size* to ensure that the joints are flexed to the same degree and are equidistant from the image receptor (IR).

Localization of Joints

For the methods that require centering of the ray above the joints, the following steps should be taken:

- Localize each joint accurately, and use a skin-marking pencil to indicate the central ray centering point.
- Because both sides are examined for comparison and a discrepancy in bone length usually exists, mark the joints of each side after the patient is in the supine position.
- With the upper limb, place the marks as follows: for the *shoulder joint,* over the superior margin of the head of the humerus; for the *elbow joint,* ½ to ¾ inch (1.3 to 1.9 cm) below the plane of the epicondyles of the humerus (depending on the size of the patient); and for the wrist, midway between the styloid processes of the radius and ulna.
- With the lower limb, locate the *hip joint* by placing a mark 1 to 1¼ inches (2.5 to 3.2 cm) (depending on the size of the patient) laterodistally and at a right angle to the midpoint of an imaginary line extending from the anterior superior iliac spine to the pubic symphysis.
- Locate the *knee joint* just below the apex of the patella at the level of the depression between the femoral and tibial condyles.
- Locate the *ankle joint* directly below the depression midway between the malleoli.

In all radiographs made by a single x-ray exposure, the image is larger than the actual body part because the x-ray photons start at a small area on the target of the x-ray tube and diverge as they travel in straight lines through the body to the IR (Fig. 11-1). This magnification can be decreased by putting the body part as close to the IR as possible and making the distance between the x-ray tube and the IR as long as possible (a procedure sometimes referred to as *teleoroentgenography*). However, a radiographic technique called *orthoroentgenology* can be used to determine the exact length of a child's limb bones.

For this radiographic technique, a metal measurement ruler is placed between the patient's lower limbs and three exposures are made on the same x-ray IR. The following steps are observed:

- Using narrow collimation and careful centering of the limb parts to the upper, middle, and lower thirds of the IR, make three exposures on one IR.
- For all three exposures, place the central ray perpendicular to and passing directly through the specified joint (hence the term *orthoroentgenology,* from the Greek word *orthos,* meaning "straight").
- Do not move the limb between exposures. Because the IR is in the Bucky tray for all exposures including that of the ankle, exposure factors must be modified accordingly.
- Position the x-ray tube directly over the patient's hip, and make the first exposure (Fig. 11-2, *A*).
- Move the x-ray tube directly over the patient's knee joint, and make a second exposure (Fig. 11-2, *B*).
- Move the x-ray tube directly over the patient's tibiotalar joint, and make a third exposure (Fig. 11-2, *C*).

If the child holds the leg perfectly still while the three exposures are made, the true distance from the proximal end of the femur to the distal end of the tibia can be directly measured on the image, as follows:

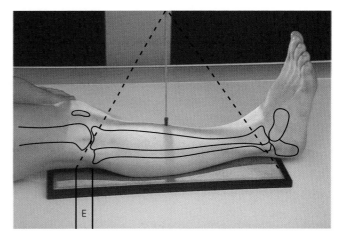

Fig. 11-1 Conventional radiographs are magnified (elongated) images. Proximal elongation in this example is equal to the distance *(E).* Similar elongation occurs distally.

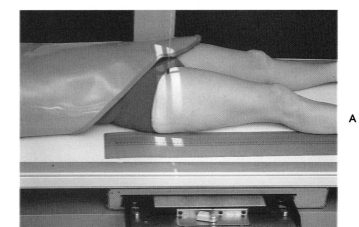

Fig. 11-2 Patient positioned for orthoroentgenographic measurement of lower limb. The central ray is centered over the hip joint **(A),** knee joint **(B),** and ankle joint **(C).** A metal ruler was placed near the lateral aspect of leg for photographic purposes. The ruler is normally placed between the limbs (see Fig. 11-4).

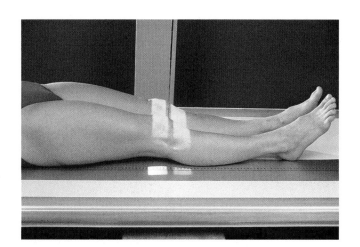

Fig. 11-3 Bilateral leg length measurement, with metal ruler placed beside leg for photographic purposes. (Proper placement of the ruler is shown in Fig. 11-4.)

- Place a special metal ruler (engraved with radiopaque centimeter or ½-inch [1.3-cm] marks that show when a radiograph is made) under the leg and on top of the table (see Fig. 11-2).
- If the IR is placed in the Bucky tray and then moved between the exposures (see Fig. 11-2), calculate the length of the femur and tibia by subtracting the numeric values projected over the two joints obtained by simultaneously exposing the patient and the metal ruler.

Another method of measuring the lengths of the femurs and tibiae is to examine both limbs simultaneously (Figs. 11-3 and 11-4):

- Center the midsagittal plane of the patient's body to the midline of the grid.
- Adjust the patient's lower limbs in the anatomic position (i.e., slight medial rotation).
- Tape the special metal ruler to the top of the table so that part of it is included in each of the exposure fields. This records the position of each joint.
- Place an IR in the Bucky tray, and shift it for centering at the three joint levels without moving the patient.

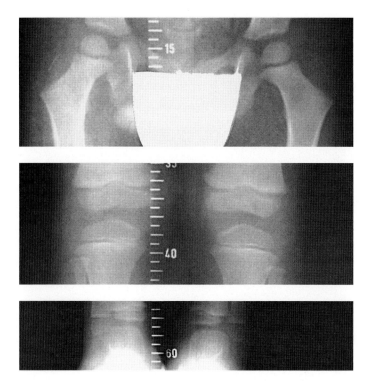

Fig. 11-4 Orthoroentgenogram for the measurement of leg length.

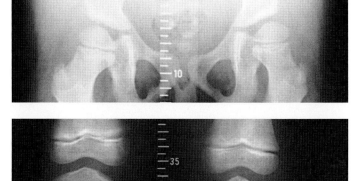

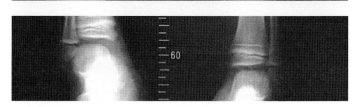

Fig. 11-5 Leg measurement showing that the right leg is shorter than the left leg.

- Center the IR and the tube successively at the previously marked level of the hip joints, the knee joints, and the ankle joints for simultaneous bilateral projections.
- When a difference in level exists between the contralateral joints, center the tube midway between the two levels.
- Make the three exposures on one 35- × 43-cm (14- × 17-inch) or 30- × 35-cm (11- × 14-inch) IR. Limb length can then be quickly determined.

The orthoroentgenographic method is reasonably accurate if the limbs are of almost the same length. When more than a slight discrepancy in limb length exists (Fig. 11-5), it is not possible to place the center of the x-ray tube exactly over both knee joints and make a single exposure or exactly over both ankle joints and make a single exposure. In such cases the tube is centered midway between the two joints. However, this results in bilateral distortion because of the diverging x-ray beam. In Fig. 11-5 the measurement obtained for the right femur is somewhat less than the actual length of the bone, whereas the measurement of the left femur is somewhat greater than the true length. The following measure can be taken to correct this problem:

- Examine each limb separately (Fig. 11-6).
- Center the limb being examined on the grid, and place the special ruler beneath the limb.

- Make a closely collimated exposure over each joint. This restriction of the exposure field not only increases the accuracy of the procedure but also considerably reduces radiation exposure (most importantly, to the gonads).
- After making joint localization marks, position the patient and apply local gonad shielding.
- Adjust the collimator to limit the exposure field as much as possible.
- With successive centering to the localization marks, make exposures of the hip, knee, and ankle.
- Repeat the procedure for the opposite limb.
- Use the same approach to measure lengths of the long bones in the upper limbs (Fig. 11-7).

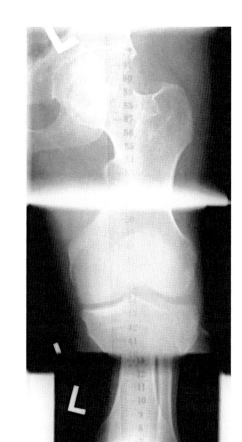

Fig. 11-6 Unilateral leg measurement.

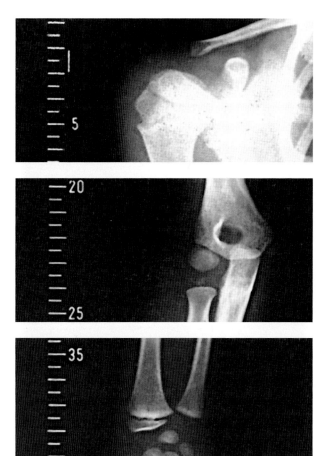

Fig. 11-7 Measurement of upper limb.

Computed Tomography Technique

Helms and McCarthy[1] reported a method for using computed tomography (CT) to measure discrepancies in leg length. Temme, Chu, and Anderson[2] compared conventional orthoroentgenograms with CT scans for long bone measurements. Both sets of investigators concluded that the CT scanogram is more consistently reproduced and that it causes less radiation exposure to the patient than the conventional radiographic approach. The CT approach is as follows:

- Take CT localizer or "scout" images of the femurs and tibias.
- Place cursors over the respective hip, knee, and ankle joints as described earlier in this chapter. To similarly study the upper limb, obtain scout images of the humerus, radius, and ulna.
- Place CT cursors over the shoulder, elbow, and wrist joints, and obtain the measurements. The measurements are displayed on the cathode ray tube (Figs. 11-8 to 11-10).

The accuracy of the CT examination depends on proper placement of the cursor. Helms and McCarthy[1] found that accuracy improved when the cursors were placed three times and the values obtained were averaged. These authors also reported that CT examinations used radiation doses that were 50 to 200 times less than those used with conventional radiography. CT examination requires about the same amount of time as conventional radiography.

---

[1]Helms CA, McCarthy S: CT scanograms for measuring leg length discrepancy, *Radiology* 252:802, 1984.

[2]Temme JB, Chu W, Anderson JC: CT scanograms compared with conventional orthoroentgenograms in long bone measurement, *Radiol Technol* 59:65, 1987.

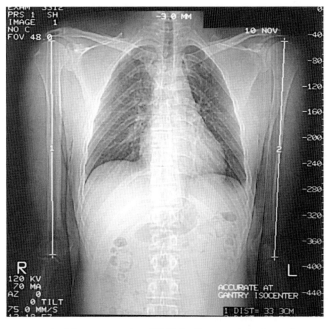

Fig. 11-8 Measurement of the arms using CT. Note the arm labels and measurements in the right lower corner.

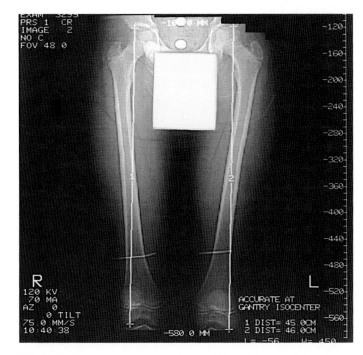

Fig. 11-9 CT measurements of femurs. The right femur is 1 cm shorter than the left femur in the same patient as in Fig. 11-8.

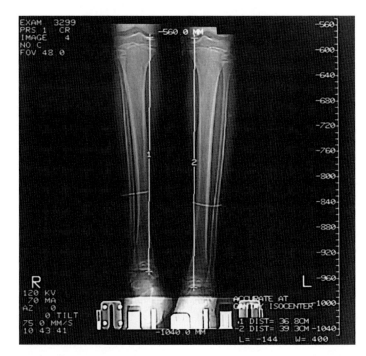

Fig. 11-10 CT measurement of the legs in the same patient as in Figs. 11-8 and 11-9.

12

CONTRAST ARTHROGRAPHY

Knee pneumoarthrogram showing normal lateral meniscus
(arrows) surrounded with air
above and below it.

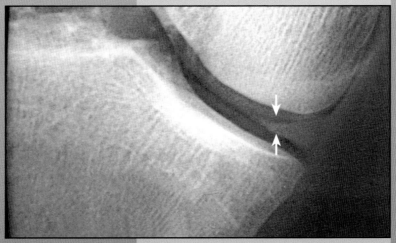

Overview

The introduction and development of magnetic resonance imaging (MRI) have significantly reduced the number of arthrograms performed in radiology departments. Because MRI is a non-invasive imaging technique, the knee, wrist, hip, shoulder, temporomandibular joint (TMJ), and other joints previously evaluated by contrast arthrography are now studied using MRI (Fig. 12-1). As a result, radiographic contrast arthrography has increasingly specialized functions.

Arthrography (Greek *arthron*, meaning "joint") is radiography of a joint or joints. *Pneumoarthrography, opaque arthrography,* and *double-contrast arthrography* are terms used to denote radiologic examinations of the soft tissue structures of joints (menisci, ligaments, articular cartilage, bursae) after the injection of one or two contrast agents into the capsular space.

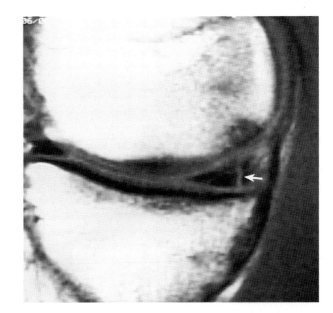

Fig. 12-1 Noninvasive MRI of knee, showing torn medial meniscus *(arrow).*

A gaseous medium is employed in pneumoarthrography, a water-soluble iodinated medium is used in opaque arthrography (Fig. 12-2), and a combination of gaseous and water-soluble iodinated media is used in double-contrast arthrography. Although contrast studies may be made on any encapsuled joint, the knee has been the most frequent site of investigation. Other joints examined by contrast arthrography include the shoulder, hip, wrist, and TMJs.

Arthrogram examinations are usually performed with a local anesthetic. The injection is made under careful aseptic conditions, usually in a combination fluoroscopic-radiographic examining room that has been carefully prepared in advance. The sterile items required, particularly the length and gauge of the needles, vary according to the part being examined. The sterile tray and the nonsterile items should be set up on a conveniently placed instrument cart or a small two-shelf table.

After aspirating any effusion, the radiologist injects the contrast agent or agents and manipulates the joint to ensure proper distribution of the contrast material. The examination is usually performed by fluoroscopy and spot images. Conventional radiographs may be taken when special images, such as an axial projection of the shoulder or an intercondyloid fossa position of the knee, are desired.

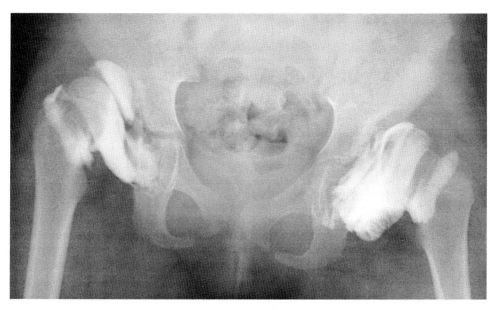

Fig. 12-2 Bilateral opaque arthrogram of bilateral congenital hip dislocations.

SUMMARY OF PATHOLOGY

Condition	Definition
Dislocation	Displacement of a bone from a joint
Joint Capsule Tear	Rupture of the joint capsule
Ligament Tear	Rupture of the ligament
Meniscus Tear	Rupture of the meniscus
Rotator Cuff Tear	Rupture of any muscle of the rotator cuff

**NEW ABBREVIATIONS
USED IN CHAPTER 12**

MRI	Magnetic resonance imaging
PA	Posteroanterior
TMJ	Temporomandibular joint

See Addendum B for a summary of all abbreviations used in Volume 2.

Contrast Arthrography of the Knee

VERTICAL RAY METHOD

Contrast arthrography of the knee by the vertical ray method requires the use of a stress device. The following steps are observed:

- Place the limb in the frame to widen or "open up" the side of the joint space under investigation. This widening, or spreading, of the intrastructural spaces permits better distribution of the contrast material around the meniscus.

- After the contrast material is injected, place the limb in the stress device (Fig. 12-3). To delineate the medial side of the joint, for example, place the stress device just above the knee and then laterally stress the lower leg.

- When contrast arthrograms are to be made by conventional radiography, turn the patient to the prone position and fluoroscopically localize the centering point for each side of the joint. The mark ensures accurate centering for closely collimated studies of each side of the joint and permits multiple exposures to be made on one IR. The images obtained of each side of the joint usually consist of an AP projection and a 20-degree right and left AP oblique projection.

- Obtain the oblique position by leg rotation or central ray angulation (Figs. 12-4 to 12-6).

- On completion of these studies, remove the frame and then perform lateral and intercondyloid fossa projections.

NOTE: Anderson and Maslin[1] recommended that tomography be used in knee arthrography. In addition, the technique can be frequently used for other contrast-filled joint capsules.

[1]Anderson PW, Maslin P: Tomography applied to knee arthrography, *Radiology* 110:271, 1974.

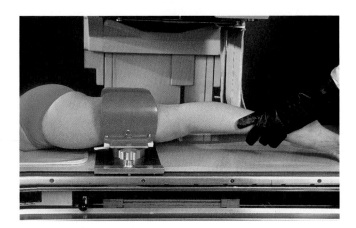

Fig. 12-3 Patient lying on lead rubber for gonad shielding and positioned in stress device on fluoroscopic table.

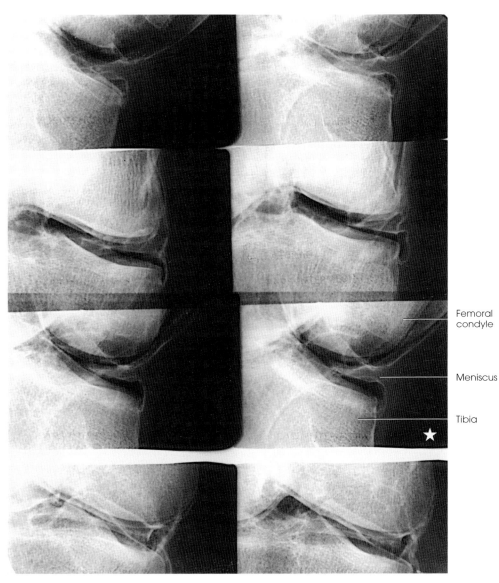

Femoral
condyle

Meniscus

Tibia

Fig. 12-4 Vertical ray double-contrast knee arthrogram.

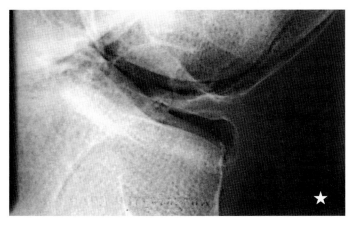

Fig. 12-5 Enlarged image of frame with star seen in Fig. 12-4.

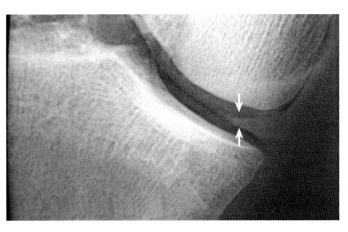

Fig. 12-6 Knee pneumoarthrogram showing normal lateral meniscus *(arrows)* surrounded with air above and below it.

Double-Contrast Arthrography of the Knee
HORIZONTAL RAY METHOD

The horizontal central ray method of performing double-contrast arthrography of the knee was described first by Andrén and Wehlin[1] and later by Freiberger, Killoran, and Cardona.[2] These investigators found that using a horizontal x-ray beam position and a comparatively small amount of each of the two contrast agents (gas-

[1]Andrén L, Wehlin L: Double-contrast arthrography of knee with horizontal roentgen ray beam, *Acta Orthop Scand* 29:307, 1960.
[2]Freiberger RH, Killoran PJ, Cardona G: Arthrography of the knee by double contrast method, *AJR* 97:736, 1966.

eous medium and water-soluble iodinated medium) improved double-contrast delineation of the knee joint structures. With this technique, the excess of the heavy iodinated solutions drains into the dependent part of the joint, leaving only the desired thin opaque coating on the gas-enveloped uppermost part, the part then under investigation.

Medial meniscus
- Adjust the patient in a semiprone position that places the posterior aspect of the medial meniscus uppermost (Figs. 12-7 and 12-8).

- To widen the joint space, manually stress the knee.
- Draw a line on the medial side of the knee, and then direct the central ray along the line and centered to the meniscus.
- With rotation toward the supine position, turn the leg 30 degrees for each of the succeeding five exposures.
- Direct the central ray along the localization line for each exposure, ensuring that it is centered to the meniscus.

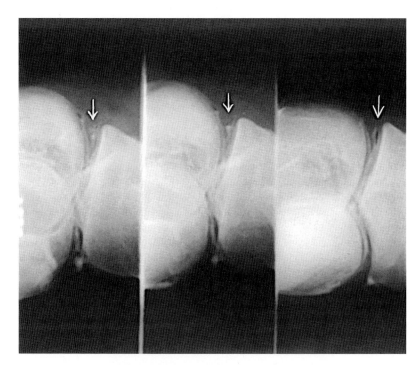

Fig. 12-7 Medial meniscus with a tear in the posterior half. Note irregular streaks of positive contrast material within the meniscal wedge *(arrows)*.

Lateral meniscus
- Adjust the patient in a semiprone position that places the posterior aspect of the lateral meniscus uppermost (Fig. 12-9).
- To widen the joint space, manually stress the knee.

- As with the medial meniscus, make six images on one IR.
- With movement toward the supine position, rotate the leg 30 degrees for each of the consecutive exposures, from the initial prone oblique position to the supine oblique position.
- Adjust the central ray angulation as required to direct it along the localization line and center it to the meniscus.

NOTE: For demonstration of the cruciate ligaments after filming of the menisci is completed,[1] the patient sits with the knee flexed 90 degrees over the side of the radiographic table. A firm cotton pillow is placed under the knee and adjusted so that some forward pressure can be applied to the leg. With the patient holding a grid IR in position, a closely collimated and slightly overexposed lateral projection is made.

[1]Mittler S, Freiberger RH, Harrison-Stubbs M: A method of improving cruciate ligament visualization in double-contrast arthrography, *Radiology* 102:441, 1972.

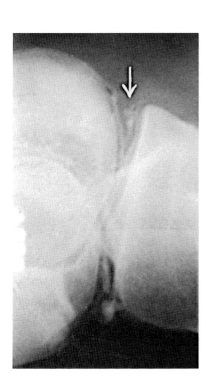

Fig. 12-8 Enlarged image showing a tear in the medial meniscus of the same patient as in Fig. 12-7.

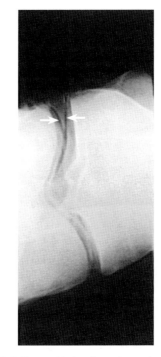

Fig. 12-9 Normal lateral meniscus *(arrows)* in the same patient as in Figs. 12-7 and 12-8.

Contrast arthrography

Wrist Arthrography

The primary indications for wrist arthrography are trauma, persistent pain, and limitation of motion. After contrast material (approximately 1.5 to 4 mL) is injected through the dorsal wrist at the articulation of the radius, scaphoid, and lunate, the wrist is gently manipulated to disperse the medium. The projections most commonly used are the PA, lateral, and both obliques (Figs. 12-10 and 12-11). Fluoroscopy or tape recording of the wrist during rotation is recommended for the exact detection of contrast medium leaks.

Hip Arthrography

Hip arthrography is performed most often in children to evaluate congenital hip dislocation before treatment (see Fig. 12-2) and after treatment (Figs. 12-12 and 12-13). In adults the primary use of hip arthrography is to detect a loose hip prosthesis or confirm the presence of infection. The cement used to fasten hip prosthesis components has barium sulfate added to make the cement and the cement-bone interface radiographically visible (Fig. 12-14). Although the addition of barium sulfate to cement is helpful in confirming proper seating of the prosthesis, it makes evaluation of the same joint by arthrography difficult.

Because both the cement and contrast material produce the same approximate radiographic density, a subtraction technique is recommended—either photographic subtraction as shown in Figs. 12-15 and 12-16 or digital subtraction as shown in Figs. 12-17 and 12-18 (see Chapter 25). A common puncture site for hip arthrography is ¾ inch (1.9 cm) distal to the inguinal crease and ¾ inch (1.9 cm) lateral to the palpated femoral pulse. A spinal needle is useful for reaching the joint capsule.

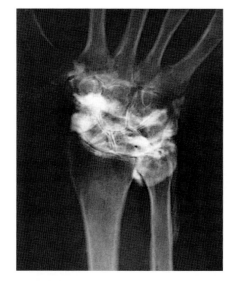

Fig. 12-10 Opaque arthrogram of wrist, demonstrating rheumatoid arthritis.

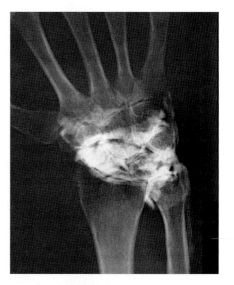

Fig. 12-11 PA arthrogram with wrist in radial deviation.

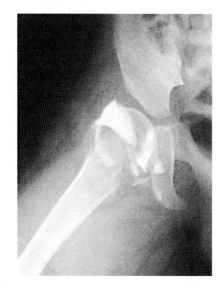

Fig. 12-12 AP opaque arthrogram showing treated congenital right hip dislocation in the same patient as in Fig. 12-2.

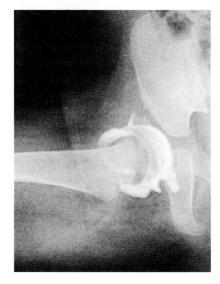

Fig. 12-13 Axiolateral "frog" right hip of patient treated for congenital dislocation of the hip.

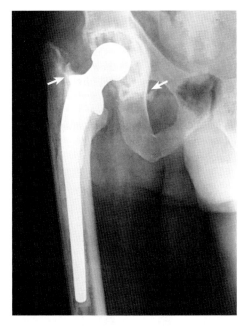

Fig. 12-14 AP hip radiograph showing radiopaque cement *(arrows)* used to secure hip prosthesis.

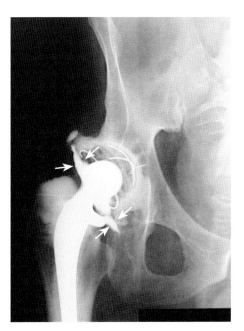

Fig. 12-15 AP hip arthrogram showing hip prosthesis in proper position. Cement with radiopaque additive is difficult to distinguish from the contrast medium used to perform arthrography *(arrows)*.

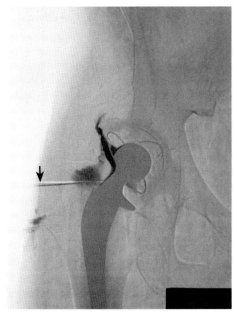

Fig. 12-16 Normal photographic subtraction AP hip arthrogram in the same patient as in Fig. 12-14. Contrast medium *(black image)* is readily distinguished from the hip prosthesis by the subtraction technique. Contrast medium does not extend inferiorly below the level of the injection needle *(arrow)*. (See Chapter 25 for a description of subtraction technique.)

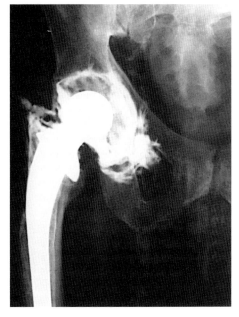

Fig. 12-17 AP hip radiograph after injection of contrast medium.

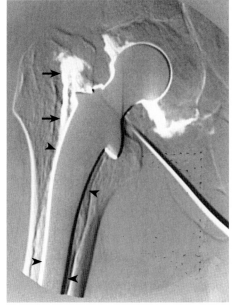

Fig. 12-18 Digital subtraction hip arthrogram in the same patient as in Fig. 12-17. Contrast medium around the prosthesis in the proximal lateral femoral shaft *(arrows)* indicates a loose prosthesis. Lines on the medial and lateral aspect of the femur *(arrowheads)* are a subtraction registration artifact caused by slight patient movement during the injection of contrast medium. (See Chapter 25 for a description of subtraction technique.)

Shoulder Arthrography

Arthrography of the shoulder is performed primarily for the evaluation of partial or complete tears in the rotator cuff or glenoidal labrum, persistent pain or weakness, and frozen shoulder. A single-contrast technique (Fig. 12-19) or a double-contrast technique (Fig. 12-20) may be used.

The usual injection site is approximately ½ inch (1.3 cm) inferior and lateral to the coracoid process. Because the joint capsule is usually deep, use of a spinal needle is recommended.

For a single-contrast arthrogram (Fig. 12-21), approximately 10 to 12 mL of positive contrast medium is injected into the shoulder.

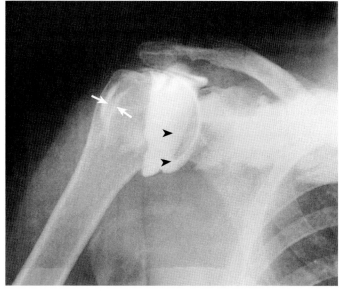

Fig. 12-19 Normal AP single-contrast shoulder arthrogram with contrast medium surrounding the biceps tendon sleeve and lying in the intertubercular (bicipital) groove *(arrows)*. The axillary recess is filled but has a normal medial filling defect *(arrowheads)* created by the glenoid labrum.

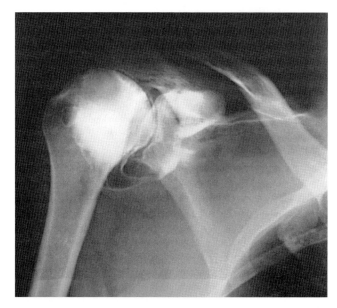

Fig. 12-20 Normal AP double-contrast shoulder arthrogram.

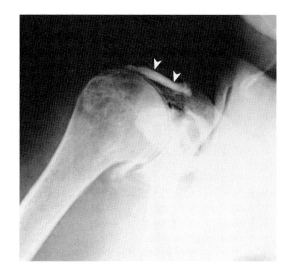

Fig. 12-21 Single-contrast arthrogram showing rotator cuff tear *(arrowheads)*.

For double-contrast examinations, approximately 3 to 4 mL of positive contrast medium and 10 to 12 mL of air are injected into the shoulder.

The projections most often used are the AP (both internal and external rotation), 30-degree AP oblique, axillary (Figs. 12-22 and 12-23), and tangential. (See Volume 1, Chapter 5, for a description of patient and part positioning.)

After double-contrast shoulder arthrography is performed, computed tomography (CT) may be used to examine some patients. CT images may be obtained at approximately 5-mm intervals through the shoulder joint. In shoulder arthrography, CT has been found to be sensitive and reliable in diagnosis. Radiographs and CT scans of the same patient are presented in Figs. 12-20 and 12-24.

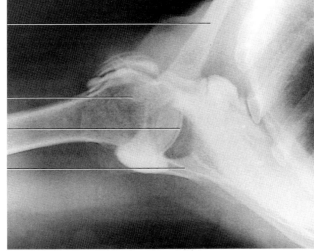

Clavicle

Humeral head

Contrast medium in glenoid cavity

Scapula

Fig. 12-22 Normal axillary single-contrast shoulder arthrogram.

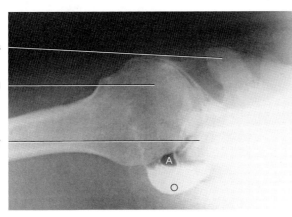

Coracoid process

Humeral head

Glenoid cavity

Fig. 12-23 Normal axillary double-contrast shoulder arthrogram projection of patient in supine position. Opaque medium (O) and air-created (A) density are seen anteriorly.

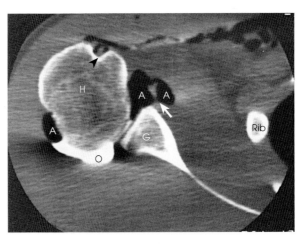

Fig. 12-24 CT shoulder arthrogram. The radiographic arthrogram in this patient was normal (see Fig. 12-20). However, the CT shoulder arthrogram shows a small chip fracture (arrow) on the anterior surface of the glenoid cavity. Head of humerus (H), air surrounding biceps tendon (arrowhead), air contrast medium (A), opaque contrast medium (O), and glenoid portion of scapula (G) are evident.

Temporomandibular Joint Arthrography

CT of the TMJ is often used instead of arthrography because CT is a noninvasive method of investigation. In many institutions, MRI has replaced CT because MRI is also a noninvasive procedure with well-established diagnostic value (Fig. 12-25).

Contrast arthrography of the TMJ is useful in diagnosing abnormalities of the articular disk, the small, oval, fibrocartilaginous or fibrous tissue plate located between the condyle of the mandible and mandibular fossa. Abnormalities of this disk can be the result of trauma or a stretched or loose posterior ligament that allows the disk to be anteriorly displaced, causing pain.

Single-contrast opaque arthrography of the TMJ, although relatively uncomfortable for the patient, is easy to perform and requires 0.5 to 1 mL of contrast medium. The puncture site is approximately ½ inch (1.3 cm) anterior to the tragus of the ear. The following steps are observed:

- Before the arthrogram is performed, take preliminary tomographic images with the patient's mouth in both the closed and open positions.
- After injection of the contrast medium, fluoroscopically observe the joint and take spot images to evaluate mandibular motion.

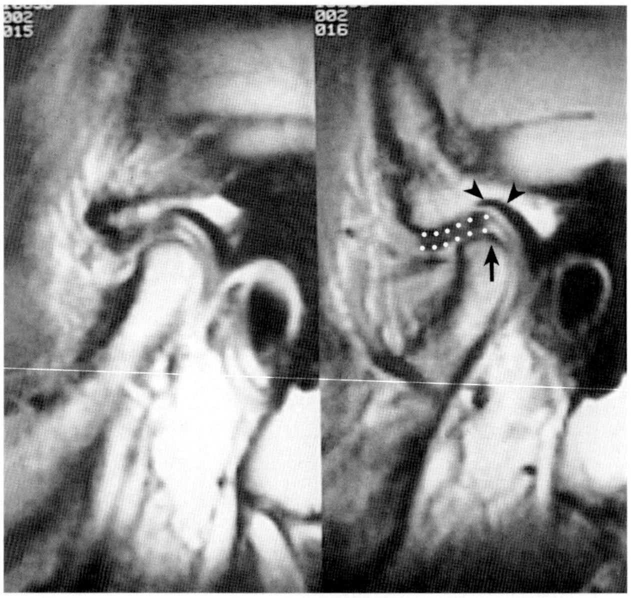

Fig. 12-25 Open-mouth lateral MRI of the TMJ, showing mandibular condyle *(arrow)*, mandibular fossa of temporal bone *(arrowheads)*, and articular disk *(dots)*.

• In general, obtain tomograms or radiographs, or both (Figs. 12-26 and 12-27), with the patient's mouth in the closed, partially open, and fully open positions.

Other Joints

Essentially any joint can be evaluated by arthrography. However, the joints discussed in this chapter—the knee, shoulder, hip, wrist, and TMJs—are the ones most often investigated.

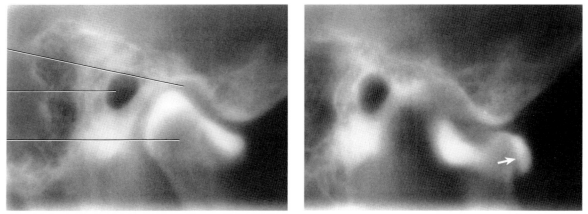

Mandibular fossa

Acoustic canal

Mandibular condyle

A

B

Fig. 12-26 Postinjection tomographic arthrogram of the TMJ taken with patient's mouth closed **(A)** and fully open **(B).** Positive contrast medium anterior to condyle *(arrow)* demonstrates anterior dislocation of the meniscus.

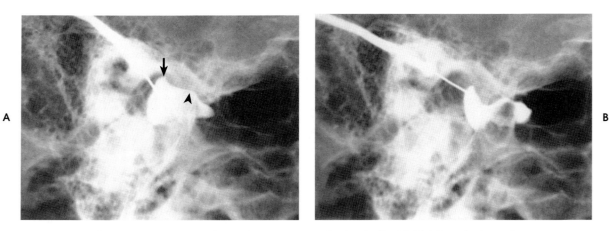

A

B

Fig. 12-27 Postinjection radiographs on same patient as in Fig. 12-26. Dislocated meniscus is shown with the mouth half open **(A)** and completely open **(B).** Mandibular fossa *(arrow)* and condyle *(arrowhead)* are shown.

13

TRAUMA RADIOGRAPHY

JEANNEAN HALL ROLLINS
SHARON A. COFFEY

AP projection of the humerus performed on a trauma patient. Fracture of the midshaft of the humerus.

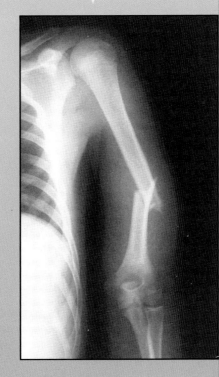

Introduction

Trauma radiography can be an exciting and challenging environment for the radiographer. For some, however, performing trauma procedures can be intimidating and stressful. The difference depends on how prepared the radiographer is to handle the situation. To reduce the stress associated with trauma radiography, the radiographer must be properly prepared for the multitude of responsibilities encountered in the emergency department (ED).

The goals of this chapter are to (1) assist the radiographer to develop an understanding of the imaging equipment used in trauma, (2) explain the role of the radiographer as a vital part of the ED team, and (3) present the common radiographic procedures performed on trauma patients. This chapter provides the information necessary to improve the skills and confidence of all radiographers caring for trauma patients.

Trauma is defined as a sudden, unexpected, dramatic, forceful, or violent event. Trauma-related injuries affect persons in all age ranges. Fig. 13-1 demonstrates the age range and peaks of patients listed in the National Trauma Database (NTDB) annual report for 2004. This database contains more than 1.1 million records from more than 400 hospitals and has received information from the vast majority of the United States. Fig. 13-2 demonstrates the distribution of trauma injuries by cause. These figures indicate that the imaging professional who chooses to work in the ED must be prepared to care for patients from every age range exhibiting a vast array of injuries.

Many types of facilities provide emergency medical care, ranging from major, metropolitan medical centers to small outpatient clinics in rural areas. The term

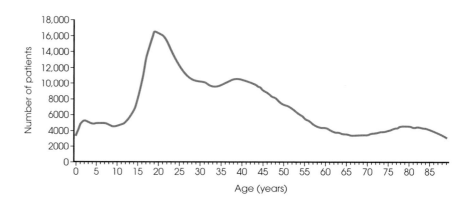

Fig. 13-1 NTDB table demonstrating number of trauma patients by age reported for 2004.

(Reprinted by permission of the American College of Surgeons.)

trauma center signifies a specific level of emergency medical care as defined by the American College of Surgeons Commission on Trauma. Trauma centers are categorized into four levels of care. Level I is the most comprehensive, and level IV is the most basic. A *level I* center is usually a university-based center, research facility, or large medical center. It provides the most comprehensive emergency medical care available with complete imaging capabilities 24 hours per day. All types of specialty physicians are available on site 24 hours per day. Radiographers are also available 24 hours per day. A *level II* center probably has all of the same spe-cialized care available but differs in that it is not a research or teaching hospital and some specialty physicians may not be available on site. *Level III* centers are usu-ally located in smaller communities where level I or level II care is not available. In general, level III centers do not have all specialists available but can resuscitate, stabilize, assess, and prepare a patient for transfer to a larger trauma center. A *level IV* center may not be a hospital at all, but rather a clinic or outpatient setting. These facilities usually provide care for minor injuries, as well as offer stabilization and arrange for transfer of more serious inju-ries to a larger trauma center.

Several types of forces, including *blunt, penetrating, explosive,* and *heat,* result in injuries. Examples of blunt trauma are motor vehicle accidents (MVAs), which include motorcycle accidents and collisions with pedestrians; falls; and aggravated assaults. Penetrating trauma includes gunshot wounds (GSWs), stab wounds, impalement injuries, and foreign body ingestion or aspiration. Explosive trauma causes injury by several mecha-nisms including pressure shock waves, high-velocity projectiles, and burns. Burns may be caused by a number of agents including fire, steam and hot water, chemicals, electricity, and frostbite.

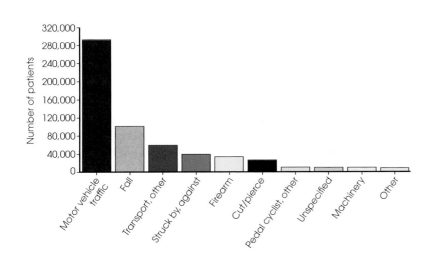

Fig. 13-2 NTDB table demonstrating number of patients injured by each mechanism in 2004.

(Courtesy American College of Surgeons.)

Preliminary Considerations

SPECIALIZED EQUIPMENT

Time is a critical element in the care of a trauma patient. To minimize the time required to acquire diagnostic x-ray images, many EDs have dedicated radiographic equipment located in the department or immediately adjacent to the department. Trauma radiographs must be taken with minimal patient movement, requiring more maneuvering of the tube and image receptor (IR). Specialized trauma radiographic systems are available and are designed to provide greater flexibility in x-ray tube and IR maneuverability (Fig. 13-3). These specialized systems help to minimize movement of the injured patient while performing imaging procedures. Additionally, some EDs are equipped with specialized beds or stretchers that have a moveable tray to hold the IR. This type of stretcher allows the use of a mobile radiographic unit and eliminates the requirement and risk of transferring an injured patient to the radiographic table.

Computed tomography (CT) is widely used for imaging of trauma patients. In many cases, CT is the first imaging modality used, now that image acquisition has become almost instantaneous. (Refer to Chapter 32 for a detailed explanation and description of CT.) The only major concern with CT imaging, compared with radiography, is the radiation dose. The debate centers on the exclusive use of CT, when lower-dose radiographs may be sufficient to make a diagnosis. Patients who are at high risk and who are not good candidates for quality radiographs, due to their injuries, may be referred to CT first.

Mobile radiography is often a necessity in the ED. Many patients will have injuries that prohibit transfer to a radiographic table, or their condition may be too critical to interrupt treatment. Trauma radiographers must be competent in performing mobile radiography on almost any part of the body and be able to use accessory devices (i.e., grids, air-gap technique) necessary to produce quality mobile images.

Mobile fluoroscopy units, usually referred to as C-arms because of their shape, are becoming more commonplace in EDs. C-arms are used for fracture reduction procedures, foreign body localization in limbs, and reduction of joint dislocations (Fig. 13-4).

An emerging imaging technology has the potential to affect trauma radiography in a significant way. The Statscan (Lodox Systems [Pty], Ltd.) is a relatively new imaging device that produces full-body imaging scans in approximately 13 seconds without moving the patient (Figs. 13-5 to 13-7). Currently there are approximately 17 of these systems worldwide. At a cost of approximately $450,000, this technology is an expensive yet exciting addition to trauma imaging.

Positioning aids are essential to quality imaging in trauma radiography. Sponges, sandbags, and the creative use of tape are often the trauma radiographer's most useful tools. Most patients who are injured cannot hold the required positions as a result of pain or impaired consciousness. Other patients cannot be moved into the proper position because to do so would exacerbate their injury. Proper use of positioning aids assists in quick adaptation of procedures to accommodate the patient's condition.

Grids and IR holders are necessities because many projections require the use of a horizontal central ray. Inspect grids routinely because a damaged grid will often cause image artifacts. IR holders enable the radiographer to perform cross-table lateral projections (dorsal decubitus position) on numerous body parts with minimal distortion. To prevent unnecessary exposure, ED personnel should not hold the IR.

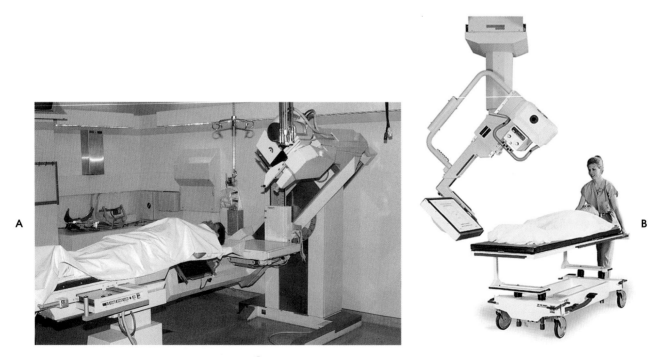

Fig. 13-3 A, Dedicated C-arm–type trauma radiographic room with patient on the table.
B, Dedicated conventional trauma radiographic room with vertical Bucky.

(**B,** Courtesy Fischer Imaging, Inc.)

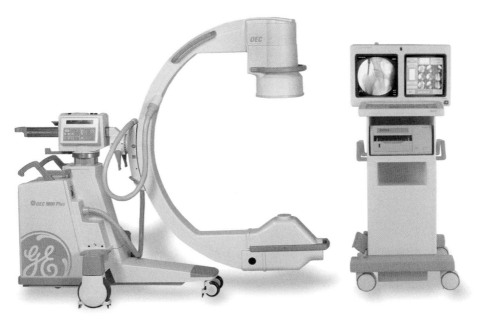

Fig. 13-4 A mobile fluoroscopic C-arm.

(Courtesy OEC Diasonics, Inc.)

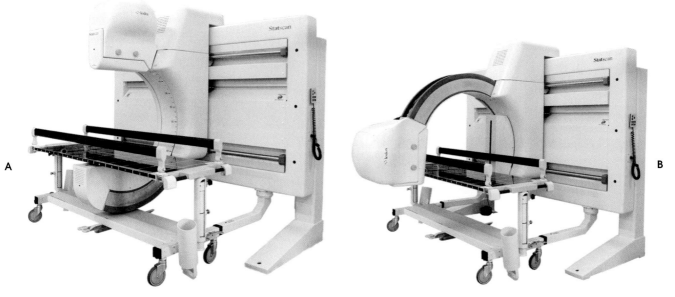

Fig. 13-5 A, Statscan system configured for AP projection. **B,** Statscan system configured for lateral projection.

(Courtesy Lodox Systems (Pty), Ltd.)

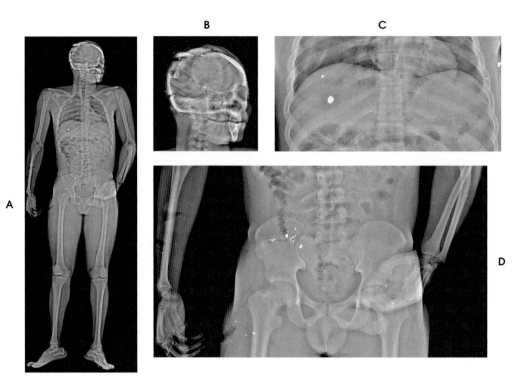

Fig. 13-6 Statscan of patient with multiple GSWs. **A,** AP full body scan—13 seconds required for acquisition. Shrapnel and projectile pathways identified by zooming in on areas of the full body scan. **B,** Skull. **C,** Diaphragm area. **D,** Pelvis.

(Courtesy Lodox Systems (Pty), Ltd.)

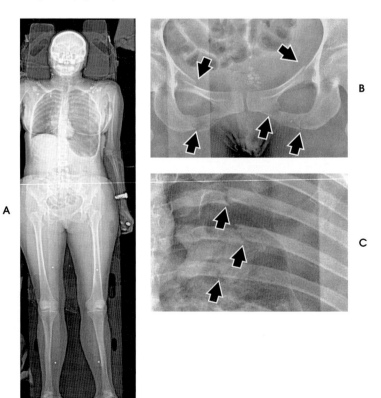

Fig. 13-7 Statscan of MVA victim with blunt trauma. **A,** AP full body scan. Tension pneumothorax demonstrated without additional processing. **B,** Zoomed lower pelvis demonstrating multiple fractures *(arrows).* **C,** Zoomed bony thorax demonstrating rib fractures *(arrows).*

(Courtesy Lodox Systems (Pty), Ltd.)

EXPOSURE FACTORS

Patient motion is always a consideration in trauma radiography. The shortest possible exposure time that can be set should be used in all procedures, except when a breathing technique is desired. Unconscious patients cannot suspend respiration for the exposure. Conscious patients are often in extreme pain and unable to cooperate for the procedure.

Radiographic exposure factor compensation may be required when making exposures through immobilization devices such as a spine board or backboard. Most trauma patients arrive at the hospital with some type of immobilization device (Fig. 13-8). Pathologic changes should also be considered when setting technical factors. For instance, internal bleeding in the abdominal cavity would absorb a greater amount of radiation than a bowel obstruction.

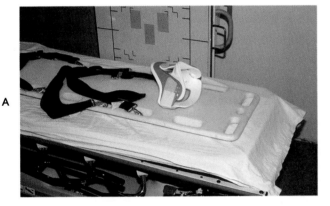

A

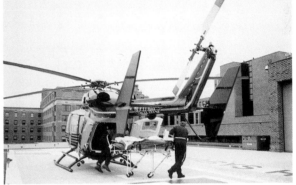

B

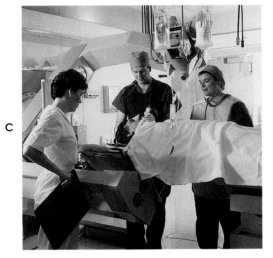

C

Fig. 13-8 A, Typical backboard and neck brace used for trauma patients. **B,** Backboard, brace, and other restraints are used on the patient throughout transport. **C,** All restraints will remain with and on the patient until all x-ray examinations are completed.

POSITIONING OF THE PATIENT

The primary challenge of the trauma radiographer is to obtain a high-quality, diagnostic image on the first attempt when the patient is unable to move into the desired position. Many methods are available to adapt a routine projection and obtain the desired image of the anatomic part. To minimize the risk of exacerbating the patient's condition, the x-ray tube and IR should be positioned, rather than the patient or the part. For example, position the stretcher adjacent to the vertical Bucky or upright table as often as the patient's condition allows (Fig. 13-9). This location enables accurate positioning with minimal patient movement for cross-table lateral images (dorsal decubitus positions) on numerous parts of the body. Additionally, the grid in the table or vertical Bucky is usually a higher ratio than that used for mobile radiography, so image contrast is improved. Another technique to increase efficiency, while minimizing patient movement, is to take all of the AP projections of the requested examinations, moving superiorly to inferiorly. Then perform all of the lateral projections of the requested examinations, moving inferiorly to superiorly. This method moves the x-ray tube in the most expeditious manner.

When taking radiographs to localize a penetrating foreign object, such as metal or glass fragments or bullets, the entrance or exit wounds, or both, should be marked with a radiopaque marker that is visible on all projections (Fig. 13-10). Two exposures at right angles to each other will demonstrate the depth, as well as the path, of the projectile.

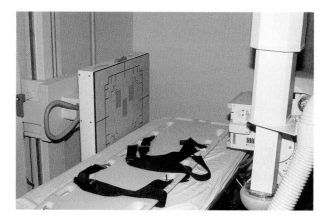

Fig. 13-9 Stretcher positioned adjacent to vertical Bucky to expedite positioning. Note x-ray tube in position for lateral projections.

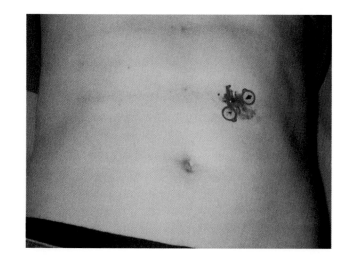

Fig. 13-10 Proper placement of radiopaque markers *(inside red circles)* on each side of a bullet entrance wound. The red circles are "stickies" that contain the radiopaque marker.

Radiographer's Role as Part of the Trauma Team

The role of the radiographer within the ED ultimately depends on the department protocol and staffing, as well as the extent of emergency care provided at the facility. Regardless of the size of the facility, the primary responsibilities of a radiographer in an emergency situation include the following:

- Perform quality diagnostic imaging procedures as requested
- Practice ethical radiation protection
- Provide competent patient care

Ranking these responsibilities is impossible because they occur simultaneously, and all are vital to quality care in the ED.

DIAGNOSTIC IMAGING PROCEDURES

Producing a high-quality, diagnostic image is one of the more obvious roles of any radiographer. A radiographer in the trauma environment has the added responsibility to perform that task efficiently. Efficiency and productivity are common and practical goals for the radiology department. In the ED, efficiency is often crucial to saving the patient's life. Diagnostic imaging in the ED is paramount to an accurate, timely, and often life-saving diagnosis.

RADIATION PROTECTION

One of the most essential duties and ethical responsibilities of the trauma radiographer is radiation protection of the patient, members of the trauma team, and self. In highly critical care situations, members of the trauma team cannot leave the patient while imaging procedures are being performed. The trauma radiographer must ensure that the other team members are protected from unnecessary radiation exposure. Common practices should minimally include the following:

- Close collimation to the anatomy of interest to reduce scatter
- Gonadal shielding for the patients of childbearing age (when doing so does not interfere with the anatomy of interest)
- Lead aprons for all personnel that remain in the room during the procedure
- Exposure factors that minimize patient dose and scattered radiation
- Announcement of impending exposure to allow unnecessary personnel to exit the room

Consideration must also be given to patients on nearby stretchers. If they are less than 6 feet away from the x-ray tube, appropriate shielding should be provided. Some of the greatest exposures to patients and medical personnel are from fluoroscopic procedures. If the C-arm fluoroscopic unit is used in the ED, special precautions should be in place to ensure that fluoroscopic exposure time is kept to a minimum and that all personnel are wearing protective aprons.

PATIENT CARE

As with all imaging procedures, trauma procedures require a patient history. The patient may provide this, if he or she is conscious, or the attending physician may inform you of the injury and the patient's status. If the patient is conscious, explain what you are doing in detail and in terms the patient can understand. Listen to the patient's rate and manner of speech, which may provide insight into his or her mental and emotional status. Make eye contact with the patient to provide comfort and reassurance. Keep in mind that a trip to the ED is an emotionally stressful event, regardless of the severity of injury or illness.

Radiographers are often responsible for the total care of the trauma patient while performing diagnostic imaging procedures. Therefore it is critical that radiographers constantly assess the patient's condition, recognize any signs of decline or distress, and report any change in the status of the patient's condition to the attending physician. The trauma radiographer must be well versed in taking vital signs and knowing normal ranges and competent in cardiopulmonary resuscitation (CPR), administration of oxygen, and dealing with all types of medical emergencies. The radiographer must be prepared to perform these procedures when covered by a standing physician's order or as departmental policy allows. Additionally, the radiographer should be familiar with the location and contents of the adult and pediatric crash carts and understand how to use the suctioning devices.

The familiar "ABCs" (airway, breathing, and circulation) of basic life support techniques must be constantly assessed during the radiographic procedures. Visual inspection and verbal questioning enables the radiographer to determine whether the status of the patient changes during the procedure. Table 13-1 serves as a guide for the trauma radiographer regarding changes in status that should be reported immediately to the attending physician. The table includes only the *common* injuries in which the radiographer may be the only health care professional with the patient during the imaging procedure. Patients with multiple trauma injuries or those in respiratory or cardiac arrest usually are imaged with a mobile radiographic unit while emergency personnel are present in the room. In these situations the primary responsibility of the trauma radiographer is to produce quality images in an efficient manner while practicing ethical radiation protection measures.

TABLE 13-1

Guide for reporting patient status change

Noted symptom	Possible cause	When to report to physician immediately
Cool, clammy skin	Shock* Vasovagal reaction†	Other symptoms of shock present
Excessive sweating (diaphoresis)	Shock*	Other symptoms of shock present
Slurred speech	Head injury Stroke (cerebrovascular accident‡) Drug or ethanol influence§	Accompanied by vomiting, especially if vomiting stops when patient is moved to different position
Agitation or confusion	Head injury Drug or ethanol influence§	Accompanied by vomiting, especially if vomiting stops when patient is moved to different position
Vomiting (without abdominal complaints) (hyperemesis)	Head injury Hyperglycemia‖ Drug or ethanol overdose	Position of patient abruptly stimulates vomiting or abruptly stops vomiting
Increased drowsiness (lethargy)	Shock* Head injury Hyperglycemia‖	Other symptoms of shock present or accompanied by vomiting
Loss of consciousness (unresponsive to voice or touch)	Shock* Head injury Hyperglycemia‖	Immediately
Pale or bluish skin pallor (cyanosis)	Airway compromise Hypovolemic shock	Immediately
Bluish nail beds	Circulatory compromise	Immediately
Patient complains of thirst	Shock* Hyperglycemia‖ Hypoglycemia	Other symptoms of shock present
Patient complains of tingling or numbness (paresthesia) or inability to move a limb	Spinal cord injury Peripheral nerve impairment	Accompanied by any symptoms of shock or altered consciousness
Seizures	Head injury	Immediately
Patient states he or she cannot feel your touch (paralysis)	Spinal cord injury Peripheral nerve impairment	Accompanied by any symptoms of shock or altered consciousness
Extreme eversion of foot	Fracture of proximal femur or hip joint	Report only if x-ray request specifies "frog leg" lateral projection of hip. This movement will exacerbate patient's injury, as well as cause intense pain. Surgical lateral position should be substituted. Watch for changes in abdominal size and firmness.
Increasing abdominal distention and firmness to palpation	Internal bleeding from pelvic fracture¶ or organ laceration	Immediately

*Hypovolemic or hemorrhagic shock is a medical condition in which there are abnormally low levels of blood plasma in the body, such that the body cannot properly maintain blood pressure, cardiac output of blood, and normal amounts of fluid in the tissues. It is the most common type of shock in trauma patients. Symptoms include diaphoresis, cool and clammy skin, decrease in venous pressure, decrease in urine output, thirst, and altered state of consciousness.

†Vasovagal reaction is also called a vasovagal attack or situational syncope, as well as vasovagal syncope. It is a reflex of the involuntary nervous system or a normal physiologic response to emotional stress. Patients may complain of nausea, feeling flushed (warm), and feeling lightheaded. They may appear pale before they lose consciousness for several seconds.

‡Cerebrovascular accident (CVA) is commonly called a stroke and may be caused by thrombosis, embolism, or hemorrhage in the vessels of the brain.

§Drugs or alcohol. Patients under the influence of drugs or alcohol, or both, are common in the emergency department. In this situation the usual symptoms of shock and head injury are unreliable. Be on guard for aggressive physical behaviors and abusive language.

‖Hyperglycemia is also known as diabetic ketoacidosis. The cause is increased blood sugar levels. The patient may exhibit any combination of symptoms noted and will have fruity-smelling breath.

¶Pelvic fractures have a high mortality rate (open fractures are as high as 50%). Hemorrhage and shock are often associated with this type of injury. Emergency cystograms are often ordered on patients with known pelvic fractures.

"Best Practices" in Trauma Radiography

Radiography of the trauma patient seldom allows the use of "routine" positions and projections. Additionally, the trauma patient requires special attention to patient care techniques while performing difficult imaging procedures. The following best practices provide some universal guidelines for the trauma radiographer.

I. **Speed**—Trauma radiographers must produce quality images in the shortest amount of time. Rapidity in performing a diagnostic examination is critical to saving the patient's life. Many practical methods that increase examination efficiency without sacrificing image quality are introduced in this chapter.

II. **Accuracy**—Trauma radiographers must provide accurate images with a minimal amount of distortion and the maximum amount of recorded detail. Alignment of the central ray, the part, and the IR applies in trauma radiography, too. Using the shortest exposure time minimizes the possibility of imaging involuntary and uncontrollable patient motion.

III. **Quality**—Quality does not have to be sacrificed to produce an image quickly. Do not fall into the trap of using the patient's condition as an excuse for careless positioning and accepting less than high-quality images.

IV. **Positioning**—Careful precautions must be taken to ensure that performance of the imaging procedure does not exacerbate the patient's injuries. The "golden rule" of two projections at right angles from one another still applies. As often as possible, position the tube and the IR, *rather than the patient,* to obtain the desired projections.

V. **Practice standard precautions**—Exposure to blood and body fluids should be expected in trauma radiography. Wear gloves, mask, and gown when appropriate. Place IR and sponges in nonporous plastic to protect them from body fluids. Wash hands frequently, especially between patients. Keep all equipment and accessory devices clean and ready for use.

VI. **Immobilization**—NEVER remove any immobilization device without physician's orders. Provide proper immobilization and support to increase patient comfort and minimize risk of motion.

VII. **Anticipation**—Anticipating required special projections or diagnostic procedures for certain injuries makes the radiographer a vital part of the ED team. For example, patients requiring surgery generally require an x-ray of the chest. In facilities where CT is not readily available for emergency patients, fractures of the pelvis often require a cystogram to determine the status of the urinary bladder. Know which procedures are often referred to CT first, or for additional images. Being prepared for and understanding the necessity of these additional procedures and images instills confidence in, and creates an appreciation for, the role of the radiographer in the emergency setting.

VIII. **Attention to detail**—NEVER leave a trauma patient (or any patient) unattended during imaging procedures. The patient's condition may change at any time, and it is the radiographer's responsibility to note these changes and report them immediately to the attending physician. If you cannot process images while maintaining eye contact with your patient, call for help. Someone must be with the injured patient at all times.

IX. **Attention to department protocol and scope of practice**—Know department protocols and practice only within your competence and abilities. The scope of practice for radiographers varies from state to state and from country to country. Be sure to study and understand the scope of your role in the emergency setting. Do not provide or offer a patient anything by mouth. Always ask the attending physician before giving the patient anything to eat or drink, no matter how persistent the patient may be.

X. **Professionalism**—Ethical conduct and professionalism in all situations and with every person is a requirement of all health care professionals, but the conditions encountered in the ED can be particularly complicated. Adhere to the Code of Ethics for Radiologic Technologists (see Chapter 1) and the Radiography Practice Standards. Be aware of the people present or nearby at all times when discussing a patient's care. The ED radiographer is exposed to a myriad of tragic conditions. Emotional reactions are common and expected but must be controlled until the emergency care of the patient is complete.

Radiographic Procedures in Trauma

The projections included in this chapter result from a telephone survey of level I trauma centers. The results indicated that the common radiographic projections ordered for initial trauma surveys are as follows[1]:

- Cervical spine, dorsal decubitus position (cross-table lateral)
- Chest, AP (mobile)
- Abdomen, AP (kidneys, ureter, and bladder [KUB] and acute abdominal series)
- Pelvis, AP
- Cervical spine, AP and obliques
- Lumbar spine
- Lower limb
- Upper limb

Skull radiographs did not rank as one of the most common imaging procedures performed in the ED of level I trauma centers. Most level I trauma centers have replaced conventional trauma skull radiographs (AP, lateral, Towne, reverse Waters, etc.) with CT of the head (Fig. 13-11). Research articles continue to delineate the advantages of CT imaging over radiography, and the results indicate that certain types of head trauma should be referred to CT first. However, smaller facilities may not have CT readily available. Therefore trauma skull positioning remains valuable knowledge for the radiographer.

---

[1]Thomas Wolfe, Methodist Medical Center, Memphis, conducted the survey as a part of his graduate practicum for Midwestern State University.

This section provides trauma positioning instructions for radiography projections of the following body areas.

- **Cervical spine**
  Lateral (dorsal decubitus position)
  Cervicothoracic (dorsal decubitus position)
  AP axial
  AP axial oblique
- **Thoracic and lumbar spine**
  Lateral (dorsal decubitus position)
- **Chest**
  AP
- **Abdomen**
  AP
  AP (left lateral decubitus position)
- **Pelvis**
  AP
- **Skull**
  Lateral (dorsal decubitus position)
  AP or PA
  AP axial (Towne method)
- **Facial bones**
  Acanthioparietal (reverse Waters method)
- **Limbs**
- **Other imaging procedures**

In addition to the dorsal decubitus positions, AP projections of the thoracic and lumbar spine are usually required for trauma radiographic surveys. The AP projections of this anatomy vary minimally in the trauma setting and therefore are not discussed in detail. Critical study and clinical practice of these procedures should adequately prepare a radiographer for work in the ED.

Certain criteria apply in all trauma imaging procedures and therefore are explained here and not included on each procedure in detail.

PATIENT PREPARATION

Remembering that the patient has endured an emotionally disturbing and distressing event in addition to the physical injuries he or she may have sustained is important. If the patient is conscious, speak calmly and look directly in the patient's eyes while explaining the procedures that have been ordered. Do not assume that the patient cannot hear you, even if he or she cannot or will not respond.

Check the patient thoroughly for items that might cause an artifact on the images. Explain what you are removing from the patient and why. Be sure to place all removed personal effects, especially valuables, in the proper container used by the facility (i.e., plastic bag) or in the designated secure area. Each facility has a procedure regarding proper storage of a patient's personal belongings. Be sure to know the procedure and follow it carefully.

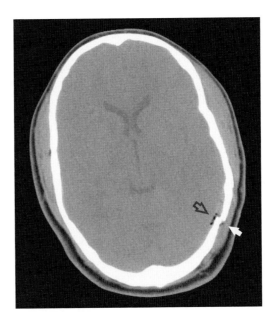

Fig. 13-11 CT of the skull demonstrating a displaced fracture *(white arrow)*. Intracranial air is present *(black open arrow)*.

(Courtesy Sunie Grossman, RT(R), St. Bernard's Medical Center, Jonesboro, Ark.)

BREATHING INSTRUCTIONS

Most injured patients have difficulty following the recommended breathing instructions for routine projections. For these patients, exposure factors should be set using the shortest possible exposure time to minimize motion on the radiograph, necessitating use of the large focal spot. The decreased resolution of the large focal spot produces greater resolution than the significant loss of resolution from patient movement. If a breathing technique is desired, this can be explained to the conscious trauma patient in the usual manner. If the patient is unconscious or unresponsive, then careful attention should be paid to the rate and degree of chest wall movement. If inspiration is desired on the image, then time the exposure to correspond to the highest point of chest expansion. Conversely, if the routine projection calls for exposure on expiration, then the exposure should be made when the patient's chest wall falls to its lowest point.

IMMOBILIZATION DEVICES

A wide variety of immobilization devices are used to stabilize injured patients. Standard protocol is to perform radiographic images without removing immobilization devices. Once injuries have been diagnosed or ruled out, the attending physician gives the order for immobilization to be removed, changed, or continued.

Many procedures necessitate the use of some sort of immobilization to prevent involuntary and voluntary motion. Many patient care textbooks discuss prudent use of such immobilization. The key issues in the use of immobilization in trauma are to neither exacerbate the patient's injury nor increase his or her discomfort.

IMAGE RECEPTOR SIZE

The IR sizes used in trauma procedures are the same as those specified for the routine projection of the anatomy of interest. Occasionally, the physician may request that more of a part be included, and then a larger IR is acceptable.

CENTRAL RAY, PART, IMAGE RECEPTOR ALIGNMENT

Unless otherwise indicated for the procedure, the central ray should be directed perpendicular to the midpoint of the grid or IR, or both. Tips for minimizing distortion are detailed on those procedures in which distortion is a potential threat to image quality.

IMAGE EVALUATION

Ideally, trauma radiographs should be of optimum quality to ensure prompt and accurate diagnosis of the patient's injuries. Evaluate images for proper positioning and technique as indicated in the routine projections. Allowances can be made when true right-angle projections (AP/PA and lateral) must be altered as a result of patient condition.

DOCUMENTATION

Deviation from routine projections is a necessity in many instances. Documenting the alterations in routine projections for the attending physician and radiologist is important so that they can properly interpret the images. Additionally, the radiographer often has to determine whether the anatomy of interest has been adequately demonstrated and perform additional projections (within the scope of the ordered examination) on an injured part to aid in proper diagnosis. Notations concerning additional projections are extremely helpful for the interpreting physicians.

NEW ABBREVIATIONS USED IN CHAPTER 13	
CPR	Cardiopulmonary resuscitation
CR	Central ray
CVA	Cerebrovascular accident
ED	Emergency department
EAM	External acoustic meatus
GSW	Gunshot wound
IOML	Infraorbitomeatal line
IVU	Intravenous urography
KUB	Kidneys, ureters, and bladder
MML	Mentomeatal line
MVA	Motor vehicle accident
OML	Orbitomeatal line
SID	Source-to-image-receptor distance

See Addendum B for a summary of all abbreviations used in Volume 2.

⚜ LATERAL PROJECTION[1]
Dorsal decubitus position

Trauma positioning tips
- *Always perform this projection first, before any other projections.*
- The attending physician or radiologist must review this image to rule out vertebral fracture or dislocation before other projections are performed.
- Use a 72-inch (183-cm) SID whenever attainable.
- Move the patient's head and neck as little as possible.
- *Shield gonads and other personnel in the room.*

[1]See mobile lateral projection in Volume 3, p. 257.

Patient position considerations
- Patient is generally immobilized on a backboard and in a cervical collar.
- Patient should relax his or her shoulders as much as possible.
- Patient should look straight ahead without any rotation of the head or neck.
- Place IR in a holder at the top of the shoulder (Fig. 13-12).
- Check that the IR is perfectly vertical.
- Ensure that the central ray is *horizontal* and centered to midpoint of IR.

Structures shown
The entire cervical spine, from sella turcica to the top of T1, must be demonstrated in profile with minimal rotation and distortion (Fig 13-13).

NOTE: If all seven cervical vertebrae including the spinous process of C7 and the C7-T1 interspace are not clearly visible, a lateral projection of the cervicothoracic region must be performed.

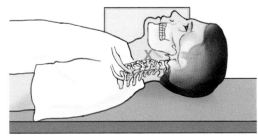

Horizontal CR to C4

Fig. 13-12 Patient and IR positioned for a trauma lateral projection of the cervical spine using the dorsal decubitus position.

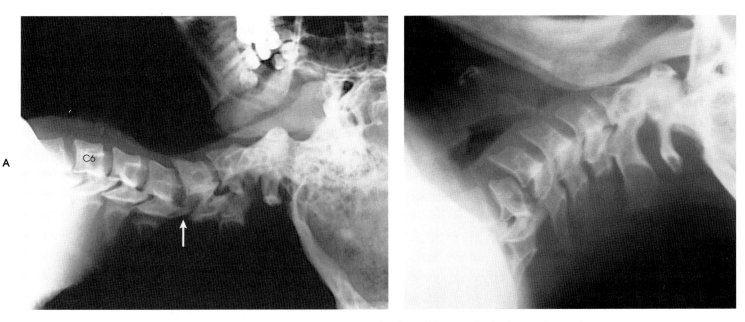

Fig. 13-13 Dorsal decubitus position lateral projection of the cervical spine performed on a trauma patient. **A,** Dislocation of the C3 and C4 articular processes *(arrow).* Note that C7 is not well demonstrated, and thus a lateral projection of the cervicothoracic vertebrae should also be performed. **B,** Fracture of the pedicles with dislocation of C5 and C6. Note superior portion of C7 shown on this image.

Trauma radiography

✹ LATERAL PROJECTION
Dorsal decubitus position

This projection is often called the "swimmer's" technique. (See Chapter 8, p. 413 for a complete description.)

Trauma positioning tips

- *This projection should be performed if the entire cervical spine including C7 and the interspace between C7 and T1 is not demonstrated on the dorsal decubitus lateral projection. The patient must be able to move both arms. Do not move the patient's arms without permission from the attending physician and review of the lateral projection.*
- Collimate the width of the x-ray beam closely to reduce scatter radiation.
- If the patient is in stable condition, position his or her stretcher adjacent to the vertical Bucky to increase efficiency and obtain optimum image quality.
- *Shield gonads and other personnel in the room.*

Patient position considerations

- Supine, usually on a backboard and in a cervical collar
- Have patient depress the shoulder closest to the tube as much as possible. *Do not push on the patient's shoulder.*
- Instruct the patient to raise the arm opposite the tube over his or her head. Assist the patient as needed, but *do not use force or move the limb too quickly* (Fig. 13-14).
- Ensure that the patient is looking straight ahead without any rotation of the head or neck.
- The central ray is *horizontal* and perpendicular to the IR entering the side of the neck just above the clavicle, passing through the C7-T1 interspace.
- Instruct the patient to breathe normally, if he or she is conscious.
- If possible, use a long exposure time technique to blur the rib shadows.

Structures shown

The lower cervical and upper thoracic vertebral bodies and spinous processes should be seen in profile between the shoulders. Contrast and density should demonstrate bony cortical margins and trabeculation (Fig. 13-15).

▼ COMPENSATING FILTER

The use of a compensating filter can improve image quality due to the extreme difference in thickness between the upper thorax and lower cervical spine.

NOTE: A grid is required to improve image contrast. If a breathing technique cannot be used, then make the exposure with respiration suspended.

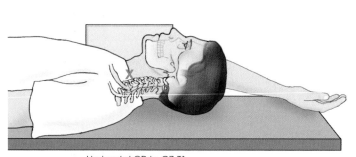

Horizontal CR to C7-T1

Fig. 13-14 Patient and IR positioned for trauma lateral projection of the cervicothoracic vertebrae using the dorsal decubitus position.

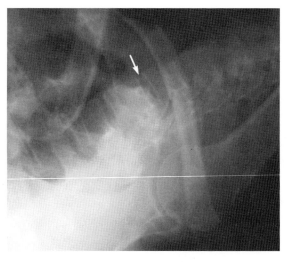

Fig. 13-15 Dorsal decubitus position lateral projection of the cervicothoracic region performed on a trauma patient. Negative examination. Note excellent image of the C7-T1 joint with use of the Ferlic swimmer's filter (*arrow*).

🔥 AP AXIAL PROJECTION[1]

Trauma positioning tips

- *Do not perform this projection until the attending physician has reviewed the lateral projection.*
- This projection is usually performed after the lateral projection.
- If the patient is on a backboard, either on a stretcher or an x-ray table, gently and slowly lift the backboard and place the IR in position under the patient's neck.
- Move the patient's head and neck as little as possible.
- Collimate the width of the x-ray beam closely to reduce scatter radiation.
- *Shield gonads and other personnel in the room.*

---

[1]See standard projection, Volume 1, p. 398.

Patient position considerations

- Supine, usually on a backboard and in a cervical collar
- Have the patient relax his or her shoulders as much as possible.
- Ensure the patient is looking straight ahead without any rotation of the head or neck.
- Place the IR under the backboard, if present, centered to approximately C4 (Fig. 13-16).
- The central ray is directed 15 to 20 degrees cephalad to the center of the IR and entering at C4.

Structures shown

C3 through T1 or T2 including interspaces and surrounding soft tissues should be demonstrated with minimal rotation and distortion. Density and contrast should demonstrate cortical margins and soft tissue shadows (Fig. 13-17).

NOTE: If the patient is not on a backboard or an x-ray table, then preferably the attending physician should lift the patient's head and neck while the radiographer positions the IR under the patient.

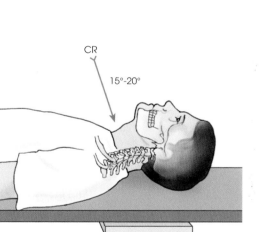

Fig. 13-16 Patient and IR positioned for a trauma AP axial projection of cervical vertebrae.

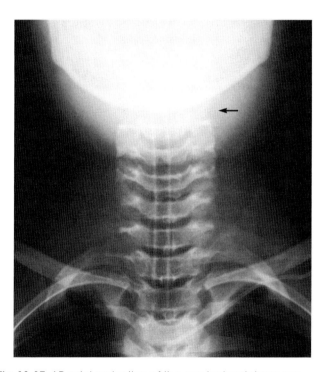

Fig. 13-17 AP axial projection of the cervical vertebrae performed on an 11-year-old trauma patient. Note cervical spine completely dislocated between C2 and C3 *(arrow).* The patient died on the x-ray table after the x-ray examinations were performed.

✦ AP AXIAL OBLIQUE PROJECTION

Trauma positioning tips

- *Do not perform this projection until the attending physician has reviewed the lateral projection.*
- If the patient is on a backboard, gently and slowly lift the board and place the IR in position.
- Move the patient's head and neck as little as possible.
- Do *not* use a grid IR because the compound central-ray angle results in grid cut-off. However, many radiography machines do not allow the x-ray tube-head to move in a compound angle. On these machines, only the 45 degree angle is used and a grid IR may then be used to improve contrast.
- Collimate the width of the x-ray beam closely to reduce scatter radiation.
- *Shield gonads and other personnel in the room.*

Patient position considerations

- Supine, usually on a backboard and in a cervical collar
- Have the patient relax his or her shoulders as much as possible.
- Ensure that the patient is looking straight ahead without any rotation of the head or neck.
- Place the IR under the immobilization device, if present, centered at the level of C4 and the adjacent mastoid process (about 3 inches [7.6 cm] lateral to mid-sagittal plane of neck) (Fig. 13-18). If a grid IR is used with one central-ray angle, the grid lines should be perpendicular to the long axis of the spine.
- The central ray is directed 45 degrees lateromedially. When a double angle is used, angle 15 to 20 degrees cephalad.
- The central ray enters slightly lateral to the midsagittal plane at the level of the thyroid cartilage and passing through C4.
- The central ray exit point should coincide with the center of the IR.

Structures shown

Cervical and upper thoracic vertebral bodies, pedicles, open intervertebral disk spaces, and open intervertebral foramina of the side opposite the central-ray entrance point are shown. This projection provides excellent detail of the facet joints, and it is important in detecting subluxations and dislocations (Fig. 13-19). If the 15-degree cephalic angle is not used, the intervertebral foramina will be foreshortened.

NOTE: If the patient is not on a backboard or an x-ray table, then preferably the attending physician should lift the patient's head and neck while the radiographer positions the IR under the patient.

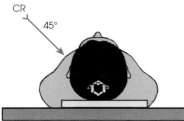

Fig. 13-18 Patient and IR positioned for a trauma AP axial oblique projection of the cervical vertebrae. The central ray *(CR)* is positioned 45 degrees mediolaterally and, if possible, 15 to 20 degrees cephalad.

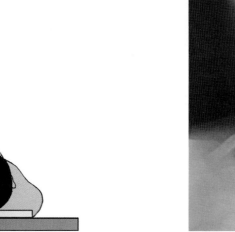

Fig. 13-19 AP axial oblique projection of the cervical vertebrae performed on a trauma patient using a 45-degree angle. Radiograph was made using a non–grid exposure technique. Negative image. Note excellent alignment of the vertebral bodies and intervertebral foramen.

✸ LATERAL PROJECTIONS
Dorsal decubitus positions

Trauma positioning tips
- *Always* perform these dorsal decubitus positions before the AP projections of the spine because the *attending physician* should review the dorsal decubitus lateral projections *to rule out vertebral fracture or dislocation* before other *projections are performed.*
- Move the patient as little as possible.
- Use of a grid is necessary to improve image contrast. Use the vertical Bucky if possible to maximize positioning and for optimal image quality.
- *Shield gonads and other personnel in the room.*

Patient position considerations
- The patient is generally immobilized and on a backboard.
- Have the patient cross the arms over chest to remove them from the anatomy of interest.
- Place the IR 1½ to 2 inches (3.8 to 5 cm) above the patient's relaxed shoulders for the thoracic spine and at the level of the iliac crests for the lumbar spine (Fig. 13-20).
- If not using the vertical Bucky, ensure that the IR is perfectly vertical.
- The central ray is *horizontal*, perpendicular to the longitudinal center of the IR, and going through the spine.
- Collimate closely to the spine to reduce scattered radiation and patient dose.

Structures shown
For the thoracic spine, the image should include T3 or T4-L1. The lumbar spine image should, at a minimum, include T12 to the sacrum. The vertebral bodies should be seen in profile with minimal rotation and distortion. Density and contrast should be sufficient to demonstrate cortical margins and bony trabeculation (Fig. 13-21).

NOTE: A lateral projection of the cervicothoracic spine must be performed to visualize the upper thoracic spine in profile.

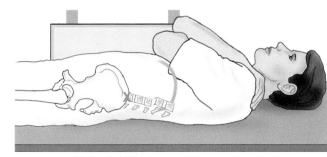

Horizontal CR to top
of iliac crest

Fig. 13-20 Patient and IR positioned for trauma lateral projection of the lumbar spine using the dorsal decubitus position and using a vertical Bucky device.

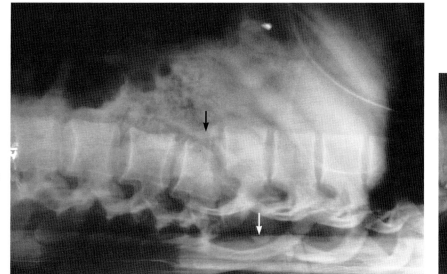
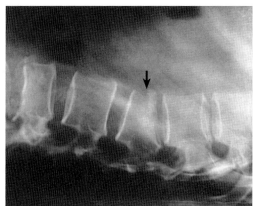

Fig. 13-21 Dorsal decubitus position lateral projection of the lumbar spine performed on a trauma patient. **A,** Fracture and dislocation of L2 *(black arrow).* Note backboard *(white arrow).* **B,** Compression fracture of the body of L2 *(arrow).* This coned-down image provides better detail of the fracture area.

🔥 AP PROJECTION[1,2]

Trauma positioning tips

- Most trauma patients must be radiographed in the supine position. If it is necessary to see air-fluid levels, a cross-table lateral x-ray beam (dorsal decubitus position) can be performed.
- Obtain help in lifting the patient to position the IR if the stretcher is not equipped with an IR tray.
- Check for signs of respiratory distress or changes in level of consciousness during radiographic examination, and *report any changes to the attending physician immediately.*

---

[1]See standard projection, Volume 1, p. 532.
[2]See mobile projection, Volume 3, p. 242.

- Assess the patient's ability to follow breathing instructions.
- Use the maximum SID possible to minimize magnification of the heart shadow.
- Use universal precautions if wounds or bleeding, or both, are present, and protect the IR with plastic covering.
- Mark entrance or exit wounds, or both, with radiopaque indicators if evaluating a penetrating injury.
- Use of a grid improves image contrast.
- *Shield gonads and other personnel in the room.*

Patient position considerations

- Position the top of the IR about 1½ to 2 inches (3.8 to 5 cm) above the patient's shoulders.
- Move the patient's arms away from the thorax and out of the collimated field.
- Ensure that the patient is looking straight ahead with his or her chin extended out of the collimated field.
- Check for rotation by determining whether the shoulders are equidistant to the IR or stretcher. This position places the midcoronal plane parallel to the IR, minimizing image distortion.
- The central ray should be directed perpendicular to the center of the IR at a point 3 inches (7.6 cm) below the jugular notch (Fig. 13-22).

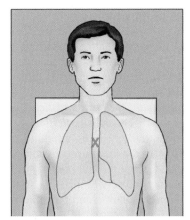

CR to center of IR

Fig. 13-22 Patient and IR positioned for a trauma AP projection of the chest.

Structures shown

An AP projection of the thorax is demonstrated. The lung fields should be included in their entirety, with minimal rotation and distortion present. Adequate aeration of the lungs must be imaged to demonstrate the lung parenchyma (Fig. 13-23).

NOTE: Ribs are somewhat visible on an AP projection, necessitating the use of a grid IR to increase image contrast. Use proper breathing instructions and techniques to ensure adequate visualization of ribs of interest.

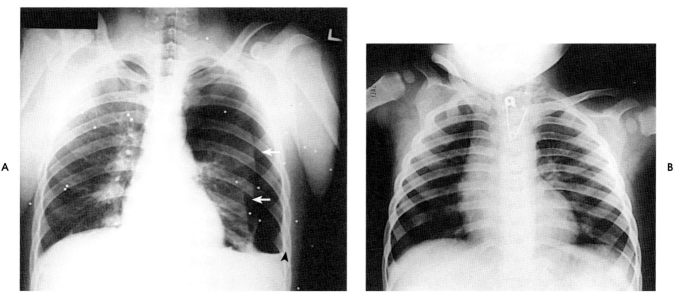

Fig. 13-23 AP upright projection of the chest performed on a trauma patient. **A,** Multiple buckshot in chest caused a hemopneumothorax. Arrows show the margin of the collapsed lung with free air laterally. Arrowhead shows fluid level at the costophrenic angle, left lung. **B,** Open safety pin lodged in esophagus of a 13-month-old baby.

🔥 AP PROJECTION[1,2]

Trauma positioning tips

- Use of a radiographic table and a Bucky provides optimum image quality. Before moving the patient, verify transfer to table with the attending physician.
- If transfer is not possible, use of a grid IR is required.
- Determine the possibility of fluid accumulation within the abdominal cavity to establish appropriate exposure factors.
- For patients with blunt force or projectile injuries, check for signs of internal bleeding during radiographic examination and *report any changes to the attending physician immediately.*

---

[1]See standard projection, Volume 2, p. 102.
[2]See mobile projection, Volume 3, p. 246.

- Mark entrance or exit wounds, or both, with radiopaque markers if evaluating projectile injuries.
- Assess the ability of the patient to follow breathing instructions.
- Use standard precautions if wounds or bleeding are present, and protect IR with plastic covering.
- *Shield gonads, if possible, and other personnel in the room.*

Patient position considerations

- Ask ED personnel to assist in transferring the patient to the radiographic table, if possible.
- If transfer is not advisable, obtain assistance to carefully lift the patient to position the grid IR under him or her.

- Center the grid IR at the level of the iliac crests, and ensure that the pubic symphysis is included (Fig. 13-24). On patients with a long torso, a second AP projection of the upper abdomen may be required to demonstrate the diaphragm and lower ribs.
- If the patient is on a stretcher, check that the grid IR is parallel with the patient's midcoronal plane. Correct tilting with sponges, sandbags, rolled towels, etc. The grid IR must be perfectly horizontal to prevent grid cut-off and image distortion. If you are unable to correct tilt on grid IR, then angle the central ray to maintain part–IR–central ray alignment.
- The central ray is directed to the center of the IR.

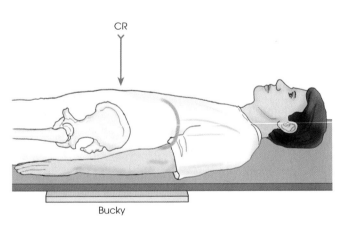

CR

Bucky

Fig. 13-24 Patient and IR positioned for a trauma AP projection of the abdomen.

Structures shown

An AP projection of the abdomen is demonstrated. The entire abdomen including the pubic symphysis and diaphragm should be included without distortion or rotation. Density and contrast should be adequate to demonstrate tissue interfaces, such as the lower margin of the liver, kidney shadows, psoas muscles, and cortical margins of bones (Fig. 13-25).

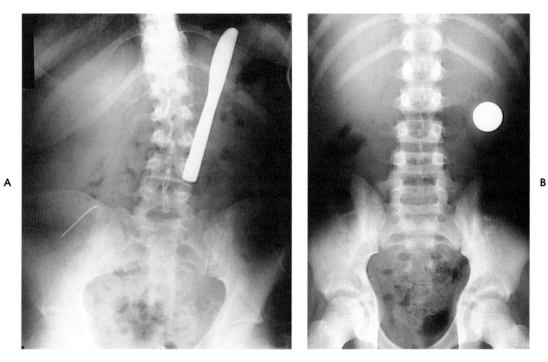

Fig. 13-25 AP projection of abdomen performed on a trauma patient. **A,** Table knife in the stomach along with other small metallic foreign bodies swallowed by the patient. **B,** Coin in the stomach swallowed by patient.

♠ AP PROJECTION[1,2]
Left lateral decubitus position

Trauma positioning tips

- Use of the vertical Bucky provides optimum image quality. If the patient must be imaged using a mobile radiographic unit, a grid IR is required.
- Verify with the *attending physician* that patient movement is possible and whether the image is necessary to assess fluid accumulation or free air in the abdominal cavity.
- The *left lateral* decubitus position demonstrates free air in the abdominal cavity because the density of the liver provides good contrast for visualization of any free air.
- If fluid accumulation is of primary interest, the side down, or dependent side, must be elevated off the stretcher or table to be completely demonstrated.
- Check for signs of internal bleeding during the radiographic examination, and *report any changes to the attending physician immediately.*

[1]See standard projection, Volume 2, p. 104.
[2]See mobile projection, Volume 3, p. 248.

- Use universal precautions if wounds or bleeding are present, and protect the IR with plastic covering. Mark all entrance and exit wounds with radiopaque markers when imaging for penetrating injuries.
- *Shield gonads, if possible, and personnel in the room.*

Patient position considerations

- Carefully and slowly turn the patient into the recumbent left lateral position. Flex the knees to provide stability.
- If the image is being taken for visualization of fluid, carefully place a block under the length of the abdomen to ensure that the entire right side is visualized.
- Ensure that the midcoronal plane is vertical to prevent image distortion.
- Center the IR 2 inches (5 cm) above the iliac crests to include the diaphragm (Fig. 13-26).

- The patient should be in the lateral position at least 5 minutes before the exposure to allow any free air to rise and be visualized.
- The central ray is directed *horizontal* and perpendicular to the center of the IR.

Structures shown

Air and fluid levels within the abdominal cavity are demonstrated. This projection is especially helpful in assessing free air in the abdomen when an upright position cannot be used. Density and contrast should be adequate to demonstrate tissue interfaces, such as the lower margin of the liver, kidney shadows, psoas muscles, and cortical margins of bones (Fig. 13-27).

NOTE: A lateral projection using the dorsal decubitus position may be substituted for this projection if the patient is too ill or injured to be properly positioned in a left lateral position. (The position will be identical to the dorsal decubitus position, lateral projection of the lumbar spine. See Fig. 13-20.)

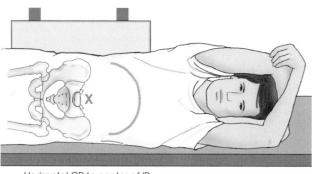

Horizontal CR to center of IR

Fig. 13-26 Patient and IR positioned for a trauma AP projection of the abdomen using the left lateral decubitus position and using a vertical Bucky device.

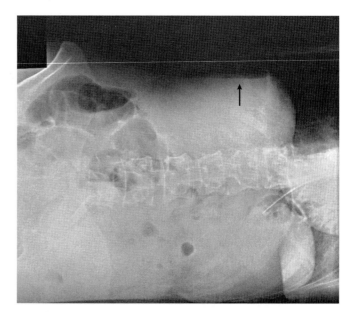

Fig. 13-27 Left lateral decubitus position AP projection of the abdomen performed on a trauma patient. Free intraperitoneal air is seen on the upper or right side of the abdomen *(arrow).* The radiograph is slightly underexposed to demonstrate the free air more easily.

🦅 AP PROJECTION[1,2]

Trauma positioning tips

- Up to 50% of pelvic fractures are fatal as a result of vascular damage and shock. The mortality risk increases with the energy of the force and the health of the victim.
- Pelvic fractures have a high incidence of internal hemorrhage. *Alert the attending physician immediately if the abdomen becomes distended and firm.*
- Hemorrhagic shock is common with pelvic and abdominal injuries. *Reassess the patient's level of consciousness repeatedly while performing radiographic examinations.*
- *Do not* attempt to internally rotate limbs for true AP projection of proximal femurs on this projection.
- Collimate closely to reduce scatter radiation.
- *Shield gonads, if possible, and other personnel in the room.*

---

[1]See standard projection, Volume 1, p. 345.
[2]See mobile projection, Volume 3, p. 250.

Patient position considerations

- The patient is supine, possibly on a backboard or in trauma pants.
- Carefully and slowly transfer the patient to the radiographic table to allow the use of a Bucky.
- If unable to transfer the patient, use a grid IR positioned under the immobilization device or patient. Ensure that the grid is horizontal and parallel to the patient's midcoronal plane to minimize distortion and rotation. Carefully align it to the central ray to minimize distortion and rotation.
- Position the IR so that the center is 2 inches (5 cm) inferior to the anterior superior iliac spine or 2 inches (5 cm) superior to the pubic symphysis.
- The central ray is directed perpendicular to the center of the IR (Fig. 13-28).
- Check the collimated field to ensure that the iliac crests and hip joints are included.

Structures shown

The pelvis and proximal femora should be demonstrated in their entirety with minimal rotation and distortion. Femoral necks will be foreshortened, and lesser trochanters will be seen. Optimum density and contrast should demonstrate bony trabeculation and soft tissue shadows (Fig. 13-29).

NOTE: Diagnosis of pelvic fractures in the ED is often immediately followed by an emergency cystogram procedure. The necessary ancillary equipment and contrast media should be readily available.

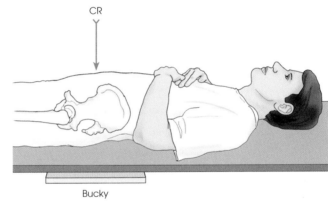

Fig. 13-28 Patient and IR positioned for a trauma AP projection of the pelvis.

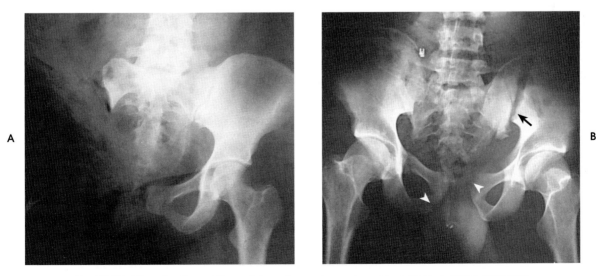

Fig. 13-29 AP projection of the pelvis performed on a trauma patient. **A,** Entire right limb torn off after being hit by a car. The pelvic bone was disarticulated at the pubic symphysis and sacroiliac joint. The patient survived. **B,** Separation of the pubic bones (*arrowheads*) anteriorly and associated fracture of the left ilium (*arrow*).

☀ LATERAL PROJECTION[1]
Dorsal decubitus position

Trauma positioning tips

- Because the scalp and face are vascular, these areas tend to bleed profusely. Protect IRs with plastic covering and practice universal precautions.
- A grid IR is used for this projection. Elevate the patient's head on a radiolucent sponge *only after cervical injury, such as fracture or dislocation, has been ruled out.*

[1]See standard projection, Volume 2, p. 308.

- Vomiting is a symptom of intracranial injury. *If a patient begins to vomit, log-roll him or her to a lateral position to prevent aspiration and alert the attending physician immediately.*
- *Alert the attending physician immediately if there is any change in the patient's level of consciousness or if the pupils are unequal.*
- Collimate closely to reduce scatter radiation.
- *Shield gonads and other personnel in the room.*

Patient position considerations

- Have the patient relax his or her shoulders.
- After cervical spine injury has been ruled out, the patient's head may be positioned to align interpupillary line perpendicular to the IR and the midsagittal plane vertical.
- If the patient is wearing a cervical collar, carefully minimize rotation and tilt of the cranium.
- Ensure that the IR is vertical.
- Direct the central ray *horizontal* entering perpendicular to a point 2 inches (5 cm) above the EAM (Fig. 13-30).

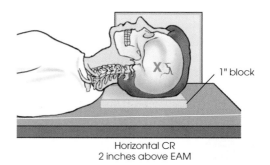

Horizontal CR
2 inches above EAM

Fig. 13-30 Patient and IR positioned for a trauma lateral projection of the cranium using the dorsal decubitus position. Note sponge in place to raise head to demonstrate posterior cranium (after checking lateral cervical spine radiograph).

Structures shown

A profile image of the superimposed halves of the cranium is seen with detail of the side closer to the IR demonstrated (Fig. 13-31). With some injuries, air-fluid levels can be demonstrated in the sphenoid sinuses.

NOTE: The supine lateral position may be used on a patient without a cervical spine injury. See Volume 2, p. 308.

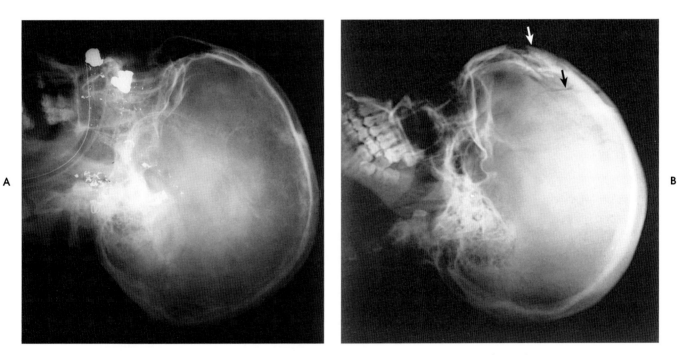

Fig. 13-31 Dorsal decubitus position lateral projection of the cranium performed on a trauma patient. **A,** Two GSWs entering at the level of C1 and traveling forward to the face and lodging in the area of the zygomas. Note bullet fragments in the EAM area. **B,** Multiple frontal skull fractures *(arrows)* caused by hitting the windshield during an auto accident.

✿ AP PROJECTION[1]
AP AXIAL PROJECTION—
TOWNE METHOD[2]

Trauma positioning tips

- Profuse bleeding should be anticipated with head and facial injuries. Use universal precautions and protect IRs and sponges with plastic.
- *Cervical spine injury should be ruled out before attempting to position the head.*
- AP projection is used for injury to the anterior cranium. The AP axial projection, Towne method, demonstrates the posterior cranium.

---

[1]See standard projection, Volume 2, p. 314.
[2]See standard projection, Volume 2, p. 316.

- Vomiting is a symptom of an intracranial injury. *If a patient begins to vomit, logroll him or her to a lateral position to prevent aspiration and alert the attending physician immediately.*
- *Alert the attending physician if the patient's level of consciousness decreases or if pupils are unequal.*
- Collimate closely to reduce scatter radiation.
- A grid IR or Bucky should be used to ensure proper image contrast.
- *Shield gonads and other personnel in the room.*

Patient position considerations

- If available and the patient's condition allows, carefully and slowly transfer the patient to the x-ray table using the immobilization device and proper transfer techniques. Transfer allows the use of the Bucky and minimizes risk of injury to the patient when positioning the IR.

- If the patient is not transferred to the radiographic table, the grid IR should be placed under the immobilization device. If no such device is present, the *attending physician* should carefully lift the patient's head and neck while the radiographer positions the grid IR under the patient.
- After a cervical spine injury has been ruled out, the patient's head may be positioned to place the OML or IOML and midsagittal plane perpendicular to the IR.
- If the patient is wearing a cervical collar, the OML or IOML cannot be positioned perpendicularly. For the AP axial projection, Towne method, the central-ray angle may have to be increased up to 60 degrees caudad, maintaining a 30-degree angle to the OML.

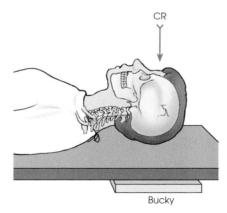

Fig. 13-32 Patient and IR positioned for a trauma AP projection of the cranium.

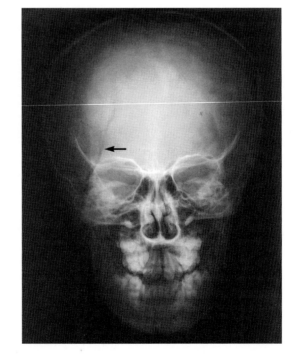

Fig. 13-33 AP projection of the cranium performed on a trauma patient. Fracture of the occipital bone *(arrow)*.

- For an AP projection, the central ray enters perpendicular to the nasion (Fig. 13-32). An AP axial projection with the central ray directed 15 degrees cephalad is sometimes performed in place of, or to accompany, the AP projection.
- For the AP axial projection, Towne method, position the top of the IR at the level of the cranial vertex. The central ray is then directed 30 degrees caudad to the OML or 37 degrees to the IOML (Fig. 13-33). The central ray passes through the EAM and exits the foramen magnum.

Structures shown

The AP projection demonstrates the anterior cranium (Fig. 13-34). The AP axial projection, Towne method, demonstrates the posterior cranium and foramen magnum (Fig. 13-35).

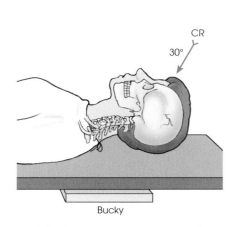

Fig. 13-34 Patient and IR positioned for a trauma AP axial projection, Towne method, of the cranium using a 30-degree central ray *(CR)* angulation.

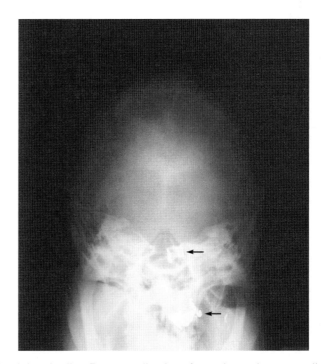

Fig. 13-35 AP axial projection, Towne method, performed on a trauma patient. GSW to the head. Metal clip *(upper arrow)* indicates entrance of the bullet on the anterior cranium. Flattened bullet and fragments *(lower arrow)* are lodged in the area of C2.

Trauma radiography

♠ ACANTHIOPARIETAL PROJECTION[1]

REVERSE WATERS METHOD

Trauma positioning tips

- Anticipate profuse bleeding with facial trauma. Protect IRs with plastic covering and practice universal precautions.
- Cervical spine injury should be ruled out before attempting to position the head.
- *Alert the attending physician if the patient's level of consciousness decreases or if pupils are unequal.*
- A grid IR or Bucky is used to ensure proper image contrast.
- Collimate closely to reduce scatter radiation.
- *Shield gonads and other personnel in the room.*

[1]See standard projection, Volume 2, p. 356.

Patient position considerations

- If available and the patient's condition allows, carefully and slowly transfer the patient to the x-ray table using the immobilization device and proper transfer techniques. Transfer allows the use of the Bucky and minimizes the risk of injury to the patient when positioning the IR.
- If the patient is not transferred to the radiographic table, the grid IR should be placed under the immobilization device. If no such device is present, the *attending physician* should carefully lift the patient's head and neck while the radiographer positions the grid IR under the patient.
- If possible, the IOML should be positioned approximately perpendicular to the IR. Note the angle of the MML.
- The midsagittal plane should be perpendicular to prevent rotation.
- The central ray is angled cephalad until it is parallel with the MML. The central ray enters the acanthion (Fig. 13-36).
- Center the IR to the central ray.

Structures shown

The superior facial bones are demonstrated (Fig. 13-37). The image should be similar to the parietoacanthial projection or routine Waters method and demonstrate symmetry of the face.

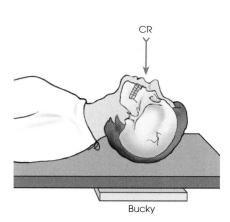

Fig. 13-36 Patient and IR positioned for a trauma acanthioparietal projection, reverse Waters method, of the cranium.

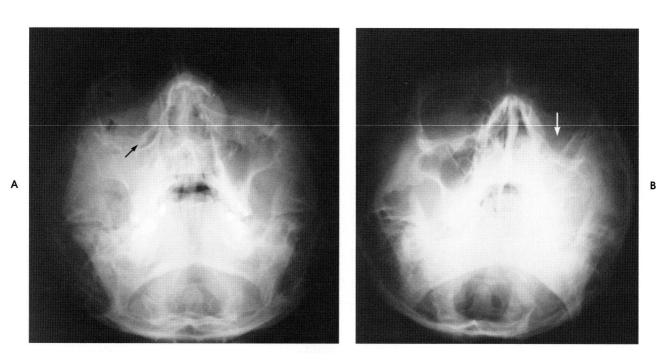

Fig. 13-37 Acanthioparietal projections, reverse Water's method, performed on trauma patients for demonstration of the facial bones. **A,** Fracture of the right orbital floor *(arrow)* with blood-filled maxillary sinus (note, no air in the sinus). Patient hit face on steering wheel during auto accident. **B,** Blowout fracture of the left orbital floor *(arrow)* with blood-filled maxillary sinus (note, no air in the sinus). Patient was hit with a fist.

Trauma positioning tips

- Use standard precautions and cover IRs and positioning aides in plastic if wounds are present.
- When lifting an injured limb, *support it at both joints and lift slowly. Lift only enough to place the IR under the part—sometimes only 1 to 2 inches (2.5 to 5 cm).* Always obtain help in lifting injured limbs and positioning the IRs to minimize patient discomfort.
- If the limb is severely injured, *do not attempt to position for true AP or lateral projections. Expose the two projections, 90 degrees apart, moving the injured limb as little as possible.*

- Check the patient's status during radiographic examination. Be aware that shock can occur from crushing injuries to extremities.
- Long bone radiographs must include both joints on the image.
- Separate examinations of the adjacent joints *may be required* if injury indicates. Do not attempt to "short cut" by only performing one projection of the long bone.
- *Shield gonads and other personnel in the room.*

Patient position considerations

- If possible, demonstrate the desired position for the conscious patient. Assist the patient in attempting to assume the position, rather than moving the injured limb.
- If the patient is unable to position the limb close to that required, move the IR and x-ray tube to obtain the desired projection (Figs. 13-38 to 13-41).

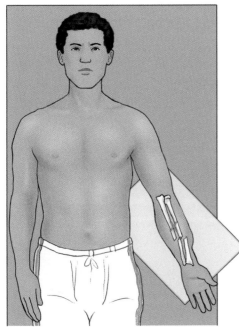

CR to center of IR

Fig. 13-38 Patient and IR positioned for a trauma AP projection of forearm.

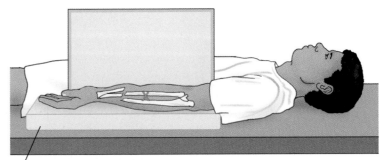

2-inch block   Horizontal CR to center of IR

Fig. 13-39 Patient and IR positioned for a trauma cross-table lateral projection of forearm.

Trauma radiography

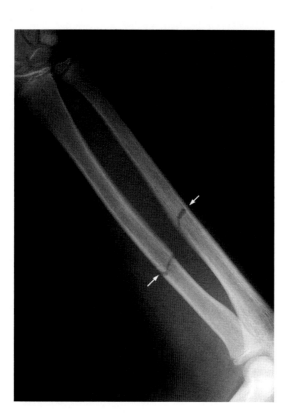

Fig. 13-40 AP projection of the forearm performed on a trauma patient. Fracture of the midportion of the radius and ulna *(arrows)*.

- Shoulder injuries should be initially imaged "as is" without rotating the limb. The "reverse" PA oblique projection of the scapular Y (an AP oblique) is useful in demonstrating dislocation of the glenohumeral joint with minimal patient movement. The patient is turned up 45 degrees and supported in position (Figs. 13-42 and 13-43).
- If imaging while the patient is still on a stretcher, check to make sure the IR is perfectly horizontal to minimize image distortion.
- The central ray must be directed perpendicular to the IR to minimize distortion.
- Immobilization techniques for the IR and upper limb are useful in obtaining an optimal image with minimal patient discomfort.

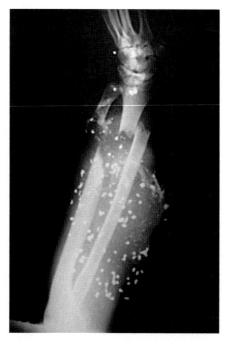

Fig. 13-41 Cross-table lateral projection of the forearm performed on a trauma patient. GSW to the forearm with fracture of the radius and ulna and extensive soft tissue damage.

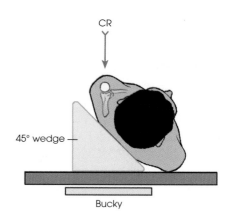

Fig. 13-42 Patient and IR positioned for a trauma AP oblique projection of the shoulder to demonstrate the scapular Y. (Reverse of the PA oblique, scapular Y—see Chapter 5.)

Structures shown

Images of the anatomy of interest, 90 degrees from one another, should be demonstrated. Density and contrast should be sufficient to visualize cortical margins, bony trabeculation, and surrounding soft tissues. Both joints should be included in projections of long bones. Projections of adjacent joints must be centered to the joint to properly demonstrate the articular ends (Figs. 13-44 and 13-45).

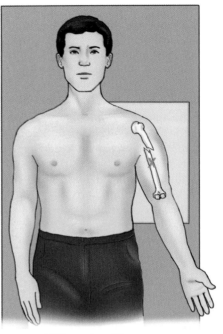

CR to center of IR

Fig. 13-44 Patient and IR positioned for a trauma AP projection of humerus.

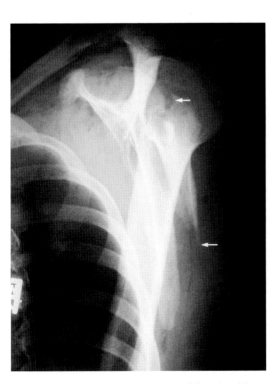

Fig. 13-43 AP oblique projection of the shoulder (reverse of the PA oblique, scapular Y) performed on a trauma patient. Several fractures of the scapula *(arrows)* with significant displacement.

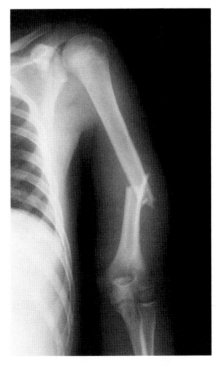

Fig. 13-45 AP projection of the humerus performed on a trauma patient. Fracture of the midshaft of the humerus.

Trauma positioning tips

- Use standard precautions, and cover IRs and positioning aids in plastic if open wounds are present.
- Immobilization devices are often present with injuries to the lower limbs, especially in cases with suspected femur fractures. *Perform image procedures with immobilization in place, unless directed to remove them by the attending physician.*
- When lifting an injured limb, *support at both joints and lift slowly. Lift only enough to place the IR under the part— sometimes only 1 to 2 inches (2.5 to 5 cm).* Always obtain help in lifting injured limbs and positioning IRs to minimize patient discomfort (Fig. 13-46).

- If the limb is severely injured, *do not* attempt to position it for true AP and lateral projections. Take two projections, 90 degrees apart, moving the injured limb as little as possible.
- Long bone examinations must include both joints. Separate images may be required.
- Examinations of the adjacent joints may be required if the condition indicates. The central ray and IR must be properly centered to the joint of interest to properly demonstrate the anatomy.
- Check on patient status during radiographic examination. Be aware that shock can occur with severe injuries to the lower extremities.
- A grid IR should be used on thicker anatomic parts, such as the femur.
- *Shield gonads and other personnel in the room.*

Patient position considerations

- Demonstrate or describe the desired position for the patient and allow him or her to attempt to assume the position, rather than moving the injured limb. Assist the patient as needed.
- If the patient is unable to position the limb close to the required true position, move the IR and x-ray tube to obtain projection (Figs. 13-47 and 13-48).
- If imaging while the patient is still on a stretcher, check to make sure the IR is perfectly horizontal to minimize image distortion.
- The central ray must be directed perpendicular to the IR to minimize distortion.
- Immobilization techniques for the IR and lower limb are extremely useful to obtain optimum quality with minimal patient discomfort.

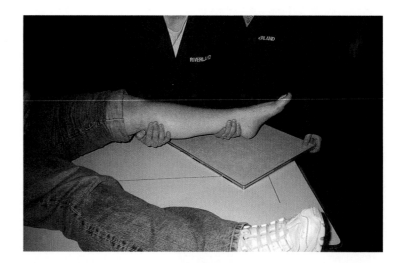

Fig. 13-46 Proper method of lifting the lower limb for placement of the IR (for AP projection) or placement of elevation blocks (for cross-table lateral). Lift only high enough to place the IR or blocks underneath. Note two hands used to gently lift this patient with a broken leg.

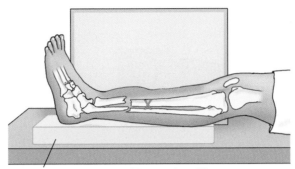

2-inch block   Horizontal CR to center of IR

Fig. 13-47 Patient and IR positioned for a trauma cross-table lateral projection of the lower leg. IR and central ray *(CR)* may be moved superiorly or inferiorly to center for other portions of the lower limb. Note positioning blocks placed under the limb to elevate it so that all of the anatomy of interest is seen.

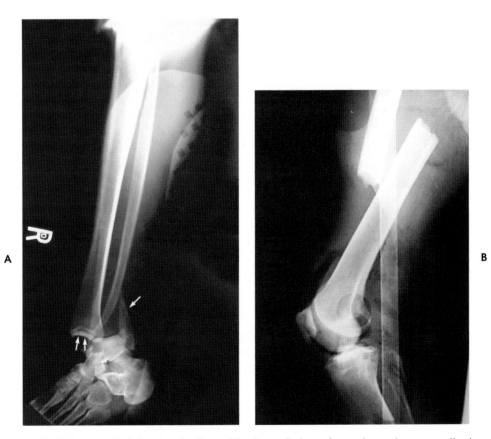

Fig. 13-48 Cross-table lateral projection of the lower limb performed on a trauma patient. **A,** Dislocation of the tibia from the talus *(double arrows)* and fracture of the fibula *(arrow).* **B,** Complete fracture and displacement of the femur. The proximal femur is seen in the AP projection, and the distal femur is rotated 90 degrees at the fracture point, resulting in a lateral projection. Note artifacts caused by immobilization devices.

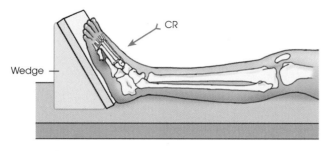

Fig. 13-49 Patient and IR positioned for a trauma AP projection of the foot or toes. Note that the IR is supported with sandbags for positioning against the foot.

Structures shown

Images of the anatomy of interest, 90 degrees from each other, should be demonstrated. Density and contrast should be sufficient to visualize cortical margins, bony trabeculation, and surrounding soft tissues. Both joints should be included in examinations of long bones. Images of articulations must be properly centered to demonstrate anatomy properly (Figs. 13-49 and 13-50).

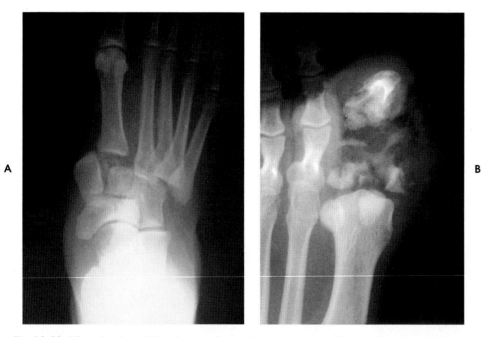

Fig. 13-50 AP projection of the foot performed on a trauma patient. **A,** Fracture and dislocation of the tarsal bones with exposure technique adjusted for optimal image of this area. **B,** GSW to the great toe.

Many injuries, once diagnosed, may require additional follow-up evaluation via a special procedure or additional imaging modality. CT is used extensively to further investigate fractures (Figs. 13-51 to 13-53) and head injuries. CT is also useful in revealing the extent of injuries sustained from blunt traumas. In penetrating trauma, CT is invaluable in helping to trace the ballistic path and to determine the organs affected by the projectile (Fig. 13-54). Angiography may be used to evaluate vascular damage. The role of ultrasound in emergency diagnosis is also increasing. These specialized imaging modalities may require a scout radiograph before the patient is referred to a different modality.

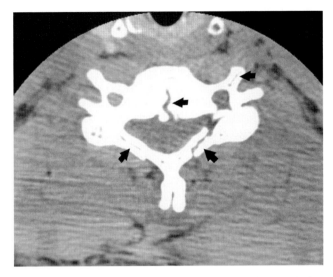

Fig. 13-51 CT of fifth cervical vertebra demonstrating multiple fractures *(arrows)*, resulting from a fall from a tree.

(Courtesy Sunie Grossman, RT(R), St. Bernard's Medical Center, Jonesboro, Ark.)

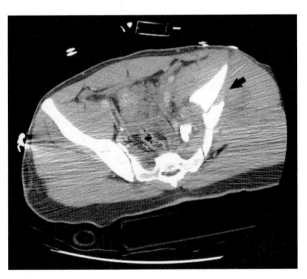

Fig. 13-52 CT of the pelvis demonstrating a fracture of the left ilium *(arrow)* with fragment displacement. Clothing and backboard artifacts are evident.

(Courtesy St. Bernard's Medical Center, Jonesboro, Ark.)

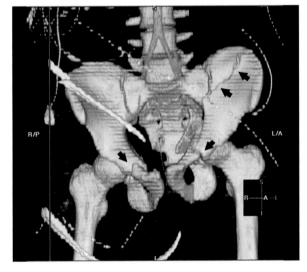

Fig. 13-53 Three-dimensional reconstruction of the pelvis from the patient in Fig. 13-52. Multiple pelvic fractures are well visualized *(arrows)*.

(Courtesy St. Bernard's Medical Center, Jonesboro, Ark.)

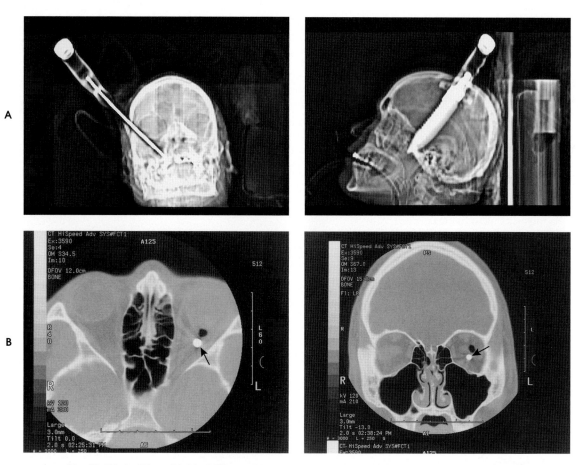

Fig. 13-54 A, AP and lateral CT scout images of the cranium. Note knife placement in the cranium. Conventional cranium radiographs were not obtained on this trauma patient. Patient was sent directly to the CT scanner for these images and sectional images before going to surgery. Patient recovered and returned home. **B,** Axial and coronal CT sectional images of the cranium at the level of the eye. Patient was shot in the left eye with a BB gun. Note BB *(arrow).* Adjacent black area is air. Patient now has monocular vision.

(**A,** Courtesy Tony Hofmann, RT(R)(CT), Shands Hospital School of Radiologic Technology, Jacksonville, Fla. **B,** Courtesy Mark H. Layne, RT(R).)

Cystography

Within the trauma radiographer's role falls the responsibility of performing ED special procedures requiring the administration of contrast media. For example, once an initial abdominal or pelvis radiograph has demonstrated a fracture of the pelvis, cystography is often ordered by the emergency physician to determine injury to the bladder (Fig. 13-55). The trauma radiographer must be prepared to alter the routine procedure to fit the condition of the patient. Optimal images are obtained if the patient is stable enough to be moved to the radiographic table. Assistance is necessary to properly transfer the patient to the table. If the examination must be performed using a mobile radiographic unit, obtain assistance to properly lift the patient to center the IR. Ensure that all personnel and nearby patients are properly shielded.

Intravenous Urography

Additionally, intravenous urography (IVU) may be ordered to assess blunt or penetrating trauma that may affect the kidneys. Generally, the procedure is abbreviated, with only one or two images taken after the contrast is administered to determine if the contrast media is being properly excreted (Fig. 13-56). The trauma radiographer must again be prepared to alter the procedure to accommodate the patient's condition.

Critical to the performance of special procedures on trauma patients is *preparedness*. The availability of all necessary ancillary equipment and contrast media should be inventoried at the beginning of each shift. Time is of the essence, and having all necessary materials available is critical to producing the images in the most efficient manner.

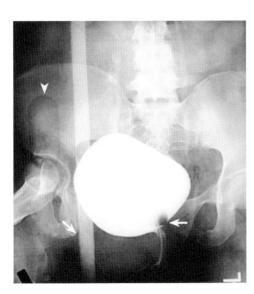

Fig. 13-55 AP pelvis for trauma cystogram of the urinary bladder. Pelvic trauma from auto accident. Note separation of the pubic symphysis *(arrows)*. Patient survived after surgery. Vertical line near right side of image and ovoid area *(arrowhead)* are from the backboard.

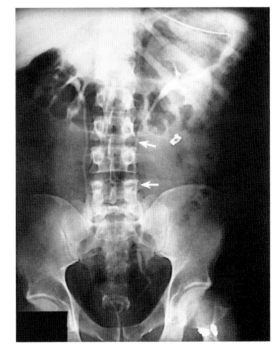

Fig. 13-56 AP abdomen performed during a trauma IVU on a gunshot victim. Bullet entered the point marked by a surgical clip in the upper left quadrant and stopped in the left hip (see bullet fragments on left femoral neck). Note medial displacement of the contrast-filled left ureter *(arrows)* caused by retroperitoneal hemorrhage.

Selected bibliography

Berquist TH, editor: *Imaging of orthopedic trauma and surgery,* ed 2, New York, 1992, Raven Press.

Bishop and Associates: *Trauma care* (website): www.traumacare.com/Terms.html. Accessed May 29, 2001.

Cwinn A: Pelvis and hip. In Rosen P, editor: *Emergency medicine: concepts and clinical practice,* ed 4, St Louis, 1998, Mosby.

Drafke M: *Trauma and mobile radiography,* Philadelphia, 1990, FA Davis.

Forbes C et al, editors: *ABC of emergency radiology,* London, 1995, BMJ.

Keats TE, editor: *Emergency radiology,* Chicago, 1984, Mosby.

Mancini ME, Klein J: *Decision-making in trauma management: a multidisciplinary approach,* Philadelphia, 1991, Decker.

McCort JJ, Mindelzun RE, editors: *Trauma radiology,* New York, 1990, Churchill-Livingstone.

Office of Statistics and Programming, National Centers for Injury Prevention and Control, CDC. Data source: National Center for Health Statistics Vital Statistics System (1998): *10 leading causes of death, United States, all races, both sexes* (website): www.cdc.gov/ncipc/wisqars/default.htm. Accessed August 8, 2001.

Online Medical Dictionary (n.d.): www.graylab.ac.uk/cgi-bin/omd. Accessed June 27, 2001.

Rosen P, editor: *Diagnostic radiology in emergency medicine,* St Louis, 1992, Mosby.

Texas Department of Health: *Essential general trauma facility criteria defined* (website): www.tdh.state.tx.us/hcqs/ems/filelib.htm. Accessed August 2001.

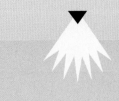

14

MOUTH AND SALIVARY GLANDS

Lateral submandibular gland showing opacification of sub-mandibular duct *(arrow).*

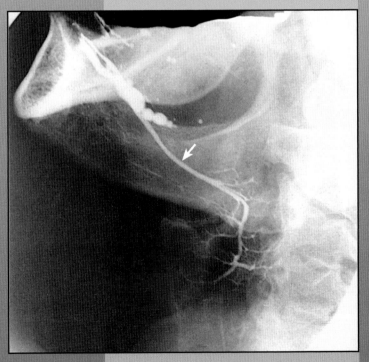

SUMMARY OF PROJECTIONS

PROJECTIONS, POSITIONS, AND METHODS

Page	Essential	Anatomy	Projection	Position	Method
68		Parotid gland	Tangential		
70		Parotid and submandibular glands	Lateral	R or L	

Mouth

The *mouth,* or *oral cavity,* is the first division of the digestive system (Fig. 14-1). It encloses the dental arches and receives the saliva secreted by the salivary glands. The cavity of the mouth is divided into (1) the *oral vestibule,* the space between the teeth and the cheeks; and (2) the *oral cavity,* or mouth proper, the space within the dental arches. The roof of the oral cavity is formed by the hard and soft palates. The floor is formed principally by the tongue, and it communicates with the pharynx posteriorly via the *oropharynx.*

The *hard palate* is the most anterior portion of the roof of the oral cavity. The hard palate is formed by the horizontal plates of the maxillae and palatine bones. The anterior and lateral boundaries are formed by the inner wall of the maxillary alveolar processes, which extend superiorly and medially to blend with the horizontal processes. The height of the hard palate varies considerably, and it determines the angulation of the inner surface of the alveolar process. The angle is less when the palate is high and is greater when the palate is low.

The *soft palate* begins behind the last molar and is suspended from the posterior border of the hard palate. Highly sensitive to touch, the soft palate is a movable musculomembranous structure that functions chiefly as a partial septum between the mouth and the pharynx. At the center of the inferior border the soft palate is prolonged into a small, pendulous process called the *uvula.* On each side of the uvula, two arched folds extend laterally and inferiorly. The *anterior arches* project forward to the sides of the base of the tongue. The *posterior arches* project posteriorly to blend with the posterolateral walls of the pharynx. The triangular space between the anterior and the posterior arches is occupied by the palatine *tonsil.*

The *tongue* is situated in the floor of the oral cavity, with its base directed posteriorly and its *apex* directed anteriorly (see Figs. 14-1 and 14-2). The tongue is freely movable. The tongue is composed of numerous muscles and is covered with a mucous membrane that varies in complexity in the different regions of the organ. The extrinsic muscles of the tongue form the greater part of the oral

floor. The mucous membrane covering the undersurface of the tongue is reflected laterally over the remainder of the floor to the gums. This part of the floor lies under the free anterior and lateral portions of the tongue and is called the *sublingual space.* Posterior movement of the free anterior part of the tongue is restricted by a median vertical band, or fold, of mucous membrane called the *frenulum of the tongue,* which extends between the undersurface of the tongue and the sublingual space. On each side of the frenulum, extending around the outer limits of the sublingual space and over the underlying salivary glands, the mucous membrane is elevated into a crestlike ridge called the *sublingual fold.* In the relaxed state the two folds are quite prominent and are in contact with the gums.

The *teeth* serve the function of *mastication,* the process of chewing and grinding food into small pieces. During mastication the teeth cut, grind, and tear the food, which is then mixed with saliva, swallowed, and later digested. The saliva softens the food, keeps the mouth moist, and contributes digestive enzymes.

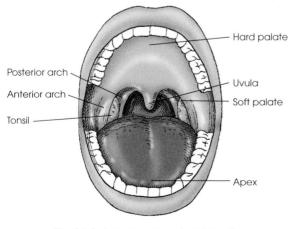

Fig. 14-1 Anterior view of oral cavity.

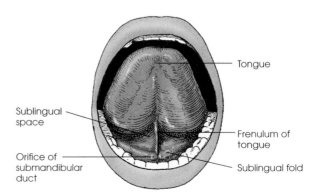

Fig. 14-2 Anterior view of undersurface of tongue and floor of mouth.

Salivary Glands

The three pairs of salivary glands produce approximately 1 L of saliva each day. The glands are named the *parotid,* the *submandibular,* and the *sublingual* (Fig. 14-3). Each gland is composed of numerous lobes, with each lobe containing small lobules. The whole gland is held together by connective tissue and a fine network of blood vessels and ducts. The minute ducts of the lobules merge into larger tributaries, which unite and form the large efferent duct that conveys the saliva from the gland to the mouth.

The *parotid glands,* the largest of the salivary glands, each consist of a flattened superficial portion and a wedge-shaped deep portion (Fig. 14-4). The superficial part lies immediately anterior to the external ear and extends inferiorly to the mandibular ramus and posteriorly to the mastoid process. The deep, or retromandibular, portion extends medially toward the pharynx. The *parotid duct* runs anteriorly and medially to open into the oral vestibule opposite the second upper molar.

The *submandibular glands* are fairly large, irregularly shaped glands. On each side a submandibular gland extends posteriorly from a point below the first molar almost to the angle of the mandible (Fig. 14-5). Although the upper part of the gland rests against the inner surface of the mandibular body, its greater portion projects below the mandible. The *submandibular duct* extends anteriorly and superiorly to open into the mouth on a small papilla at the side of the frenulum of the tongue.

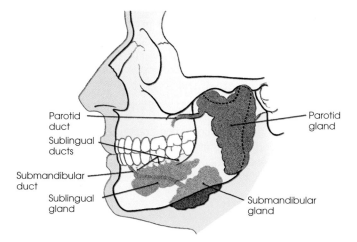

Parotid duct
Sublingual ducts
Submandibular duct
Sublingual gland
Parotid gland
Submandibular gland

Fig. 14-3 Salivary glands from the left lateral aspect.

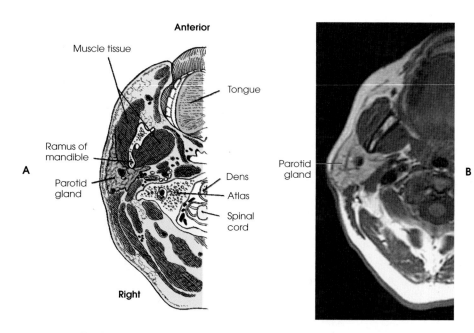

Anterior

Muscle tissue
Tongue
Ramus of mandible
Parotid gland
Dens
Atlas
Spinal cord

A

Parotid gland

B

Right

Fig. 14-4 A, Horizontal section of face, showing relation of parotid gland to mandibular ramus. Auricle is not shown. **B,** Axial MRI of parotid gland.

(**B,** Courtesy J. Louis Rankin, BS, RT(R)(MR).)

The *sublingual glands,* the smallest pair, are narrow and elongated in form (see Fig. 14-5). These glands are located in the floor of the mouth beneath the sublingual fold. Each is in contact with the mandible laterally and extends posteriorly from the side of the frenulum of the tongue to the submandibular gland. Numerous small *sublingual ducts* exist. Some of these ducts open into the floor of the mouth along the crest of the sublingual fold, and others open into the submandibular duct. The main sublingual duct opens beside the orifice of the submandibular duct.

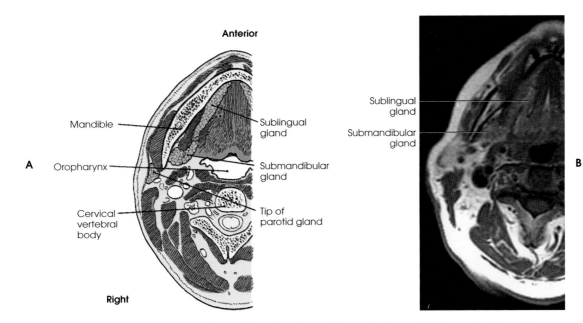

Fig. 14-5 A, Horizontal section of face, showing relation of submandibular and sublingual glands to surrounding structures. Auricle is not shown. **B,** Axial MRI of submandibular and sublingual glands.

(**B,** Courtesy J. Louis Rankin, BS, RT(R)(MR).)

SUMMARY OF ANATOMY

Mouth	Salivary glands
oral vestibule	parotid glands
oral cavity	parotid ducts
oropharynx	submandibular glands
hard palate	submandibular ducts
soft palate	sublingual glands
uvula	sublingual ducts
anterior arches	
posterior arches	
tonsil	
tongue	
apex	
sublingual space	
frenulum of the tongue	
sublingual fold	
teeth	

SUMMARY OF PATHOLOGY

Condition	Definition
Calculus	Abnormal concretion of mineral salts, often called a stone
Fistula	Abnormal connection between two internal organs or between an organ and the body surface
Foreign Body	Foreign material in the airway
Salivary Duct Obstruction	Condition preventing the passage of saliva through the duct
Stenosis	Narrowing or contraction of a passage
Tumor	New tissue growth where cell proliferation is uncontrolled

PROJECTION REMOVED

The following projection has been removed from this edition of the atlas. See previous editions of the atlas for a description of this projection.

Submandibular and sublingual glands
* Axial projection, Intraoral method

Sialography

Sialography is the term applied to radiologic examination of the salivary glands and ducts with the use of a contrast material, usually one of the water-soluble iodinated media. Because of improvements in computed tomography (CT) and magnetic resonance imaging (MRI) techniques, sialography is performed less often than it once was. When the presence of a salivary stone or lesion is suspected, CT or MRI is often the modality of choice. However, sialography remains a viable tool when a definitive diagnosis is necessary for a problem related to one of the salivary ducts.

The procedure is used to demonstrate such conditions as inflammatory lesions and tumors, determine the extent of salivary fistulae, and localize diverticulae, strictures, and calculi. Because the glands are paired and the pairs are in such close proximity, only one gland at a time can be examined by the sialographic method (Fig. 14-6).

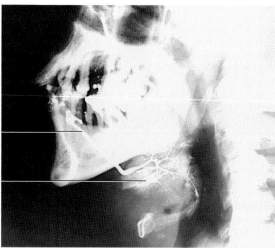

Submandibular duct

Submandibular gland

Fig. 14-6 Sialogram showing opacified submandibular gland.

Sialography involves the following steps:

- Inject the radiopaque medium into the main duct. From there the contrast flows into the intraglandular ductules, making it possible to demonstrate the surrounding glandular parenchyma, as well as the duct system (Fig. 14-7).
- Obtain preliminary radiographs to detect any condition demonstrable without the use of a contrast medium and to establish the optimum exposure technique.

- About 2 or 3 minutes before the sialographic procedure, give the patient a secretory stimulant to open the duct for ready identification of its orifice and for easier passage of a cannula or catheter. For this purpose, have the patient suck on a wedge of fresh lemon. On completion of the examination, have the patient suck on another lemon wedge to stimulate rapid evacuation of the contrast medium.
- Take a radiograph about 10 minutes after the procedure to verify clearance of the contrast medium, if necessary.

Most physicians inject the contrast medium by manual pressure (i.e., with a syringe attached to the cannula or catheter). Other physicians advocate delivery of the medium by hydrostatic pressure only. The latter method requires the use of a water-soluble iodinated medium, with the contrast solution container (usually a syringe barrel with the plunger removed) attached to a drip stand and set at a distance of 28 inches (70 cm) above the level of the patient's mouth. Some physicians perform the filling procedure under fluoroscopic guidance and obtain spot radiographs.

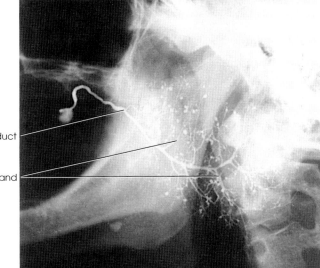

Parotid duct

Parotid gland

Fig. 14-7 Sialogram showing parotid gland in patient without teeth.

Parotid Gland

TANGENTIAL PROJECTION

Image receptor: 8 × 10 inch (18 × 24 cm) lengthwise

Position of patient
- Place the patient in either a recumbent or seated position.
- Because the parotid gland lies midway between the anterior and posterior surfaces of the skull, obtain the tangential projection of the glandular region from either the posterior or the anterior direction.

Position of part
Supine body position
- With the patient supine, rotate the head slightly toward the side being examined so that the parotid area is perpendicular to the plane of the IR.
- Center the IR to the parotid area.
- With the patient's head resting on the occiput, adjust the head so that the mandibular ramus is parallel with the longitudinal axis of the IR (Fig. 14-8).

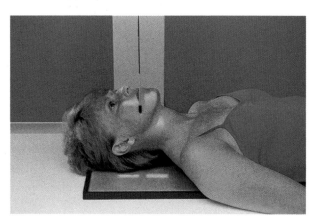

Fig. 14-8 Tangential parotid gland, supine position.

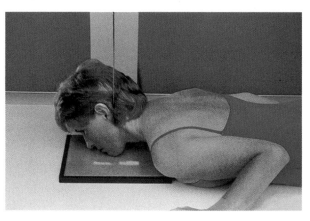

Fig. 14-9 Tangential parotid gland, prone position.

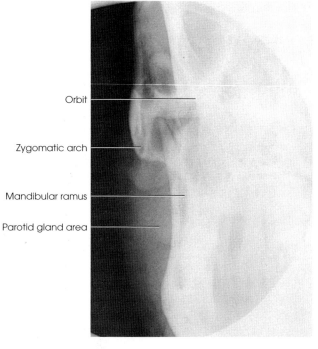

Orbit

Zygomatic arch

Mandibular ramus

Parotid gland area

Fig. 14-10 Tangential parotid gland. An examination of the right cheek area to rule out tumor reveals soft tissue fullness and no calcification.

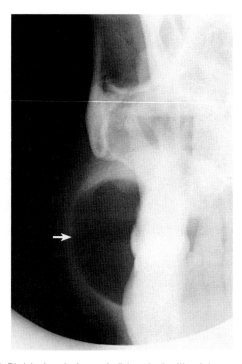

Fig. 14-11 Right cheek *(arrow)* distended with air in mouth (same patient as in Fig. 14-10). No abnormal finding in region of parotid gland.

Prone body position

- With the patient prone, rotate the head so that the parotid area being examined is perpendicular to the plane of the IR.
- Center the IR to the parotid region.
- With the patient's head resting on the chin, adjust the flexion of the head so that the mandibular ramus is parallel with the longitudinal axis of the IR (Fig. 14-9).
- When the parotid (Stensen's) duct does not have to be demonstrated, rest the patient's head on the forehead and nose.
- *Shield gonads.*
- *Respiration:* Improved radiographic quality can be obtained, particularly for the demonstration of calculi, by having the patient fill the mouth with air and then puff the cheeks out as much as possible. When this cannot be done, ask the patient to suspend respiration for the exposure.

Central ray

- Perpendicular to the plane of the IR, directed along the lateral surface of the mandibular ramus

Structures shown

A tangential projection demonstrates the region of the parotid gland and duct. These structures are clearly outlined when an opaque medium is used (Figs. 14-10 to 14-14).

EVALUATION CRITERIA

The following should be clearly demonstrated:

- Soft tissue density
- Most of the parotid gland lateral to and clear of the mandibular ramus
- Mastoid overlapping only the upper portion of the parotid gland

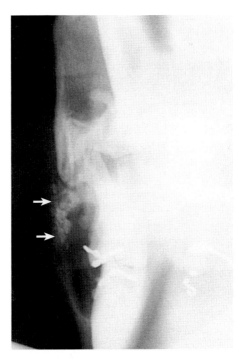

Fig. 14-12 Tangential parotid gland, with right cheek distended with air. Considerable calcification is seen in region of parotid gland (*arrows*).

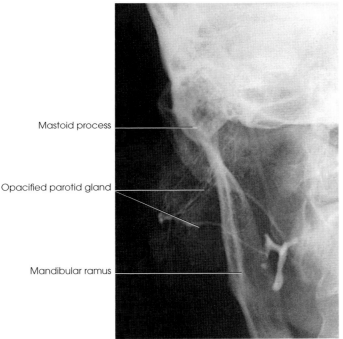

Mastoid process

Opacified parotid gland

Mandibular ramus

Fig. 14-13 Tangential parotid gland showing opacification.

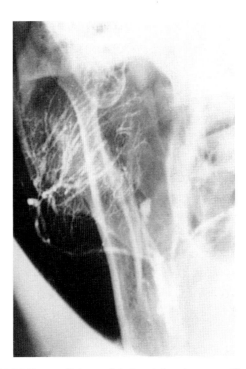

Fig. 14-14 Tangential parotid gland showing opacification.

Mouth and salivary glands

LATERAL PROJECTION
R or L position

Image receptor: 8 × 10 inch (18 × 24 cm) lengthwise

Position of patient
- Place the patient in a semiprone or seated and upright position.

Position of part
Parotid gland
- With the affected side closest to the IR, extend the patient's neck so that the space between the cervical area of the spine and the mandibular rami is cleared.
- Center the IR to a point approximately 1 inch (2.5 cm) superior to the mandibular angle.
- Adjust the head so that the midsagittal plane is rotated approximately 15 degrees toward the IR from a true lateral position.
Submandibular gland
- Center the IR to the inferior margin of the angle of the mandible.
- Adjust the patient's head in a true lateral position (Fig. 14-15).

- Iglauer[1] suggested depressing the floor of the mouth to displace the submandibular gland below the mandible. When the patient's throat is not too sensitive, accomplish this by having the patient place an index finger on the back of the tongue on the affected side.
- *Shield gonads.*
- *Respiration:* Suspend.

Central ray
- Perpendicular to the center of the IR and directed (1) at a point 1 inch (2.5 cm) superior to the mandibular angle to demonstrate the parotid gland or (2) at the inferior margin of the mandibular angle to demonstrate the submandibular gland

---

[1]Iglauer S: A simple maneuver to increase the visibility of a salivary calculus in the roentgenogram, *Radiology* 21:297, 1933.

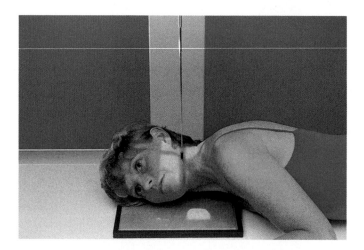

Fig. 14-15 Lateral submandibular gland.

Structures shown

A lateral image demonstrates the bony structures and any calcific deposit or swelling in the unobscured areas of the parotid (Figs. 14-16 and 14-17) and submandibular glands (Fig. 14-18). The glands and their ducts are well outlined when an opaque medium is used.

EVALUATION CRITERIA

The following should be clearly demonstrated:

- Mandibular rami free of overlap from the cervical vertebrae to best show the parotid gland superimposed over the ramus
- Superimposed mandibular rami and angles, if no tube angulation or head rotation is used for the submandibular gland
- Oblique position for the parotid gland

NOTE: An oblique projection is often necessary to obtain an image of the deeper portions of the parotid and submandibular glands. Any of the axiolateral projections of the mandible (see Fig. 14-18) can be used for this purpose (see Chapter 21).

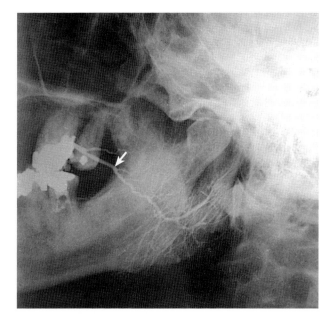

Fig. 14-16 Lateral parotid gland showing opacified gland and parotid duct *(arrow)*.

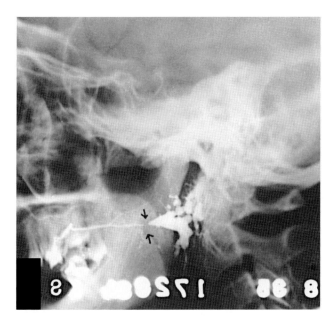

Fig. 14-17 Lateral parotid gland showing opacification and partial blockage of parotid duct *(arrows)*.

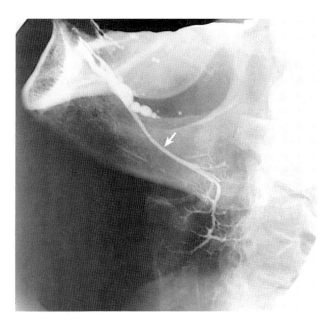

Fig. 14-18 Axial lateral submandibular gland showing opacification of submandibular duct *(arrow)*.

15

ANTERIOR PART OF NECK
Pharynx • Larynx • Thyroid Gland

Lateral projection showing calcified hematoma of thyroid gland (*arrows*).

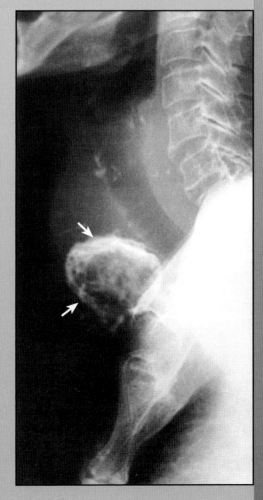

SUMMARY OF PROJECTIONS

PROJECTIONS, POSITIONS, AND METHODS

Page	Essential	Anatomy	Projection	Position	Method
86		Pharynx and larynx	AP		
88		Soft palate, pharynx, and larynx	Lateral	R or L	

Neck

The *neck* occupies the region between the skull and the thorax (Figs. 15-1 and 15-2). For radiographic purposes the neck is divided into posterior and anterior portions in accordance with the tissue composition and function of the structures. The procedures that are required to dem-onstrate the osseous structures occupying the posterior division of the neck are described in the discussion of the cervical vertebrae in Chapter 8. The portions of the central nervous system and circulatory system that pass through the neck are described in Chapters 24 and 25.

The portion of the neck that lies in front of the vertebrae is composed largely of soft tissues. The upper parts of the respiratory and digestive systems are the principal structures. The thyroid and parathyroid glands, as well as the larger part of the submandibular glands, are also located in the anterior portion of the neck.

Thyroid Gland

The *thyroid gland* consists of two lateral lobes connected at their lower thirds by a narrow median portion called the *isthmus* (Fig. 15-3). The lobes are approximately 2 inches (5 cm) long, 1¼ inches (3 cm) wide, and ¾ inch (1.9 cm) thick. The isthmus lies at the front of the upper part of the trachea, and the lobes lie at the sides. The lobes reach from the lower third of the thyroid cartilage to the level of the first thoracic vertebra. Although the thyroid gland is normally suprasternal in position, it occasionally extends into the superior aperture of the thorax.

Parathyroid Glands

The *parathyroid glands* are small ovoid bodies, two on each side, *superior* and *inferior.* These glands are situated one above the other on the posterior aspect of the adjacent lobe of the thyroid gland.

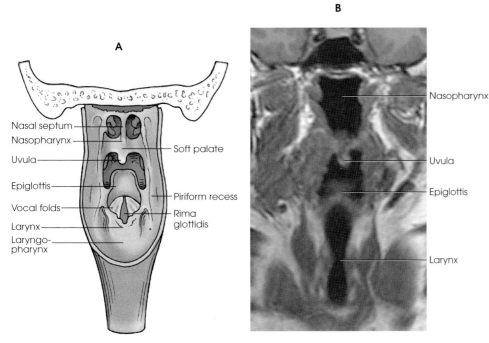

Fig. 15-1 **A,** Interior posterior view of the neck. **B,** Coronal MRI of the neck.

(**B,** Courtesy J. Louis Rankin, BS, RT(R)(MR).)

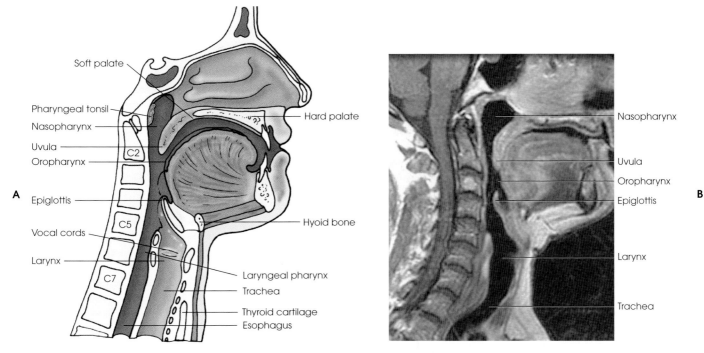

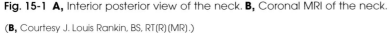

Fig. 15-2 Sagittal section of the face and neck. **B,** Sagittal MRI of the neck.

(**B,** Courtesy J. Louis Rankin, BS, RT(R)(MR).)

Pharynx

The *pharynx* serves as a passage for both air and food and thus is common to the respiratory and digestive systems (see Fig. 15-2). The pharynx is a musculo-membranous, tubular structure situated in front of the vertebrae and behind the nose, mouth, and larynx. Approximately 5 inches (13 cm) in length, the pharynx extends from the undersurface of the body of the sphenoid bone and the basilar part of the occipital bone inferiorly to the level of the disk between the sixth and seventh cervical vertebrae, where it becomes continuous with the esophagus. The pharyngeal cavity is subdivided into nasal, oral, and laryngeal portions.

The *nasopharynx* lies posteriorly above the *soft* and *hard* palates. (The upper part of the hard palate forms the floor of the nasopharynx.) Anteriorly, the naso-pharynx communicates with the posterior apertures of the nose. Hanging from the posterior aspect of the soft palate is a small conical process, the *uvula.* On the roof and posterior wall of the nasopharynx, between the orifices of the auditory tubes,

the mucosa contains a mass of lymphoid tissue known as the *pharyngeal tonsil* (or *adenoids* when enlarged). Hypertrophy of this tissue interferes with nasal breathing and is common in children. This condition is well demonstrated in a lateral radiograph of the nasopharynx.

The *oropharynx* is the portion extending from the soft palate to the level of the *hyoid bone.* The base, or root, of the tongue forms the anterior wall of the oropharynx. The *laryngeal pharynx* lies posterior to the larynx, its anterior wall being formed by the posterior surface of the larynx. The laryngeal pharynx extends inferiorly and is continuous with the esophagus.

The air-containing nasal and oral pharynges are well visualized in lateral images except during the act of phona-tion, when the soft palate contracts and tends to obscure the nasal pharynx. An opaque medium is required for demon-stration of the lumen of the laryngeal pharynx, although it can be distended with air during the *Valsalva's maneuver* (an increase in intrathoracic pressure pro-duced by forcible expiration effort against the closed glottis).

Larynx

The *larynx* is the organ of voice (Figs. 15-1 through 15-5). Serving as the air pas-sage between the pharynx and the trachea, the larynx is also one of the divisions of the respiratory system.

The larynx is a movable, tubular struc-ture; is broader above than below; and is approximately 1½ inches (3.8 cm) in length. Situated below the root of the tongue and in front of the laryngeal pharynx, the larynx is suspended from the hyoid bone and extends from the level of the superior margin of the fourth cervical vertebra to its junction with the trachea at the level of the inferior margin of the sixth cervical vertebra. The thin, leaf-shaped *epiglottis* is situated behind the root of the tongue and the hyoid bone and above the laryngeal entrance. It has been stated that the epiglottis serves as a trap to prevent leakage into the larynx between acts of swallowing. The *thyroid cartilage* forms the laryngeal prominence, or *Adam's apple.*

The inlet of the larynx is oblique, slant-ing posteriorly as it descends. A pouchlike fossa called the *piriform recess* is located on each side of the larynx and external to its orifice. The piriform recesses are well shown as triangular areas on fron-tal projections when insufflated with air (Valsalva's maneuver) or when filled with an opaque medium.

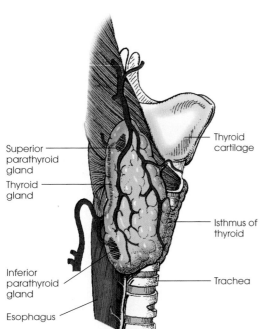

Superior parathyroid gland

Thyroid gland

Inferior parathyroid gland

Esophagus

Thyroid cartilage

Isthmus of thyroid

Trachea

Fig. 15-3 Lateral aspect of laryngeal area demonstrating the thyroid gland and the isthmus that connects its two lobes.

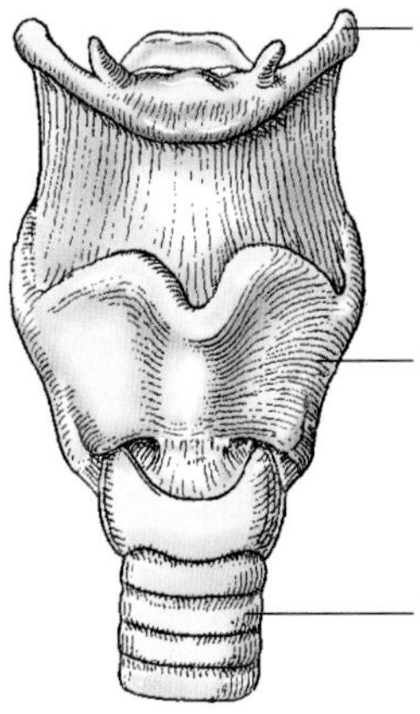

Hyoid bone

Thyroid cartilage

Trachea

Fig. 15-4 Anterior aspect of larynx.

The entrance of the larynx is guarded superiorly and anteriorly by the epiglottis and laterally and posteriorly by folds of mucous membrane. These folds, which extend around the margin of the laryngeal inlet from their junction with the epiglottis, function as a sphincter during swallowing. The *laryngeal cavity* is subdivided into three compartments by two pairs of mucosal folds that extend anteroposteriorly from its lateral walls. The superior pair of folds are the *vestibular folds,* or false vocal cords. The space above them is called the *laryngeal vestibule.* The lower two folds are separated from each other by a median fissure called the *rima glottidis.* They are known as the *vocal folds,* or true vocal folds (see Fig. 15-5). The vocal cords are vocal ligaments that are covered by the vocal folds. The ligaments and the rima glottidis comprise the vocal apparatus of the larynx and are collectively referred to as the *glottis.*

PROCEDURES REMOVED

The following procedures have been removed from this edition of the atlas. See previous editions of the atlas for a description of these procedures.

Thyroid gland: methods of examinations

SUMMARY OF ANATOMY

Thyroid gland	Pharynx	Larynx
isthmus	nasopharynx	epiglottis
	soft palate	thyroid cartilage
Parathyroid glands	hard palate	piriform recess
superior	uvula	laryngeal cavity
inferior	pharyngeal tonsil	vestibular folds (false
	oropharynx	vocal cords)
	hyoid bone	laryngeal vestibule
	laryngeal pharynx	rima glottides
		vocal folds (true vocal
		cords)
		glottis

NEW ABBREVIATION USED IN CHAPTER 15

SMV   Submentovertical

See Addendum B for a summary of all abbreviations used in Volume 2.

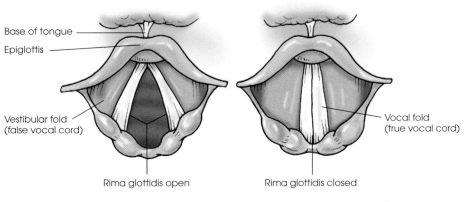

Base of tongue
Epiglottis
Vestibular fold (false vocal cord)
Rima glottidis open
Vocal fold (true vocal cord)
Rima glottidis closed

Fig. 15-5 Superior aspect of larynx (open and closed true vocal folds).

Soft Palate, Pharynx, and Larynx: Methods of Examination

The throat structures may be examined with or without an opaque contrast medium. The technique employed depends on the abnormality being investigated. Computed tomography (CT) studies are often performed to radiographically demonstrate areas of the palate, pharynx, and larynx with little or no discomfort to the patient. Magnetic resonance imaging (MRI) is also used to evaluate the larynx. The radiologic modality selected is often determined by the institution and physician. The radiologic examinations discussed in the following sections are performed less often than in the past.

PALATOGRAPHY

Bloch and Quantrill[1] used a positive-contrast technique to investigate suspected tumors of the soft palate. The technique involves the following steps:

- Seat the patient laterally before a vertical grid device with the nasopharynx centered to the image receptor (IR).
- For the first palatogram, have the patient swallow a small amount of a thick, creamy barium sulfate suspension to coat the inferior surface of the soft palate and the uvula.

[1]Bloch S, Quantrill JR: The radiology of nasopharyngeal tumors, including positive contrast nasopharyngography, *S Afr Med J* 42:1030, 1968.

- Obtain a second lateral image after 0.5 mL of the creamy barium suspension is injected into each nasal cavity to coat the superior surface of the soft palate and the posterior wall of the nasopharynx.

Morgan et al.[1] described a technique for evaluating abnormalities of chewing and swallowing in children. In this technique the chewing and swallowing function is injected with cineradiography as the child chews barium-impregnated chocolate fudge. (The fudge recipe was included in their article.)

Cleft palate studies are performed in the following manner:

- Seat the patient laterally upright with the IR centered to the nasopharynx.
- Make the exposures during phonation to demonstrate the range of movement of the soft palate and the position of the tongue during each of the following sounds[2,3]: *d-a-h, m-m-m, s-s-s,* and *e-e-e.*

[1]Morgan JA et al: Barium-impregnated chocolate fudge for the study of chewing mechanism in children, *Radiology* 94:432, 1970.
[2]Randall P, O'Hara AE, Bakes FP: A simple roentgen examination for the study of soft palate function in patients with poor speech, *Plast Reconstr Surg* 21:345, 1958.
[3]O'Hara AE: Roentgen evaluation of patients with cleft palate, *Radiol Clin North Am* 1:1, 1963.

NASOPHARYNGOGRAPHY

Hypertrophy of the pharyngeal tonsil or adenoids is clearly delineated in a direct lateral projection centered to the nasopharynx, ¾ inch (1.9 cm) directly anterior to the external acoustic meatus, as shown in Fig. 15-6. The image must be exposed during the intake of a deep breath through the nose to ensure filling of the nasopharynx with air. Mouth breathing moves the soft palate posteriorly to near approximation with the posterior wall of the nasopharynx and thus causes inspired air to bypass the nasopharynx as it is directed inferiorly into the larynx.

Positive-contrast nasopharyngography is performed to assess the extent of nasopharyngeal tumors (Fig. 15-7). Some examiners recommend an iodized oil for this examination.[1] Others prefer finely ground barium sulfate, either in paste form[2] or applied dry with a pressure blower.

Preliminary radiographs commonly consist of a submentovertical (SMV) projection of the skull and an upright lateral projection centered to the nasopharynx, ¾ inch (1.9 cm) directly anterior to the external acoustic (auditory) meatus.

[1]Johnson TH, Green AE, Rice EN: Nasopharyngography: its technique and uses, *Radiology* 88:1166, 1967.
[2]Khoo FY, Chia KB, Nalpon J: A new technique of contrast examination of the nasopharynx with cinefluorography and roentgenography, *AJR* 99:238, 1967.

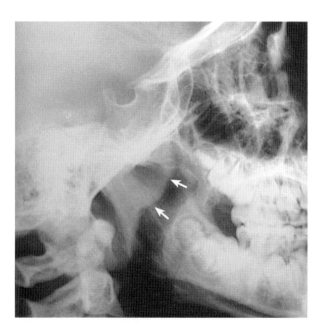

Fig. 15-6 Lateral pharyngeal tonsil demonstrating hypertrophy *(arrows).*

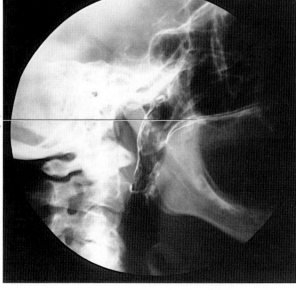

Roof of contrast-coated palate

Fig. 15-7 Lateral nasopharyngogram.

When using an iodized oil or a barium paste, follow these steps:

• Place the patient on the examining table in the supine position after local anesthetization.
• Elevate the shoulders to extend the neck enough to permit the orbitomeatal line to be adjusted at an angle of 40 to 45 degrees to a horizontal plane.
• Keep the head in this position throughout the examination.

• Both before and after instillation of contrast medium into the nasal cavities, obtain basal projections with the central ray directed midway between the mandibular angles at an angle of 15 to 20 degrees cephalad.
• Obtain lateral projections with a horizontal central ray centered to the nasopharynx.
• On completion of this phase of the examination, have the patient sit up

and blow the nose. This act evacuates most of the contrast medium, and the remainder will be swallowed. Reports indicate that none of the contrast medium is aspirated because the swallowing mechanism is triggered before the material reaches the larynx.

Additional studies in the upright position are then made as directed by the examining physician (Figs. 15-8 to 15-11).

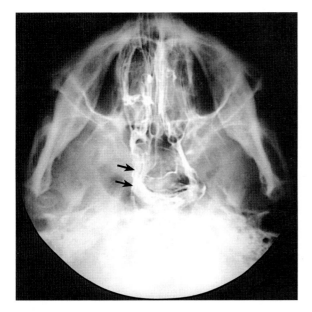

Fig. 15-8 SMV nasopharyngography, right ninth nerve sign. Note the asymmetry of the nasopharynx, with flattening on the right and presence of irregularity *(arrows)*.

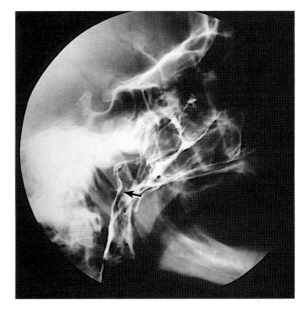

Fig. 15-9 Lateral nasopharyngography, right ninth nerve sign, lateral projection shows a mass in the posterior aspect of the nasopharynx *(arrow)* with an umbilication in the same patient as in Fig. 15-8.

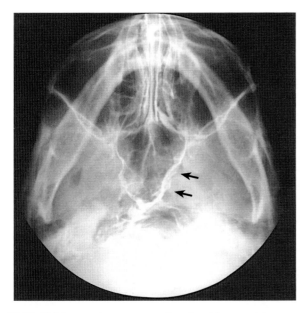

Fig. 15-10 SMV nasopharyngography of a 69-year-old woman with a long history of decreased hearing on left side and left facial paresthesia (burning, prickling). Nasopharynx is asymmetric with blunting of cartilage at opening of auditory tube *(arrows)*.

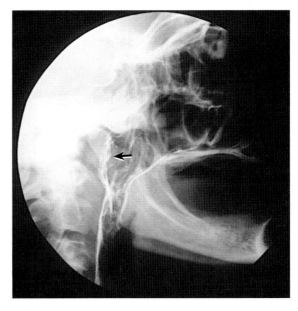

Fig. 15-11 Lateral nasopharyngography showing a shallow niche at C1 level of axis. Niche may represent an ulcer *(arrow)*.

Chittinand, Patheja, and Wisenberg[1] described an opaque-contrast nasopharyngographic procedure in which the patient is not required to keep the neck in an uncomfortable extended position for the entire examination. The following steps are observed:

- Seat the patient before a vertical grid device.
- Obtain preliminary lateral and SMV projections.
- Do not use topical anesthetization. (According to the originators, the procedure does not require anesthesia.)
- Using a standard spray bottle, introduce water into each nasal cavity. Then spray Micropaque powder into each nostril with a powder blower connected to a pressure unit.
- Take two SMV projections—one at rest and one during a modified Valsalva's maneuver—and one lateral projection.
- Have the patient blow the nose. Medium not expelled is swallowed. Immediate chest radiographs should not reveal barium in the lungs, and 24-hour follow-up radiographs should reveal complete clearing of the nasopharynx.

PHARYNGOGRAPHY

Opaque studies of the pharynx are made with an ingestible contrast medium, usually a thick, creamy mixture of water and barium sulfate. This examination is frequently carried out using fluoroscopy with spot-film images only. These or conventional projections are made during deglutition (swallowing).

Deglutition

The act of swallowing is performed by the rapid and highly coordinated action of many muscles. The following points are important in radiography of the pharynx and upper esophagus:

1. The middle area of the tongue becomes depressed to collect the mass, or bolus, of material to be swallowed.
2. The base of the tongue forms a central groove to accommodate the bolus and then moves superiorly and inferiorly along the roof of the mouth to propel the bolus into the pharynx.

[1]Chittinand S, Patheja SS, Wisenberg MJ: Barium nasopharyngography, *Radiology* 98:387, 1961.

3. Simultaneously with the posterior thrust of the tongue, the larynx moves anteriorly and superiorly under the root of the tongue, the sphincteric folds nearly closing the laryngeal inlet (orifice).
4. The epiglottis divides the passing bolus and drains the two portions laterally into the piriform recesses as it lowers over the laryngeal entrance.

The bolus is projected into the pharynx at the height of the anterior movement of the larynx (Figs. 15-12 to 15-14). Synchronizing a rapid exposure with the peak of the act is necessary.

The shortest exposure time possible must be used for studies made during deglutition. The following steps should be observed:

- Ask the patient to hold the barium sulfate bolus in the mouth until signaled and then to swallow the bolus in one movement.
- If a mucosal study is to be attempted, ask the patient to refrain from swallowing again.
- Take the mucosal study during the modified Valsalva's maneuver for double-contrast delineation.

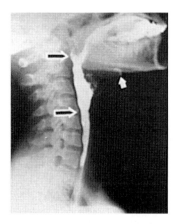

Fig. 15-12 Lateral projection with exposure made at peak of laryngeal elevation. Hyoid bone *(white arrow)* is almost at level of mandible. Pharynx *(between large arrows)* is completely distended with barium.

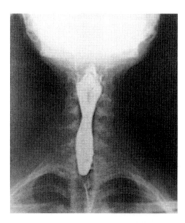

Fig. 15-13 AP projection of the same patient as in Fig. 15-12. Epiglottis divides bolus into two streams, filling the piriform recess below. Barium can also be seen entering upper esophagus.

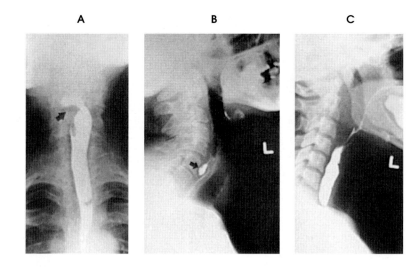

A   B   C

Fig. 15-14 AP projection of pharynx and upper esophagus with barium. **A,** Head was turned to right, with resultant asymmetric filling of pharynx. Bolus is passing through left piriform recess, leaving right side unfilled *(arrow)*. **B,** Lateral projection after patient swallowed barium, showing a diverticulum *(arrow)*. **C,** Lateral projection made slightly later, showing only filling of upper esophagus.

Some fluoroscopic equipment can expose up to 12 frames per second using the 100-mm or 105-mm cut or roll film. Many institutions with such equipment use it to spot-radiograph patients in rapid sequence during the act of swallowing. Another technique is to record the fluoroscopic image on videotape or cine film. The recorded image may then be studied to identify abnormalities during the active progress of deglutition.

Gunson method

Gunson[1] offered a practical suggestion for synchronizing the exposure with the height of the swallowing act in deglutition studies of the pharynx and superior esophagus. Gunson's method consists of tying a dark-colored shoestring (metal tips removed) snugly around the patient's throat above the thyroid cartilage (Fig. 15-15). Anterior and superior movements of the larynx are then shown by the elevation of the shoestring as the thyroid cartilage moves anteriorly and immediately thereafter by the displacement of the shoestring as the cartilage passes superiorly.

Having the exposure coincide with the peak of the anterior movement of the larynx, the instant at which the bolus of contrast material is projected into the pharynx, is desirable. However, as stated by Templeton and Kredel,[2] the action is so rapid that satisfactory filling is usually obtained if the exposure is made as soon as anterior movement is noted.

[1]Gunson EF: Radiography of the pharynx and upper esophagus: shoestring method, *Xray Tech* 33:1, 1961.
[2]Templeton FE, Kredel RA: The cricopharyngeal sphincter, *Laryngoscope* 53:1, 1943.

LARYNGOPHARYNGOGRAPHY

Stationary or tomographic negative-contrast studies of the air-containing laryngopharyngeal structures are made in both AP and lateral projections. AP projections are made with the patient in either the supine or seated and upright position, with the head extended enough to prevent superimposition of the mandibular shadow on that of the larynx. Lateral projections are made with a soft tissue radiograph technique and the patient in the upright position.

Negative-contrast studies of the laryngopharyngeal structures provide considerable information about alterations in the normal anatomy and function of laryngopharyngeal structures. Both negative- and positive-contrast AP projections are made during the respiratory and stress maneuvers discussed in the following sections.

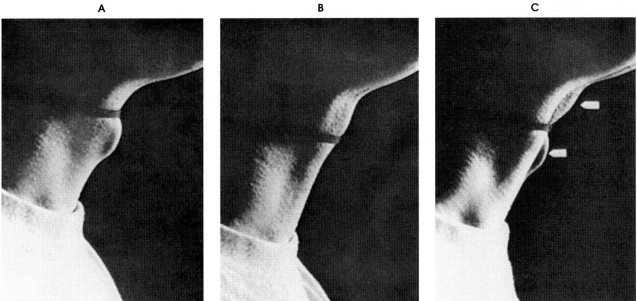

A   B   C

Fig. 15-15 A, An ordinary dark shoelace has been tied snugly around the patient's neck above the Adam's apple. **B,** The exposure was made at the peak of superior and anterior movement of the larynx during swallowing. At this moment the pharynx is completely filled with barium, which is the ideal instant for making an x-ray exposure. **C,** Double-exposure photograph emphasizing movement of Adam's apple during swallowing. Note extent of anterior and superior excursion *(arrows)*.

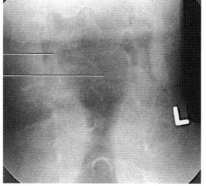

Fig. 15-16 AP projection during inspiration.

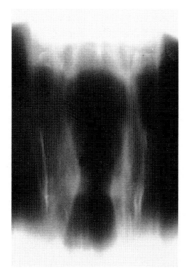

Fig. 15-17 AP projection linear tomogram during inspiration.

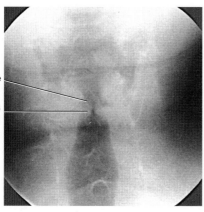

Fig. 15-18 AP projection during phonation of *e-e-e*.

Quiet inspiration

Quiet inspiration tests abduction of the vocal cords. The resultant radiograph should show the cords open (abducted), with an uninterrupted column of air extending from the laryngeal vestibule inferiorly into the trachea (Figs. 15-16 and 15-17).

Normal (expiratory) phonation

Normal (expiratory) phonation tests adduction of the vocal cords. The patient is asked to take a deep breath and, while exhaling slowly, to phonate either a high-pitched *e-e-e* or a low-pitched *a-a-h*. The resultant image should show the closed (adducted) vocal cords just above the break in the air column at the closed rima glottidis (Figs. 15-18 and 15-19). Phonation is normally performed during expiration. This test is now generally referred to as *normal* or *expiratory phonation* to distinguish it from the inspiratory phonation.

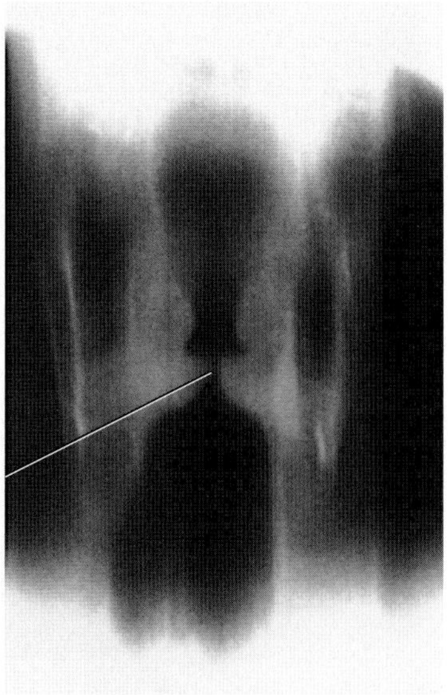

Fig. 15-19 AP projection linear tomogram during phonation of *e-e-e*.

Inspiratory phonation

Powers, Holtz, and Ogura[1] introduced the use of inspiratory phonation for demonstration of the laryngeal ventricle. This maneuver is also called *reverse phonation* and *aspirate* or *aspirant maneuver.*

The patient is asked to exhale completely and then inhale slowly while making a harsh, stridulous sound with the phonation of *e-e-e* or another high-pitched sound. This test adducts the vocal cords, moves them inferiorly, and balloons the ventricle for clear delineation (Fig. 15-20).

Valsalva's maneuver

Valsalva's maneuver shows complete closure of the glottis. This maneuver tests the elasticity and functional integrity of the glottis (Fig. 15-21).

For the true Valsalva's maneuver, the patient is asked to take a deep breath and hold the breath in while bearing down as if trying to move the bowels. This act forces the breath against the closed glottis, which increases both intrathoracic and intraabdominal pressure.

[1]Powers WE, Holtz S, Ogura J: Contrast examination of the larynx and pharynx: inspiratory phonation, *AJR* 92:40, 1964.

Modified Valsalva's maneuver

The modified Valsalva's maneuver tests the elasticity of the laryngeal pharynx (hypopharynx) and the piriform recesses. The resultant radiograph should show the glottis closed and the laryngeal pharynx and piriform recesses distended with air (Fig. 15-22).

For the modified Valsalva's maneuver, the patient pinches the nostrils together with the thumb and forefinger of one hand. Keeping the mouth closed, the patient makes and sustains a slight effort to blow the nose. Alternatively, the patient can blow the cheeks outward against the closed nostrils and mouth as if blowing into a horn or balloon.

The selected respiratory and stress maneuver employed must be carefully explained and demonstrated just before its use. The patient should perform the maneuver one or more times until able to perform it correctly.

TOMOLARYNGOGRAPHY

Tomographic studies of the laryngopharyngeal structures, either before or after the introduction of a radiopaque contrast medium, are made in the frontal plane. One set is usually made during quiet inspiration (see Fig. 15-17) and one during normal (expiratory) phonation (see Fig. 15-19), but the stress maneuvers are used as indicated. The rapid-travel linear sweep is generally considered to be the technique of choice for these studies, and the exposures are made during the first half of a wide arc (40 to 50 degrees) to prevent overlap streaking by the facial bones and teeth.

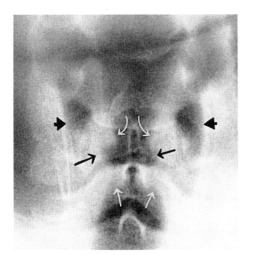

Fig. 15-20 AP projection, inspiratory phonation, showing laryngeal ventricle *(horizontal black arrows),* true vocal folds *(white arrows),* and piriform recesses *(black arrowheads).*

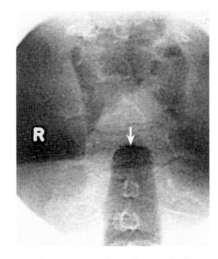

Fig. 15-21 AP projection demonstrating true Valsalva's maneuver and showing closed glottis *(arrow).*

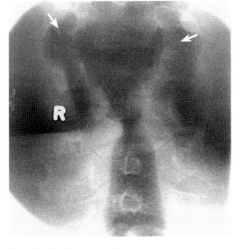

Fig. 15-22 AP projection demonstrating modified Valsalva's maneuver and showing air-filled piriform recesses *(arrows).*

POSITIVE-CONTRAST LARYNGOPHARYNGOGRAPHY

Positive-contrast examinations of the larynx and laryngopharynx are usually performed to determine the exact site, size, and extent of tumor masses. The examination is conducted using fluoroscopy with spot radiographs or cineradiographic recordings, or both. In conjunction with the examination procedure described by Powers, McGee, and Seaman,[1] iodized oil is the medium most commonly used, although other radiopaque media are employed. A mild sedative may be administered before the examination. The following steps are then observed:

- After satisfactory preliminary radiographs are obtained, seat the patient upright and then anesthetize the laryngopharyngeal structures with a topical anesthetic to inhibit the gag, cough, and deglutition reflexes if necessary.
- Give the patient explicit instructions on each of the test maneuvers to be used.
- Caution the patient to avoid coughing and swallowing after the introduction of the radiopaque medium (Figs. 15-23 to 15-25).
- For the administration of the medium, attach a syringe loaded with the specified amount of iodized oil to a curved metal cannula.
- With the patient seated upright, slowly drip the iodized oil over the back of the tongue or directly into the larynx, coating all structures of the larynx and laryngopharynx.
- Examine the patient fluoroscopically, making spot radiographs at the height of each of the various test maneuvers. Some examiners obtain cineradiographic recordings with a continuous catheter drip of thin barium or iodized oil into the larynx.

[1]Powers WE, McGee HH, Seaman WB: Contrast examination of the larynx and pharynx, *Radiology* 68:169, 1957.

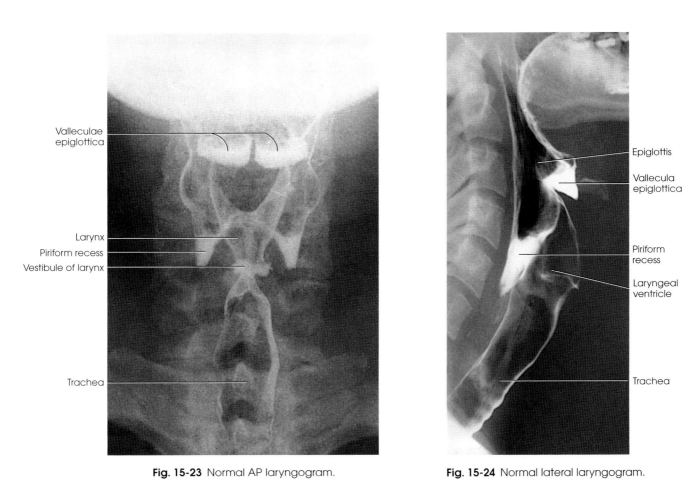

Valleculae
epiglottica

Larynx

Piriform recess

Vestibule of larynx

Trachea

Fig. 15-23 Normal AP laryngogram.

Epiglottis

Vallecula
epiglottica

Piriform
recess

Laryngeal
ventricle

Trachea

Fig. 15-24 Normal lateral laryngogram.

A

B

C

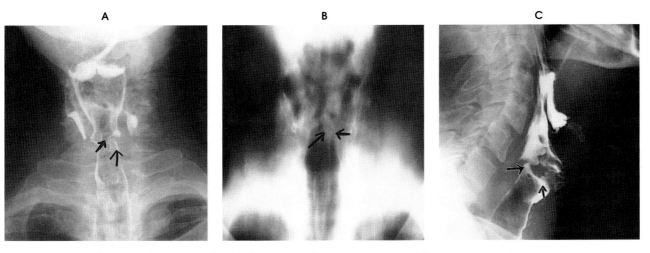

Fig. 15-25 A, AP projection. **B,** Tomogram showing rounded soft tissue mass involving two thirds of left cord hanging down into subglottic larynx *(arrows)*. **C,** On lateral projection, this is best demonstrated with Valsalva's maneuver.

AP PROJECTION

Radiographic studies of the pharyngolaryngeal structures are made during breathing, phonation, stress maneuvers, and swallowing. To minimize the incidence of motion, the shortest possible exposure time must be used in the examinations. For the purpose of obtaining improved contrast on the AP projections, use of a grid is recommended.

Image receptor: 8 × 10 inch (18 × 24 cm) or 24 × 30 cm lengthwise

Position of patient

- Except for tomographic studies, which require a recumbent body position (Fig. 15-26), place the patient in the upright position, either seated or standing, whenever possible.

Position of part

- Center the midsagittal plane of the body to the midline of the vertical grid device.
- Ask the patient to sit or stand straight. If the standing position is used, have the patient distribute the weight of the body equally on the feet.
- Adjust the patient's shoulders to lie in the same horizontal plane to prevent rotation of the head and neck and resultant obliquity of the throat structures.
- Center the IR at the level of or just below the laryngeal prominence.
- Extend the patient's head only enough to prevent the mandibular shadow from obscuring the laryngeal area.
- *Shield gonads.*
- *Respiration:* Obtain preliminary radiographs (both AP and lateral) during the inspiratory phase of quiet nasal breathing to ensure that the throat passages are filled with air. To determine the optimum time for the exposure, watch the breathing movements of the chest. Make the exposure *just before* the chest comes to rest at the end of one of its inspiratory expansions (Figs. 15-27 and 15-28).

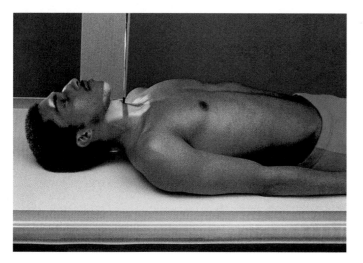

Fig. 15-26 AP pharynx and larynx with patient in supine position for tomography.

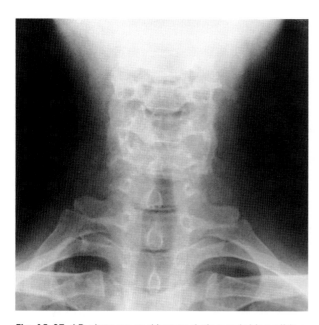

Fig. 15-27 AP pharynx and larynx during quiet breathing.

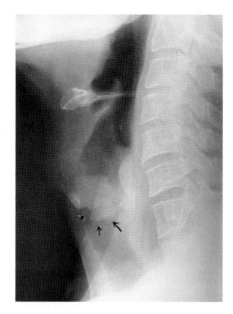

Fig. 15-28 Lateral pharynx and larynx showing polypoid mass of right false fold hanging into subglottic larynx *(arrows)*.

Central ray

- Perpendicular to the laryngeal prominence

Additional studies

Further necessary studies of the pharynx and larynx are usually determined fluoroscopically. These studies may be made at the following times:

1. During the Valsalva's or modified Valsalva's stress maneuvers, or both (Fig. 15-29)
2. At the height of the act of swallowing a bolus of 1 tablespoon of creamy barium sulfate suspension. The patient holds the barium sulfate bolus in the mouth until signaled and then swallows it in one movement. The patient is asked to refrain from swallowing again if a double-contrast study is to be attempted.

3. During the modified Valsalva's maneuver, immediately after the barium swallow for double-contrast delineation of the piriform recesses
4. During phonation and with the larynx in the rest position after its opacification with an iodinated contrast medium

Tomographic studies of the larynx are made during phonation of a high-pitched *e-e-e*. After these studies, one or more sectional studies may be made at the selected level or levels with the larynx at rest (Figs. 15-30 and 15-31).

The following should be clearly demonstrated:

- ■ Area from the superimposed mandible and base of the skull to the lung apices and superior mediastinum
- ■ No overlap of the laryngeal area by the mandible
- ■ No rotation of neck
- ■ Throat filled with air in preliminary studies
- ■ Radiographic density permitting visualization of the pharyngolaryngeal structures

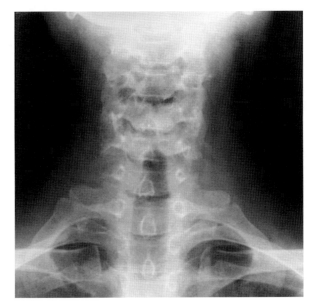

Fig. 15-29 AP pharynx and larynx demonstrating Valsalva's maneuver.

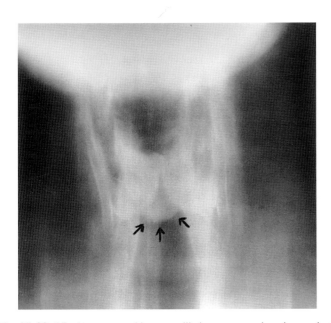

Fig. 15-30 AP pharynx and larynx with tomogram showing polypoid laryngeal mass *(arrows)*.

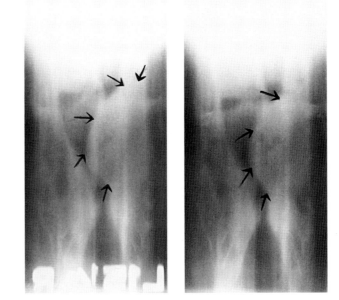

Fig. 15-31 AP pharynx and larynx. These tomograms demonstrate large cyst of left aryepiglottic fold and piriform recess *(arrows)*.

Soft Palate, Pharynx, and Larynx

LATERAL PROJECTION
R or L position

Image receptor: 8 × 10 inch (18 × 24 cm) lengthwise

Position of patient
- Ask the patient to sit or stand laterally before the vertical grid device.
- Adjust the patient so that the coronal plane passing through or just anterior to the temporomandibular joints is centered to the midline of the IR.

Position of part
- Ask the patient to sit or stand straight, with the adjacent shoulder resting firmly against the stand for support.
- Adjust the body so that the midsagittal plane is parallel with the plane of the IR.
- Depress the shoulders as much as possible, and adjust them to lie in the same transverse plane. If necessary, have the patient clasp the hands in back to posteriorly rotate the shoulders.
- Extend the patient's head slightly.
- Immobilize the head by having the patient look at an object in line with the visual axis.

Central ray
- Perpendicular to the IR, centering the IR (1) 1 inch (2.5 cm) below the level of the external acoustic (auditory) meatuses for demonstration of the nasopharynx and for cleft palate studies; (2) at the level of the mandibular angles for demonstration of the oropharynx; or (3) at the level of the laryngeal prominence for demonstration of the larynx, laryngeal pharynx, and upper end of the esophagus (Fig. 15-32)

Procedure
Preliminary studies of the pharyngolaryngeal structures are made during the inhalation phase of quiet nasal breathing to ensure filling of the passages with air (Fig. 15-33).

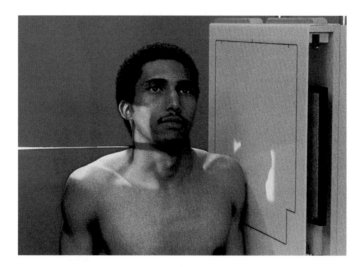

Fig. 15-32 Lateral pharynx and larynx.

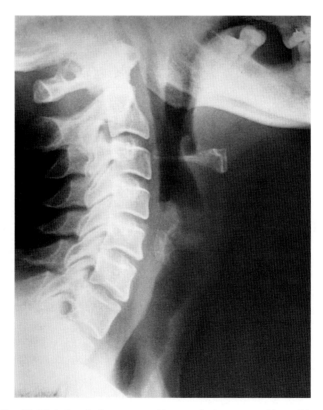

Fig. 15-33 Lateral pharynx and larynx during normal breathing.

According to the site and nature of the abnormality, further studies may be made. Each of the selected maneuvers must be explained to the patient and practiced just before actual use. The studies are obtained at one or more of the following:

1. During phonation of specified vowel sounds for demonstration of the vocal cords and for cleft palate studies (Fig. 15-34)
2. During the Valsalva's maneuver to distend the subglottic larynx and trachea with air (Fig. 15-35)
3. During the modified Valsalva's maneuver to distend the supraglottic larynx and the laryngeal pharynx with air

4. At the height of the act of swallowing a bolus of 1 tablespoon of creamy barium sulfate suspension for demonstration of the pharyngeal structures
5. With the larynx at rest or during phonation after opacification of the structure with an iodinated medium
6. During the act of swallowing a tuft or pledget of cotton (or food) saturated with a barium sulfate suspension for demonstration of nonopaque foreign bodies located in the pharynx or upper esophagus

EVALUATION CRITERIA

The following should be clearly demonstrated:

- Soft tissue density of the pharyngolaryngeal structures
- Area from the nasopharynx to the uppermost part of the lungs in preliminary studies
- Specific area of interest centered in detailed examinations
- No superimposition of the trachea by the shoulders
- Closely superimposed mandibular shadows
- Throat filled with air in preliminary studies

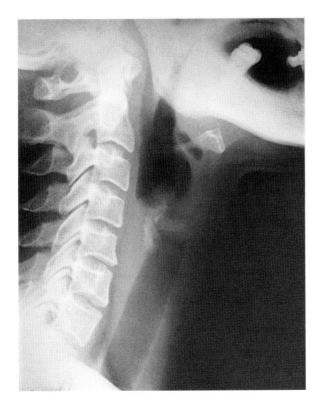

Fig. 15-34 Lateral pharynx and larynx during phonation of *e-e-e*.

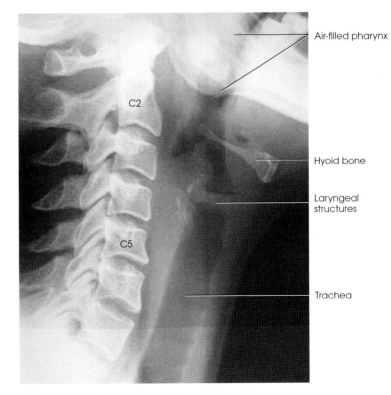

Fig. 15-35 Lateral pharynx and larynx during Valsalva's maneuver.

Air-filled pharynx

C2

Hyoid bone

Laryngeal structures

C5

Trachea

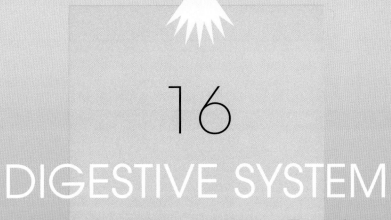

16

DIGESTIVE SYSTEM
Abdomen • Biliary Tract

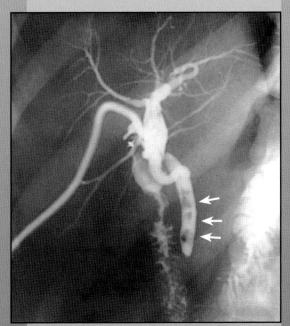

AP oblique postoperative cholangiogram, RPO position, showing multiple stones in common bile duct (arrows).

SUMMARY OF PROJECTIONS

PROJECTIONS, POSITIONS, AND METHODS

Page	Essential	Anatomy	Projection	Position	Method
102	♠	Abdomen	AP	Supine; upright	
104	♠	Abdomen	PA	Upright	
104	♠	Abdomen	AP	L lateral decubitus	
108	♠	Abdomen	Lateral	R or L	
109	♠	Abdomen	Lateral	R or L dorsal decubitus	
112		Percutaneous transhepatic cholangiography	AP/AP oblique	Supine/RPO	
114		Postoperative (T-tube) cholangiography	AP/AP oblique	Supine/RPO	
116		Endoscopic retrograde cholangiopancreatography	AP/AP oblique	Supine/RPO	

Icons in the Essential column indicate projections frequently performed in the United States and Canada. Students should be competent in these projections.

Digestive System

The *digestive system* consists of the alimentary tract (described in Chapter 17) and certain accessory organs that contribute to the digestive process.

The radiologically important accessory organs of the digestive system are the *teeth,* which serve to masticate the food; the *salivary glands,* which secrete fluid into the mouth for the salivation of food; and the *liver* and *pancreas,* which secrete specialized digestive juices into the small intestine. The anatomy and positioning of the thoracic, oral, and cervical portions of the digestive system are described in Chapters 10, 14, and 15, respectively.

Peritoneum

The *abdominopelvic* cavity consists of two parts: (1) a large superior portion, the *abdominal cavity;* and (2) a smaller inferior part, the pelvic cavity. The abdominal cavity extends from the diaphragm to the superior aspect of the bony pelvis. The abdominal cavity contains the stomach, small and large intestines, liver, gallbladder, spleen, pancreas, and kidneys. The *pelvic cavity* lies within the margins of the bony pelvis and contains the rectum and sigmoid of the large intestine, the urinary bladder, and the reproductive organs.

The abdominopelvic cavity is enclosed in a double-walled seromembranous sac called the *peritoneum.* The outer portion of this sac, termed the *parietal peritoneum,* is in close contact with the abdominal wall, the greater (false) pelvic wall, and most of the undersurface of the diaphragm. The inner portion of the sac, known as the *visceral peritoneum,* is positioned over or around the contained organs. The peritoneum forms folds called the *mesentery* and *omenta,* which serve to support the viscera in position. The space between the two layers of the peritoneum is called the *peritoneal cavity* and contains serous fluid (Fig. 16-1, *A*). Because there are no mesenteric attachments of the intestines in the pelvic cavity, pelvic surgery can be performed without entry into the peritoneal cavity.

The *retroperitoneum* is the cavity behind the peritoneum. Organs such as the kidneys and pancreas lie in the retroperitoneum.

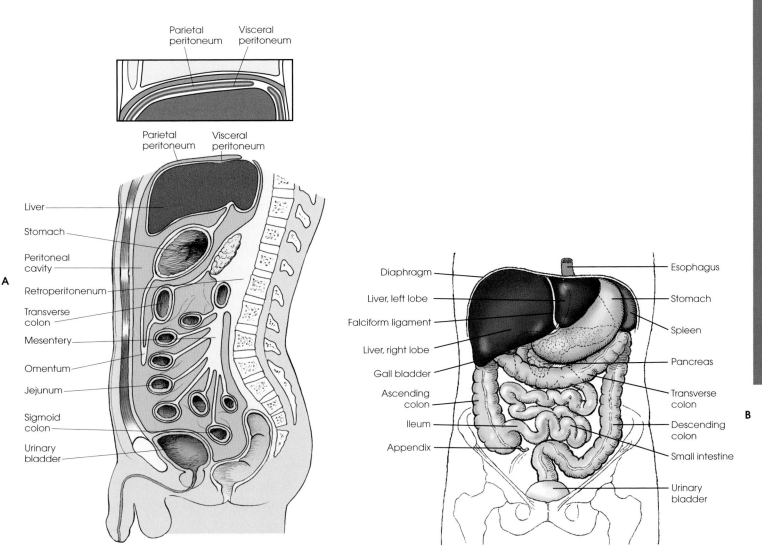

Parietal peritoneum   Visceral peritoneum

Parietal peritoneum   Visceral peritoneum

Liver
Stomach
Peritoneal cavity
Retroperitonenum
Transverse colon
Mesentery
Omentum
Jejunum
Sigmoid colon
Urinary bladder

A

Diaphragm
Liver, left lobe
Falciform ligament
Liver, right lobe
Gall bladder
Ascending colon
Ileum
Appendix

Esophagus
Stomach
Spleen
Pancreas
Transverse colon
Descending colon
Small intestine
Urinary bladder

B

Fig. 16-1 A, Lateral aspect of abdomen demonstrating the peritoneal sac and its components. **B,** Anterior aspect of abdominal viscera in relation to surrounding structures.

Liver and Biliary System

The *liver,* the largest gland in the body, is an irregularly wedge-shaped gland. It is situated with its base on the right and its apex directed anteriorly and to the left (Figs. 16-1 and 16-2). The deepest point of the liver is the inferior aspect just above the right kidney. The diaphragmatic surface of the liver is convex and conforms to the undersurface of the diaphragm. The visceral surface is concave and molded over the viscera on which it rests. Almost all of the right hypochondrium and a large part of the epigastrium are occupied by the liver. The right portion extends inferiorly into the right lateral region as far as the fourth lumbar vertebra, and the left extremity extends across the left hypochondrium.

At the *falciform ligament,* the liver is divided into a large *right lobe* and a much smaller *left lobe.* Two minor lobes are located on the medial side of the right lobe: the *caudate lobe* on the posterior surface and the *quadrate lobe* on the inferior surface (Fig. 16-3). The hilum of the liver, called the *porta hepatis,* is situated transversely between the two minor lobes.

The *portal vein* and the *hepatic artery,* both of which convey blood to the liver, enter the porta hepatis and branch out through the liver substance (see Fig. 16-3, *C*). The portal vein ends in the sinusoids, and the hepatic artery ends in capillaries that communicate with sinusoids. Thus in addition to the usual arterial blood supply, the liver receives blood from the portal system.

The portal system, of which the portal vein is the main trunk, consists of the veins arising from the walls of the stomach, from the greater part of the intestinal tract and the gallbladder, and from the pancreas and the spleen. The blood circulating through these organs is rich in nutrients and is carried to the liver for modification before being returned to the heart. The *hepatic veins* convey the blood from the liver sinusoids to the inferior vena cava.

The liver has numerous physiologic functions. The primary consideration from the radiographic standpoint is the formation of *bile.* The gland secretes bile at the rate of 1 to 3 pints (½ to 1½ L) each day. Bile, the channel of elimination for the waste products of red blood cell destruction, is an excretion as well as a secretion. As a secretion, it is an important aid in the emulsification and assimilation of fats. The bile is collected from the liver cells by the ducts and either carried to the gallbladder for temporary storage or poured directly into the duodenum through the common bile duct.

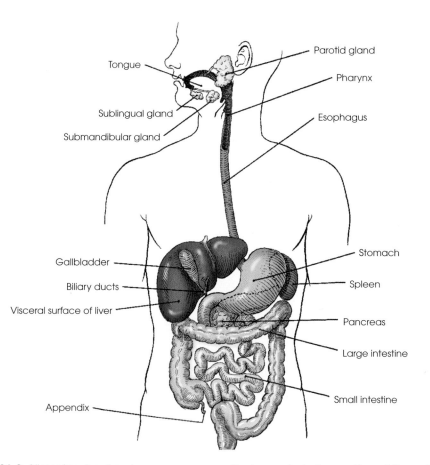

Fig. 16-2 Alimentary tract and accessory organs. To demonstrate the position of the gallbladder in relation to the liver, the liver is shown with the inferior portion pulled anteriorly and superiorly, thus placing the liver in an atypical position. The true relationship of the liver and gallbladder is seen in Fig. 16-1.

The biliary, or excretory, system of the liver consists of the bile ducts and gallbladder (Figs. 16-3 and 16-4). Beginning within the lobules as bile capillaries, the ducts unite to form larger and larger passages as they converge, finally forming two main ducts, one leading from each major lobe. The two main *hepatic ducts* emerge at the porta hepatis and join to form the *common hepatic duct,* which in turn unites with the *cystic duct* to form the *common bile duct.* The hepatic and cystic ducts are each about 1½ inches (3.8 cm) in length. The common bile duct passes inferiorly for a distance of approximately 3 inches (7.6 cm). The common bile duct joins the pancreatic duct, and they enter together or side by side into an enlarged chamber known as the *hepatopancreatic ampulla,* or *ampulla of Vater.* The ampulla opens into the descending portion of the duodenum. The distal end of the common bile duct is controlled by the *choledochal sphincter* as it enters the duodenum. The

hepatopancreatic ampulla is controlled by a circular muscle known as the *sphincter of the hepatopancreatic ampulla,* or *sphincter of Oddi.* During interdigestive periods the sphincter remains in a contracted state, thus routing most of the bile into the gallbladder for concentration and

temporary storage; during digestion it relaxes to permit the bile to flow from the liver and gallbladder into the duodenum. The hepatopancreatic ampulla opens on an elevation on the duodenal mucosa known as the *major duodenal papilla.*

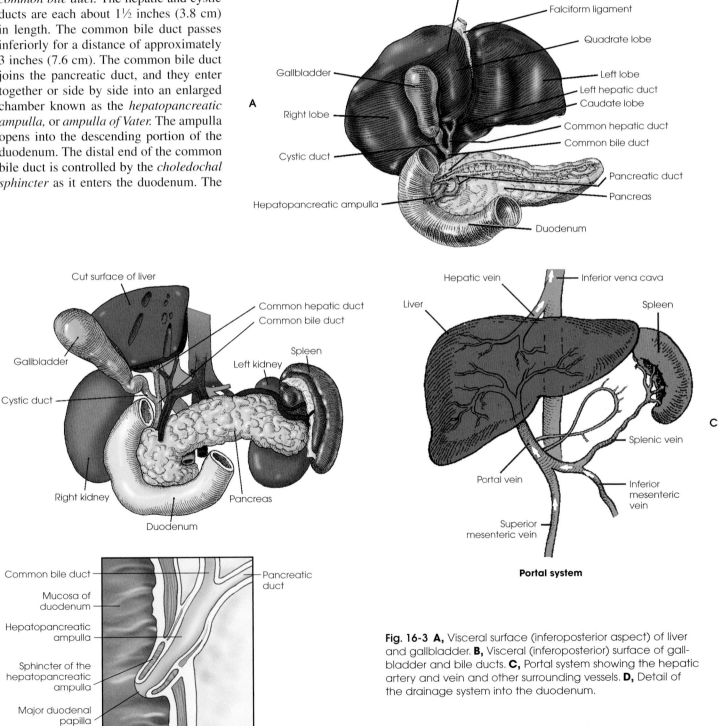

Portal system

Fig. 16-3 A, Visceral surface (inferoposterior aspect) of liver and gallbladder. **B,** Visceral (inferoposterior) surface of gallbladder and bile ducts. **C,** Portal system showing the hepatic artery and vein and other surrounding vessels. **D,** Detail of the drainage system into the duodenum.

The *gallbladder* is a thin-walled, more or less pear-shaped, musculomembranous sac with a capacity of approximately 2 oz. The gallbladder functions to concentrate bile by absorption of the water content; store bile during interdigestive periods; and, by contraction of its musculature, evacuate the bile during digestion. The muscular contraction of the gallbladder is activated by a hormone called *cholecystokinin*. This hormone is secreted by the duodenal mucosa and released into the blood when fatty or acid chyme passes into the intestine. The organ consists of a narrow neck that is continuous with the *cystic duct;* a body or main portion; and a fundus, which is its broad lower portion. The gallbladder is usually lodged in a fossa on the visceral (inferior) surface of the right lobe of the liver, where it lies in an oblique plane inferiorly and anteriorly. Measuring about 1 inch (2.5 cm) in width at its widest part and 3 to 4 inches (7.5 to 10 cm) in length, the gallbladder extends from the lower right margin of the porta hepatis to a variable distance below the anterior border of the liver. The position of the gallbladder varies with body habitus, being high and well away from the midline in hypersthenic persons and low and near the spine in asthenic individuals (see Fig. 16-4). The gallbladder is sometimes embedded in the liver and frequently hangs free below the inferior margin of the liver.

Pancreas and Spleen

The *pancreas* is an elongated gland situated across the posterior abdominal wall. Extending from the duodenum to the spleen (Figs. 16-3 and 16-5), the pancreas is about 5½ inches (14 cm) in length and consists of a head, neck, body, and tail. The *head,* which is the broadest portion of the organ, extends inferiorly and is enclosed within the curve of the duodenum at the level of the second or third lumbar vertebra. The *body* and *tail* of the pancreas pass transversely behind the stomach and in front of the left kidney, with the narrow tail terminating near the spleen. The pancreas cannot be visualized on plain radiographic studies.

The pancreas is both an *exocrine* and an *endocrine* gland. The exocrine cells of the pancreas are arranged in lobules with a highly ramified duct system. This exocrine portion of the gland produces *pancreatic juice,* which acts on proteins, fats, and carbohydrates. The endocrine portion of the gland consists of clusters of islet cells, or islets of Langerhans, which are randomly distributed throughout the pancreas. Each islet consists of clusters of cells surrounding small groups of capillaries. These cells produce the hormones *insulin* and *glucagon,* which are responsible for sugar metabolism. The islet cells do not communicate directly with the ducts but release their secretions directly into the blood through a rich capillary network.

The digestive juice secreted by the exocrine cells of the pancreas is conveyed into the *pancreatic duct* and from there into the duodenum. The pancreatic duct often unites with the common bile duct to form a single passage via the hepatopancreatic ampulla, which opens directly into the descending duodenum.

The *spleen* is included in this section only because of its location; it belongs to the lymphatic system. The spleen is a glandlike but ductless organ that functions to produce lymphocytes and to store and remove dead or dying red blood cells. The spleen is more or less bean shaped and measures about 5 inches (13 cm) in length, 3 inches (7.6 cm) in width, and 1½ inches (3.8 cm) in thickness. Situated obliquely in the left upper quadrant, the spleen is just below the diaphragm and behind the stomach. It is in contact with the abdominal wall laterally, with the left suprarenal gland and left kidney medially, and with the left colic flexure of the colon inferiorly. The spleen is visualized both with and without contrast media.

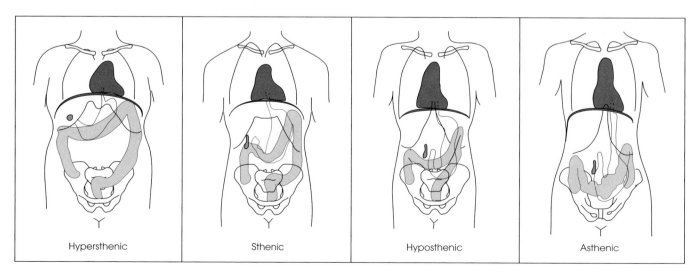

| Hypersthenic | Sthenic | Hyposthenic | Asthenic |

Fig. 16-4 Gallbladder *(green)* position varies with body habitus. Note the extreme difference in position of the gallbladder between the hypersthenic and asthenic habitus.

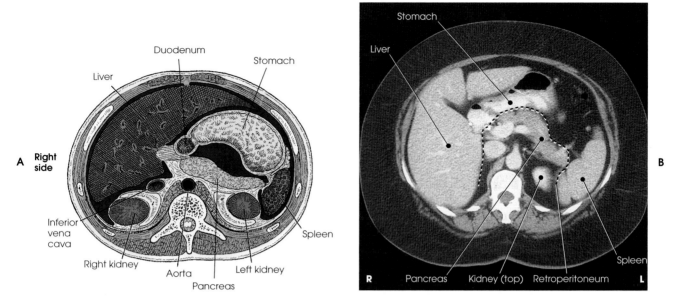

Fig. 16-5 Sectional image of upper abdomen (viewed from the patient's feet upward), showing relationship of digestive system components. **B,** Axial CT image of the same area of the abdomen as in **A.**

(From Kelley LL, Petersen CM: *Sectional anatomy for imaging professionals,* St Louis, 1997, Mosby.)

SUMMARY OF ANATOMY

Peritoneum	Liver and biliary system	Pancreas and spleen
abdominopelvic cavity	falciform ligament	pancreas
abdominal cavity	right lobe	head
pelvic cavity	left lobe	body
peritoneum	caudate lobe	tail
parietal	quadrate lobe	exocrine gland
peritoneum	porta hepatis	pancreatic juice
visceral	hepatic artery	endocrine gland
peritoneum	portal vein	islet cells
mesentery	hepatic veins	pancreatic duct
omenta	hepatic ducts	spleen
peritoneal cavity	bile	
retroperitoneum	common hepatic duct	
	cystic duct	
	common bile duct	
	hepatopancreatic am-pulla	
	sphincter of the hepa-topancreatic ampulla	
	major duodenal papilla	
	gallbladder	
	cystic duct	

SUMMARY OF PATHOLOGY

Condition	Definition
Abdominal Aortic Aneurysm	Localized dilatation of the abdominal aorta
Biliary Stenosis	Narrowing of the bile ducts
Bowel Obstruction	Blockage of the bowel lumen
Cholecystitis	Acute or chronic inflammation of the gallbladder
Choledocholithiasis	Calculus in the common bile duct
Cholelithiasis	The presence of gallstones
Ileus	Failure of bowel peristalsis
Metastases	Transfer of a cancerous lesion from one area to another
Pancreatitis	Acute or chronic inflammation of the pancreas
Pancreatic Pseudocyst	Collection of debris, fluid, pancreatic enzymes, and blood as a complication of acute pancreatitis
Pneumoperitoneum	Presence of air in the peritoneal cavity
Tumor	New tissue growth where cell proliferation is uncontrolled

EXPOSURE TECHNIQUE CHART ESSENTIAL PROJECTIONS

DIGESTIVE SYSTEM

Part	cm	kVp*	tm	mA	mAs	AEC	SID	IR	Dose† (mrad)
Abdomen‡—AP	21	75		200s		●● ●	48″	35 × 43 cm	185
PA	21	75		200s		●● ●	48″	35 × 43 cm	185
AP (decubitus)	24	80		200s		○○ ●	48″	35 × 43 cm	300
Lateral	30	90		200s		○○ ●	48″	35 × 43 cm	916
Lateral (decubitus)	30	95		200s		○○ ●	48″	35 × 43 cm	1040

s, Small focal spot.
*kVp values are for a three-phase, 12-pulse generator.
†Relative doses for comparison use. All doses are skin entrance for average adult at cm indicated.
‡Bucky, 16:1 grid. Screen/film speed 300.

NEW ABBREVIATIONS USED IN CHAPTER 16

AAA	Abdominal aortic aneurysm
ERCP	Endoscopic retrograde cholangiopancreatography
NPO	nil per os (nothing by mouth)
PTC	Percutaneous transhepatic cholangiography
RUQ	Right upper quadrant

See Addendum B for a summary of all abbreviations used in Volume 2.

Abdominal Radiographic Procedures

PRELIMINARY PROCEDURES AND POSITIONS

Preparation

Careful preliminary preparation of the intestinal tract is important in radiologic investigations of the abdominal viscera. In the presence of nonacute conditions the preparation can consist of any combination of controlled diet, laxative, and enemas. The preparation ordered is generally determined by the medical facility in which the examination is to be performed.

Although many patients referred for an examination of the abdomen are well enough to undergo routine preparation, a number have or are suspected of having some condition that removes them from the "routine" classification even though they are not acutely ill. In such patients the referring physician is consulted as to the presumptive diagnosis, and the procedure is varied as needed. Preliminary preparation is never administered to ill patients who are acutely ill or have a condition such as visceral rupture or intestinal obstruction or perforation.

Exposure technique

In examinations without a contrast medium, it is imperative to obtain maximum soft tissue differentiation throughout the different regions of the abdomen. Because of the wide range in the thickness of the abdomen and the delicate differences in physical density between the contained viscera, it is necessary to use a more critical exposure technique than is required to demonstrate the difference in density between an opacified organ and the structures adjacent to it. The exposure factors should therefore be adjusted to produce a radiograph with moderate gray tones and less black-and-white contrast. If the kilovolt peak (kVp) is too high, the possibility of not demonstrating small or semiopaque gallstones increases (Fig. 16-6, *A*).

Sharply defined outlines of the psoas muscles, the lower border of the liver, the kidneys, the ribs, and the transverse processes of the lumbar vertebrae are the best criteria for judging the quality of an abdominal radiograph.

Immobilization

One of the prime requisites in abdominal examinations is the prevention of movement, both voluntary and involuntary. The following steps are observed:

- To prevent muscle contraction caused by tension, adjust the patient in a comfortable position so that he or she can relax.
- Explain the breathing procedure, and make sure the patient understands exactly what is expected.
- If necessary, apply a compression band across the abdomen for *immobilization* but not compression.
- Do not start the exposure for 1 to 2 seconds after the suspension of respiration to allow the patient to come to rest and involuntary movement of the viscera to subside.

Voluntary motion produces a blurred outline of the structures that do not have involuntary movement, such as the liver, psoas muscles, and spine. Patient breathing during exposure results in blurring of bowel gas outlines in the upper abdomen as the diaphragm moves (Fig. 16-6, *B*). Involuntary motion caused by peristalsis may produce either a localized or generalized haziness of the image. Involuntary contraction of the abdominal wall or the muscles around the spine may cause movement of the entire abdominal area and produce generalized radiographic haziness.

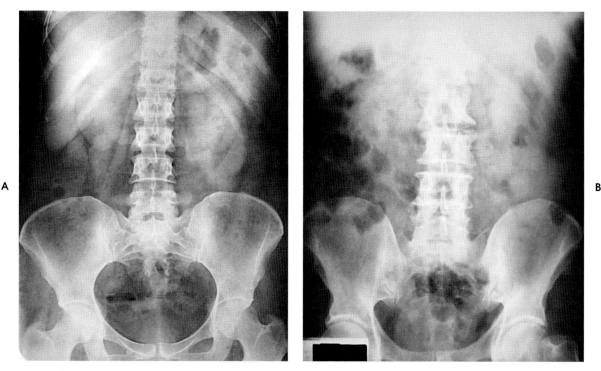

Fig. 16-6 A, AP abdomen showing proper positioning and collimation. **B,** AP abdomen demonstrating blurred bowel gas in the right upper quadrant (RUQ), caused by patient breathing during exposure.

Radiographic projections

Radiography of the abdomen may include one or more radiographic projections. The most commonly performed is the supine AP projection, often called a KUB because it includes the *k*idneys, *u*reters, and *b*ladder. Projections used to complement the supine AP may include an upright AP abdomen or an AP projection in the lateral decubitus position (the left lateral decubitus is most often preferred), or both. Both radiographs are useful in assessing the abdomen in patients with free air (pneumoperitoneum) and in determining presence and location of air-fluid levels. Other abdominal projections may include a lateral projection or a lateral projection in the supine (dorsal decubitus) body position. Many institutions also obtain a PA chest radiograph to include the upper abdomen and diaphragm. The PA chest radiograph is indicated because any air escaping from the gastrointestinal tract into the peritoneal space rises to the highest level, usually just beneath the diaphragm.

POSITIONING PROTOCOLS

Radiographs obtained to evaluate the patient's abdomen vary considerably depending on the institution and physician. For example, some consider the preliminary evaluation radiograph to consist of only the AP (supine) projection. Others obtain two projections: a supine and an upright AP abdomen (often called a *flat* and an *upright*). A three-way or acute abdomen series may be requested to rule out free air, bowel obstruction, and infections. The three projections usually include (1) an AP with the patient supine, (2) an AP with the patient upright, and (3) a PA chest. If the patient cannot stand for the upright AP projection, the projection is performed using the left lateral decubitus position. The PA chest projection can be used to detect free air that may accumulate under the diaphragm.

Positioning for radiographs of the abdomen is described in the following pages. (For a description of positioning for the PA chest, see Chapter 10.)

Radiation Protection

General radiation protection techniques must be used. Gonadal shielding is required in the following situations:
1. If the gonads lie in close proximity (2 inches [5 cm]) to the primary x-ray field despite proper beam limitation
2. If the clinical objectives of the examination will not be compromised. The concern is whether the use of gonadal shielding will cover an area of interest on the radiograph.
3. If the patient has a reasonable reproductive potential

Regardless of whether gonad shielding is used, close and accurate collimation is necessary to limit the x-ray beam. In addition to reducing the amount of radiation exposure to an unnecessary area, this practice also improves the quality of radiographs.

ꙮ AP PROJECTION
Supine; upright

Image receptor: 35 × 43 cm lengthwise

Position of patient
- For the AP abdomen, or KUB, projection, place the patient either in the supine or upright position. The supine position is preferred for most initial examinations of the abdomen.

Position of part
- Center the midsagittal plane of the body to the midline of the grid device.
- If the patient is upright, distribute the weight of the body equally on the feet.
- Place the patient's arms where they will not cast shadows on the image.
- With the patient supine, place a support under the knees to relieve strain.
- For the *supine position,* center the IR at the level of the iliac crests and ensure that the pubic symphysis is included (Fig. 16-7).

- For the *upright position,* center the IR 2 inches (5 cm) above the level of the iliac crests or high enough to include the diaphragm (Fig. 16-8).
- If the bladder is to be included on the upright radiograph, center the IR at the level of the iliac crests.
- If a patient is too tall to include the entire pelvic area, obtain a second radiograph to include the bladder on a 24- × 30-cm IR if necessary. The 24- × 30-cm IR is placed crosswise and centered 2 to 3 inches (5 to 7.6 cm) above the upper border of the pubic symphysis.
- If necessary, apply a compression band across the abdomen with moderate pressure for immobilization.
- *Shield gonads:* Use local gonad shielding for examinations of male patients (not shown for illustrative purposes).
- *Respiration:* Suspend at the end of expiration so that the abdominal organs are not compressed.

Central ray
- Perpendicular to the IR at the level of the iliac crests for the supine position
- Horizontal and 2 inches (5 cm) above the level of the iliac crests to include the diaphragm for the upright position

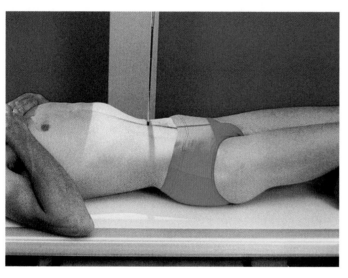

Fig. 16-7 AP abdomen, supine.

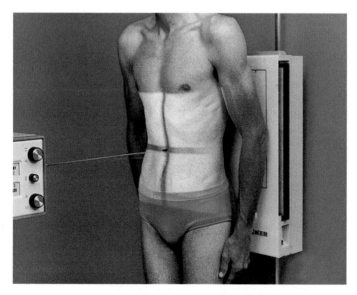

Fig. 16-8 AP abdomen, upright.

Structures shown

An AP projection of the abdomen shows the size and shape of the liver, the spleen and the kidneys, and intraabdominal calcifications or evidence of tumor masses (Fig. 16-9). Additional examples of supine and upright abdomen projections are shown in Figs. 16-15 and 16-16.

EVALUATION CRITERIA

The following should be clearly demonstrated:
- Area from the pubic symphysis to the upper abdomen (Two radiographs may be necessary if the patient is tall.)
- Proper patient alignment is ensured by the following:
  - Centered vertebral column
  - Ribs, pelvis, and hips equidistant to the edge of the radiograph on both sides
- No rotation of patient, as indicated by the following:
  - Spinous processes in the center of the lumbar vertebrae
  - Ischial spines of the pelvis symmetric, if visible
  - Alae or wings of the ilia symmetric
- Soft tissue gray tones should demonstrate the following:
  - Lateral abdominal wall and properitoneal fat layer (flank stripe)
  - Psoas muscles, lower border of the liver, and kidneys
  - Inferior ribs
  - Transverse processes of the lumbar vertebrae
  - Right or left marker visible but not lying over the abdominal contents
- Diaphragm without motion on upright abdomen examinations (Crosswise IR placement is appropriate if the patient is large.)
- Density on upright abdomen examination, similar to supine examination. However, reduce density if pneumoperitoneum is suspected.
- Upright abdomen identified with an appropriate marker

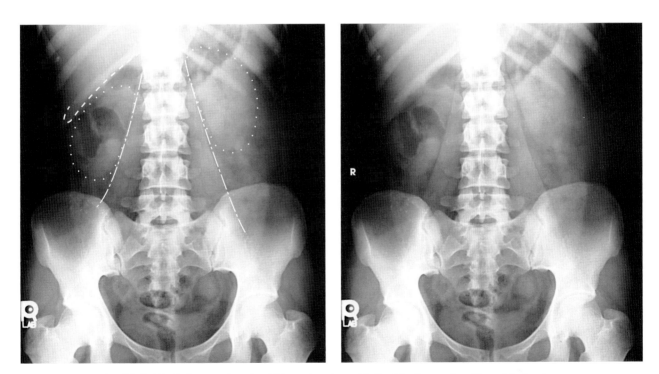

Fig. 16-9 AP abdomen showing kidney shadows *(dotted line)*, margin of liver *(dashed line)*, and psoas muscles *(dot-dash lines)*.

♠ PA PROJECTION
Upright

When the kidneys are not of primary interest, the upright PA projection should be considered. Compared with the AP projection, the PA projection of the abdomen greatly reduces patient gonadal dose.

Image receptor: 35 × 43 cm lengthwise

Position of patient

- With the patient in the upright position, place the anterior abdominal surface in contact with the vertical grid device.
- Center the abdominal midline to the midline of the IR.
- Center the IR 2 inches (5 cm) above the level of the iliac crests (Fig. 16-10), as previously described for the upright AP projection. The central ray, structures shown, and evaluation criteria are the same as for the upright AP projection.

♠ AP PROJECTION
L lateral decubitus position

Image receptor: 35 × 43 cm

Position of patient

- If the patient is too ill to stand, place him or her in a lateral recumbent position lying on a radiolucent pad on a transportation cart. Use a left lateral decubitus position in most situations.
- If possible, have the patient lie on the side for several minutes before the exposure to allow air to rise to its highest level within the abdomen.
- Place the patient's arms above the level of the diaphragm so that they are not projected over any abdominal contents.
- Flex the patient's knees slightly to provide stabilization.
- *Exercise care* to ensure that the patient does not fall off the cart; if a cart is used, *lock all wheels* securely in position.

Position of part

- Adjust the height of the vertical grid device so that the long axis of the IR is centered to the midsagittal plane.
- Position the patient so that the level of the iliac crests is centered to the IR. A slightly higher centering point, 2 inches (5 cm) above the iliac crests, may be necessary to ensure that the diaphragms are included in the image (Fig. 16-11).
- Adjust the patient to ensure that a true lateral position is attained.
- *Shield gonads.*
- *Respiration:* Suspend at the end of expiration.

▼ COMPENSATING FILTER

For patients with large abdomens, a compensating filter will improve image quality by preventing overexposure of the upper-side abdominal area.

Central ray

- Directed *horizontal* and perpendicular to the midpoint of the IR

NOTE: A right lateral decubitus position is often requested or may be required when the patient cannot lie on the left side.

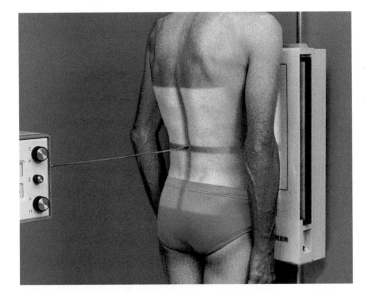

Fig. 16-10 PA abdomen, upright position. This projection is suggested for survey examination of the abdomen when the kidneys are not of primary interest.

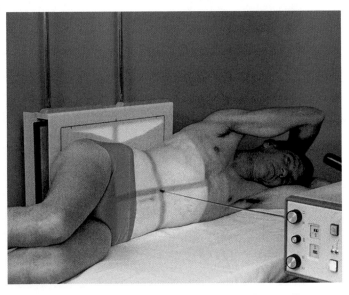

Fig. 16-11 AP abdomen, left lateral decubitus position.

Structures shown

In addition to showing the size and shape of the liver, spleen, and kidneys, the AP abdomen with the patient in the left decubitus position is most valuable for demonstrating free air and air-fluid levels when an upright abdomen projection cannot be obtained (Fig. 16-12).

The following should be clearly demonstrated:

- Diaphragm without motion
- Both sides of the abdomen. If this is not possible, do the following:
  - ☐ Elevate and demonstrate the side down when fluid is suspected.
  - ☐ Demonstrate the side up when free air is suspected.
- Abdominal wall, flank structures, and diaphragm
- No rotation of patient
- Proper identification visible, including patient side and marking to indicate which side is up

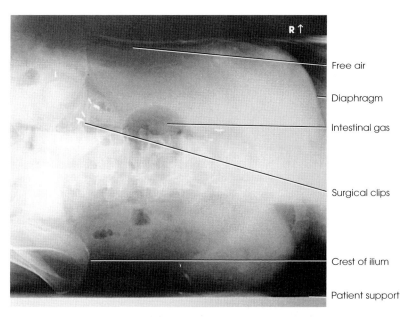

Free air

Diaphragm

Intestinal gas

Surgical clips

Crest of ilium

Patient support

Fig. 16-12 AP abdomen, left lateral decubitus position demonstrating free air collection along right flank. Note correct marker placement.

Abdominal sequencing

To demonstrate small amounts of intraperitoneal gas in acute abdominal cases, Miller[1,2] recommended that the patient be kept in the left lateral position on a stretcher for 10 to 20 minutes before abdominal radiographs are obtained. This position allows gas to rise into the area under the right hemidiaphragm, where the image will not be superimposed by the gastric gas bubble. If larger amounts of free air are present, many radiology departments suggest that the patient lie on the side for a minimum of 5 minutes before the radiograph is produced. Projections of the abdomen are then taken as follows:

- Perform an AP or PA projection of the chest and upper abdomen with the patient in the left lateral decubitus position.
- Use the chest exposure technique for this radiograph (Fig. 16-13).
- Maintain the patient in the left lateral decubitus position while the patient is being moved onto a horizontally placed table. Tilt the table and patient to the upright position.
- Turn the patient to obtain AP or PA projections of the chest and abdomen (Figs. 16-14 and 16-15).
- Return the table back to the horizontal position for a supine AP or PA projection of the abdomen (Fig. 16-16).

[1]Miller RE, Nelson SW: The roentgenologic demonstration of tiny amounts of free intraperitoneal gas: experimental and clinical studies, *AJR* 112:574, 1971.
[2]Miller RE: The technical approach to the acute abdomen, *Semin Roentgenol* 8:267, 1973.

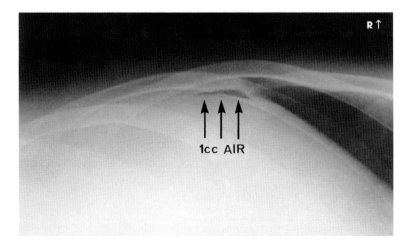

Fig. 16-13 Enlarged portion of an AP abdomen, left lateral decubitus position in a patient injected with 1 mL of air into the abdominal cavity.

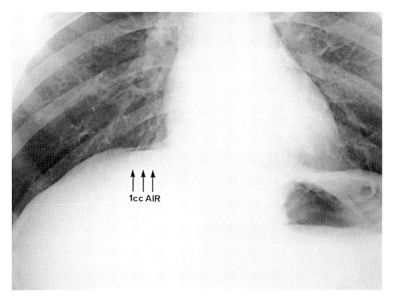

Fig. 16-14 Enlarged portion of an upright AP chest showing free air in same patient as in Fig. 16-13.

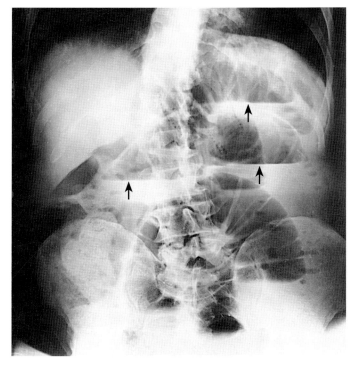

Fig. 16-15 AP abdomen, upright position, showing air-fluid levels *(arrows)* in intestine (same patient as in Fig. 16-16).

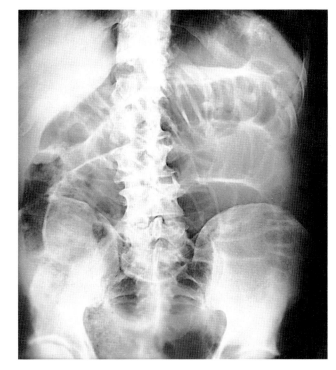

Fig. 16-16 AP abdomen. Supine study showing intestinal obstruction in same patient as in Fig. 16-15.

Digestive system

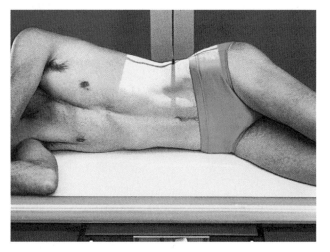

Fig. 16-17 Right lateral abdomen.

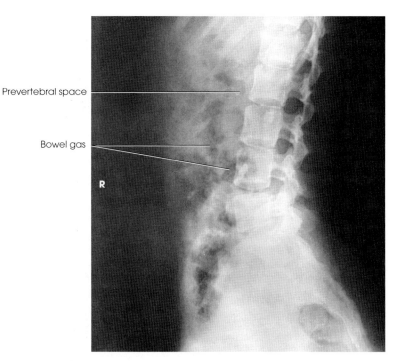

Prevertebral space

Bowel gas

Fig. 16-18 Right lateral abdomen.

🔥 LATERAL PROJECTION
R or L position

Image receptor: 35 × 43 cm lengthwise

Position of patient
- Turn the patient to a lateral recumbent position on either the right or left side.

Position of part
- Flex the patient's knees to a comfortable position, and adjust the body so that the midcoronal plane is centered to the midline of the grid.
- Place supports between the knees and the ankles.
- Flex the elbows, and place the hands under the patient's head (Fig. 16-17).
- Center the IR at the level of the iliac crests or 2 inches (5 cm) above the crests to include the diaphragm.
- Place a compression band across the pelvis for stability if necessary.
- *Shield gonads.*
- *Respiration:* Suspend at the end of expiration.

Central ray
- Perpendicular to the IR and entering the midcoronal plane at the level of the iliac crest or 2 inches (5 cm) above the iliac crest if the diaphragm is included

Structures shown
A lateral projection of the abdomen demonstrates the prevertebral space occupied by the abdominal aorta, as well as any intraabdominal calcifications or tumor masses (Fig. 16-18).

EVALUATION CRITERIA

The following should be clearly demonstrated:
- Abdominal contents visible with soft tissue gray tones
- No rotation of patient, indicated by the following:
  - ☐ Superimposed ilia
  - ☐ Superimposed lumbar vertebrae pedicles and open intervertebral foramina
- As much of the remaining abdomen as possible when the diaphragm is included

⚘ LATERAL PROJECTION
R or L dorsal decubitus position

Image receptor: 35 × 43 cm

Position of patient
- When the patient cannot stand or lie on the side, place the patient in the supine position on a transportation cart or other suitable support with the right or left side in contact with the vertical grid device.
- Place the patient's arms across the upper chest to ensure they are not projected over any abdominal contents, or place them behind the patient's head.
- Flex the patient's knees slightly to relieve strain on the back.
- *Exercise care* to ensure that the patient does not fall from the cart or table; if a cart is used, *lock all wheels* securely in position.

Position of part
- Adjust the height of the vertical grid device so that the long axis of the IR is centered to the midcoronal plane.
- Position the patient so that a point approximately 2 inches (5 cm) above the level of the iliac crests is centered to the IR (Fig. 16-19).
- Adjust the patient to make sure no rotation from the supine position occurs.
- *Shield gonads.*
- *Respiration:* Suspend at the end of expiration.

Central ray
- Directed *horizontal* and perpendicular to the center of the IR, entering the midcoronal plane 2 inches (5 cm) above the level of the iliac crests

Structures shown
The lateral projection of the abdomen is valuable in demonstrating the prevertebral space and is quite useful in determining air-fluid levels in the abdomen (Fig. 16-20).

EVALUATION CRITERIA

The following should be clearly demonstrated:
- Diaphragm without motion
- Abdominal contents visible with soft tissue gray tones
- Patient elevated so that entire abdomen is demonstrated

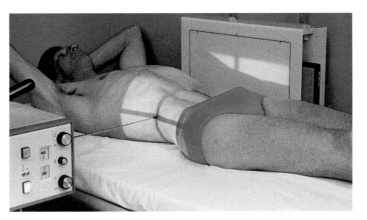

Fig. 16-19 Lateral abdomen, left dorsal decubitus position.

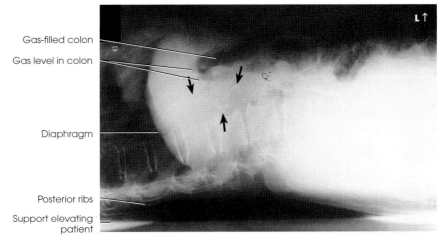

Gas-filled colon
Gas level in colon
Diaphragm
Posterior ribs
Support elevating patient

Fig. 16-20 Lateral abdomen, left dorsal decubitus position, demonstrating a calcified aorta *(arrows)*. Note correct marker placement.

Abdominal Fistulae and Sinuses

For radiographic demonstration of the origin and extent of fistulae (abnormal passages, usually between two internal organs) and sinuses (abnormal channels leading to abscesses), the following steps are observed:

- Fill the tract with a radiopaque contrast medium, usually under fluoroscopic control.
- Obtain right-angle projections. Oblique projections are occasionally required to demonstrate the full extent of a sinus tract.
- To explore fistulae and sinuses in the abdominal region, have the intestinal tract as free of gas and fecal material as possible.
- Unless the injection is made under fluoroscopic control, take a scout radiograph of the abdomen to check the condition of the intestinal tract before beginning the examination.
- When more than one sinus opening is present, occlude each accessory opening with sterile gauze packing to prevent reflux of the contrast substance and identify every opening with a specific lead marker placed over the dressing (Figs. 16-21 to 16-23).
- Dress and identify the primary sinus opening in a similar manner if the catheter is removed after the injection.
- When a reflux of the contrast medium occurs, cleanse the skin thoroughly before making an exposure.

When fluoroscopy is not employed, place the patient in position for the first projection before the injection to prevent drainage of the opaque substance by unnecessary movement. An initial radiograph is taken and evaluated before the examination is started or the patient's position is changed.

For demonstration of a fistula involving the colon, barium is instilled by enema. If a fistula involving the small bowel is suspected, the patient ingests a thin barium suspension, which is followed by fluoroscopy/radiography until it reaches the suspected region. The bladder is filled with an iodinated contrast media when involvement of this structure is evaluated. Cutaneous fistulas and sinus tracts are opacified by introduction of an iodinated contrast media through a small diameter catheter. The procedures are performed using fluoroscopic observation, with images taken as indicated.

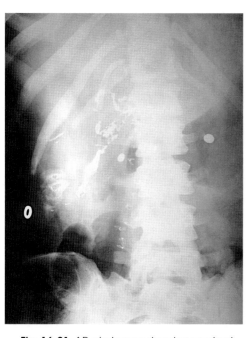

Fig. 16-21 AP abdomen showing contrast-filled sinus tract with a lead circular ring on body surface.

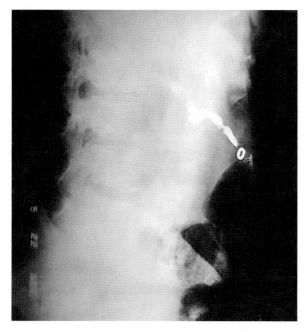

Fig. 16-22 Lateral abdomen showing sinus tract with a lead circular ring on body surface.

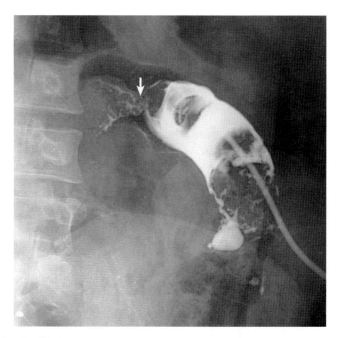

Fig. 16-23 Oblique abdomen, LPO position, showing fistula (arrow).

Biliary Tract and Gallbladder

Several techniques can be used to examine the gallbladder and the biliary ductal system. In many institutions, sonography is the modality of choice. This section of the atlas discusses the radiographic techniques currently available.

Table 16-1 lists some of the prefixes associated with the biliary system. *Cholegraphy* is the general term for a radiographic study of the biliary system. More specific terms can be used to describe the portion of the biliary system under investigation. For example, *cholecystography* is the radiographic investigation of the gallbladder, and *cholangiography* is the radiographic study of the biliary ducts.

Advances in sonography, CT, MRI, and nuclear medicine have reduced the radiographic examination of the biliary tract primarily to direct injection procedures including percutaneous transhepatic cholangiography (PTC), postoperative (T-tube) cholangiography, and endoscopic retrograde cholangiopancreatography (ERCP). The contrast agent selected for use in the direct-injection techniques may be any one of the water-soluble iodinated compounds employed for intravenous urography.

PROJECTIONS REMOVED

Biliary tract and gallbladder
- PA projection
- PA oblique projection, LAO position
- Lateral projection (right)
- AP projection, right lateral decubitus position

Intravenous cholangiography
- AP oblique projection, RPO position

TABLE 16-1

Biliary system combining forms

Root forms	Meaning
chole-	Relationship with bile
cysto-	Bag or sac
choledocho-	Common bile duct
cholangio-	Bile ducts
cholecyst-	Gallbladder

Percutaneous Transhepatic Cholangiography

Percutaneous transhepatic cholangiography (PTC)[1] is another technique employed for preoperative radiologic examination of the biliary tract. This technique is used for patients with jaundice when the ductal system has been shown to be dilated by CT or sonography but the cause of the obstruction is unclear. The performance of this examination has greatly increased because of the availability of the Chiba ("skinny") needle. In addition, PTC is often used to place a drainage catheter for the treatment of obstructive jaundice. When a drainage catheter is used, both diagnostic and drainage techniques are performed at the same time.

[1]Evans JA et al: Percutaneous transhepatic cholangiography, *Radiology* 78:362, 1962.

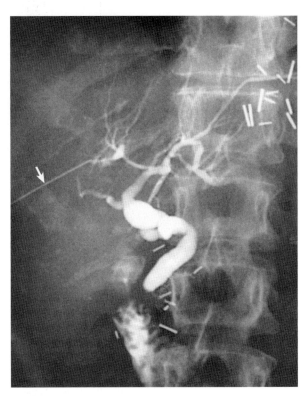

Fig. 16-24 PTC with Chiba needle *(arrow)* in position, showing dilated biliary ducts.

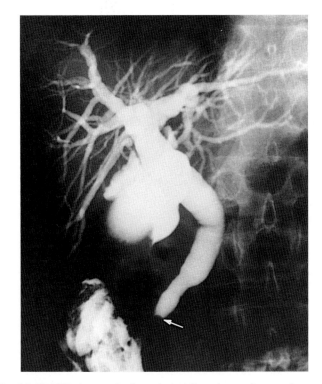

Fig. 16-25 PTC demonstrating obstruction stone at ampulla *(arrow)*.

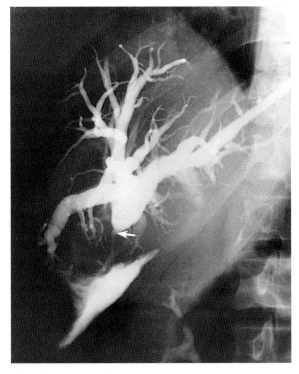

Fig. 16-26 PTC demonstrating stenosis *(arrow)* of common hepatic duct caused by trauma.

PTC is performed by placing the patient on the radiographic table in the supine position. The patient's right side is surgically prepared and appropriately draped. After a local anesthetic is administered, the Chiba needle is held parallel to the floor and inserted through the right lateral intercostal space and advanced toward the liver hilum. The stylet of the needle is withdrawn, and a syringe filled with contrast medium is attached to the needle. Under fluoroscopic control, the needle is slowly withdrawn until the contrast medium is seen to fill the biliary ducts. In most instances the biliary tree is readily located because the ducts are generally dilated. After the biliary ducts are filled, the needle is completely withdrawn and serial or spot AP projections of the biliary area are taken (Figs. 16-24 to 16-26).

BILIARY DRAINAGE PROCEDURE AND STONE EXTRACTION

If dilated biliary ducts are identified by CT, PTC, or sonography, the radiologist, after consultation with the referring physician, may elect to place a drainage catheter in the biliary duct.[1,2] A needle larger than the Chiba needle used in the PTC procedure is inserted through the lateral abdominal wall and into the biliary duct. A guidewire is then passed through the lumen of the needle, and the needle is removed. Once the catheter is passed over

[1]Molnar W, Stockum AE: Relief of obstructive jaundice through percutaneous transhepatic catheter—a new therapeutic method, *AJR* 122:356, 1974.
[2]Hardy CH, Messner JM, Crawley LC: Percutaneous transhepatic biliary drainage, *Radiol Technol* 56:8, 1984.

the guidewire, the wire is then removed, leaving the catheter in place.

The catheter can be left in place for prolonged drainage, or it can be used for attempts to extract retained stones if they are identified. Retained stones are extracted using a wire basket and a small balloon catheter under fluoroscopic control. This extraction procedure is usually attempted after the catheter has been in place for some time (Figs. 16-27 and 16-28).

Percutaneous transhepatic cholangiography

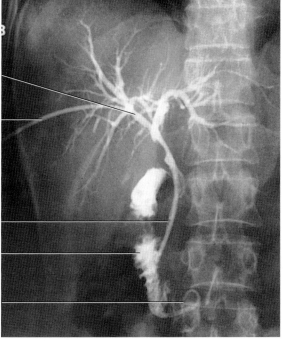

Right hepatic duct

Catheter

Drainage catheter in common bile duct

Contrast "spill" into duodenum

Tip of catheter

Fig. 16-27 PTC with drainage catheter in place.

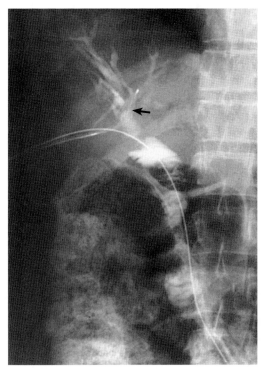

Fig. 16-28 Post-PTC image showing wire basket (*arrow*) around retained stone.

Postoperative (T-Tube) Cholangiography

Postoperative, delayed, *and* T-tube cholangiography are radiologic terms applied to the biliary tract examination that is performed by way of the T-shaped tube left in the common hepatic and common bile ducts for postoperative drainage. This examination is performed to demonstrate the caliber and patency of the ducts, the status of the sphincter of the hepatopancreatic ampulla, and the presence of residual or previously undetected stones or other pathologic conditions.

Postoperative cholangiography is performed in the radiology department. Preliminary preparation usually consists of the following:
1. The drainage tube is clamped the day preceding the examination to let the tube fill with bile as a preventive measure against air bubbles entering the ducts, where they would simulate cholesterol stones.
2. The preceding meal is withheld.
3. When indicated, a cleansing enema is administered about 1 hour before the examination. Premedication is not required.

The contrast agent used is one of the water-soluble iodinated contrast media. The density of the contrast medium used in postoperative cholangiograms is recommended to be no more than 25% to 30% because small stones may be obscured with a higher concentration.

After a preliminary radiograph of the abdomen has been obtained, the patient is adjusted in the RPO position (AP oblique projection) with the RUQ of the abdomen centered to the midline of the grid (Figs. 16-29 and 16-30).

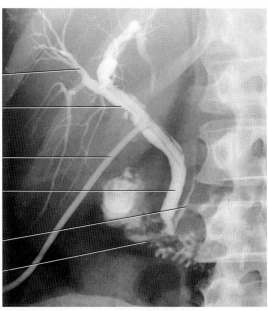

Right hepatic duct

Hepatic duct

T-tube

Common bile duct

Pancreatic duct

Contrast medium in duodenum

Fig. 16-29 AP oblique postoperative cholangiogram, RPO position.

With universal precautions employed, the contrast medium is injected under fluoroscopic control, and spot and conventional radiographs are made as indicated. Otherwise, 24- × 30-cm IRs are exposed serially after each of several fractional injections of the medium and then at specified intervals until most of the contrast solution has entered the duodenum.

Stern, Schein, and Jacobson[1] stressed the importance of obtaining a lateral projection to demonstrate the anatomic branching of the hepatic ducts in this plane and to detect any abnormality not otherwise demonstrated (Fig. 16-31). The clamp generally is not removed from the T-tube before the examination is completed. Therefore the patient may be turned onto the right side for this study.

[1]Stern WZ, Schein CJ, Jacobson HG: The significance of the lateral view in T-tube cholangiography, *AJR* 87:764, 1962.

Postoperative (T-tube) cholangiography

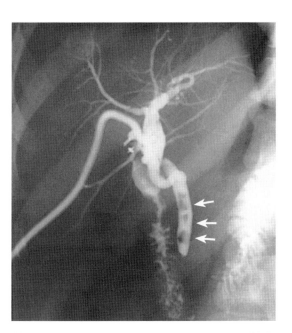

Fig. 16-30 AP oblique postoperative cholangiogram, RPO position, showing multiple stones in common bile duct *(arrows)*.

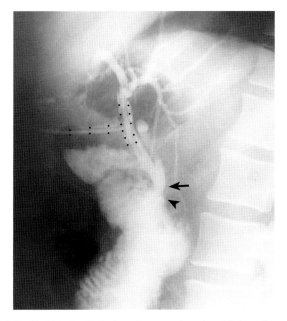

Fig. 16-31 Right lateral cholangiogram showing AP location of T-tube *(dots)*, common bile duct *(arrow)*, and hepatopancreatic ampulla (duct of Vater) *(arrowhead)*.

Endoscopic Retrograde Cholangiopancreatography

Endoscopic retrograde cholangiopancreatography (ERCP) is a procedure used to diagnose biliary and pancreatic pathologic conditions. ERCP is a useful diagnostic method when the biliary ducts are not dilated and when no obstruction exists at the ampulla.

ERCP is performed by passing a fiberoptic endoscope through the mouth into the duodenum under fluoroscopic control. To ease passage of the endoscope, the patient's throat is sprayed with a local anesthetic. Because this causes temporary pharyngeal paresis, food and drink are usually prohibited for at least 1 hour after the examination. Food may be withheld for up to 10 hours after the procedure to minimize irritation to the stomach and small bowel.

After the endoscopist locates the hepatopancreatic ampulla (ampulla of Vater), a small cannula is passed through the endoscope and directed into the ampulla (Fig. 16-32). Once the cannula is properly placed, the contrast medium is injected into the common bile duct. The patient may then be moved, fluoroscopy performed, and spot radiographs taken (Figs. 16-33 and 16-34). Oblique spot radiographs may be taken to prevent overlap of the common bile duct and the pancreatic duct. Because the injected contrast material should drain from normal ducts within approximately 5 minutes, radiographs must be exposed immediately.

The contrast medium that is used depends on the preference of the radiologist or gastroenterologist. Dense contrast agents opacify small ducts well, but they may obscure small stones. If small stones are suspected, use of a more dilute contrast medium is suggested.[1] A history of patient sensitivity to an iodinated contrast medium in another examination (e.g., intravenous urography) does not necessarily contraindicate its use for ERCP. However, the patient must be watched carefully for a reaction to the contrast medium during ERCP.

ERCP is often indicated when both clinical and radiographic findings indicate abnormalities in the biliary system or pancreas. Sonography of the upper part of the abdomen before endoscopy is often recommended to assure the physician that no pancreatic pseudocysts are present. This step is important because contrast medium injected into pseudocysts may lead to inflammation or rupture.

---

[1]Cotton P, William C: *Practical gastrointestinal endoscopy,* Oxford, England, 1980, Blackwell.

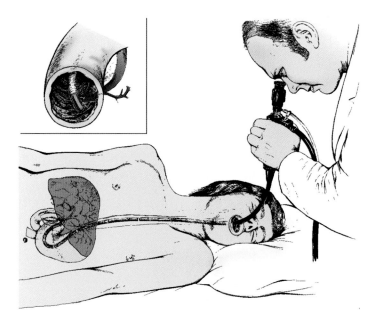

Fig. 16-32 Cannulation procedure. Procedure is begun with patient in left lateral position. This schematic diagram gives an overview of the location of the examiner and the position of the scope and its relationship to various internal organs. *Inset:* Magnified view of the tip of the scope with cannula in papilla.

(From Stewart ET, Vennes JA, Gennen JE: *Atlas of endoscopic retrograde cholangiopancreatography,* St Louis, 1977, Mosby.)

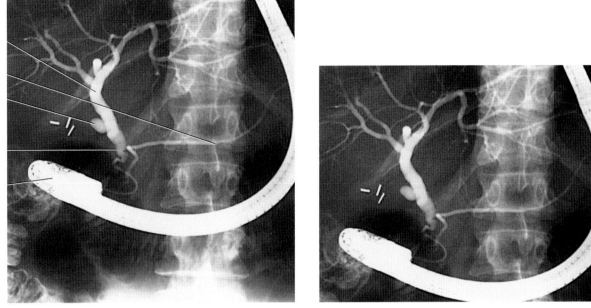

Common hepatic duct

Pancreatic duct

Cystic stump

Common bile duct

Endoscope

Fig. 16-33 ERCP spot radiograph, PA projection.

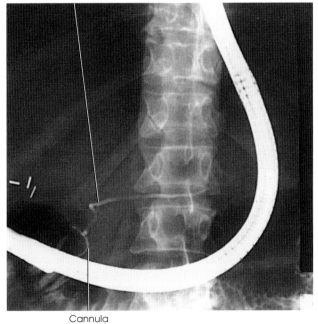

Pancreatic duct

Cannula

Fig. 16-34 ERCP spot radiograph, PA projection.

17

DIGESTIVE SYSTEM
Alimentary Canal

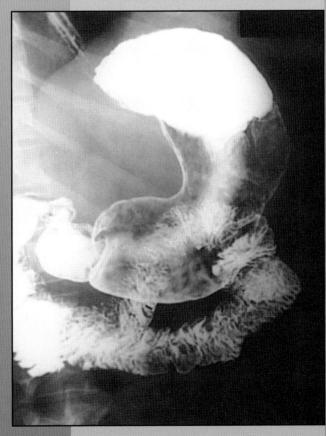

Double-contrast AP oblique stomach and duodenum, LPO position.

SUMMARY OF PROJECTIONS

PROJECTIONS, POSITIONS, AND METHODS

Page	Essential	Anatomy	Projection	Position	Method
138	🌲	Esophagus	AP or PA		
138	🌲	Esophagus	AP or PA oblique	RAO or LPO	
138	🌲	Esophagus	Lateral	R or L	
144	🌲	Stomach and duodenum	PA		
146		Stomach and duodenum	PA axial		
148	🌲	Stomach and duodenum	PA oblique	RAO	
150	🌲	Stomach and duodenum	AP oblique	LPO	
152	🌲	Stomach and duodenum	Lateral	R only	
154	🌲	Stomach and duodenum	AP		
156		Superior stomach and distal esophagus	PA oblique	RAO	WOLF
158		Stomach and duodenum serial and mucosal studies	PA oblique	RAO	
160	🌲	Small intestine	PA or AP		
176	🌲	Large intestine	PA		
178	🌲	Large intestine	PA axial		
179	🌲	Large intestine	PA oblique	RAO	
180	🌲	Large intestine	PA oblique	LAO	
181	🌲	Large intestine	Lateral	R or L	
182	🌲	Large intestine	AP		
183	🌲	Large intestine	AP axial		
184	🌲	Large intestine	AP oblique	LPO	
185	🌲	Large intestine	AP oblique	RPO	
187	🌲	Large intestine	AP or PA	R lateral decubitus	
188	🌲	Large intestine	PA or AP	L lateral decubitus	
189		Large intestine	Lateral	R or L ventral decubitus	
190	🌲	Large intestine	AP, PA, oblique, lateral	Upright	
191		Large intestine	Axial		CHASSARD-LAPINÉ

Icons in the Essential column indicate projections frequently performed in the United States and Canada. Students should be competent in these projections.

Digestive System

The *digestive system* consists of two parts: the *accessory glands* and the *alimentary canal*. The accessory glands, which include the *salivary glands, liver, gallbladder,* and *pancreas,* secrete digestive enzymes into the alimentary canal. (These glands are described in Chapter 16.) The alimentary canal is a musculomembranous tube that extends from the mouth to the anus. The regions of the alimentary canal vary in diameter according to functional requirements. The greater part of the canal, which is about 29 to 30 feet (8.6 to 8.9 m) in length, lies in the abdominal cavity. The component parts of the alimentary canal (Fig. 17-1) are the *mouth,* in which food is masticated and converted into a bolus by insalivation; the *pharynx* and *esophagus,* which are the organs of swallowing; the *stomach,* in which the digestive process begins; the *small intestine,* in which the digestive process is completed; and the *large intestine,* which is an organ of egestion and water absorption that terminates at the *anus.*

Esophagus

The *esophagus* is a long, muscular tube that carries food and saliva from the laryngopharynx to the stomach (see Fig. 17-1). The adult esophagus is approximately 10 inches (24 cm) in length and ¾ inch (1.9 cm) in diameter. Similar to the rest of the alimentary canal, the esophagus has a wall composed of four layers. Beginning with the outermost layer and moving in, the layers are as follows:

- Fibrous layer
- Muscular layer
- Submucosal layer
- Mucosal layer

The *esophagus* lies in the midsagittal plane. It originates at the level of the sixth cervical vertebra, or the upper margin of the thyroid cartilage. The esophagus enters the thorax from the superior portion of the neck. In the thorax the esophagus passes through the mediastinum, anterior to the vertebral bodies and posterior to the trachea and heart (see Fig. 17-1, *B*). In the lower thorax the esophagus passes through the diaphragm at T10. Inferior to the diaphragm the esophagus curves sharply left, increases in diameter, and joins the stomach at the *esophagogastric junction,* which is at the level of the xiphoid tip (T11). The expanded portion of the terminal esophagus, which lies in the abdomen, is called the *cardiac antrum.*

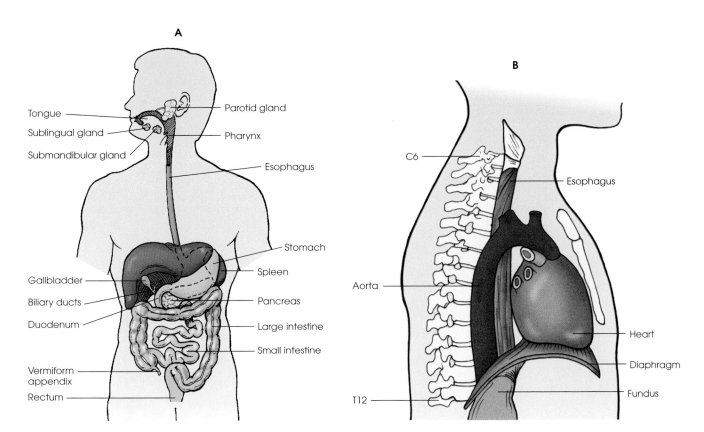

Fig. 17-1 A, Alimentary canal and its accessory organs, with the liver lifted to show the gallbladder. **B,** Lateral view of the thorax, showing the esophagus positioned anterior to the vertebral bodies and posterior to the trachea and heart.

Stomach

The *stomach* is the dilated, saclike portion of the digestive tract extending between the esophagus and the small intestine (Fig. 17-2). Its wall is composed of the same four layers as the esophagus.

The stomach is divided into four parts:
- Cardia
- Fundus
- Body
- Pyloric portion

The *cardia* of the stomach is the section immediately surrounding the esophageal opening. The *fundus* is the superior portion of the stomach that expands superiorly and fills the dome of the left hemidiaphragm. When the patient is in the upright position, the fundus is usually filled with gas and in radiography is referred to as the *gas bubble.* Descending from the fundus and beginning at the level of the cardiac notch is the *body* of the stomach. The inner mucosal layer of the body of the stomach contains numerous longitudinal folds called *rugae.* When the stomach is full, the rugae are smooth. The body of the stomach ends at a vertical plane passing through the *angular notch.* Distal to this plane is the *pyloric portion* of the stomach, which consists of the *pyloric antrum* and the narrow *pyloric canal* to the immediate right of the angular notch.

The stomach has anterior and posterior surfaces. The right border of the stomach is marked by the *lesser curvature.* The lesser curvature begins at the esophagogastric junction, is continuous with the right border of the esophagus, and is a concave curve ending at the pylorus. The left and inferior borders of the stomach are marked by the *greater curvature.* The greater curvature begins at the sharp angle at the esophagogastric junction, the *cardiac notch,* and follows the superior curvature of the fundus and then the convex curvature of the body down to the pylorus. The greater curvature is four to five times longer than the lesser curvature.

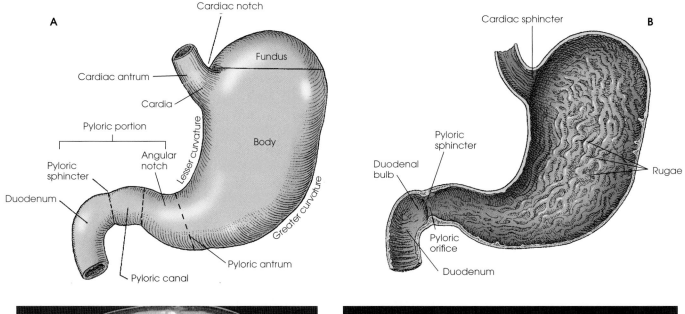

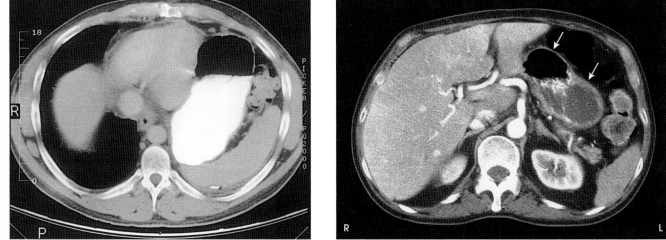

Fig. 17-2 A, Anterior surface of stomach. **B,** Interior view. **C,** Axial CT image of the upper abdomen showing the position of the stomach in relation to surrounding organs. Note contrast media *(white)* and air *(black)* in the stomach. **D,** Axial CT image showing stomach without contrast. Note air *(upper arrow)* and empty stomach *(lower arrow).*

(D, Modified from Kelley LL, Petersen CM: *Sectional anatomy for imaging professionals,* St Louis, 1997, Mosby.)

The entrance to and the exit from the stomach are each controlled by a muscle sphincter. The esophagus joins the stomach at the esophagogastric junction through an opening termed the *cardiac orifice.* The muscle controlling the cardiac orifice is called the *cardiac sphincter.* The opening between the stomach and the small intestine is the *pyloric orifice,* and the muscle controlling the pyloric orifice is called the *pyloric sphincter.*

The size, shape, and position of the stomach depend on body habitus and vary with posture and the amount of stomach contents (Fig. 17-3). In persons of hypersthenic habitus the stomach is almost horizontal and is high, with its most dependent portion well above the umbilicus. In persons of asthenic habitus the stomach is vertical and occupies a low position, with its most dependent portion extending well below the transpyloric, or interspinous, line. Between these two extremes are the intermediate types of bodily habitus with corresponding variations in the shape and position of the stomach. Note that the habitus of 85% of the population is either sthenic or hyposthenic. Radiographers should become familiar with the various positions of the stomach in the different types of body habitus so that accurate positioning of the stomach is ensured.

The stomach has several functions in the digestive process. The stomach serves as a storage area for food until it can be further digested. It is also where food is broken down. Acids, enzymes, and other chemicals are secreted to chemically break down food. Food is also mechanically broken down through churning and peristalsis. Food that has been mechanically and chemically altered in the stomach is transported to the duodenum as a material called *chyme.*

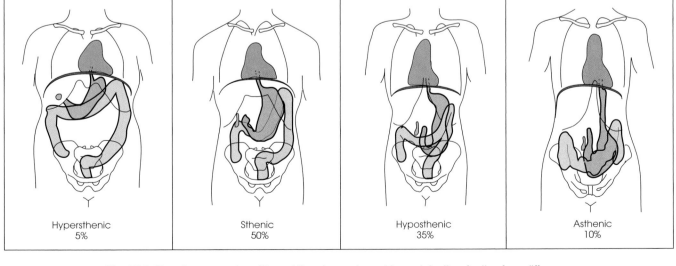

Hypersthenic 5%	Sthenic 50%	Hyposthenic 35%	Asthenic 10%

Fig. 17-3 Size, shape, and position of the stomach and large intestine for the four different types of body habitus. Note the extreme difference between the hypersthenic and asthenic types.

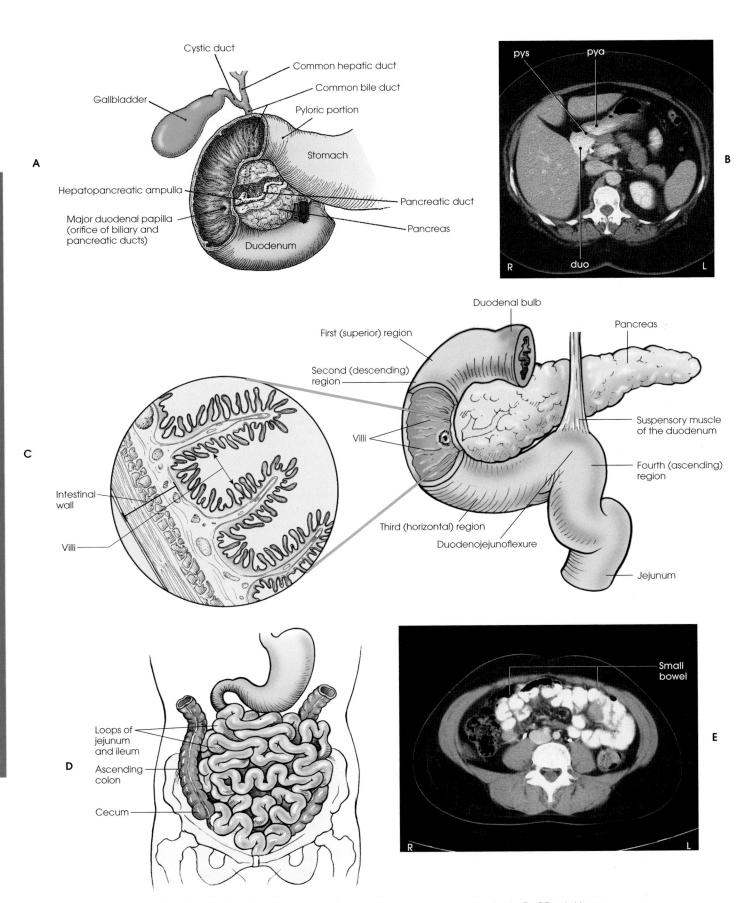

Fig. 17-4 A, Duodenal loop in relation to biliary and pancreatic ducts. **B,** CT axial image of pyloric antrum *(pya),* pyloric sphincter *(pys),* and duodenal bulb *(duo).* **C,** Anatomic areas of the duodenum. *Inset:* Cross-section of duodenum, showing villi. **D,** Loops of small intestine lying in central and lower abdominal cavity. **E,** CT axial image of small bowel loops with contrast.

(**B** and **E,** Modified from Kelley LL, Petersen CM: *Sectional anatomy for imaging professionals,* St Louis, 1997, Mosby.)

Small Intestine

The *small intestine* extends from the pyloric sphincter of the stomach to the ileocecal valve, where it joins the large intestine at a right angle. Digestion and absorption of food occur in this portion of the alimentary canal. The length of the adult small intestine averages about 22 feet (6.5 m), and its diameter gradually diminishes from approximately 1½ inches (3.8 cm) in the proximal part to approximately 1 inch (2.5 cm) in the distal part. The wall of the small intestine contains the same four layers as the walls of the esophagus and stomach. The mucosa of the small intestine contains a series of fingerlike projections called *villi,* which assist the process of digestion and absorption.

The small intestine is divided into three portions:
- Duodenum
- Jejunum
- Ileum

The *duodenum* is 8 to 10 inches (20 to 24 cm) in length and is the widest portion of the small intestine (Fig. 17-4). It is retroperitoneal and relatively fixed in position. Beginning at the pylorus, the duodenum follows a C-shaped course. Its four regions are described as the *first* (superior), *second* (descending), *third* (horizontal or inferior), and *fourth* (ascending) portions. The segment of the first portion is called the *duodenal bulb* because of its radiographic appearance when it is filled with an opaque contrast medium. The second portion is about 3 or 4 inches (7.6 to 10 cm) long. This segment passes inferiorly along the head of the pancreas and in close relation to the undersurface of the liver. The common bile duct and the pancreatic duct usually unite to form the *hepatopancreatic ampulla,* which opens on the summit of the *greater duodenal papilla* in the duodenum. The third portion passes toward the left at a slight superior inclination for a distance of about 2½ inches (6 cm) and continues as the fourth portion on the left side of the vertebrae. This portion joins the jejunum at a sharp curve called the *duodenojejunal flexure* and is supported by the *suspensory muscle of the duodenum* (ligament of Treitz). The duodenal loop, which lies in the second portion, is the most fixed part of the small intestine and normally lies in the upper part of the umbilical region of the abdomen; however, its position varies with body habitus and with the amount of gastric and intestinal contents.

The remainder of the small intestine is arbitrarily divided into two portions, with the upper two fifths referred to as the *jejunum* and the lower three fifths as the *ileum.* The jejunum and ileum are gathered into freely movable loops, or gyri, and are attached to the posterior wall of the abdomen by the mesentery. The loops lie in the central and lower part of the abdominal cavity within the arch of the large intestine.

Large Intestine

The *large intestine* begins in the right iliac region, where it joins the ileum of the small intestine, forms an arch surrounding the loops of the small intestine, and ends at the anus (Fig. 17-5). The large intestine has four main parts:

- Cecum
- Colon
- Rectum
- Anal canal

The large intestine is about 5 feet (1.5 m) long and is greater in diameter than the small intestine. The wall of the large intestine contains the same four layers as the walls of the esophagus, stomach, and small intestine. The muscular portion of the intestinal wall contains an external band of longitudinal muscle that forms into three thickened bands called *taeniae coli.* One band is positioned anteriorly, and two are positioned posteriorly. These bands create a pulling muscle tone that forms a series of pouches called the *haustra.* The main functions of the large intestine are reabsorption of fluids and elimination of waste products.

The *cecum* is the pouchlike portion of the large intestine and is below the junction of the ileum and the colon. The cecum is approximately 2½ inches (6 cm) in length and 3 inches (7.6 cm) in diameter. The *vermiform appendix* is attached to the posteromedial side of the cecum. The appendix is a narrow, wormlike tube that is about 3 inches (7.6 cm) long. The *ileocecal valve* is just below the junction of the ascending colon and the cecum. The valve projects into the lumen of the cecum and guards the opening between the ileum and the cecum.

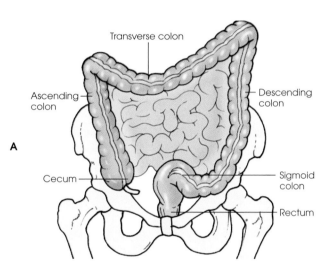

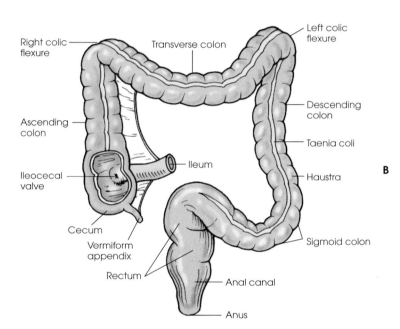

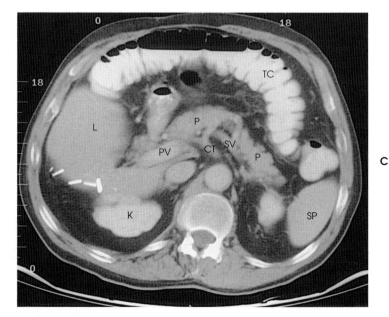

Fig. 17-5 A, Anterior aspect of large intestine positioned in abdomen. **B,** Anterior aspect of large intestine. **C,** Axial CT of the upper abdomen showing an actual image of the transverse colon positioned in the anterior abdomen.

The *colon* is subdivided into ascending, transverse, descending, and sigmoid portions. The *ascending colon* passes superiorly from its junction with the cecum to the undersurface of the liver, where it joins the transverse portion at an angle called the *right colic flexure* (formerly hepatic flexure). The *transverse colon,* which is the longest and most movable part of the colon, crosses the abdomen to the undersurface of the spleen. The transverse portion then makes a sharp curve, called the *left colic flexure* (formerly splenic flexure), and ends in the descending portion. The *descending colon* passes inferiorly and medially to its junction with the sigmoid portion at the superior aperture of the lesser pelvis. The *sigmoid colon* curves to form an S-shaped loop and ends in the rectum at the level of the third sacral segment.

The *rectum* extends from the sigmoid colon to the anal canal. The *anal canal* terminates at the *anus,* which is the external aperture of the large intestine (Fig. 17-6). The rectum is approximately 6 inches (15 cm) long. The distal portion, about 1 inch (2.5 cm) in length, is constricted to form the anal canal. Just above the anal canal is a dilation called the *rectal ampulla.* Following the sacrococcygeal curve, the rectum passes inferiorly and posteriorly to the level of the pelvic floor and then bends sharply anteriorly and inferiorly into the anal canal, which extends to the anus. The rectum and anal canal thus have two AP curves, a fact that must be remembered when an enema tube is inserted.

The size, shape, and position of the large intestine vary greatly, depending on body habitus (see Fig. 17-3). In hypersthenic patients the large intestine is positioned around the periphery of the abdomen and therefore may require more radiographs to demonstrate its entire length. At the other extreme is the asthenic patient's large intestine, which is bunched together and positioned low in the abdomen.

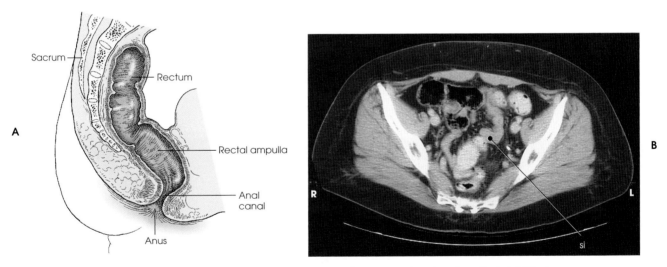

Fig. 17-6 A, Sagittal section showing direction of anal canal and rectum. **B,** Axial CT of the lower pelvis showing the rectum and sigmoid colon *(si)* in relation to surrounding organs.

(**B,** From Kelley LL, Petersen CM: *Sectional anatomy for imaging professionals,* St Louis, 1997, Mosby.)

Digestive system

DIGESTIVE SYSTEM, ALIMENTARY CANAL

Part	cm	kVp*	tm	mA	mAs	AEC	SID	IR	Dose† (mrad)
Esophagus‡									
AP and PA	16	110		300s		○○ ●	48″	35 × 43 cm	60
Obliques	21	110		300s		○○ ●	48″	35 × 43 cm	75
Lateral	30	110		300s		○○ ●	48″	35 × 43 cm	160
Stomach and Duodenum‡									
PA and AP	21	100		300s		●● ●	48″	30 × 35 cm	329
PA Axial	24	100		300s		●● ●	48″	35 × 43 cm	395
PA and AP Oblique	24	100		300s		●● ●	48″	30 × 35 cm	460
Lateral	27	110		300s		●● ●	48″	30 × 35 cm	597
Small Intestine‡									
PA and AP	21	100		300s		●● ●	48″	35 × 43 cm	329
Large Intestine‡									
PA and AP	21	100		300s		●● ●	48″	35 × 43 cm	329
PA and AP Axial	24	100		300s		●● ●	48″	35 × 43 cm	460
PA and AP Oblique	24	100		300s		●● ●	48″	35 × 43 cm	460
Lower Lateral	31	120		300s		●● ●	48″	24 × 30 cm	853
AP and PA Decubitus	24	110		300s		●● ●	48″	35 × 43 cm	362

s, Small focal spot.
*kVp values are for a three-phase, 12-pulse generator.
†Relative doses for comparison use. All doses are skin entrance for average adult at cm indicated.
‡Bucky, 16:1 grid. Screen/film speed 300.

SUMMARY OF ANATOMY

Digestive system
Alimentary canal
mouth
pharynx
esophagus
stomach
small intestine
large intestine (colon)
anus

Accessory glands
salivary glands
liver
gallbladder
pancreas

Esophagus
fibrous layer
muscular layer
submucosal layer
mucosal layer
esophagogastric junction
cardiac antrum
cardiac notch

Stomach
cardia
fundus
body
 rugae
angular notch
pyloric portion
 pyloric antrum
 pyloric canal
lesser curvature
cardiac notch
greater curvature

cardiac orifice
cardiac sphincter
pyloric orifice
pyloric sphincter
chyme

Small intestine
villi
duodenum (four regions)
 first (superior)
  duodenal bulb
 second (descending)
  major duodenal papilla
 third (horizontal)
 fourth (ascending)
  duodenojejunal flexure
  suspensory muscle of
   the duodenum
jejunum
ileum

Large intestine
taeniae coli
haustra
cecum
vermiform appendix
ileocecal valve
colon
 ascending colon
 right colic flexure
 transverse colon
 left colic flexure
 descending colon
 sigmoid colon
rectum
 rectal ampulla
 anal canal
 anus

SUMMARY OF PATHOLOGY

Condition	Definition
Achalasia	Failure of the smooth muscle of the alimentary canal to relax
Appendicitis	Inflammation of the appendix
Barrett's Esophagus	Peptic ulcer of the lower esophagus, often with stricture
Bezoar	Mass in the stomach formed by material that does not pass into the intestine
Carcinoma	Malignant new growth composed of epithelial cells
Colitis	Inflammation of the colon
Diverticulitis	Inflammation of diverticula in the alimentary canal
Diverticulosis	Diverticula in the colon without inflammation or symptoms
Diverticulum	Pouch created by the herniation of the mucous membrane through the muscular coat
Esophageal Varices	Enlarged tortuous veins of the lower esophagus, resulting from portal hypertension
Gastritis	Inflammation of the lining of the stomach
Gastroesophageal Reflux	Backward flow of the stomach contents into the esophagus
Hiatal Hernia	Protrusion of the stomach through the esophageal hiatus of the diaphragm
Hirschsprung's or Congenital Aganglionic Megacolon	Absence of parasympathetic ganglia, usually in the distal colon, resulting in the absence of peristalsis
Ileus	Failure of bowel peristalsis
Inguinal Hernia	Protrusion of the bowel into the groin
Intussusception	Prolapse of a portion of the bowel into the lumen of an adjacent part
Malabsorption Syndrome	Disorder in which subnormal absorption of dietary constituents occurs
Celiac Disease or Sprue	Malabsorption disease caused by a mucosal defect in the jejunum
Meckel's Diverticulum	Diverticulum of the distal ileum, similar to the appendix
Polyp	Growth or mass protruding from a mucous membrane
Pyloric Stenosis	Narrowing of the pyloric canal causing obstruction
Regional Enteritis or Crohn's	Inflammatory bowel disease, most commonly involving the distal ileum
Ulcer	Depressed lesion on the surface of the alimentary canal
Ulcerative Colitis	Recurrent disorder causing inflammatory ulceration in the colon
Volvulus	Twisting of a bowel loop on itself
Zenker's Diverticulum	Diverticulum located just above the cardiac portion of the stomach

Large intestine

NEW ABBREVIATIONS USED IN CHAPTER 17

BE	Barium enema
CTC	CT colonography
M-A	Miller-Abbott
MPR	Multiplanar reconstruction
UGI	Upper gastrointestinal
VC	Virtual colonoscopy

See Addendum B for a summary of all abbreviations used in Volume 2.

Technical Considerations

GASTROINTESTINAL TRANSIT

Peristalsis is the term applied to the contraction waves by which the digestive tube propels its contents toward the rectum. Normally three or four waves per minute occur in the filled stomach. The waves begin in the upper part of the organ and travel toward the pylorus. The average emptying time of the normal stomach is 2 to 3 hours.

Peristaltic action in the intestines is greatest in the upper part of the canal and gradually decreases toward the lower portion. In addition to peristaltic waves, localized contractions occur in the duodenum and the jejunum. These contractions usually occur at intervals of 3 to 4 seconds during digestion. The first part of a "barium meal" normally reaches the ileocecal valve in 2 to 3 hours and the last

portion in 4 to 5 hours. The barium usually reaches the rectum within 24 hours.

The specialized procedures commonly used in radiologic examinations of the esophagus, stomach, and intestines are discussed in this section. The esophagus extends between the pharynx and the cardiac end of the stomach and occupies a constant position in the posterior part of the mediastinum, where its radiographic demonstration presents little difficulty when a contrast medium is used. On the other hand, the stomach and intestines vary in size, shape, position, and muscular tonus according to the body habitus (see Fig. 17-3). In addition to the normal structural and functional differences, an extensive variety of gastrointestinal abnormalities can cause further changes in location and motility. These variations make the gastrointestinal investigation of every patient an individual study, and meticulous attention must be given to each detail in the examination procedure.

EXAMINATION PROCEDURE

The alimentary canal is usually examined using a combination of fluoroscopy and radiography. Fluoroscopy makes it possible to observe the canal in motion, perform special mucosal studies, and determine the subsequent procedure required for a complete examination. Images are obtained, as indicated, during and after the fluoroscopic examination to provide a permanent record of the findings.

Contrast media

Because the thin-walled alimentary canal does not have sufficient density to be demonstrated through the surrounding structures, its radiographic demonstration requires the use of an artificial contrast medium. *Barium sulfate,* which is a water-insoluble salt of the metallic element barium, is the contrast medium universally used in examinations of the alimentary canal (Fig. 17-7). The barium sulfate used for this purpose is a specially prepared, chemically pure product to which various chemical substances have been added. Barium sulfate is available as either a dry powder or liquid. The powdered barium has different concentrations and is mixed with plain water. The concentration depends on the part to be examined and the preference of the physician.

A number of special barium sulfate products are also available. Those with finely divided barium sulfate particles tend to resist precipitation and remain in suspension longer than the regular barium preparations. Some barium preparations contain gums or other suspending or dispersing agents and are referred to as *suspended* or *flocculation-resistant* preparations.

The speed with which the barium mixture passes through the alimentary canal depends on the suspending medium, the temperature of the medium, and the consistency of the preparation, as well as the motile function of the alimentary canal.

In addition to barium sulfate, *water-soluble, iodinated contrast media* suitable for opacification of the alimentary canal are available (Fig. 17-8). These preparations are modifications of basic intravenous urographic media, such as diatrizoate sodium and diatrizoate meglumine.

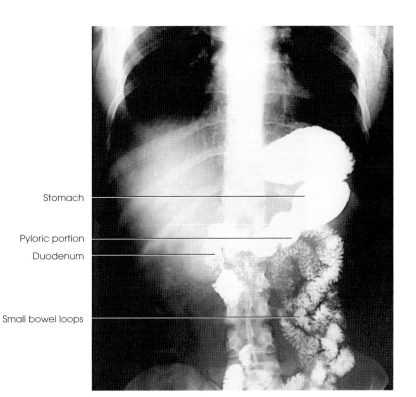

Fig. 17-7 Barium sulfate suspension in the stomach, sthenic body habitus.

Stomach

Pyloric portion

Duodenum

Small bowel loops

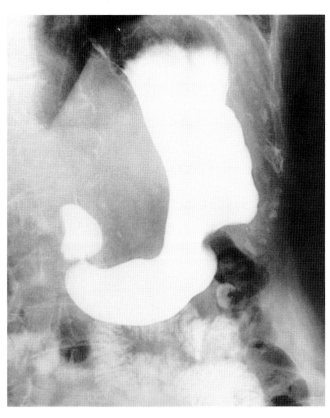

Fig. 17-8 Water-soluble, iodinated solution in the stomach.

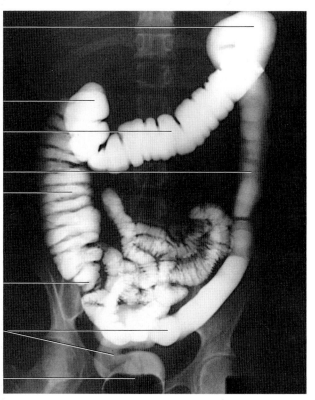

Left colic flexure

Right colic flexure

Transverse colon

Descending colon

Ascending colon

Cecum

Sigmoid colon

Rectum

Fig. 17-9 Barium sulfate suspension administered by rectum, sthenic body habitus.

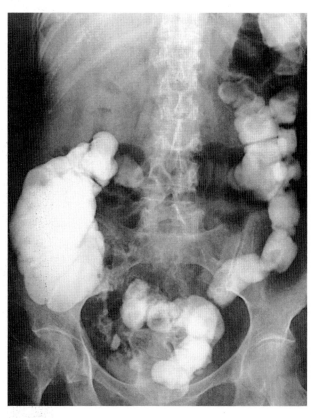

Fig. 17-10 Water-soluble, iodinated solution administered by mouth.

Iodinated solutions move through the gastrointestinal tract quicker than barium sulfate suspensions (Figs. 17-9 and 17-10). An iodinated solution normally clears the stomach in 1 to 2 hours, and the entire iodinated contrast column reaches and outlines the colon in about 4 hours. An orally administered iodinated medium differs from barium sulfate in the following ways:

1. It outlines the esophagus, but it does not adhere to the mucosa as well as a barium sulfate suspension does.
2. It affords an entirely satisfactory examination of the stomach and duodenum including mucosal delineation.
3. It permits rapid survey of the entire small intestine but fails to provide clear anatomic detail of this portion of the alimentary canal. This failure results from the dilution of the contrast medium and the resultant decrease in opacification.
4. Because of the normal rapid absorption of water through the colonic mucosa, the medium again becomes densely concentrated in the large intestine. Consequently, the entire large intestine is opacified with retrograde filling using a barium sulfate suspension. As a result of its increased concentration and accelerated transit time, a reasonably rapid investigation of the large intestine can be performed by the oral route when a patient cannot cooperate for a satisfactory enema study.

A great advantage of water-soluble media is that they are easily removed by aspiration either before or during surgery. Furthermore, if a water-soluble, iodinated medium escapes into the peritoneum through a preexisting perforation of the stomach or intestine, no ill effects result. The medium is readily absorbed from the peritoneal cavity and excreted by the kidneys. This is a definite advantage when perforated ulcers are under investigation.

A disadvantage of iodinated preparations is their strongly bitter taste, which can be masked only to a limited extent. Patients should be forewarned so that they can more easily tolerate ingesting these agents.

In addition, these iodinated contrast media are hyperosmolar, encouraging movement of excess fluid into the gastrointestinal tract lumen.

Radiologic apparatus

Fluoroscopic equipment used today contains highly sophisticated image intensification systems (Fig. 17-11). These systems can be connected to accessory units, such as cine film recorders, television systems, spot-film cameras, digital-image cameras, and video recorders. Remote-control fluoroscopic rooms are also available and are used by the fluoroscopist located in an adjacent control area (Fig. 17-12). Although conventional IR-loaded spot-image devices are still used with image intensification, digital fluoroscopic units that permit the recording of multiple fluoroscopic images are common.

Compression and palpation of the abdomen are often performed during an examination of the alimentary canal. Many types of compression devices are available. The fluoroscopic unit pictured in Fig. 17-11 shows a compression cone in contact with the patient's abdomen. This device is often used during general fluoroscopic examinations.

Other types of commercial compression devices include the pneumatic compression paddle shown in Fig. 17-13. This device is often placed under the duodenal bulb and then inflated to place pressure on the abdomen. The air is then slowly released, and the compression on the body part is eliminated.

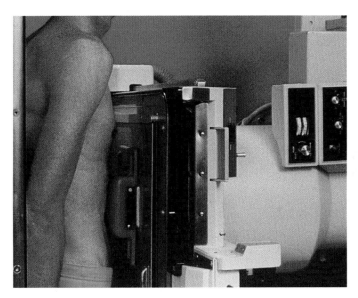

Fig. 17-11 Image intensification system, with compression cone in contact with abdomen.

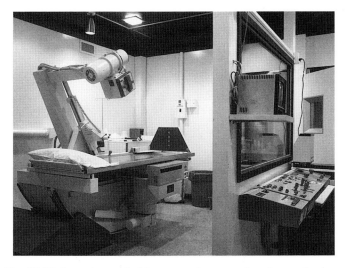

Fig. 17-12 Remote-control fluoroscopic room, showing patient fluoroscopic table (left) and fluoroscopist's control console (right). The fluoroscopist views the patient through the large window.

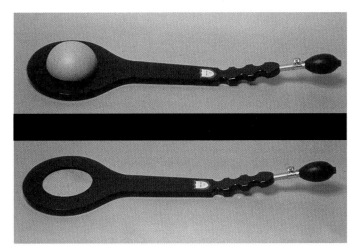

Fig. 17-13 Compression paddle: inflated (above) and noninflated (below).

Preparation of examining room

The examining room should be completely prepared before the patient enters. In preparing the room, the radiographer should observe the following steps:

- Adjust the equipment controls to the appropriate settings.
- Have the footboard and shoulder support available.
- Check the mechanism of the spot-film device or spot-film camera, or both, and ensure that sufficient films are available.
- Prepare the required type and amount of contrast medium.

Before beginning the examination, the radiographer should do the following:

- Explain to the patient that the barium sulfate mixture may taste chalky.
- Inform the patient that the room may be somewhat darkened during fluoroscopy.
- When the fluoroscopist enters the examining room, introduce the patient and the fluoroscopist to each other.

Exposure time

One of the most important considerations in gastrointestinal radiography is the elimination of motion. The highest degree of motor activity is normally found in the stomach and proximal part of the small intestine. The activity gradually decreases along the intestinal tract until it becomes fairly slow in the distal part of the large bowel. Peristaltic speed also depends on the individual patient's body habitus and is influenced by pathologic changes, use of narcotic pain killers, body position, and respiration. The amount of exposure time for each region must be based on these factors.

In esophageal examinations the radiographer should observe the following guidelines:

- Use an exposure time of 0.1 second or less for upright radiographs. The time may be slightly longer for recumbent images because the barium descends more slowly when patients are in recumbent positions.

- Remember that barium passes through the esophagus fairly slowly if it is swallowed at the end of full inspiration. The rate of passage is increased if the barium is swallowed at the end of moderate inspiration. However, the barium is delayed in the lower part for several seconds if it is swallowed at the end of full expiration.
- Keep in mind that respiration is inhibited for several seconds after the beginning of deglutition, which allows sufficient time for the exposure to be made without instructing the patient to hold his or her breath after swallowing.

In examinations of the stomach and small intestine, the radiographer should observe the following guidelines:

- Use an exposure time of no longer than 0.2 second for patients with normal peristaltic activity and never more than 0.5 second; the exposure time should be 0.1 second or less for those with hypermotility.
- Make exposures of the stomach and intestines at the end of expiration in the routine procedure.

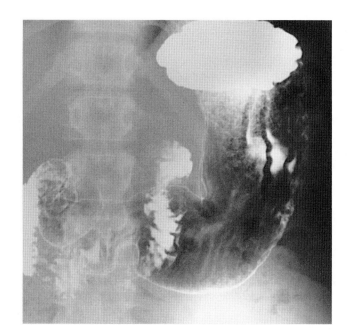

Fig. 17-14 AP spot radiograph of barium-filled fundus of stomach.

Radiation Protection

During fluoroscopy, spot filming (Figs. 17-14 and 17-15), and radiographic filming for either a partial or a complete gastrointestinal examination, the patient will receive radiation. It is taken for granted that properly added filtration is in place at all times in each x-ray tube in the radiology department. It is further assumed that based on the capacity of the machines and the best available accessory equipment, the exposure factors are adjusted to deliver the least possible radiation to the patient.

Protection of the patient from unnecessary radiation is a professional responsibility of the radiographer. (See Chapter 1 of this atlas for specific guidelines.) In this chapter the *Shield gonads* statement at the end of the *Position of part* section indicates that the patient is to be protected from unnecessary radiation by restricting the radiation beam using proper collimation. Placing lead shielding between the gonads and the radiation source when the clinical objectives of the examination are not compromised is also appropriate.

Esophagus
CONTRAST STUDIES

The esophagus may be examined by performing a *full-column, single-contrast* study in which only barium or water-soluble, iodinated contrast agent is used to fill the esophageal lumen. A *double-contrast* procedure also may be used. For this study, high-density barium and carbon dioxide crystals (which liberate carbon dioxide when exposed to water) are the two contrast agents. No preliminary preparation of the patient is necessary.

Barium sulfate mixture

A 30% to 50% weight/volume suspension[1] is useful for the full-column, single-contrast technique. A low-viscosity, high-density barium developed for double-contrast gastric examinations may be used for a double-contrast examination. Whatever the weight/volume concentration of the barium, the most important criterion is that the barium flows sufficiently to coat the walls of the esophagus. The barium manufacturer's mixing instructions must be closely followed to attain optimum performance of the contrast medium.

---

[1]Scukas J: Contrast media. In Margulis AR, Burhenne HJ, editors: *Alimentary tract radiology,* vol 1, ed 4, St Louis, 1989, Mosby.

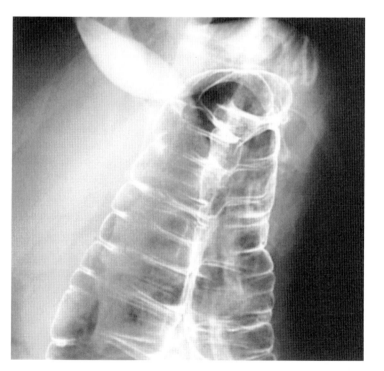

Fig. 17-15 Spot radiograph of air-contrast colon, showing left colic flexure.

Examination procedures

For a single-contrast examination (Figs. 17-16 to 17-18), the following steps are observed:

- Start the fluoroscopic and spot-film examinations with the patient in the upright position whenever possible.

- Use the horizontal and Trendelenburg positions as indicated.
- After the fluoroscopic examination of the heart and lungs and when the patient is upright, instruct the patient to take the cup containing the barium suspension in the left hand and to drink it on request.

The radiologist asks the patient to swallow several mouthfuls of the barium so that the act of deglutition can be observed to determine whether any abnormality is present. The radiologist instructs the patient to perform various breathing maneuvers under fluoroscopic observation so that spot radiographs of areas or lesions not otherwise demonstrated can be obtained.

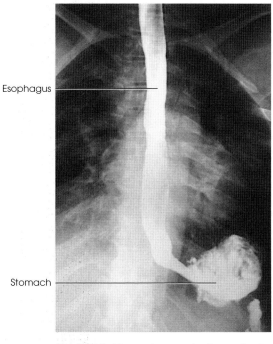

Esophagus

Stomach

Fig. 17-16 AP esophagus, single-contrast study.

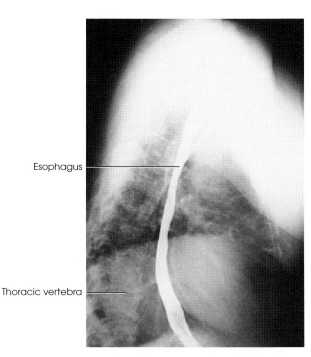

Esophagus

Thoracic vertebra

Fig. 17-17 Lateral esophagus, single-contrast study.

The performance of the *double-contrast* esophageal examination (Fig. 17-19) is similar to that of a single-contrast examination. For a double-contrast examination, a free-flowing, high-density barium must be used. A gas-producing substance, usually carbon dioxide crystals, can be added to the barium mixture or given by mouth immediately *before* the barium suspension is ingested. Spot radiographs are taken during the examination, and delayed images may be obtained on request.

OPAQUE FOREIGN BODIES

Opaque foreign bodies lodged in the pharynx or in the upper part of the esophagus can usually be demonstrated without the use of a contrast medium. A soft tissue neck or lateral projection of the retrosternal area may be taken for this purpose. Obtain a lateral neck radiograph at the height of swallowing for the delineation of opaque foreign bodies in the upper end of the intrathoracic esophagus. Swallowing elevates the intrathoracic esophagus a distance of two cervical segments, placing it above the level of the clavicles.

Tufts or pledgets of cotton saturated with a thin barium suspension are sometimes used to demonstrate an obstruction or to detect *nonopaque foreign bodies* in the pharynx and upper esophagus (Fig. 17-20).

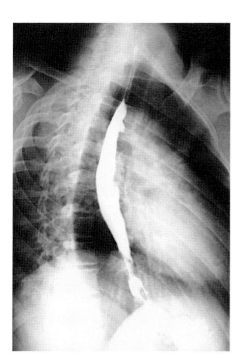

Fig. 17-18 PA oblique esophagus, RAO position, single-contrast study.

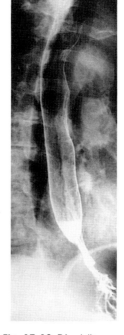

Fig. 17-19 PA oblique distal esophagus, RAO position, double-contrast spot image.

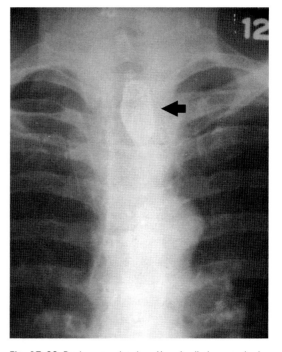

Fig. 17-20 Barium-soaked cotton ball demonstrating nonopaque foreign body in upper esophagus *(arrow)*.

AP, PA, OBLIQUE, AND LATERAL PROJECTIONS

Image receptor: 35 × 43 cm lengthwise and centered so that the top of the IR is positioned at the level of the mouth for inclusion of the entire esophagus

Position of patient

• Position the patient as for chest radiographs (AP, PA, oblique, and lateral; see Chapter 10). Because the RAO position of 35 to 40 degrees (Fig. 17-21, A) makes it possible to obtain a wider space for an unobstructed image of the esophagus between the vertebrae and the heart, it is usually used in preference to the LAO position. The LPO position has also been recommended.[1]
• Unless the upright position is specified (Fig. 17-21, B), place the patient in the recumbent position for esophageal studies (Figs. 17-22 and 17-23). The recumbent position is used to obtain more complete contrast filling of the esophagus (especially filling of the proximal part) by having the barium column flow against gravity. The recumbent position is routinely used for the demonstration of variceal distentions of the esophageal veins because varices (Fig. 17-24) are best filled by having the blood flow against gravity. Variceal filling is more complete during increased venous pressure, which may be applied by full expiration or by the Valsalva maneuver (see Chapter 15, p. 83).

[1]Cockerill EM et al: Optimal visualization of esophageal varices, *Am J Roentgenol* 126:512, 1976.

AP OR PA PROJECTION

The following steps are observed:
• Place the patient in the supine or prone position with the arms above the head in a comfortable position.
• Center the midsagittal plane to the grid.
• Turn the head slightly, if necessary, to assist drinking of the barium mixture.
• *Shield gonads.*

AP OR PA OBLIQUE
RAO or LAO position

The steps are as follows:
• Position the patient in the RAO or LPO position with the midsagittal plane forming an angle of 35 to 40 degrees from the grid device.
• For the RAO position, adjust the patient's side-down arm at the side and the side-up arm on the pillow by the head. For the LPO position, do the same, with the side-down arm at the side and the side-up arm on the pillow.
• Center the elevated side to the grid through a plane approximately 2 inches (5 cm) lateral to the midsagittal plane (see Figs. 17-22 and 17-23).
• *Shield gonads.*

LATERAL PROJECTION
R or L position

The procedure is as follows:
• Place the patient's arms forward, with the forearm on the pillow near the head.
• Place the patient's arms forward.
• Center the midcoronal plane to the grid.
• *Shield gonads.*

Central ray

• Perpendicular to the midpoint of the IR (The central ray will be at the level of T5-T6.)

Structures shown

The contrast medium–filled esophagus should be demonstrated from the lower part of the neck to the esophagogastric junction, where the esophagus joins the stomach.

EVALUATION CRITERIA

The following should be clearly demonstrated:

General
■ Esophagus from the lower part of the neck to its entrance into the stomach
■ Esophagus filled with barium
■ Penetration of the barium

AP or PA projection
■ Esophagus through the superimposed thoracic vertebrae
■ No rotation of the patient

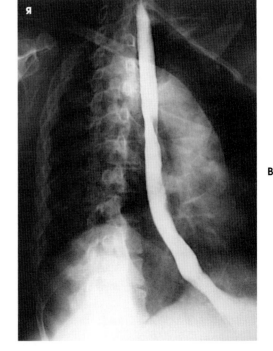

Fig. 17-21 A, PA oblique esophagus, RAO position. **B,** Upright PA oblique esophagus, RAO position.

Oblique projection
■ Esophagus between the vertebrae and the heart

Lateral projection
■ Patient's arm not interfering with visualization of the proximal esophagus
■ Ribs posterior to the vertebrae superimposed to show that the patient was not rotated

NOTE: The general criteria apply to all projections: AP or PA, oblique, and lateral.

Barium administration and respiration
• Feed the barium sulfate suspension to the patient by spoon, by cup, or through a drinking straw, depending on its consistency.
• Ask the patient to swallow several mouthfuls of barium in rapid succession and then to hold a mouthful until immediately before the exposure.

• For the demonstration of esophageal varices, instruct the patient (1) to fully expire and then to swallow the barium bolus and avoid inspiration until the exposure has been made or (2) to take a deep breath and, while holding the breath, to swallow the bolus and then perform the Valsalva maneuver (see Fig. 17-24, *A*).
• For other conditions, instruct the patient simply to swallow the barium bolus, which is normally done during moderate inspiration (see Fig. 17-24, *B*). Because respiration is inhibited for about 2 seconds after swallowing, the patient does not have to hold his or her breath for the exposure. If the contrast medium is swallowed at the end of full inspiration, make two or three exposures in rapid succession before the contrast medium passes into the stomach. For demonstration of the entire esophagus, it is sometimes necessary to make the exposure while the patient is drinking the barium suspension through a straw in rapid and continuous swallows.
• The patient may be asked to swallow a barium tablet to evaluate the degree of lumen narrowing with esophageal structure.

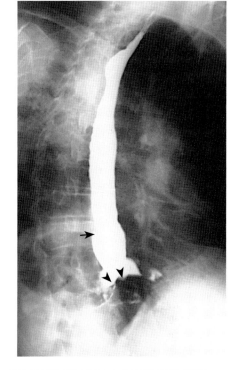

Fig. 17-22 PA oblique esophagus, RAO position, single-contrast study showing tear in esophageal lumen *(arrow)* and lesion partially obstructing esophagus *(arrowheads)*.

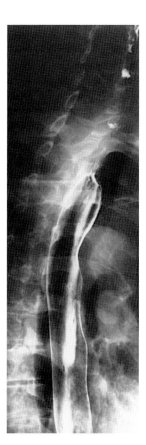

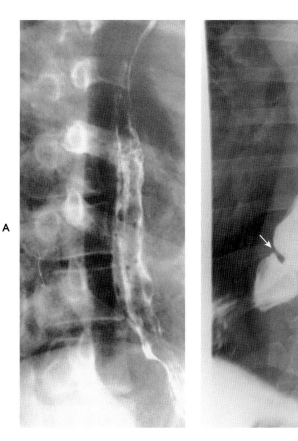

Fig. 17-23 PA oblique proximal esophagus, RAO position, double-contrast spot film.

Fig. 17-24 A, Spot-film studies showing esophageal varices. **B,** Barium bolus clearly demonstrates Schatzki's ring *(arrows)*.

(Courtesy Michael J. Kudlas, MEd, RT(R)(QM).)

Stomach: Gastrointestinal Series

Upper gastrointestinal (UGI) tract radiographs are used to evaluate the distal esophagus, stomach, and some or all of the small intestine. A UGI examination (Fig. 17-25), usually called a *gastrointestinal* or an *upper gastrointestinal* (UGI) series, may include the following:

1. A preliminary radiograph of the abdomen to delineate the liver, spleen, kidneys, psoas muscles, and bony structures and to detect any abdominal or pelvic calcifications or tumor masses. The detection of calcifications and tumor masses requires that the survey radiograph of the abdomen be taken after preliminary cleansing of the intestinal tract but before administration of the contrast medium.
2. An examination consisting of fluoroscopic and serial radiographic studies of the esophagus, stomach, and duodenum using an ingested opaque mixture, usually barium sulfate.
3. When requested, a small intestine study consisting of radiographs obtained at frequent intervals during passage of the contrast column through the small intestine, at which time the vermiform appendix and the ileocecal region may be examined.

Ambulatory outpatients or acutely ill patients, such as those with a bleeding ulcer, are usually examined in the supine position using a fluoroscopic and spot-film procedure. Everything possible should be done to expedite the procedure. Any contrast preparation must be ready, and the examination room must be fully prepared before the patient is brought into the radiology department.

PRELIMINARY PREPARATION
Preparation of patient

Because a gastrointestinal series is time consuming, the patient should be told the approximate time required for the procedure before being assigned an appointment for an examination. The patient also needs to understand the reason for preliminary preparation so that full cooperation can be given.

The stomach must be empty for an examination of the UGI tract (the stomach and small intestine). It is also desirable to have the colon free of gas and fecal material. When the patient is constipated, a non–gas-forming laxative may be administered 1 day before the examination.

An empty stomach is ensured by withholding both food and water after midnight for a period of 8 to 9 hours before the examination. When a small intestine study is to be made, food and fluid are withheld after the evening meal.

Because it is believed that nicotine and chewing gum stimulate gastric secretion and salivation, some physicians tell patients not to smoke or chew gum after midnight on the night before the examination. This restriction is made to prevent excessive fluid from accumulating in the stomach and diluting the barium suspension enough to interfere with its coating property.

Barium sulfate suspension

The contrast medium generally used in routine gastrointestinal examinations is barium sulfate mixed with water. The preparation must be thoroughly mixed according to the manufacturer's instructions. Specially formulated, high-density barium is also available. Advances in the production of barium have all but eliminated the use of a single barium formula for most gastrointestinal examinations performed in the radiology department.

Most physicians use one of the many commercially prepared barium suspensions. These products are available in several flavors, and some are conveniently packaged in individual cups containing the dry ingredients. To these products, the radiographer merely has to add water, recap the cup, and shake it to obtain a smooth suspension. Other barium suspensions are completely mixed and ready to use.

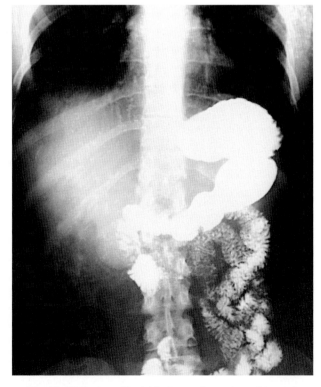

Fig. 17-25 Barium-filled AP stomach and small bowel.

Contrast Studies

Two general procedures are routinely used to examine the stomach: the *single-contrast* method and the *double-contrast* method. A *biphasic* examination is a combination of the single-contrast and double-contrast methods during the same procedure. *Hypotonic duodenography* is another, less commonly used examination.

SINGLE-CONTRAST EXAMINATION

In the single-contrast method (Fig. 17-26), a barium sulfate suspension is administered during the initial fluoroscopic examination. The barium suspension used for this study is usually in the 30% to 50% weight/volume range.[1] The following steps are observed:

- Whenever possible, begin the examination with the patient in the upright position.
- The radiologist may first examine the heart and lungs fluoroscopically and observe the abdomen to determine whether food or fluid is in the stomach.
- Give the patient a glass of barium and instruct the patient to drink it as requested by the radiologist. If the patient is in the recumbent position, administer the suspension through a drinking straw.
- The radiologist asks the patient to swallow two or three mouthfuls of the barium. During this time, examine and expose any indicated spot films of the esophagus. By manual manipulation of the stomach through the abdominal wall, the radiologist then coats the gastric mucosa.
- Obtain images with the spot-film device or another compression device to demonstrate a mucosal lesion of the stomach or duodenum.
- After studying the rugae and as the patient drinks the remainder of the barium suspension, observe the filling of the stomach and further examine the duodenum. Based on this examination, the following can be accomplished:
  1. Determine the size, shape, and position of the stomach.
  2. Examine the changing contour of the stomach during peristalsis.
  3. Observe the filling and emptying of the duodenal bulb.

[1]Skucas J: Contrast media. In Margulis AR, Burhenne HJ, editors: *Alimentary tract radiology,* vol 1, ed 4, St Louis, 1989, Mosby.

4. Detect any abnormal alteration in the function or contour of the esophagus, stomach, and duodenum.
5. Take spot films as indicated.

The contrast medium normally begins to pass into the duodenum almost immediately. However, nervous tension of the patient may delay transit of the contrast material.

Fluoroscopy is performed with the patient in the upright and recumbent positions while the body is rotated and the table is angled so that all aspects of the esophagus, stomach, and duodenum are demonstrated. Spot films are exposed as indicated. If esophageal involvement is suspected, a study is usually made with a thick barium suspension.

Subsequent radiographs of the stomach and duodenum should be obtained immediately after fluoroscopy before any considerable amount of the barium suspension passes into the jejunum.

Position of patient

The stomach and duodenum may be examined using PA, AP, oblique, and lateral projections with the patient in the upright and recumbent positions, as indicated by the fluoroscopic findings.

One variation of the supine positions is the LPO position. In another variation, the head end of the table is lowered 25 to 30 degrees for the demonstration of a hiatal hernia. Finally, for the demonstration of esophageal regurgitation and hiatal hernias, the head end of the table is lowered 10 to 15 degrees and the patient is rotated slightly toward the right side to place the esophagogastric (gastroesophageal) junction in profile to the right of the spine. The medical significance of diagnosing hiatal hernias is a topic that has received much attention in recent years. Some authors report little correlation between the presence of a hiatal hernia and gastrointestinal symptoms. If little correlation exists, radiographic evaluation is of little value in the majority of hiatal hernias.

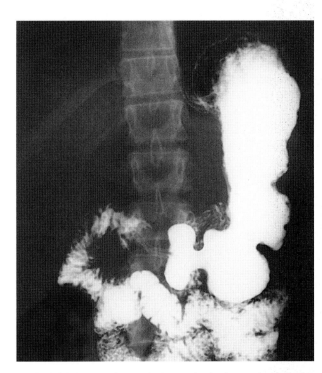

Fig. 17-26 Barium-filled PA stomach, single-contrast study.

DOUBLE-CONTRAST EXAMINATION

A second approach to the examination of the gastrointestinal tract is the *double-contrast* technique (Fig. 17-27). The principal advantages of this method over the single-contrast method are that small lesions are less easily obscured and the mucosal lining of the stomach can be more clearly visualized. However, for successful results, the patient must be able to move with relative ease throughout the examination.

For double-contrast studies, the following steps are observed:

- To begin the examination, place the patient on the fluoroscopic table in the upright position.
- Give the patient a gas-producing substance in the form of a powder, crystals, pills, or a carbonated beverage. (An older technique involved placing pinholes in the sides of a drinking straw so that the patient ingested air while drinking the barium suspension during the examination.)
- Give the patient a small amount of commercially available, high-density barium suspension. For even coating of the stomach walls, the barium must flow freely and have a low viscosity. Many high-density barium products are available; these suspensions have weight/volume ratios of up to 250%.
- Place the patient in the recumbent position, and instruct him or her to turn from side to side or to roll over a few times. This movement serves to coat the mucosal lining of the stomach as the carbon dioxide continues to expand. The patient may feel the need to belch but should refrain from doing so until the examination is finished to ensure that an optimum amount of contrast material (gas) remains for the duration of the examination.

- Just before the examination, the patient may be given glucagon or other anticholinergic medications intravenously or intramuscularly to relax the gastrointestinal tract. These medications improve visualization by inducing greater distention of the stomach and intestines. Before administering these agents, the radiologist must consider a number of factors including side effects, contraindications, availability, and cost.

Radiographic imaging procedure

The conventional images obtained after the fluoroscopic examination may be the same as those obtained for the single-contrast examination. Often the radiographs with the greatest amount of diagnostic information are the spot images taken during fluoroscopy. Therefore the radiologist will, in most cases, have already obtained most of the necessary diagnostic radiographs. Nonfluoroscopic images may not be necessary.

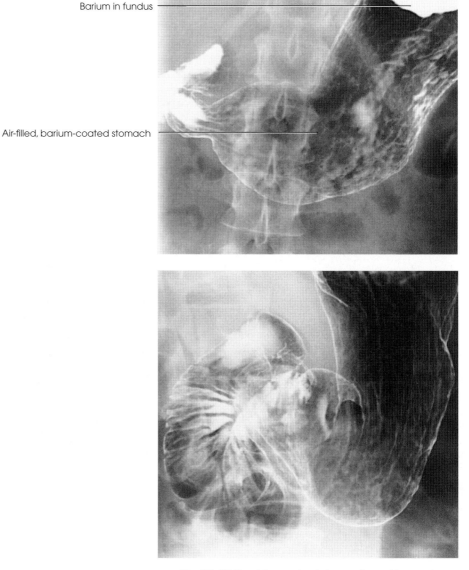

Barium in fundus

Air-filled, barium-coated stomach

Fig. 17-27 Double-contrast stomach spot images.

BIPHASIC EXAMINATION

The *biphasic* gastrointestinal examination incorporates the advantages of both the single-contrast and double-contrast UGI examinations, with both examinations performed during the same procedure. The patient first undergoes a double-contrast examination of the UGI tract. When this study is completed, the patient is given an approximately 15% weight/volume barium suspension and a single-contrast examination is performed. This biphasic approach increases the accuracy of diagnosis without significantly increasing the cost of the examination.

HYPOTONIC DUODENOGRAPHY

The use of *hypotonic duodenography* as a primary diagnostic tool has decreased in recent years. When lesions beyond the duodenum are suspected, the double-contrast gastrointestinal examination described can aid in the diagnosis. When pancreatic disease is suspected, computed tomography (CT) or needle biopsy can also be used. Thus hypotonic duodenography is necessary less frequently.

First described by Liotta,[1] hypotonic duodenography requires intubation (Figs. 17-28 and 17-29) and is used for the evaluation of postbulbar duodenal lesions and the detection of pancreatic disease. A newer tubeless technique requires temporary drug-induced duodenal paralysis so that a double-contrast examination can be performed without interference from peristaltic activity. During the atonic state when the duodenum is distended with the contrast medium to two or three times its normal size, it presses against and outlines any abnormality in the contour of the head of the pancreas.

[1]Liotta D: Pour le diagnostic des tumeus du pancréas: la duodénographic hypotonique, *Lyon Chir* 50:445, 1955.

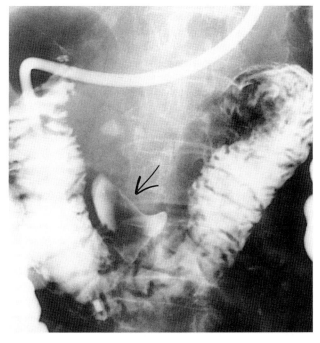

Fig. 17-28 Hypotonic duodenogram showing deformity of duodenal diverticulum by small carcinoma of head of pancreas (*arrow*).

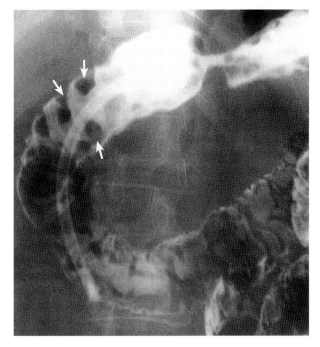

Fig. 17-29 Hypotonic duodenogram showing multiple defects (*arrows*) in duodenal bulb and proximal duodenum, caused by hypertrophy of Brunner's glands.

⚜ PA PROJECTION

Image receptor: 30 × 35 cm lengthwise

Position of patient

- For radiographic studies of the stomach and duodenum, place the patient in the recumbent position. However, the upright position is sometimes used to demonstrate the relative position of the stomach.

- When adjusting thin patients in the prone position, support the weight of the body on pillows or other suitable pads positioned under the thorax and pelvis. This adjustment keeps the stomach or duodenum from pressing against the vertebrae, with resultant pressure-filling defects.

Position of part

- Adjust the patient's position either recumbent or upright, so that the midline of the grid coincides with a sagittal plane passing halfway between the vertebral column and the left lateral border of the abdomen (Fig. 17-30).

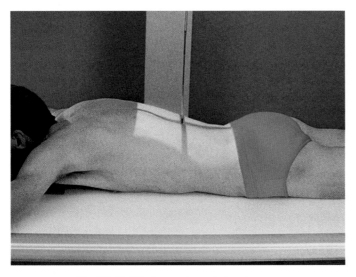

Fig. 17-30 PA stomach and duodenum.

- Center the IR about 1 to 2 inches above the lower rib margin at the level of L1-L2 when the patient is prone (Figs. 17-31 and 17-32).
- For upright images, center the IR 3 to 6 inches (7.6 to 15 cm) lower than L1-L2. The greatest visceral movement between the prone and upright positions occurs in asthenic patients.
- Do not apply an immobilization band for standard radiographic projections of the stomach and intestines because the pressure is likely to cause filling defects and because it interferes with emptying and filling of the duodenal bulb, factors that are important in serial studies.
- *Shield gonads.*
- *Respiration:* Suspend at the end of expiration unless otherwise requested.

Central ray

- Perpendicular to the center of the IR

Structures shown

A PA projection of the contour of the barium-filled stomach and duodenal bulb is demonstrated. The upright projection shows the size, shape, and relative position of the filled stomach, but it does not give an adequate demonstration of the unfilled fundic portion of the organ. In the prone position the stomach moves superiorly 1½ to 4 inches (3.8 to 10 cm) according to the patient's body habitus (Figs. 17-33 to 17-36). At the same time the stomach spreads horizontally, with a comparable decrease in its length. (Note that the fundus usually fills in asthenic patients.)

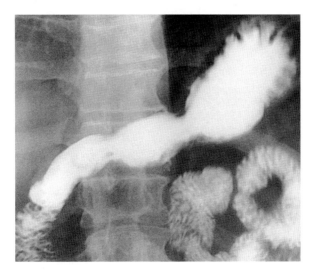

Fig. 17-31 Single-contrast PA stomach and duodenum.

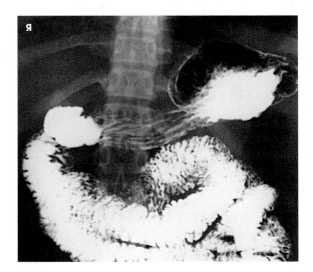

Fig. 17-32 Double-contrast PA stomach and duodenum.

The pyloric canal and duodenal bulb are well demonstrated in patients with an asthenic or a hyposthenic habitus. These structures are often partially obscured in patients with a sthenic habitus and, except in the PA axial projection, are completely obscured by the prepyloric portion of the stomach in patients with a hypersthenic habitus.

The following should be clearly demonstrated:
- Entire stomach and duodenal loop
- Stomach centered at the level of the pylorus
- No rotation of the patient
- Exposure technique that demonstrates the anatomy

NOTE: A 35- × 43-cm IR is often used when the distal esophagus or the small bowel is to be visualized along with the stomach.

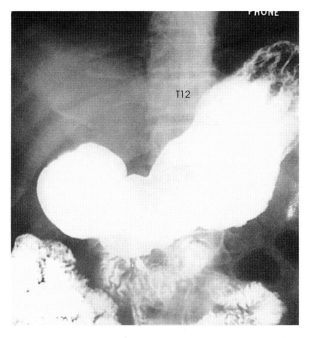

Fig. 17-33 Hypersthenic patient.

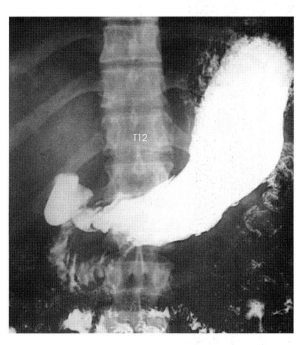

Fig. 17-34 Sthenic patient.

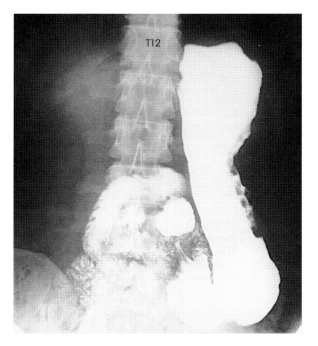

Fig. 17-35 Hyposthenic patient.

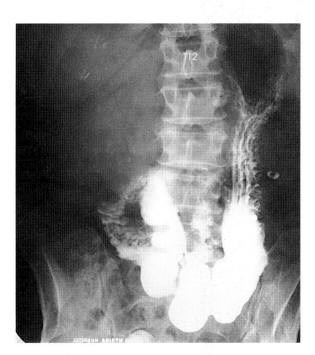

Fig. 17-36 Asthenic patient.

PA AXIAL PROJECTION

Image receptor: 35 × 43 cm lengthwise

Position of patient
- Place the patient in the prone position.

Position of part
- Adjust the patient's body so that the midsagittal plane is centered to the grid.

- For the sthenic patient, center the IR at the level of L2 (Fig. 17-37); center it somewhat higher for the hypersthenic patient and somewhat lower for the asthenic patient. L2 will lie about 1 to 2 inches above the lower rib margin.
- *Shield gonads.*
- *Respiration:* Suspend respiration at the end of expiration unless otherwise requested.

Central ray
- Directed to the midpoint of the IR at an angle of 35 to 45 degrees cephalad. Gugliantini[1] recommended a cephalic angulation of 20 to 25 degrees for demonstration of the stomach in infants.

---

[1]Gugliantini P: Utilitá delle incidenze oblique caudo-craniali nello studio radiologico della stenosi congenita ipertrofica del piloro, *Ann Radiol [Diagn]* 34:56, 1961. Abstract, *Am J Roentgenol* 87:623, 1962.

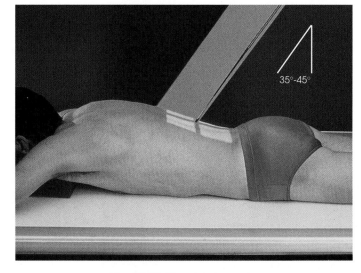

Fig. 17-37 PA axial stomach.

Structures shown

Gordon[1] developed the PA axial projection to "open up" the high, horizontal (hypersthenic-type) stomach for demonstration of the greater and lesser curvatures, the antral portion of the stomach, the pyloric canal, and the duodenal bulb. The resultant image gives the hypersthenic stomach much the same configuration as the average sthenic type of stomach (Fig. 17-38).

---

[1]Gordon SS: The angled posteroanterior projection of the stomach: an attempt at better visualization of the high transverse stomach, *Radiology* 69:393, 1957.

The following should clearly be demonstrated:

- Entire stomach and proximal duodenum
- Stomach centered at the level of the pylorus
- Exposure technique that demonstrates the anatomy

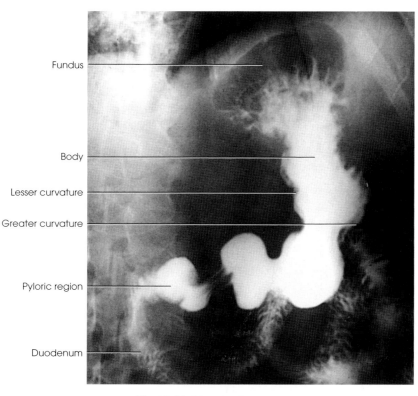

Fig. 17-38 PA axial stomach, sthenic habitus.

Fundus

Body

Lesser curvature

Greater curvature

Pyloric region

Duodenum

♠ PA OBLIQUE PROJECTION
RAO position

Image receptor: 30 × 35 cm lengthwise

Position of patient
- Place the patient in the recumbent position.

Position of part
- After the PA projection, instruct the patient to rest the head on the right cheek and to place the right arm along the side of the body.
- Have the patient raise his or her left side and support the body on the left forearm and flexed left knee.
- Adjust the patient's position so that a sagittal plane passing midway between the vertebrae and the lateral border of the elevated side coincides with the midline of the grid (Fig. 17-39).
- Center the IR about 1 to 2 inches above the lower rib margin, at the level of L1-L2, when the patient is prone.

- Make the final adjustment in body rotation. The approximately 40 to 70 degrees of rotation required to give the best image of the pyloric canal and duodenum depend on the size, shape, and position of the stomach. In general, hypersthenic patients require a greater degree of rotation than do sthenic and asthenic patients.
- The RAO position is used for serial studies of the pyloric canal and the duodenal bulb because gastric peristalsis is usually more active when the patient is in this position.
- *Shield gonads.*
- *Respiration:* Suspend at the end of expiration unless otherwise requested.

Central ray
- Perpendicular to the center of the IR

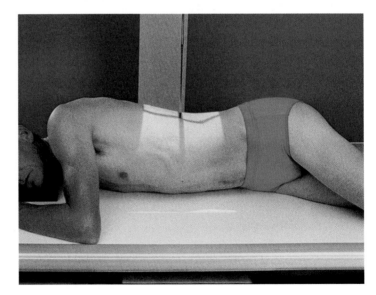

Fig. 17-39 PA oblique stomach and duodenum, RAO position.

Stomach and Duodenum

Structures shown

A PA oblique projection of the stomach and entire duodenal loop is presented. This projection gives the best image of the pyloric canal and the duodenal bulb in patients whose habitus approximates the sthenic type (Figs. 17-40 and 17-41).

Because gastric peristalsis is generally more active with the patient in the RAO position, a serial study of several exposures is sometimes obtained at intervals of 30 to 40 seconds for delineation of the pyloric canal and duodenal bulb.

EVALUATION CRITERIA

The following should be clearly demonstrated:
- Entire stomach and duodenal loop
- No superimposition of the pylorus and duodenal bulb
- Duodenal bulb and loop in profile
- Stomach centered at the level of the pylorus
- Exposure technique that demonstrates the anatomy

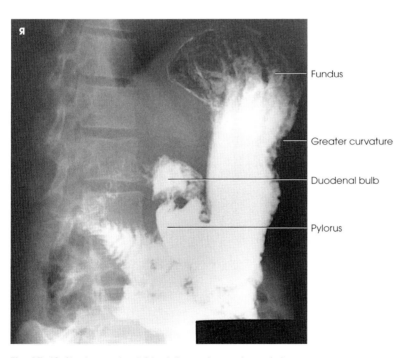

Fundus

Greater curvature

Duodenal bulb

Pylorus

Fig. 17-40 Single-contrast PA oblique stomach and duodenum, RAO position.

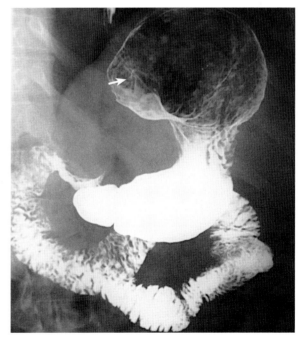

Fig. 17-41 Double-contrast PA oblique stomach and duodenum. Note esophagus entering stomach *(arrow)*.

⚘ AP OBLIQUE PROJECTION
LPO position

Image receptor: 30 × 35 cm lengthwise

Position of patient
• Place the patient in the supine position.

Position of part
• Have the patient abduct the left arm and place the hand near the head, or place the extended arm alongside the body.
• Place the right arm alongside the body or across the upper chest, as preferred.
• Have the patient turn toward the left, resting on the left posterior body surface.
• Flex the patient's right knee, and rotate the knee toward the left for support.
• Place a positioning sponge against the patient's elevated back for immobilization.
• Adjust the patient's position so that a sagittal plane passing approximately midway between the vertebrae and the left lateral margin of the abdomen is centered to the IR.

• Adjust the center of the IR at the level of the body of the stomach. The centering will be at a point midway between the xiphoid process and the lower margin of the ribs (Fig. 17-42).
• The degree of rotation required to best demonstrate the stomach depends on the patient's body habitus. An average angle of 45 degrees should be sufficient for the sthenic patient, but the degree of angulation can vary from 30 to 60 degrees.
• *Shield gonads.*
• *Respiration:* Suspend at the end of expiration unless otherwise instructed.

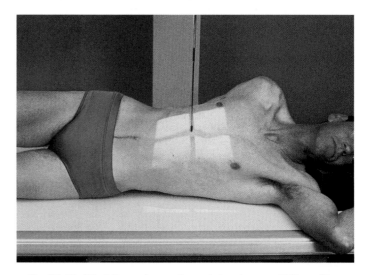

Fig. 17-42 AP oblique stomach and duodenum, LPO position.

Central ray
• Perpendicular to the center of the IR

Structures shown

The AP oblique projection demonstrates the fundic portion of the stomach (Fig. 17-43). Because of the effect of gravity, the pyloric canal and duodenal bulb are not as filled with barium as they are in the opposite and complementary position (the RAO position; see Figs. 17-39 to 17-41).

The following should be clearly demonstrated:
▪ Entire stomach and duodenal loop
▪ Fundic portion of stomach
▪ No superimposition of the pylorus and duodenal bulb
▪ Body of the stomach centered to the radiograph
▪ Exposure technique that demonstrates the anatomy
▪ Body and pylorus with double-contrast visualization

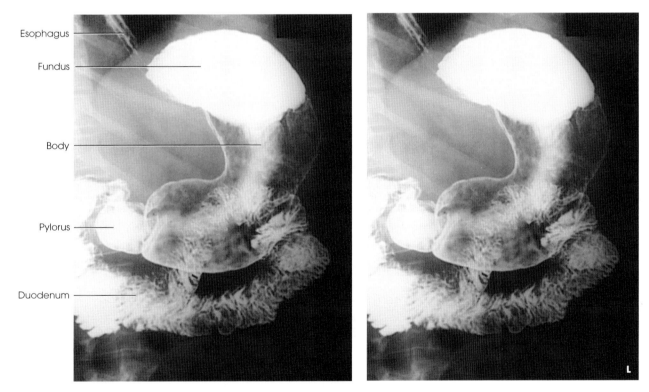

Fig. 17-43 Double-contrast AP oblique stomach and duodenum, LPO position.

Esophagus
Fundus
Body
Pylorus
Duodenum

Stomach and duodenum

♠ LATERAL PROJECTION
R position

Image receptor: 30 × 35 cm lengthwise

Position of patient

- Place the patient in the *upright left-lateral position* for demonstration of the left retrogastric space and in the *recumbent right-lateral position* for demonstration of the right retrogastric space, duodenal loop, and duodenojejunal junction.

Position of part

- With the patient in either the upright or recumbent position, adjust the body so that a plane passing midway between the midcoronal plane and the anterior surface of the abdomen coincides with the midline of the grid.
- Center the IR at the level of L1-L2 for the recumbent position (about 1 to 2 inches above the lower rib margin) and at L3 for the upright position.
- Adjust the body in a true lateral position (Fig. 17-44).
- *Shield gonads.*
- *Respiration:* Suspend at the end of expiration unless otherwise requested.

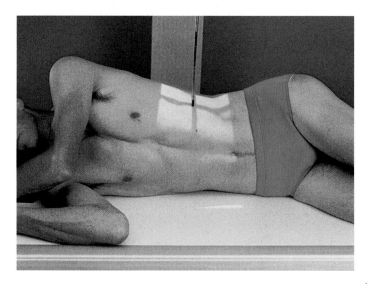

Fig. 17-44 Right lateral stomach and duodenum.

Central ray

• Perpendicular to the center of the IR

Structures shown

A lateral projection shows the anterior and posterior aspects of the stomach, the pyloric canal, and the duodenal bulb (Figs. 17-45 and 17-46). The right lateral projection commonly affords the best image of the pyloric canal and the duodenal bulb in patients with a hypersthenic habitus.

EVALUATION CRITERIA

The following should be clearly demonstrated:

■ Entire stomach and duodenal loop
■ No rotation of the patient, as demonstrated by the vertebrae
■ Stomach centered at the level of the pylorus
■ Exposure technique that demonstrates the anatomy

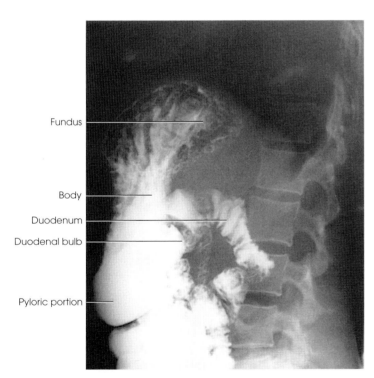

Fundus
Body
Duodenum
Duodenal bulb
Pyloric portion

Fig. 17-45 Single-contrast right lateral stomach and duodenum.

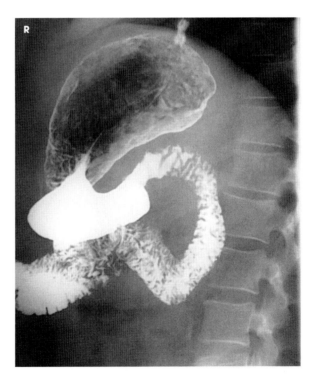

Fig. 17-46 Double-contrast right lateral stomach and duodenum.

▲ AP PROJECTION

Image receptor: 30 × 35 cm crosswise for the stomach and duodenum, lengthwise for small hiatal hernias; 35 × 43 cm lengthwise for large diaphragmatic herniations or for the stomach and small bowel

Position of patient

- Place the patient in the supine position. The stomach moves superiorly and to the left in this position, and except in thin patients, its pyloric end is elevated so that the barium flows into and fills its cardiac or fundic portions, or both. The filling of the fundus displaces the gas bubble into the pyloric end of the stomach, where it allows double-contrast delineation of posterior wall lesions when a single-contrast examination is performed. If the patient is thin, the intestinal loops do not move superior enough to tilt the stomach for fundic filling. Therefore rotating the patient's body toward the left or angling the head end of the table downward is necessary.
- Tilt the table to full or partial Trendelenburg angulation for the demonstration of diaphragmatic herniations (Fig. 17-47). In the Trendelenburg position, the involved organ or organs, which may appear to be normally located in all other body positions, shift upward and protrude through the hernial orifice (most commonly through the esophageal hiatus).

Position of part

- Adjust the position of the patient so that the midline of the grid coincides (1) with the midline of the body when a 35- × 43-cm IR is used (Figs. 17-47 and 17-48) or (2) with a sagittal plane passing midway between the midline and the left lateral margin of the abdomen when a 30- × 35-cm IR is used. Longitudinal centering of the large IR depends on the extent of hernial protrusion into the thorax and is determined during fluoroscopy.
- For the stomach and duodenum, center the 30- × 35-cm IR at a level midway between the xiphoid process and the lower rib margin (approximately L1-L2). For the 35- × 43-cm IR, center it at the same level and adjust up or down slightly, depending on whether the diaphragm or small bowel needs to be seen.
- *Shield gonads.*
- *Respiration:* Suspend at the end of expiration unless otherwise requested.

Central ray

- Perpendicular to the center of the IR

Structures shown

Stomach

An AP projection of the stomach shows a well-filled fundic portion and usually a double-contrast delineation of the body, pyloric portion, and duodenum (Fig. 17-49). Because of the elevation and superior displacement of the stomach, this projection affords the best AP projection of the retrogastric portion of the duodenum and jejunum.

Diaphragm

An AP projection of the abdominothoracic region demonstrates the organ or organs involved in, and the location and extent of, any gross hernial protrusion through the diaphragm (Figs. 17-50 and 17-51).

EVALUATION CRITERIA

The following should be clearly demonstrated:

- Entire stomach and duodenal loop
- Double-contrast visualization of the gastric body, pylorus, and duodenal bulb
- Retrogastric portion of the duodenum and jejunum
- Lower lung fields on 35- × 43-cm radiographs for demonstration of diaphragmatic hernias
- Stomach centered at the level of the pylorus on 30- × 35-cm radiographs
- No rotation of the patient
- Exposure technique that demonstrates the anatomy

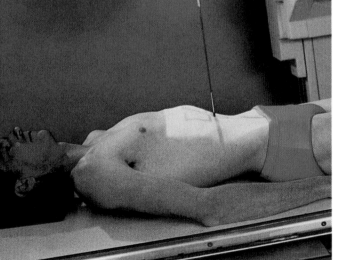

Fig. 17-47 AP stomach and duodenum with table in partial Trendelenburg position.

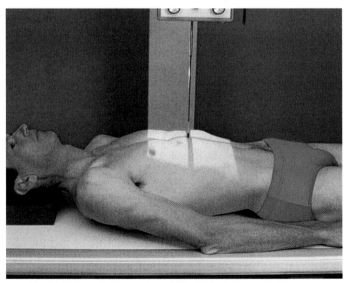

Fig. 17-48 AP stomach and duodenum.

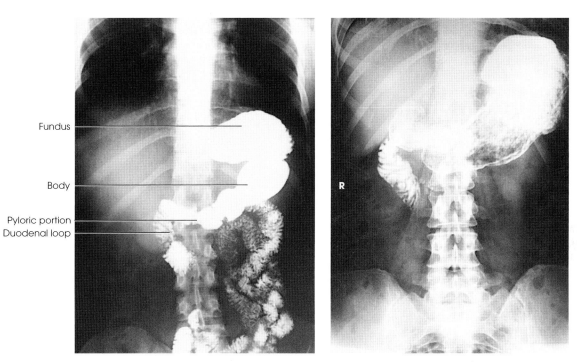

Fundus

Body

Pyloric portion
Duodenal loop

R

Fig. 17-49 AP stomach and duodenum, sthenic habitus.

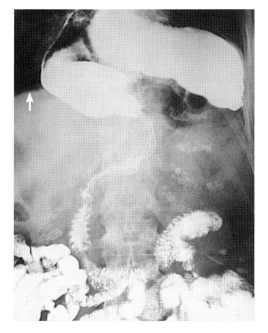

Fig. 17-50 AP stomach and duodenum, showing hiatal hernia above the level of the diaphragm *(arrow)*.

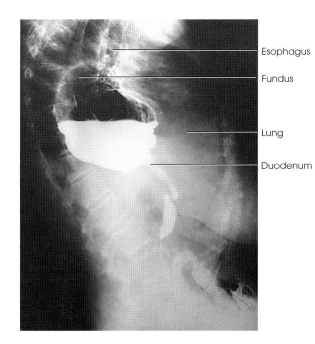

Esophagus

Fundus

Lung

Duodenum

Fig. 17-51 Upright left lateral stomach showing hiatal hernia. (Comparison lateral radiographs are shown in Figs. 17-45 and 17-46.)

Digestive system

PA OBLIQUE PROJECTION
WOLF METHOD[1] (FOR HIATAL HERNIA)
RAO position

> **Image receptor:** 35 × 43 cm lengthwise

The Wolf method[1] is a modification of the Trendelenburg position. The technique was developed for the purpose of applying greater intraabdominal pressure than is provided by body angulation alone and thereby ensuring more consistent results in the radiographic demonstration of small, sliding gastroesophageal herniations through the esophageal hiatus.

The Wolf method requires the use of a semicylindric radiolucent compression device measuring 22 inches (55 cm) in length, 10 inches (24 cm) in width, and 8 inches (20 cm) in height. (The compression sponge depicted in Fig. 17-52 is slightly smaller than the one described by Wolf.)

[1]Wolf BS, Guglielmo J: Method for the roentgen demonstration of minimal hiatal herniation, *J Mt Sinai Hosp NY* 23:738, 741, 1956.

Wolf and Guglielmo[1] stated that this compression device not only provides Trendelenburg angulation of the patient's trunk but also increases intraabdominal pressure enough to permit adequate contrast filling and maximum distention of the entire esophagus. A further advantage of the device is that it does not require angulation of the table; thus the patient can hold the barium container and ingest the barium suspension through a straw with comparative ease.

[1]Wolf BS, Guglielmo J: The roentgen demonstration of minimal hiatus hernia, *Med Radiogr Photogr* 33:90, 1957.

Position of patient
- Place the patient in the prone position on the radiographic table.

Position of part
- Instruct the patient to assume a modified knee-chest position during placement of the compression device.
- Place the compression device horizontally under the abdomen and just below the costal margin.
- Adjust the patient in a 40- to 45-degree RAO position, with the thorax centered to the midline of the grid.
- Instruct the patient to ingest the barium suspension in rapid, continuous swallows.
- To allow for complete filling of the esophagus, make the exposure during the third or fourth swallow (see Fig. 17-52).
- *Shield gonads.*
- *Respiration:* Suspend at the end of expiration.

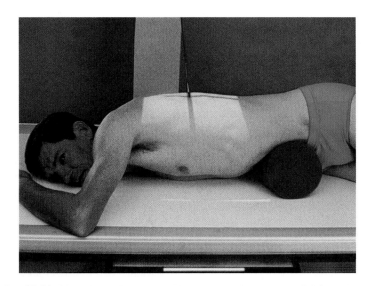

Fig. 17-52 PA oblique stomach with compression sponge, RAO position.

Central ray

- Perpendicular to the long axis of the patient's back and centered at the level of either T6 or T7. This position usually results in a 10- to 20-degree caudad angulation of the central ray.

Structures shown

The Wolf method demonstrates the relationship of the stomach to the diaphragm and is useful in diagnosing a hiatal hernia (Fig. 17-53).

EVALUATION CRITERIA

The following should be clearly demonstrated:

- Middle or distal aspects of the esophagus and the upper aspect of the stomach
- Esophagus visible between the vertebral column and the heart

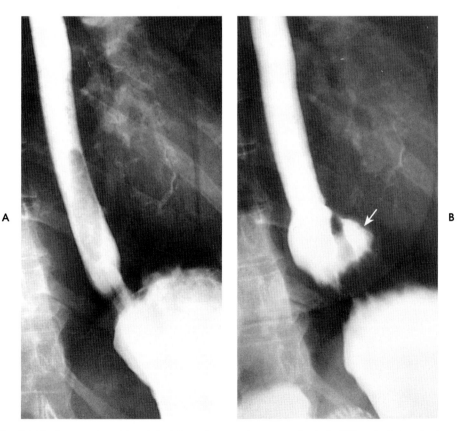

Fig. 17-53 Comparison PA axial oblique images in one patient. **A,** Without abdominal compression: no evidence of hernia. **B,** With abdominal compression: obvious large sliding hernia *(arrow).*

Digestive system

PA OBLIQUE PROJECTION
RAO position

Some institutions obtain radiographs specifically to demonstrate the gastric mucosa after the fluoroscopic examination. A pneumatic paddle may be used (Fig. 17-54). The paddle is fluoroscopically positioned under the area of the pyloric sphincter and duodenal bulb. A radiograph is obtained with the pneumatic paddle inflated, and additional radiographs are taken as the paddle is deflated. The fluoroscopic portion of this examination is performed by the radiologist.

Position of patient
- Place the patient in a prone and slightly RAO position, and center the region to be studied to approximately the midline of the grid.
- Place an inflatable paddle under the area of interest.

Position of part
- Under fluoroscopic control, adjust the patient so that the area of the duodenal bulb is centered to the paddle.
- For a mucosal study, inflate the compression bladder of the paddle to provide the desired degree of pressure (Figs. 17-54 and 17-55).

- After the fluoroscopic adjustments, position the x-ray tube over the patient, and expose postfluoroscopic images.
- Place the IR in the Bucky tray, and center it to the paddle.
- For subsequent exposures, change the IR.
- *Shield gonads.*
- *Respiration:* Suspend at the end of expiration unless otherwise requested.

Central ray
- Perpendicular to the IR

Structures shown

This method demonstrates a compression and a noncompression study of the pyloric end of the stomach and the duodenal bulb at different stages of filling and emptying. A compression study of the mucosa of a localized area of the gastrointestinal tract is also shown (Fig. 17-56).

EVALUATION CRITERIA

The following should be clearly demonstrated:
- Pylorus and duodenal bulb centered, free of superimposition, and in profile

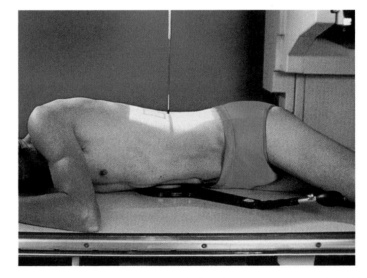

Fig. 17-54 PA oblique pylorus and duodenal bulb with compression paddle, RAO position.

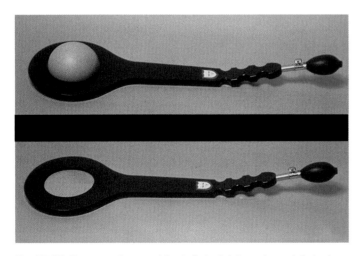

Fig. 17-55 Compression paddle: inflated *(above)*; noninflated *(below)*.

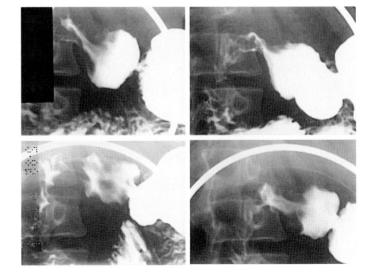

Fig. 17-56 Serial compression study showing varying degrees of compression and the value of the compression paddle in demonstrating the duodenal bulb.

Small Intestine

Radiologic examinations of the small intestine are performed by administering a barium sulfate preparation (1) by *mouth;* (2) by complete *reflux filling* with a large-volume barium enema (BE); or (3) by direct injection into the bowel through an intestinal tube, a technique that is called *enteroclysis,* or small intestine enema. The latter two methods are used when the oral method fails to provide conclusive information.[1] The enteroclysis is technically difficult, so its use is usually limited to larger medical facilities.

PREPARATION FOR EXAMINATION

Preferably, the patient will have a soft or low-residue diet for 2 days before the small intestine study. Because of economics, however, it often is not possible to delay the examination for 2 days. Therefore food and fluid are usually withheld after the evening meal of the day before the examination, and breakfast is withheld on the day of the study. A cleansing enema may be administered to clear the colon; however, an enema is not always recommended for enteroclysis because enema fluid may be retained in the small intestine. The barium formula varies depending on the method of examination. The patient's bladder should be empty before and during the procedure to avoid displacing or compressing the ileum.

[1]Fitch D: The small-bowel see-through: an improved method of radiographic small bowel visualization, *Can J Med Rad Technol* 26:167, 1995.

ORAL METHOD OF EXAMINATION

The radiographic examination of the small intestine is usually termed a *small bowel series* because several identical radiographs are done at timed intervals. The oral examination, or ingestion of barium through the mouth, is usually preceded by a preliminary radiograph of the abdomen. Each radiograph of the small intestine is identified with a time marker indicating the interval between its exposure and the ingestion of barium. The studies are made with the patient in either the supine or prone position. The supine position is used (1) to take advantage of the superior and lateral shift of the barium-filled stomach for visualization of the retrogastric portions of the duodenum and jejunum and (2) to prevent possible compression overlapping of loops of the intestine. The prone position is used to compress the abdominal contents, which increases radiographic quality. For the final radiographs in thin patients, it may be necessary to angle the table into the Trendelenburg position to "unfold" low-lying and superimposed loops of the ileum.

The first small intestine radiograph is usually taken 15 minutes after the patient drinks the barium. The interval to the next exposure varies from 15 to 30 minutes depending on the average transit time of the barium sulfate preparation used. Regardless of the barium preparation used, the radiologist inspects the radiographs as they are processed and varies the procedure according to the requirements for the individual patient. Fluoroscopic and radiographic studies (spot or conventional) may be made of any segment of the bowel as the loops become opacified.

Some radiologists request that a glass of ice water (or another routinely used food stimulant) be given to the patient with hypomotility after 3 or 4 hours of administrating barium sulfate to accelerate peristalsis. Others give patients a water-soluble gastrointestinal contrast medium, tea, or coffee to stimulate peristalsis. Still others administer peristaltic stimulants every 15 minutes through the transit time. With these methods, the transit of the medium is demonstrated fluoroscopically, spot and conventional radiographs are exposed as indicated, and the examination is usually completed in 30 to 60 minutes.

Digestive system

⚜ PA OR AP PROJECTION

Image receptor: 35 × 43 cm lengthwise

Position of patient
- Place the patient in the prone or supine position.

Position of part
- Adjust the patient so that the midsagittal plane is centered to the grid.
- For the sthenic patient, center the IR at the level of L2 for radiographs taken within 30 minutes after the contrast medium is administered (Fig. 17-57).
- For delayed radiographs, center the IR at the level of the iliac crests.
- *Shield gonads.*
- *Respiration:* Suspend at the end of expiration unless otherwise requested.

Central ray
- Perpendicular to the midpoint of the IR (L2) for early radiographs or at the level of the iliac crests for delayed sequence exposures

Structures shown
The PA or AP projection demonstrates the small intestine progressively filling until the barium reaches the ileocecal valve (Figs. 17-58 to 17-65).

When the barium has reached the ileocecal region, fluoroscopy may be performed and compression radiographs obtained (Fig. 17-66).

The examination is usually completed when the barium is visualized in the cecum, typically in about 2 hours for a patient with normal intestinal motility.

The following should be clearly demonstrated:
- Entire small intestine on each image
- Stomach on initial images
- Time marker
- Vertebral column centered on the radiograph
- No rotation of the patient
- Exposure technique that demonstrates the anatomy
- Complete examination when barium reaches the cecum

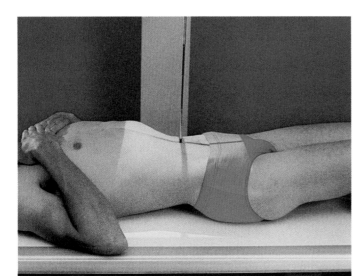

Fig. 17-57 AP small intestine.

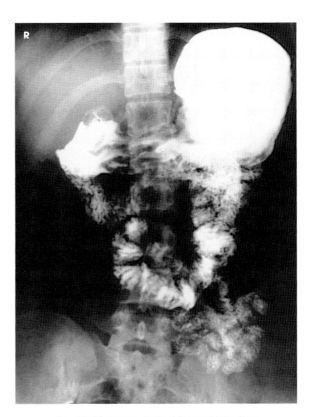

Fig. 17-58 Immediate AP small intestine.

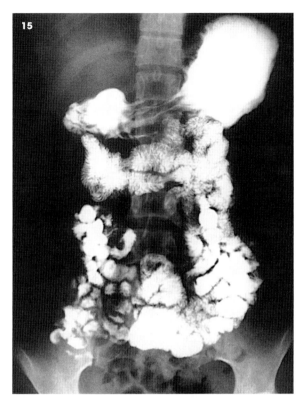

Fig. 17-59 AP small intestine at 15 minutes.

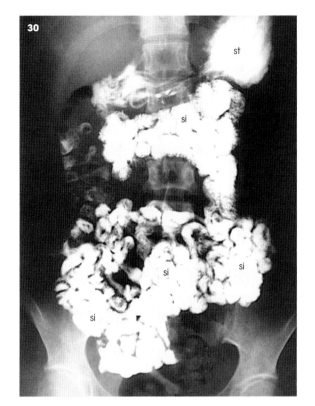

Fig. 17-60 AP small intestine at 30 minutes, showing stomach *(st)* and small intestine *(si)*.

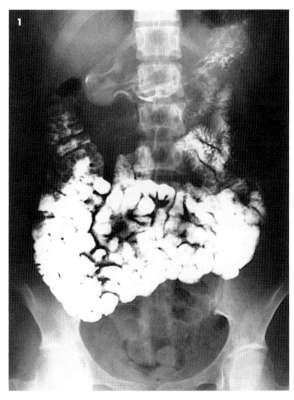

Fig. 17-61 AP small intestine at 1 hour, demonstrating barium-filled cecum.

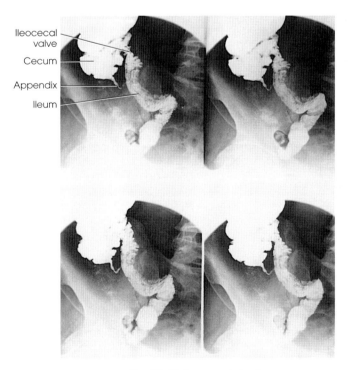

Fig. 17-62 Ileocecal studies.

COMPLETE REFLUX EXAMINATION

For a complete reflux examination of the small intestine,[1,2] the patient's colon and small intestine are filled by administering a BE to demonstrate the colon and small bowel. Before the examination, glucagon may be administered to relax the intestine. Diazepam (Valium) may also be given to diminish patient discomfort during the initial filling of the bowel. A 15% ± 5% weight/volume barium suspension is often used, and a large amount of the suspension (about 4500 mL) is required to fill the colon and small intestine.

A retention enema tip is used, and the patient is placed in the supine position for the examination. The barium suspension is allowed to flow until it is observed in the duodenal bulb. The enema bag is then lowered to the floor to drain the colon before radiographs of the small intestine are obtained (see Fig. 17-63).

[1]Miller RE: Complete reflux small bowel examination, *Radiology* 84:457, 1965.
[2]Miller RE: Localization of the small bowel hemorrhage; complete reflex small bowel examination, *Am J Dig Dis* 17:1019, 1972.

ENTEROCLYSIS PROCEDURE

Enteroclysis (the injection of nutrient or medicinal liquid into the bowel) is a radiographic procedure in which contrast medium is injected into the duodenum under fluoroscopic control for examination of the small intestine. The contrast medium is injected through a specially designed enteroclysis catheter, historically a Bilbao or Sellink tube.

Before the procedure is begun, the patient's colon must be thoroughly cleansed. Enemas are not recommended as preparation for enteroclysis because some enema fluid may be retained in the small intestine. Under fluoroscopic control, the enteroclysis catheter with a stiff guidewire is advanced to the end of the duodenum at the duodenojejunal flexure, near the ligament of Treitz. The retention balloon, if present, is filled with sterile water or saline. Barium is then instilled through the tube at a rate of approximately 100 mL/min (Fig. 17-64). Spot radiographs, with and without compression, are taken as required. In some patients, air is injected after the contrast fluid has reached the distal small intestine (Fig. 17-65). When CT is to be performed, an iodinated contrast medium (Figs. 17-66 and 17-67) or tap water (Figs. 17-68 and 17-69) may be used.

After fluoroscopic examination of the patient's small intestine, radiographs of the small intestine may be requested. The projections most often requested include the AP, PA, obliques, and lateral. Both recumbent and upright images may be requested. (Positioning descriptions involving the abdomen are presented in Chapter 16.)

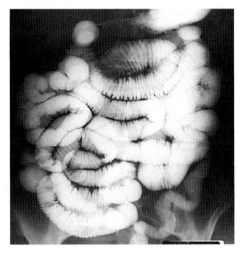

Fig. 17-63 Normal retrograde reflux examination of small intestine.

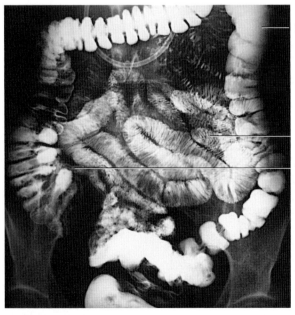

Fig. 17-64 Enteroclysis procedure with barium visualized in colon.

Barium in colon

Small intestine

Terminal ileum

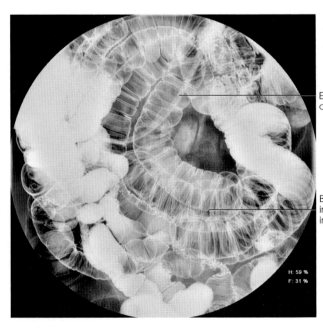

Fig. 17-65 Air-contrast enteroclysis.

Enteroclysis catheter

Barium air in small intestine

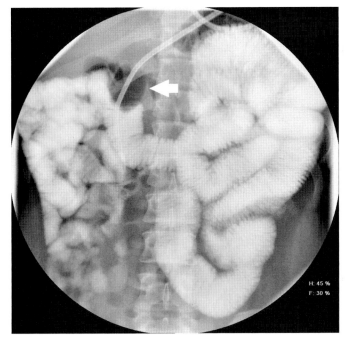

Fig. 17-66 Enteroclysis with iodinated contrast medium. Filled retention balloon is seen in duodenum *(arrow)*.

(Courtesy Michelle Alting, AS, RT(R).)

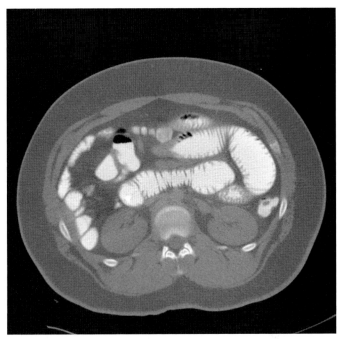

Fig. 17-67 Axial CT enteroclysis of patient in Fig. 17-66.

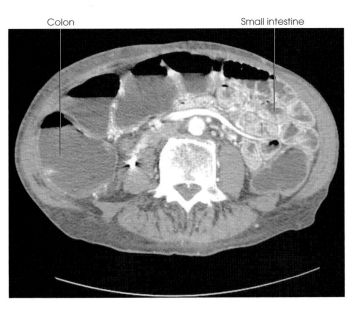

Colon   Small intestine

Fig. 17-68 Axial CT enteroclysis with tap water and intravenous iodinated contrast medium. The intraluminal water *(dark gray)* is clearly delineated from the bowel wall *(light gray)*.

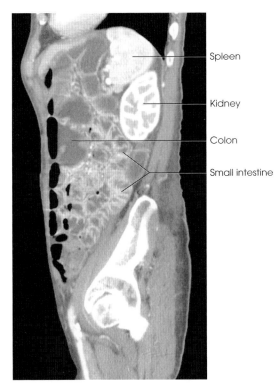

Spleen

Kidney

Colon

Small intestine

Fig. 17-69 Sagittal reconstruction of CT enteroclysis from Fig. 17-68.

163

INTUBATION EXAMINATION PROCEDURES

Gastrointestinal intubation is the procedure in which a long, specially designed tube is inserted through the nose and passed into the stomach. From there the tube is carried inferiorly by peristaltic action. Gastrointestinal intubation is used for both therapeutic and diagnostic purposes.

When gastrointestinal intubation is used therapeutically, the tube is connected to a suction system for continuous siphoning of the gas and fluid contents of the gastrointestinal tract. The purpose of the maneuver is to prevent or relieve postoperative distention or to deflate or decompress an obstructed small intestine.

Although used much less frequently than in the past, a *Miller-Abbott* (M-A) double-lumen, single-balloon tube (or other similar tubing) can be used to intubate the small intestine. Just above the tip of the M-A tube is a small, thin rubber balloon. Marks on the tube, beginning at the distal end, indicate the extent of the tube's passage and are read from the edge of the nostril. The marks are graduated in centimeters up to 85 cm and are given in feet thereafter. The lumen of the tube is asymmetrically divided into the following: (1) a small balloon lumen that communicates with the balloon only and is used for the inflation and deflation of the balloon and for the injection of mercury to weight the balloon and (2) a large aspiration lumen that communicates with the gastrointestinal tract through perforations near and at the distal end of the tube. Gas and fluids are withdrawn through the aspiration lumen, and liquids are injected through it.

The introduction of an intestinal tube is an unpleasant experience for the patient, especially one who is acutely ill. Depending on the condition of the patient, the tube is more readily passed if the patient can sit erect and lean slightly forward or if the patient can be elevated almost to a sitting position.

With the intestinal tube in place, the patient is turned to an RAO position, a syringe is connected to the balloon lumen, and the mercury is poured into the syringe and allowed to flow into the balloon. The air is then slowly withdrawn from the balloon. The tube is secured with an adhesive strip beside the nostril to prevent regurgitation or advancement of the tube. The stomach is aspirated, either by syringe or by attaching the large position of the lumen to the suction apparatus.

With the tip of the tube situated close to the pyloric sphincter and the patient in the RAO position (a position in which gastric peristalsis is usually more active), the tube should pass into the duodenum in a reasonably short time. Without intervention, however, this process sometimes takes many hours. Having the patient drink ice water to stimulate peristalsis is often successful. When this measure fails, the examiner guides the tube into the duodenum by manual manipulation under fluoroscopic observation. After the tube enters the duodenum, it is again inflated to provide a bolus that the peristaltic waves can more readily move along the intestine.

When the tube is inserted for decompression of an intestinal obstruction and possible later radiologic investigation, the adhesive strip is removed and replaced with an adhesive loop attached to the forehead. The tube can slide through the loop without tension as it advances toward the obstructed site. The patient is then returned to the hospital room. Radiographs of the abdomen may be taken to check the progress of the tube and the effectiveness of decompression. Simple obstructions are sometimes relieved by suction; others require surgical intervention.

If the passage of the intestinal tube is arrested, the suction is discontinued and the patient is returned to the radiology department for an M-A tube study. The contrast medium used for studies of a localized segment of the small intestine may be either a water-soluble, iodinated solution (Fig. 17-70) or a thin barium sulfate suspension. Under fluoroscopic observation the contrast agent is injected through the large lumen of the tube with a syringe. Spot and conventional radiographs are obtained as indicated.

When the intestinal tube is introduced for the purpose of performing a small intestine enema, the tube is advanced into the proximal loop of the jejunum and then secured at this level with an adhesive strip taped beside the nose. Medical opinion varies as to the quantity of barium suspension required for this examination (Fig. 17-71). The medium is injected through the aspiration lumen of the tube in a continuous, low-pressure flow. Spot and conventional radiographs are exposed as indicated. Except for the presence of the tube in the upper jejunum, the resultant radiographs resemble those obtained by the oral method.

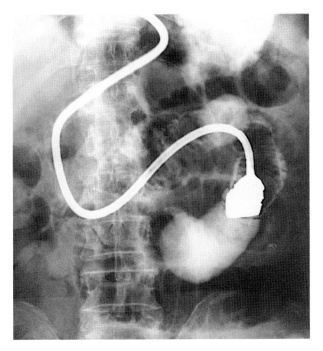

Fig. 17-70 M-A tube study with water-soluble medium.

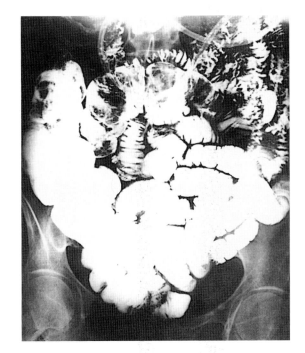

Fig. 17-71 Small bowel examination by M-A tube with injection of barium sulfate.

Large Intestine
CONTRAST STUDIES

The two basic radiologic methods of examining the large intestine by means of diagnostic or contrast enemas are (1) the *single-contrast* method (Fig. 17-72), in which the colon is examined with a barium sulfate suspension or water-soluble iodide only, and (2) the *double-contrast* method (Fig. 17-73), which may be performed as a two-stage or single-stage procedure. In the *two-stage, double-contrast procedure,* the colon is examined with a barium sulfate suspension and then, immediately after evacuation of the barium suspension, with an air enema or another gaseous enema. In the *single-stage, double-contrast procedure* the fluoroscopist selectively injects the barium suspension and the gas.

The contrast medium demonstrates the anatomy and tonus of the colon and most of the abnormalities to which it is subject. The gaseous medium serves to distend the lumen of the bowel and to render visible, through the transparency of its shadow, all parts of the barium-coated mucosal lining of the colon and any small intraluminal lesions, such as polypoid tumors.

A recent development in radiographic examination of the large intestine is computed tomography colonography (CTC), also called *virtual colonoscopy* (VC), a procedure used as a primary screening tool for colorectal cancer or after a failed conventional colonoscopy. This software-driven technique combines helical CT and virtual-reality software to create 3D and multiplanar images of the colonic mucosa. Examples of currently available CTC techniques include the perspective filet or virtual dissection view, 3D topographic view, multiplanar reformatted (MPR) view, and the colonoscopic-like endoluminal view (Figs. 17-74, 17-75, and 17-76).

Contrast media

Commercially prepared barium sulfate products are generally used for routine retrograde examinations of the large intestine. Some of these products are referred to as *colloidal preparations* because they have finely divided barium particles that resist precipitation, whereas others are referred to as suspended or *flocculation-resistant preparations* because they contain some form of suspending or dispersing agent.

The newest barium products available are referred to as *high-density barium sulfate.* These products absorb a greater percentage of radiation, similar to the older "thick" barium products. High-density barium is particularly useful for double-contrast studies of the alimentary canal in which uniform coating of the lumen is required.

Air is the gaseous medium usually used in the double-contrast enema study. Therefore the procedure is generally called an *air-contrast study.* Carbon dioxide may also be used because it is more rapidly absorbed than the nitrogen in air when evacuation of the gaseous medium is incomplete. Use of air as a contrast medium for radiographic evaluation of the colon is not limited to the double-contrast enema procedure. Air or CO_2 insufflation of the colon is used to perform CTC or VC.

Water-soluble, iodinated contrast media enemas are performed when colon

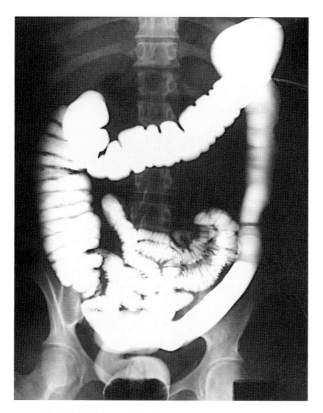

Fig. 17-72 Large intestine, single-contrast study.

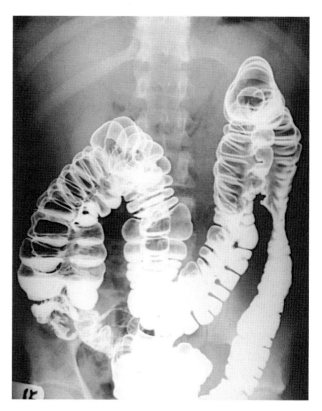

Fig. 17-73 Large intestine, double-contrast study.

perforation or leak is suspected. These iodinated contrast agents are administered orally to selected patients when retrograde filling of the colon with barium is not possible or is contraindicated. A disadvantage of the iodinated solutions is that evacuation often is insufficient for satisfactory double-contrast visualization of the mucosal pattern. However, when a patient is unable to cooperate for a successful enema study, orally administered iodinated medium allows satisfactory examination of the colon. With these oral agents, transit time from ingestion to colonic filling is fast, averaging 3 to 4 hours. Furthermore, iodinated solutions are practically nonabsorbable from the gastrointestinal mucosa. As a result, the oral dose reaches and outlines the entire large bowel. Unlike an ingested barium sulfate suspension, this medium is not subject to drying, flaking, and unequal distribution in the colon. Therefore it frequently delineates the intestine almost as well as the BE does.

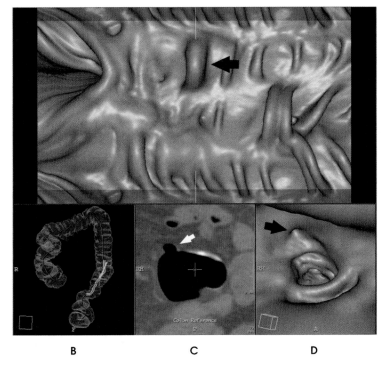

Fig. 17-74 Examples of CTC or VC. **A,** Perspective filet or virtual dissection view, demonstrating diverticulum *(arrow)*. **B,** 3D topographic view: Purple line in the sigmoid shows length of filet in **A. C,** Axial MPR, demonstrating same diverticulum as in **A** *(arrow)*. **D,** Endoluminal view showing opening *(arrow)* of diverticulum from **A.**

(**D,** Courtesy J. Louis Rankin, BS, RT(R)(MR).)

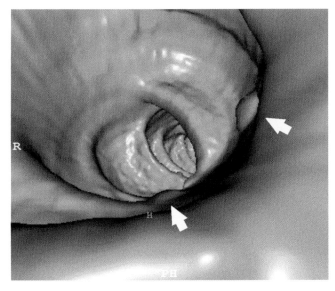

Fig. 17-75 Endoluminal CTC image, demonstrating two tubular adenomas *(arrows)*.

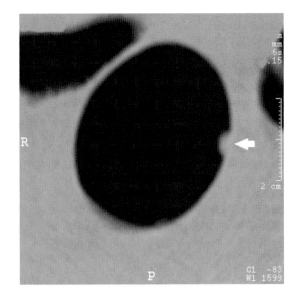

Fig. 17-76 Axial MPR image of the upper tubular adenoma *(arrow)* from Fig. 17-75.

Preparation of intestinal tract

Medical opinion about preparation measures varies. However, members of the medical profession usually agree that the large intestine must be completely emptied of its contents to render all portions of its inner wall visible for inspection. When coated with a barium sulfate suspension, retained fecal masses are likely to simulate the appearance of polypoid or other small tumor masses (Fig. 17-77). This makes thorough cleansing of the entire colon a matter of prime importance. Preliminary preparation of the intestinal tract of patients who have a condition such as severe diarrhea, gross bleeding, or symptoms of obstruction is, of course, limited. Other patients are prepared, with modification as indicated, according to the specifications established by the examining physician. The preliminary preparation usually includes dietary restrictions and a bowel cleaning regimen. The methods of bowel-cleansing include the following:
- Complete intestinal tract cleansing kits
- Gastrointestinal lavage preparations
- Cleansing enema

Standard barium enema apparatus

Disposable soft plastic enema tips and enema bags are commercially available in different sizes. A soft rubber rectal catheter of small caliber should be used in patients who have inflamed hemorrhoids, fissures, a stricture, or other abnormalities of the anus.

Disposable rectal *retention tips* (Fig. 17-78) have replaced the older retention catheters, such as the Bardex or Foley catheter. The retention tip is a double-lumen tube with a thin balloon at its distal end. Because of the danger of intestinal wall damage, the retention tip must be inserted with extreme care. The enema retention tip is used in the patient who has a relaxed anal sphincter or another condition that makes it difficult or impossible to retain an enema. Some radiologists routinely use retention enema tips and inflate them if necessary.

The disposable rectal retention tip has a balloon cuff that fits snugly against the enema nozzle both before inflation and after deflation so that it can be inserted and removed with little discomfort to the patient. A reusable squeeze inflator is recommended to limit the air capacity to approximately 90 mL. One complete squeeze of the inflator provides adequate distention of the retention balloon without danger of overinflation. Disposable retention tips are available for both double-contrast and single-contrast enemas. For the safety of the patient, any retention balloon must be inflated with caution, using fluoroscopy, just before the examination.

For the performance of a double-contrast BE examination, a special rectal tip is necessary to instill air in the colon (Fig. 17-79). Alternatively, air can simply be pumped into the colon using a sphygmomanometer bulb. Double-contrast retention tips are also available.

Most enema bags have a capacity of 3 quarts (3000 mL) when completely filled and have graduated quantity markings on the side. A filter may be incorporated within the bag to prevent the passage of any unmixed lumps of barium. The tubing is approximately 6 feet long. Smaller enema bags (500 mL) with short, large-diameter tubing have been developed for double-contrast BE procedures.

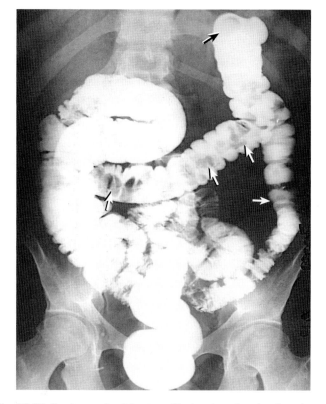

Fig. 17-77 Single-contrast, barium-filled colon, showing fecal material that simulates or masks pathologic condition *(arrows)*.

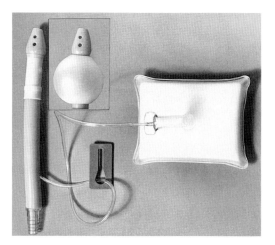

Fig. 17-78 Disposable retention enema tip. Uninflated balloon fits snugly. *Inset:* Balloon cuff inflated with 90 mL of air (one complete squeeze of inflator).

Preparation of barium suspensions

The concentration of the barium sulfate suspensions used for single-contrast colonic enemas varies considerably. The often recommended range is between 12% and 25% for weight/volume. For double-contrast examinations, a relatively high-density barium product is used. A 75% to 95% weight/volume ratio is common.

Commercial BE preparations are available as premixed liquids that can be poured into the disposable enema kit bag. Powdered barium is also available in single-contrast disposable kit bags. Water is added, and the solution is mixed by shaking the bag.

Instructions for mixing a barium preparation vary according to the manufacturer and the type of barium used. The best recommendation is to follow the manufacturer's instructions precisely.

If warm BEs are administered, the temperature should be somewhat below body temperature—about 85° to 90° F (29° to 30° C). In addition to being unpleasant and debilitating, an enema that is too warm is injurious to intestinal tissues and produces so much irritation that it is difficult, if not impossible, for the patient to retain the enema long enough for a satisfactory examination.

Preparation and care of patient

In no radiologic examination is the full cooperation of the patient more essential to success than in the retrograde examination of the colon. Few patients who are physically able to retain the enema fail to do so when they understand the procedure and realize that in large measure the success of the examination depends on them. The radiographer should observe the following guidelines in preparing a patient for retrograde examination of the colon:

- Take time to explain the procedural differences between an ordinary cleansing enema and a diagnostic enema: (1) With the diagnostic enema the fluoroscopist examines all portions of the bowel as it is being filled with contrast medium under fluoroscopic observation; (2) this part of the examination involves palpation of the abdomen, rotation of the body as required to visualize the different segments of the colon, and the taking of spot radiographs without and, when indicated, with compression; (3) a series of large radiographs are taken before the colon can be evacuated.
- Assure the patient that retention of the diagnostic enema preparation will be comparatively easy because its flow is controlled under fluoroscopic observation.
- Instruct the patient to (1) keep the anal sphincter tightly contracted against the tubing to hold it in position and prevent leakage, (2) relax the abdominal muscles to prevent intraabdominal pressure, and (3) concentrate on deep oral breathing to reduce the incidence of colonic spasm and resultant cramps.
- Assure the patient that the flow of the enema will be stopped for the duration of any cramping.

The patient who has not had a previous colonic examination is usually fearful of being embarrassed by inadequate draping and failure to retain the enema for the required time. The radiographer can dispel or greatly relieve the patient's anxiety by observing the following steps:

- Assure the patient that he or she will be properly covered.
- Assure the patient that although there is little chance of "mishap," he or she will be well protected but that there is no need to feel embarrassed should one occur.
- Keep a bedpan in the examining room for the patient who cannot or may not be able to make the trip to the toilet.

The preliminary preparation required for a retrograde study of the colon is strenuous for the patient. The examination itself further depletes the patient's strength. Feeble patients, particularly elderly persons, are likely to become weak and faint from the exertion of the preparation, the examination, and the effort made to expel the enema. The strenuous nature of these procedures presents an increased risk for patients with a history of heart disease. An emergency call button should be available in the lavatory so that the patient can summon help if necessary. Although the patient's privacy must be respected, the radiographer or an aide should frequently inquire to ensure that the patient is all right.

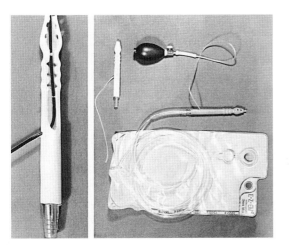

Fig. 17-79 Air-contrast enema tip shown with the air tube filled with ink to demonstrate position.

Insertion of enema tip

In preparation for insertion of the enema tip, the following steps are observed:

- Instruct the patient to turn onto the left side, roll forward about 35 to 40 degrees, and rest the flexed right knee on the table, above and in front of the slightly flexed left knee (Sims' position). This position relaxes the abdominal muscles, which decreases intra-abdominal pressure on the rectum and makes relaxation of the anal sphincter less difficult.
- Adjust the IV pole so that the enema contents are no higher than 24 inches (61 cm) above the level of the anus.
- Adjust the overlapping back of the gown or other draping to expose the anal region only, but keep the patient otherwise well covered. The anal orifice is commonly partially obscured by distended hemorrhoids or a fringe of undistended hemorrhoids. Sometimes there is a contraction or other abnormality of the orifice. Therefore it is necessary for the anus to be exposed and sufficiently well lighted for the orifice to be clearly visible so that the enema tip can be inserted without injury or discomfort.

- Run a little of the barium mixture into a waste basin to free the tubing of air, and then lubricate the rectal tube well with a water-soluble lubricant.
- Advise the patient to relax and take deep breaths so that no discomfort is felt when the tube is inserted.
- Elevate the right buttock laterally to open the gluteal fold.
- As the abdominal muscles and anal sphincter are relaxed during the expiration phase of a deep breath, insert the rectal tube gently and slowly into the anal orifice. Following the angle of the anal canal, direct the tube anteriorly 1 to 1½ inches (2.5 to 3.8 cm). Then following the curve of the rectum, direct the tube slightly superiorly.
- Insert the tube for a total distance of no more than 4 inches (10 cm). Insertion for a greater distance is not only unnecessary but may injure the rectum.
- If the tube does not enter easily, ask the patient to assist if capable.
- *Never* forcibly insert a rectal tube because the patient may have distended internal hemorrhoids or another condition that makes forced insertion of the tube dangerous.

- After the enema tip is inserted, hold it in position to prevent it from slipping while the patient turns to the supine or prone position for fluoroscopy, according to the preference of the fluoroscopist. The retention cuff may be inflated at this time.
- Adjust the protective underpadding, and relieve any pressure on the tubing so that the enema mixture will flow freely.

SINGLE-CONTRAST BARIUM ENEMA

Administration of contrast medium

After preparing the patient for the examination, the radiographer observes the following steps:

- Notify the radiologist as soon as everything is ready for the examination.
- If the patient has not been introduced to the radiologist, make the introduction at this time.
- At the radiologist's request, release the control clip and ensure the enema flow.
- When occlusion of the enema tip occurs, displace soft fecal material by withdrawing the rectal tube about 1 inch (2.5 cm). Then before reinserting the tip, temporarily elevate the enema bag to increase fluid pressure.

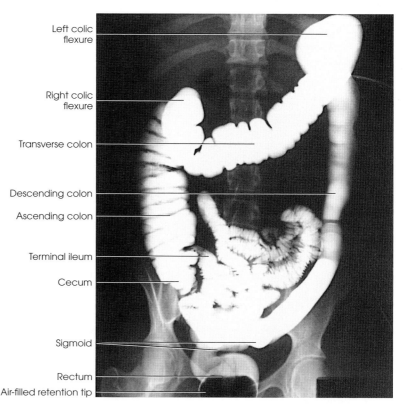

Left colic flexure
Right colic flexure
Transverse colon
Descending colon
Ascending colon
Terminal ileum
Cecum
Sigmoid
Rectum
Air-filled retention tip

Fig. 17-80 Single-contrast BE image, sthenic habitus.

The rectal ampulla fills slowly. Unless the barium flow is stopped for a few seconds once the rectal ampulla is full, the suspension will flow through the sigmoid and descending portions of the colon at a fairly rapid rate, frequently causing a severe cramp and acute stimulation of the defecation impulse. The flow of the barium suspension is usually stopped for several seconds at frequent intervals during the fluoroscopically controlled filling of the colon.

During the fluoroscopic procedure, the radiologist rotates the patient to inspect all segments of the bowel. The radiologist takes spot radiographs as indicated and determines the positions to be used for subsequent radiographic studies. On completion of the fluoroscopic examination, the enema tip is usually removed so that the patient can be maneuvered more easily and so that the tip is not accidentally displaced during the imaging procedure. A retention tube is not removed until the patient is placed on a bedpan or the toilet.

After the IRs have been exposed (Fig. 17-80), the patient is escorted to a toilet or placed on a bedpan and instructed to expel as much of the barium suspension as possible. A postevacuation radiograph is then taken (Fig. 17-81). If this radiograph shows evacuation to be inadequate for satisfactory delineation of the mucosa, the patient may be given a hot beverage (tea or coffee) to stimulate further evacuation.

Positioning of opacified colon

The most commonly obtained projections for the single-contrast BE are the PA or AP, PA obliques, an axial for the sigmoid, and a lateral for demonstration of the rectum.

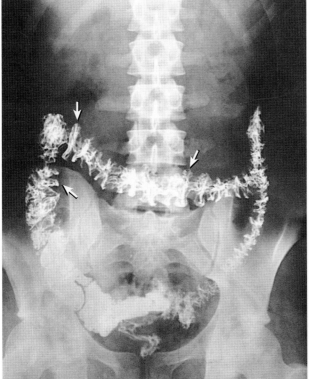

Fig. 17-81 Postevacuation image demonstrating mucosal pattern (arrows). Hyposthenic habitus.

DOUBLE-CONTRAST BARIUM ENEMA

Two approaches to administering double-contrast BEs are currently in use. The first technique is a *two-stage procedure,* described by Welin,[1] in which the entire colon is filled with a barium suspension. After the enema administration, the patient evacuates the barium and immediately returns to the fluoroscopic table where air or another gaseous medium is injected into the colon. The second approach is the *single-stage, double-contrast examination.* The popularity of this approach can be attributed primarily to recent advancements in the manufacture of high-density barium sulfate.

Single-stage procedure

In performing the single-stage, double-contrast enema, certain requirements must be met to ensure an adequate examination. The most important requirement is that the patient's colon be exceptionally clean. Residual fecal material can obscure

small polyps or tumor masses. A second requirement is that a suitable barium suspension be used. A barium mixture that clumps or flakes will neither clearly demonstrate the lumen nor properly drain from the colon.

Currently available, premixed liquid barium products are generally more uniform for radiographic use than most barium suspensions mixed in the health care institution. A barium product with a density as high as 200% weight/volume may be used for a single-stage, double-contrast examination of the colon. The most important criterion is that the barium flows sufficiently to coat the walls of the colon.

With advances in the manufacture of high-density barium, high-quality double-contrast colon radiographs can be consistently obtained during one filling of the colon. In the single-stage procedure the barium and air are instilled in a single procedure. Miller[1] described a 7-*pump* method for performing single-stage,

double-contrast examinations. This method reduces cost, saves time, and reduces radiation exposure to the patient. (A more complete description of the 7-pump method is provided in the seventh edition or earlier editions of this atlas.)

Fluoroscopy is performed to check the location of the barium, and additional air is instilled under fluoroscopic control. The patient is slowly rotated 360 degrees and placed in the supine position. Then spot radiographs and overhead radiographs are taken (Figs. 17-82 and 17-83).

In addition to the 7-pump method, a single-stage, double-contrast examination can be performed using a technique that does not employ a special air-contrast enema tip. With this technique the barium and air are instilled through the closed enema bag system (Fig. 17-84).

---

[1]Welin S: Modern trends in diagnostic roentgenology of the colon, *Br J Radiol* 31:453, 1958.

[1]Miller RE: Barium pneumocolon: technologist-performed "7-pump" method, *Am J Roentgenol* 139:1230, 1982.

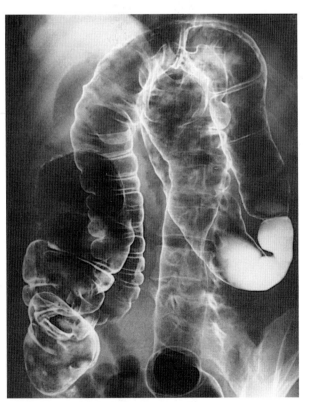

Fig. 17-82 AP oblique colon, RPO position, double-contrast study.

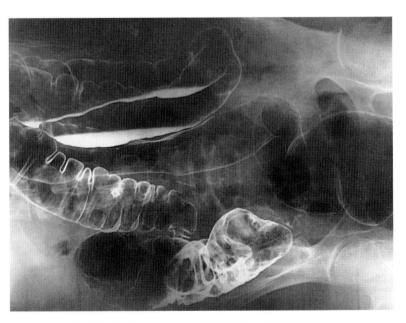

Fig. 17-83 AP colon, right lateral decubitus position.

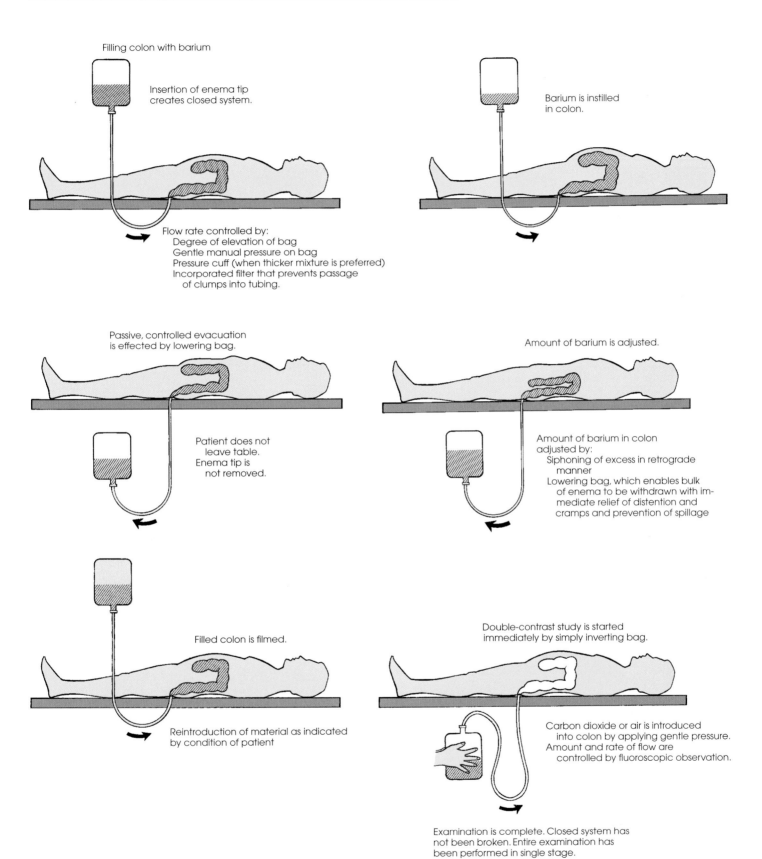

Filling colon with barium

Insertion of enema tip
creates closed system.

Flow rate controlled by:
　Degree of elevation of bag
　Gentle manual pressure on bag
　Pressure cuff (when thicker mixture is preferred)
　Incorporated filter that prevents passage
　　of clumps into tubing.

Barium is instilled
in colon.

Passive, controlled evacuation
is effected by lowering bag.

Patient does not
　leave table.
Enema tip is
　not removed.

Amount of barium is adjusted.

Amount of barium in colon
adjusted by:
　Siphoning of excess in retrograde
　　manner
　Lowering bag, which enables bulk
　　of enema to be withdrawn with im-
　　mediate relief of distention and
　　cramps and prevention of spillage

Filled colon is filmed.

Reintroduction of material as indicated
by condition of patient

Double-contrast study is started
immediately by simply inverting bag.

Carbon dioxide or air is introduced
　into colon by applying gentle pressure.
Amount and rate of flow are
　controlled by fluoroscopic observation.

Examination is complete. Closed system has
not been broken. Entire examination has
been performed in single stage.

Fig. 17-84 Conduction of single-stage, closed-system, double-contrast examination.

(From Pochaczevsky R, Sherman RS: A new technique for roentgenologic examination of the colon,
AJR 89:787, 1963.)

Welin method

Welin[1,2] developed a technique for double-contrast enemas that reveals even the smallest intraluminal lesions (Figs. 17-85 and 17-86). He stated that this method of examination is extremely valuable in the early diagnosis of conditions such as ulcerative colitis, regional colitis, and polyps.

Welin stressed the importance of preparing the intestine for the examination, stating that (1) the colon must be cleansed as thoroughly as possible, and (2) the colonic mucosa must be prepared in such a way that an extremely thin and even coating of barium can adhere to the colonic wall. He recommended regulation of evacuation so that the two stages of the examination can be carried out at short intervals to avoid unnecessary waiting time, and the patient does not have to be in the examining room for more than 20 to 25 minutes.

[1]Welin S: Modern trends in diagnostic roentgenology of the colon, *Br J Radiol* 31:453, 1958.
[2]Welin S: Results of the Malmo technique of colon examination, *JAMA* 199:369, 1967.

Stage 1

With the patient in the prone position to prevent possible ileal leak, the colon is filled to the left colic flexure, after which a conventional radiograph is taken (i.e., a right lateral projection of the barium-filled rectum). The patient is then sent to the lavatory to evacuate the barium. Afterward, if the patient feels the need to do so, he or she is allowed to lie down and rest.

Stage 2

When the patient returns to the examining table, the enema tip is inserted and the patient is again turned to the prone position. The prone position not only prevents ileal leakage with resultant opacification and overlap of the small intestine on the rectosigmoid area, but it also aids in adequate drainage of excess barium from the rectum.

The radiologist allows the barium mixture to run up to the middle of the sigmoid colon (slightly farther if the sigmoid is long). The patient is then turned onto the right side, and air is instilled through the enema tip. The air forces the barium along, distributing it throughout the colon, and the patient is turned as required for even coating of the entire colon. Spot radiographs are made as indicated. If barium flows back into the rectum, it is drained out through the enema tip. More air is then instilled. Welin stressed the importance of instilling enough air (1800 to 2000 mL or more) to obtain proper distention of the colon.

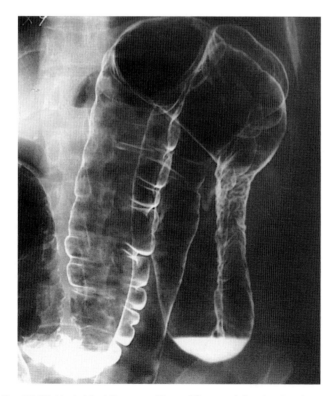

Fig. 17-85 Upright oblique position of flexure, following implementation of Welin method.

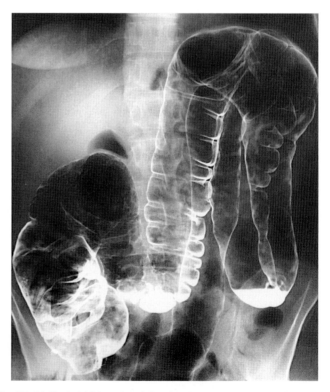

Fig. 17-86 Upright PA colon following implementation of Welin method.

When sufficient distention of the colon has been obtained, 35- × 43-cm (14- × 17-inch) radiographs are obtained (Fig. 17-87) to include the rectum, using the following sequence: a PA projection, PA oblique (LAO and RAO) projections, and a right lateral projection (24 × 30 cm [10 × 12 inches]). The patient is then turned to the supine position for an AP projection and two AP oblique (LPO and RPO) projections, all to include the transverse colon and its flexures. These studies are followed by AP projections in the right and left lateral decubitus positions to include the rectum. Finally, the patient is placed in the erect position for PA and PA oblique (RAO and LAO) projections of the horizontal colon and the left and right colic flexures.

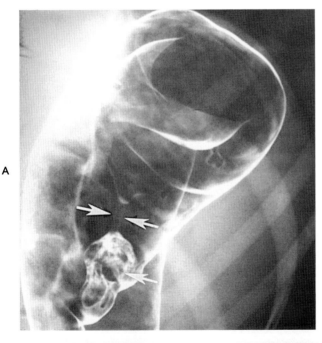

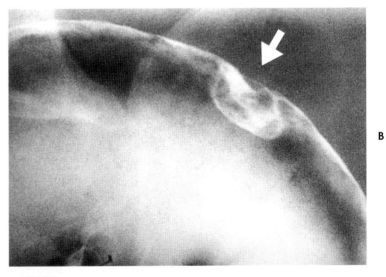

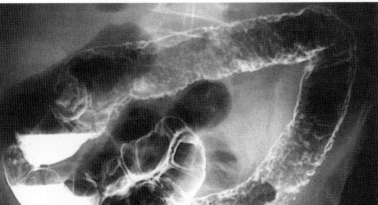

Fig. 17-87 A, Pedunculated polyps *(arrows)* during stage 2 of Welin method. **B,** Small carcinoma with intubation *(arrow)* during stage 2 of Welin method. **C,** Cobblestone appearance of granulomatous colitis in an image obtained during stage 2 of Welin method.

OPACIFIED COLON

Radiographic studies of the adult colon are made on 35- × 43-cm IRs. Except for axial projections, these IRs may be centered at the level of the iliac crests on patients of sthenic build—somewhat higher for hypersthenic patients and somewhat lower for asthenic patients. The AP and PA projections of the colon and abdomen may require two exposures, with the IRs placed crosswise: The first is centered high enough to include the diaphragm, and the second low enough to include the rectum. Localized studies of the rectum and rectosigmoid junction are often exposed on 24- × 30-cm or 30- × 35-cm IRs centered at or slightly above the level of the pubic symphysis. Preevacuation radiographs of the colon include one or more images for the demonstration of otherwise obscured flexed and curved areas of the large intestine.

Depending on the preference of the radiologist, the radiographic projections taken after fluoroscopy vary considerably. Therefore any combination of the following images may be taken to complete the examination.

▲ PA PROJECTION

Image receptor: 35 × 43 cm lengthwise

Position of patient
- Place the patient in the prone position.

Position of part
- Center the midsagittal plane to the grid.
- Adjust the center of the IR at the level of the iliac crests (Fig. 17-88).
- In addition to positioning for the PA projection, place the fluoroscopic table in a slight Trendelenburg position if necessary. This table position helps separate redundant and overlapping loops of the bowel by "spilling" them out of the pelvis.
- *Shield gonads.*
- *Respiration:* Suspend.

Central ray
- Perpendicular to the IR to enter the midline of the body at the level of the iliac crests

Structures shown

The PA projection demonstrates the entire colon with the patient prone (Figs. 17-89 to 17-91).

EVALUATION CRITERIA

The following should be clearly demonstrated:
- Entire colon including the flexures and the rectum (Two IRs may be necessary for hypersthenic patients.)
- Vertebral column centered so that the ascending and descending portions of the colon are included

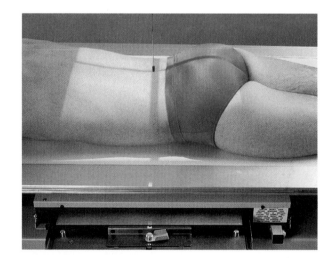

Fig. 17-88 PA large intestine.

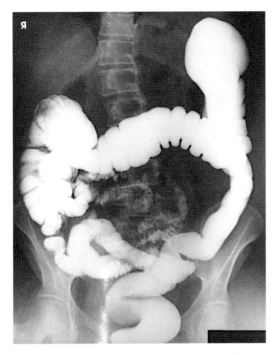

Fig. 17-89 Single-contrast PA large intestine.

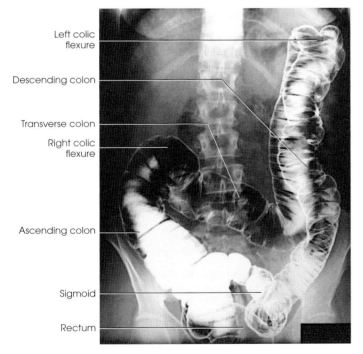

Left colic flexure

Descending colon

Transverse colon

Right colic flexure

Ascending colon

Sigmoid

Rectum

Fig. 17-90 Double-contrast PA large intestine, hyposthenic body habitus.

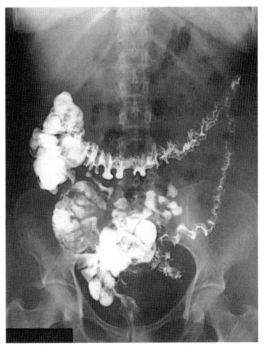

Fig. 17-91 Postevacuation PA large intestine.

✿ PA AXIAL PROJECTION

Image receptor: 35 × 43 cm or 24 × 30 cm lengthwise

Position of patient
- Place the patient in the prone position.

Position of part
- Center the midsagittal plane to the grid.
- Adjust the center of the IR at the level of the iliac crests (Fig. 17-92).
- *Shield gonads.*
- *Respiration:* Suspend.

Central ray
- Directed 30 to 40 degrees caudad to enter the midline of the body at the level of the anterior superior iliac spine (ASIS)

Structures shown
The PA axial projection best demonstrates the rectosigmoid area of the colon (Figs. 17-93 and 17-94).

The following should be clearly demonstrated:
- Rectosigmoid area centered to radiograph
- Rectosigmoid area with less superimposition than in the PA projection because of the angulation of the central ray
- Transverse colon and both flexures not necessarily included

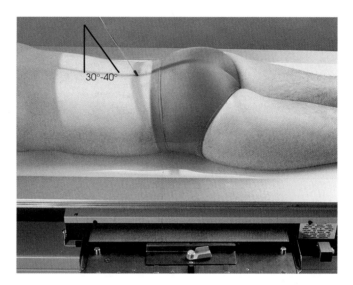

Fig. 17-92 PA axial large intestine.

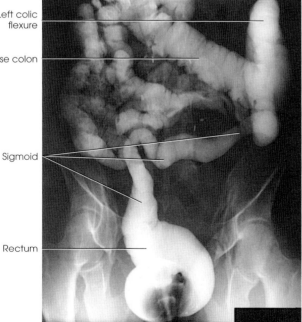

Left colic flexure

Transverse colon

Sigmoid

Rectum

Fig. 17-93 Single-contrast PA axial (30-degree angulation) large intestine.

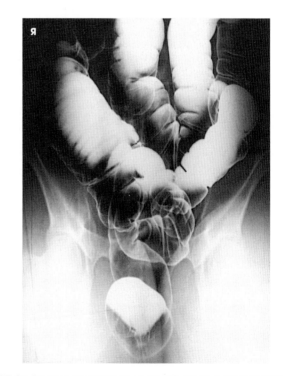

Fig. 17-94 Double-contrast PA axial (40-degree angulation) large intestine.

PA OBLIQUE PROJECTION
RAO position

Image receptor 35 × 43 cm lengthwise

Position of patient
- Place the patient in the prone position.

Position of part
- With the patient's right arm by the side of the body and the left hand by the head, have the patient roll onto the right hip to obtain a 35- to 45-degree rotation from the radiographic table.
- Flex the patient's left knee to provide stability.
- Center the patient's body to the midline of the grid.
- Adjust the center of the IR at the level of the iliac crests (Fig. 17-95).
- *Shield gonads.*
- *Respiration:* Suspend.

Central ray
- Perpendicular to the IR and entering approximately 1 to 2 inches (2.5 to 5 cm) lateral to the midline of the body on the elevated side at the level of the iliac crest

Structures shown
The RAO position best demonstrates the right colic flexure, the ascending portion of the colon, and the sigmoid portion of the colon (Figs. 17-96 and 17-97).

The following should be clearly demonstrated:
- Entire colon
- Right colic flexure less superimposed or open when compared with the PA projection
- Ascending colon, cecum, and sigmoid colon

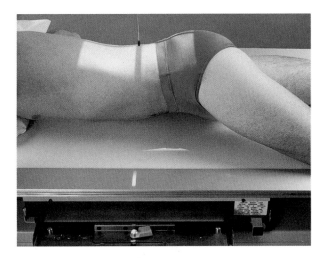

Fig. 17-95 PA oblique large intestine, RAO position.

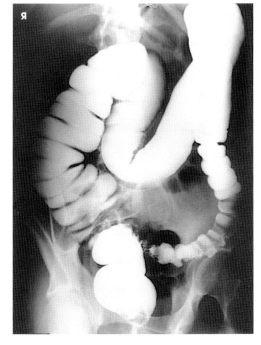

Fig. 17-96 Single-contrast PA oblique large intestine, RAO position.

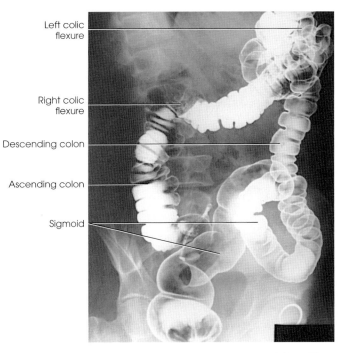

Left colic flexure

Right colic flexure

Descending colon

Ascending colon

Sigmoid

Fig. 17-97 Double-contrast PA oblique large intestine, RAO position.

♠ PA OBLIQUE PROJECTION
LAO position

Image receptor: 35 × 43 cm lengthwise

Position of patient
- Place the patient in the prone position.

Position of part
- With the patient's left arm by the side of the body and the right hand by the head, have the patient roll onto the left hip to obtain a 35- to 45-degree rotation from the radiographic table.
- Flex the patient's right knee to provide stability.
- Center the patient's body to the midline of the grid.
- Adjust the center of the IR at the level of the iliac crest (Fig. 17-98).
- *Shield gonads.*
- *Respiration:* Suspend.

Central ray
- Perpendicular to the IR and entering approximately 1 to 2 inches (2.5 to 5 cm) lateral to the midline of the body on the elevated side at the level of the iliac crest

Structures shown
The LAO position best demonstrates the left colic flexure and the descending portion of the colon (Figs. 17-99 and 17-100).

The following should be clearly demonstrated:
- Entire colon
- Left colic flexure less superimposed or open when compared with the PA projection
- Descending colon

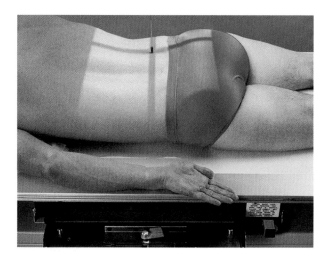

Fig. 17-98 PA oblique large intestine, LAO position.

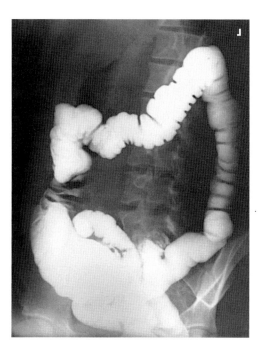

Fig. 17-99 Single-contrast PA oblique large intestine, LAO position.

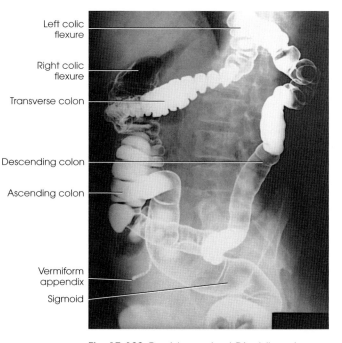

Left colic flexure

Right colic flexure

Transverse colon

Descending colon

Ascending colon

Vermiform appendix

Sigmoid

Fig. 17-100 Double-contrast PA oblique large intestine, LAO position.

▲ LATERAL PROJECTION
R or L position

Image receptor: 24 × 30 cm lengthwise

Position of patient
- Place the patient in the lateral recumbent position on either the left or right side.

Position of part
- Center the midcoronal plane to the center of the grid.
- Flex the patient's knees slightly for stability, and place a support between the knees to keep the pelvis lateral.
- Adjust the patient's shoulders and hips to be perpendicular (Fig. 17-101).
- Adjust the center of the IR to the ASIS.
- *Shield gonads.*
- *Respiration:* Suspend.

Central ray
- Perpendicular to the IR to enter the midcoronal plane at the level of the ASIS

Structures shown
The lateral projection best demonstrates the rectum and distal sigmoid portion of the colon (Figs. 17-102 and 17-103).

The following should be clearly demonstrated:
- ■ Rectosigmoid area in the center of the radiograph
- ■ No rotation of the patient
- ■ Superimposed hips and femurs
- ■ Superior portion of colon not necessarily included when the rectosigmoid region is the area of interest

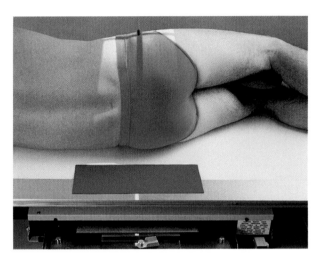

Fig. 17-101 Left lateral rectum.

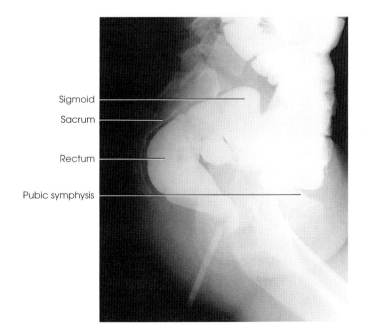

Sigmoid

Sacrum

Rectum

Pubic symphysis

Fig. 17-102 Single-contrast left lateral rectum.

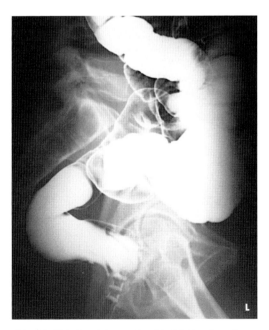

Fig. 17-103 Double-contrast left lateral rectum.

Large intestine

♠ AP PROJECTION

Image receptor: 35 × 43 cm lengthwise

Position of patient
• Place the patient in the supine position.

Position of part
• Center the midsagittal plane to the grid.
• Adjust the center of the IR at the level of the iliac crests (Fig. 17-104).
• *Shield gonads.*
• *Respiration:* Suspend.

Central ray
• Perpendicular to the IR to enter the midline of the body at the level of the iliac crests

Structures shown
The AP projection demonstrates the entire colon with the patient supine (Figs. 17-105 and 17-106).

The following should be clearly demonstrated:
■ Entire colon including the splenic flexure and the rectum (Two IRs may be necessary for hypersthenic patients.)
■ Vertebral column centered so that the ascending colon and the descending colon are completely included

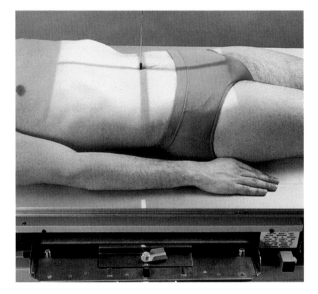

Fig. 17-104 AP large intestine.

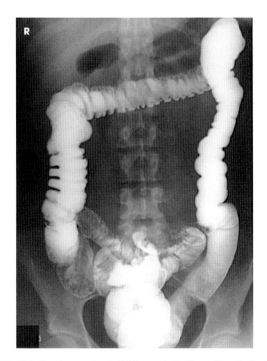

Fig. 17-105 Single-contrast AP large intestine, sthenic habitus.

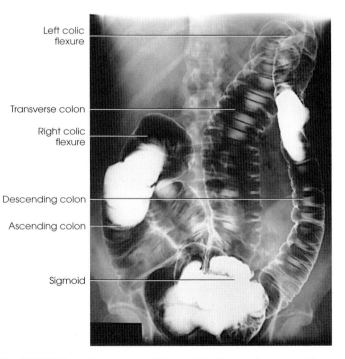

Left colic flexure

Transverse colon

Right colic flexure

Descending colon

Ascending colon

Sigmoid

Fig. 17-106 Double-contrast AP large intestine, asthenic habitus.

⚜ AP AXIAL PROJECTION

Image receptor: 35 × 43 cm or 24 × 30 cm lengthwise

Position of patient
• Place the patient in the supine position.

Position of part
• Center the midsagittal plane to the grid.
• Adjust the center of the IR at a level approximately 2 inches (5 cm) above the level of the iliac crests (Fig. 17-107).
• *Shield gonads.*
• *Respiration:* Suspend.

Central ray
• Directed 30 to 40 degrees cephalad to enter the midline of the body approximately 2 inches (5 cm) below the level of the ASIS
• Directed to enter the inferior margin of the pubic symphysis when a collimated image is desired for demonstration of the rectosigmoid region

Structures shown
The AP axial projection best demonstrates the rectosigmoid area of the colon (Figs. 17-108 and 17-109). A similar image is obtained when the patient is prone (see Fig. 17-92).

EVALUATION CRITERIA
The following should be clearly demonstrated:
■ Rectosigmoid area centered when using a 24- × 30-cm IR
■ Rectosigmoid area with less superimposition than in the AP projection because of the angulation of the central ray
■ Transverse colon and flexures not necessarily included

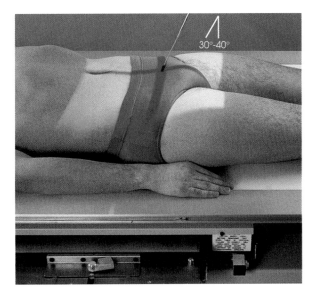

Fig. 17-107 AP axial large intestine.

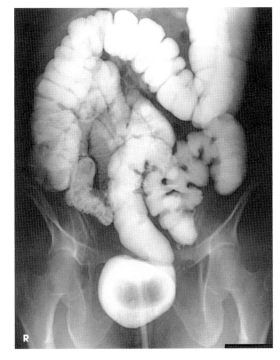

Fig. 17-108 Single-contrast AP axial large intestine.

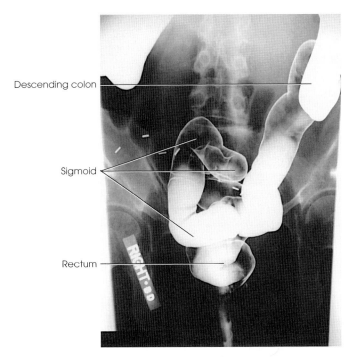

Descending colon

Sigmoid

Rectum

Fig. 17-109 Double-contrast AP axial large intestine.

♠ AP OBLIQUE PROJECTION
LPO position

Image receptor: 35 × 43 cm lengthwise

Position of patient
• Place the patient in the supine position.

Position of part
• With the patient's left arm by the side of the body and the right arm across the superior chest, have the patient roll onto the left hip to obtain a 35- to 45-degree rotation from the table.
• Use a positioning sponge and flex the patient's right knee for stability, if necessary.
• Center the patient's body to the midline of the grid.
• Adjust the center of the IR at the level of the iliac crests (Fig. 17-110).
• *Shield gonads.*
• *Respiration:* Suspend.

Central ray
• Perpendicular to the IR to enter approximately 1 to 2 inches (2.5 to 5 cm) lateral to the midline of the body on the elevated side at the level of the iliac crest

Structures shown
The LPO position best demonstrates the right colic flexure and the ascending and sigmoid portions of the colon (Figs. 17-111 and 17-112).

EVALUATION CRITERIA
The following should be clearly demonstrated:
■ Entire colon
■ Right colic flexure less superimposed or open when compared with the AP projection
■ Ascending colon, cecum, and sigmoid colon

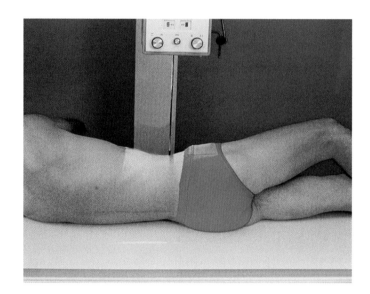

Fig. 17-110 AP oblique large intestine, LPO position.

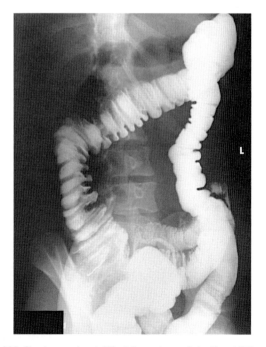

Fig. 17-111 Single-contrast AP oblique large intestine, LPO position.

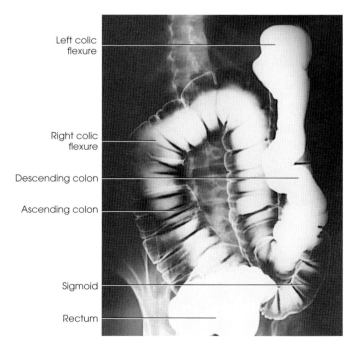

Left colic flexure
Right colic flexure
Descending colon
Ascending colon
Sigmoid
Rectum

Fig. 17-112 Double-contrast AP oblique large intestine, LPO position.

♠ AP OBLIQUE PROJECTION
RPO position

Image receptor: 35 × 43 cm lengthwise

Position of patient
- Place the patient in the supine position.

Position of part
- With the patient's right arm by the side of the body and the left arm across the superior chest, have the patient roll onto the right hip to obtain a 35- to 45-degree rotation from the radiographic table.
- Use a positioning sponge and flex the patient's right knee for stability, if needed.
- Center the patient's body to the midline of the grid.
- Adjust the center of the IR at the level of the iliac crests (Fig. 17-113).
- *Shield gonads.*
- *Respiration:* Suspend.

Central ray
- Perpendicular to the IR to enter approximately 1 to 2 inches (2.5 to 5 cm) lateral to the midline of the body on the elevated side at the level of the iliac crest

Structures shown
The RPO position best demonstrates the left colic flexure and the descending colon (Figs. 17-114 and 17-115).

The following should be clearly demonstrated:
- Entire colon
- Left colic flexure and descending colon

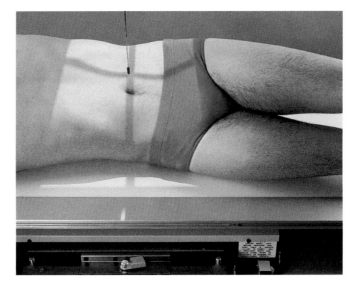

Fig. 17-113 AP oblique large intestine, RPO position.

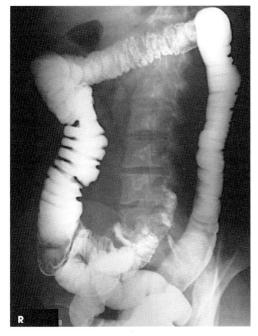

Fig. 17-114 Single-contrast AP oblique large intestine, RPO position.

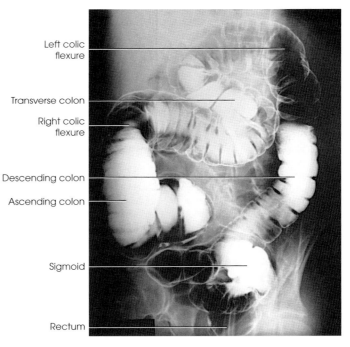

Left colic flexure

Transverse colon

Right colic flexure

Descending colon

Ascending colon

Sigmoid

Rectum

Fig. 17-115 Double-contrast AP oblique large intestine, RPO position.

Decubitus Positions

When a patient is being prepared for an examination in a decubitus position, the following general guidelines are observed:

- Take all decubitus radiographs (1) with the patient lying on the fluoroscopic table and a grid IR firmly supported behind the patient's body, (2) with the patient lying on a patient cart with the body against an upright table or chest device, or (3) with the patient lying on a table or cart and a specially designed vertical grid device behind the patient.

- To ensure demonstration of the side on which the patient is lying, elevate the patient on a suitable radiolucent support. If this is not done, the radiograph will record artifacts from the patient mattress or the table edge and superimpose these images over the portion of the patient's colon on the "down" side.

- For all decubitus procedures, *exercise extreme caution* to ensure that the wheels of the cart are securely locked so that the patient will not fall.

- For lateral decubitus radiographs, have the patient put the back or abdomen against the vertical grid device. Most patients find it more comfortable to have their back against the vertical grid device than to have their abdomen against the same device.

- If both lateral decubitus radiographs are requested (which is often the case with air-contrast examinations), take one radiograph with the patient's anterior body surface against the vertical grid device and the second radiograph with the posterior body surface against the vertical grid device.

♠ AP OR PA PROJECTION
Right lateral decubitus position

Image receptor: 35 × 43 cm lengthwise

Position of patient
- Place the patient on the right side with the back or abdomen in contact with the vertical grid device.
- *Exercise care* to ensure that the patient does not fall from the cart or table; if a cart is used, *lock all wheels* securely.

Position of part
- With the patient lying on an elevated radiolucent support, center the midsagittal plane to the grid.
- Adjust the center of the IR to the level of the iliac crests (Fig. 17-116).
- *Shield gonads.*
- *Respiration:* Suspend.

Central ray
- *Horizontal* and perpendicular to the IR to enter the midline of the body at the level of the iliac crests

Structures shown
The right lateral decubitus position demonstrates an AP or PA projection of the contrast-filled colon. This position best demonstrates the "up" medial side of the ascending colon and the lateral side of the descending colon when the colon is inflated with air (Figs. 17-117 and 17-118).

EVALUATION CRITERIA
The following should be clearly demonstrated:
- ■ Area from the left colic flexure to the rectum
- ■ No rotation of the patient, as evidenced by the ribs and pelvis
- ■ For single-contrast examinations, adequate penetration of the barium; for double-contrast examinations, the air-inflated portion of the colon is of primary importance and should not be overpenetrated.

▼ COMPENSATING FILTER
Image quality can be improved on larger patients with the use of a special decubitus filter.

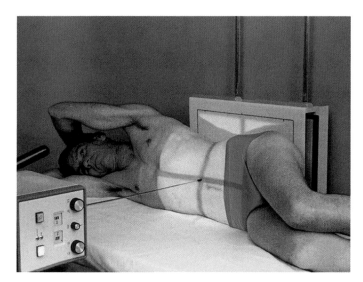

Fig. 17-116 AP large intestine, right lateral decubitus position.

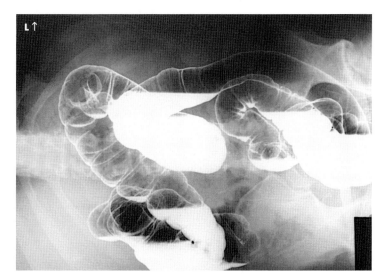

Fig. 17-117 Double-contrast AP large intestine, right lateral decubitus position.

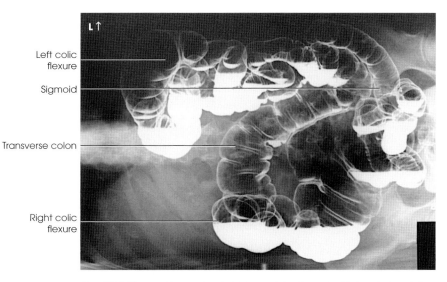

Left colic flexure

Sigmoid

Transverse colon

Right colic flexure

Fig. 17-118 Double-contrast AP large intestine, right lateral decubitus position.

🌢 PA OR AP PROJECTION
Left lateral decubitus position

Image receptor: 35 × 43 cm lengthwise

Position of patient
- Place the patient on the left side with the abdomen or back in contact with the vertical grid device.
- *Exercise care* to ensure that the patient does not fall from the cart or table; if a cart is used, *lock all wheels* securely in position.

Position of part
- With the patient lying on an elevated radiolucent support, center the midsagittal plane to the grid.
- Adjust the center of the IR at the level of the iliac crests (Fig. 17-119).
- *Shield gonads.*
- *Respiration:* Suspend.

Central ray
- *Horizontal* and perpendicular to the IR to enter the midline of the body at the level of the iliac crests

Structures shown
The left lateral decubitus position demonstrates a PA or AP projection of the contrast-filled colon. This position best demonstrates the "up" lateral side of the ascending colon and the medial side of the descending colon when the colon is inflated with air (Figs. 17-120 and 17-121).

EVALUATION CRITERIA

The following should be clearly demonstrated:
- Area from the left colic flexure to the rectum
- No rotation of the patient, as evidenced by the ribs and pelvis
- For single-contrast examinations, adequate penetration of the barium; for double-contrast examinations, the air-inflated portion of the colon is of primary importance and should not be overpenetrated.

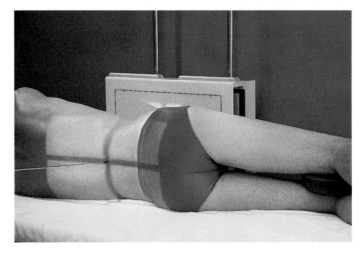

Fig. 17-119 PA large intestine, left lateral decubitus position.

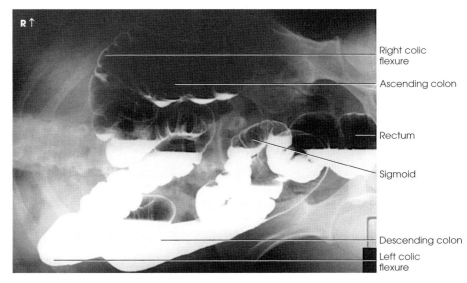

Fig. 17-120 Double-contrast PA large intestine, left lateral decubitus position.

Right colic flexure
Ascending colon
Rectum
Sigmoid
Descending colon
Left colic flexure

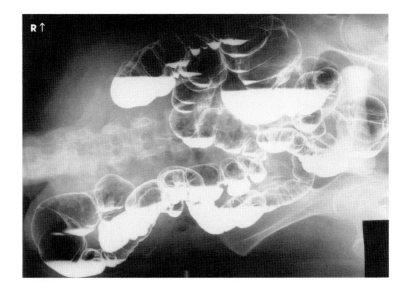

Fig. 17-121 Double-contrast PA large intestine, left lateral decubitus position.

LATERAL PROJECTION
R or L ventral decubitus position

Image receptor: 35 × 43 cm lengthwise

Position of patient
- Place the patient in the prone position with either the right or left side against the vertical grid device.

Position of part
- Elevate the patient on a radiolucent support, and center the midcoronal plane to the grid.
- Adjust the center of the IR at the level of the iliac crests.
- *Shield gonads.*
- *Respiration:* Suspend.

Central ray
- *Horizontal* and perpendicular to the IR to enter the midcoronal plane of the body at the level of the iliac crests

Structures shown
The ventral decubitus position demonstrates a lateral projection of the contrast-filled colon. This position best demonstrates the "up" posterior portions of the colon and is most valuable in double-contrast examinations (Fig. 17-122).

EVALUATION CRITERIA
The following should be clearly demonstrated:
- Area from the flexures to the rectum
- No rotation of the patient
- For single-contrast examinations, adequate penetration of the barium; for double-contrast examinations, the air-inflated portion of the colon is of primary importance and should not be overpenetrated.
- Enema tip removed for an unobstructed image of the rectum

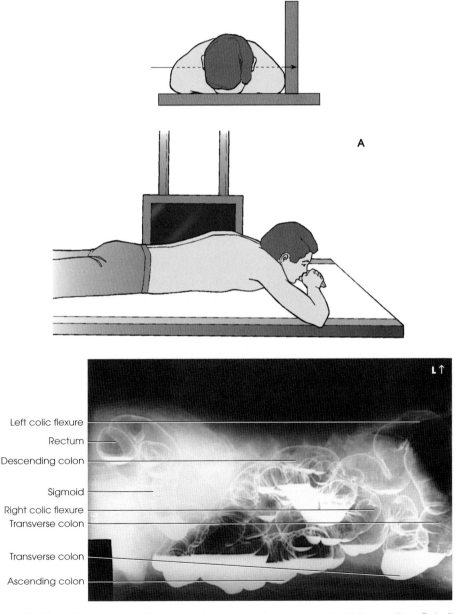

Left colic flexure
Rectum
Descending colon
Sigmoid
Right colic flexure
Transverse colon
Transverse colon
Ascending colon

Fig. 17-122 A, Patient in position for a lateral projection, ventral decubitus position. **B,** Left lateral large intestine, ventral decubitus position.

♠ AP, PA, OBLIQUE, AND LATERAL PROJECTIONS

Upright position

Upright AP, PA, oblique, and lateral projections may be taken as requested. The positioning and evaluation criteria for upright radiographs are identical to those required for the recumbent positions. However, the IR is placed at a lower level to compensate for the drop of the bowel because of the effect of gravity (Figs. 17-123 to 17-125).

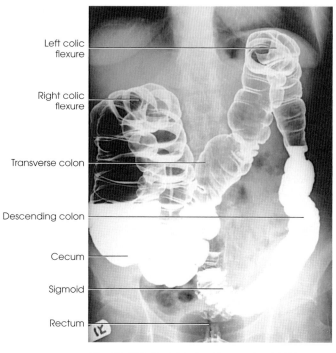

Left colic flexure

Right colic flexure

Transverse colon

Descending colon

Cecum

Sigmoid

Rectum

Fig. 17-123 Upright double-contrast AP large intestine.

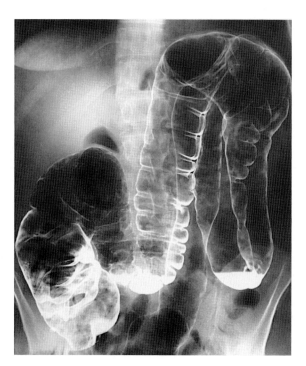

Fig. 17-124 Upright double-contrast PA large intestine.

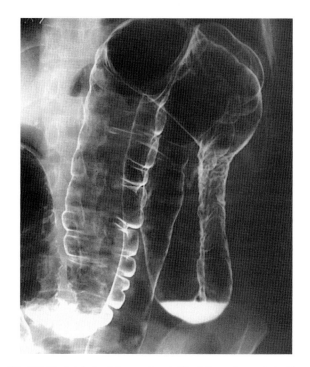

Fig. 17-125 Upright double-contrast AP oblique large intestine, RPO position.

AXIAL PROJECTION
CHASSARD-LAPINÉ METHOD

The Chassard-Lapiné method is used to demonstrate the rectum, rectosigmoid junction, and sigmoid. This projection, which is made at almost a right angle to the AP projection, demonstrates the anterior and posterior surfaces of the lower portion of the bowel and permits the coils of the sigmoid to be projected free from overlapping.[1-3] The projection may be exposed after evacuation of the large intestine, although a preevacuation radiograph can be exposed when the patient has reasonable sphincteric control.[1]

Image receptor: 30 × 35 cm lengthwise

Position of patient
- Seat the patient on the radiographic table.

Position of part
- Instruct the patient to sit well back on the side of the table so that the midcoronal plane of the body is as close as possible to the midline of the table.
- If necessary, shift the transversely placed 30- × 35-cm (11- × 14-inch) IR forward in the Bucky tray so that its transverse axis coincides as nearly as possible with the midcoronal plane of the body.

[1]Raap G: A position of value in studying the pelvis and its contents, *South Med J* 44:95, 1951.
[2]Cimmino CV: Radiography of the sigmoid flexure with the Chassard-Lapiné projection, *Med Radiogr Photogr* 30:44, 1954.
[3]Ettinger A, Elkin M: Study of the sigmoid by special roentgenographic views, *Am J Roentgenol* 72:199, 1954.

- Instruct the patient to abduct the thighs as far as the edge of the table permits so that they do not interfere with flexion of the body.
- Center the IR to the midline of the pelvis, and ask the patient to lean directly forward as far as possible (Fig. 17-126).
- Have the patient grasp the ankles for support.
- *Respiration:* Suspend.

The exposure required for this projection is approximately the same as that required for a lateral projection of the pelvis.

Central ray
- Perpendicular through the lumbosacral region at the level of the greater trochanters

Structures shown
The Chassard-Lapiné image demonstrates the rectum, rectosigmoid junction, and sigmoid in the axial projection (Fig. 17-127).

The following should be clearly demonstrated:
- Rectosigmoid area in the center of the radiograph
- Rectosigmoid area not obscured by superior area of colon
- Minimal superimposition of the rectosigmoid area
- Penetration of the lumbosacral region and the barium

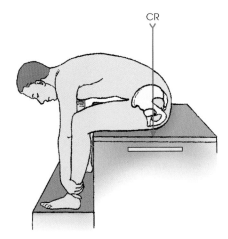

Fig. 17-126 Chassard-Lapiné method.

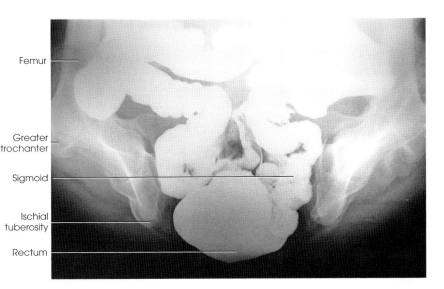

Femur

Greater trochanter

Sigmoid

Ischial tuberosity

Rectum

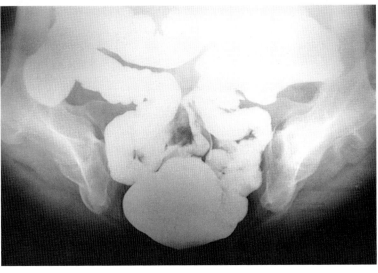

Fig. 17-127 Axial rectosigmoid: Chassard-Lapiné method.

COLOSTOMY STUDIES

Enterostomy (Gr. *enteron,* "intestine" + *stoma,* "opening") is the general term applied to the surgical procedure of forming an artificial opening to the intestine, usually through the abdominal wall, for fecal passage. The regional terms are *colostomy, cecostomy, ileostomy,* and *jejunostomy.*

The colon is the most common site of disease in the large intestine. Therefore surgical procedures are often performed on this structure. Loop colostomy is sometimes performed to divert the fecal column, either temporarily or permanently, from areas of diverticulitis or ulcerative colitis. Most colostomies, however, are performed because of malignancies of the lower bowel and rectum. When a tumor is present, the lower carcinomatous part of the bowel is resected, and the end of the remaining part of the bowel is brought to the surface through the abdominal wall. This passage, or *stoma,* has no sphincter.

Preparation of intestinal tract

Postoperative contrast enema studies are performed at suitable intervals to determine the efficacy of treatment in the patient with diverticulitis or ulcerative colitis and to detect new or recurrent lesions in the patient who has had a tumor. The demonstration of polyps and other intraluminal lesions depends on adequate cleansing of the bowel, which is as important in the presence of a colostomy as otherwise. In the patient with a colostomy, the usual preparation is irrigation of the stoma the night before the study and again on the morning of the examination.

Colostomy enema equipment

Although equipment must be scrupulously clean and nondisposable items must be sterilized after each use, sterile technique is not required because the stoma is part of the intestinal tract. Except for a suitable device to prevent stomal leakage of the contrast material, the equipment used in the patient with a colostomy is the same as that used in routine contrast enema studies. The same barium sulfate formula is used, and gas studies are made. The opaque and double-contrast studies can be performed in a single-stage examination with the use of a disposable enema kit.

A device must be used to prevent spillage of contrast enema material in the patient with a colostomy. Otherwise, because of the absence of sphincter control, the contrast enema may escape through the colostomy almost as rapidly as it is injected. If this happens, bowel filling will be unsatisfactory and shadows cast by barium soilage of the abdominal wall and the examining table will obscure areas of interest. Abdominal stomas must be effectively occluded for studies made by retrograde injection, and leakage around the stomal catheter must be prevented for studies made by injection into either an abdominal or a perineal colostomy. Numerous devices are available for this purpose.

DIAGNOSTIC ENEMA

Diagnostic enemas may be given through a colostomy stoma with the use of tips and adhesive disks designed for the patient's use in irrigating the colostomy (Fig. 17-128). The tips are available in four sizes to accommodate the usual sizes of colostomy stomas. These tips usually have a flange to prevent them from slipping through the colostomy opening. An adhesive disk is placed over the flange to minimize reflux soilage. The enema tubing is attached directly to the tip, which the patient holds in position to prevent the weight of the tubing from displacing the tip to an angled position. In addition to keeping a set of Laird tips on hand, it is recommended that the patient be asked to bring an irrigation device.

Retention catheters are also used in colostomy studies. Some radiologists use them alone, and others insert them through a device to prevent slipping and to collect leakage. Colostomy stomas are fragile and thus are subject to perforation by any undue pressure or trauma. Perforations have occurred during the insertion of an inflated bulb into a blind pouch and from overdistention of the stoma.

Preparation of patient

If the patient uses a special dressing, colostomy pouch, or stomal seal, he or she should be advised to bring a change for use after the examination. When fecal emission is such that a pouch is required, the patient should be given a suitable dressing to place over the stoma after the device has been removed.

The radiographer then observes the following steps:

- Clothe the patient in a kimono type of gown that opens in front or back, depending on the location of the colostomy.
- Place the patient on the examining table in the supine position if he or she has an abdominal colostomy and in the prone position if he or she has a perineal colostomy.
- Before taking the preliminary radiograph and while wearing disposable gloves, remove and discard any dressing.
- Cleanse the skin around the stoma appropriately.
- Place a gauze dressing over the stoma to absorb any seepage until the physician is ready to start the examination.
- Lubricate the stomal catheter or tube well (but not excessively) with a water-soluble lubricant. The catheter should be inserted by the physician or the patient. If a catheter is forced through a stoma, the colon may be perforated.

Spot radiographs are taken during the examination. Postfluoroscopy radiographs are taken as needed. The projections requested depend on the location of the stoma and the anatomy to be demonstrated (Figs. 17-129 to 17-132).

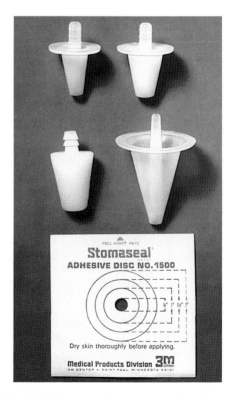

Fig. 17-128 Laird colostomy irrigation tips and Stomaseal disks.

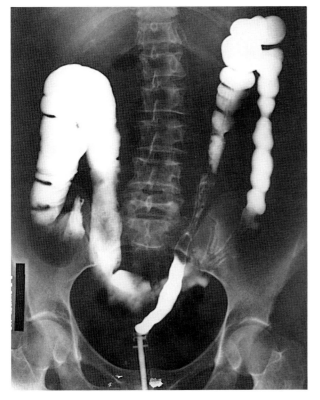

Fig. 17-129 Opaque colon by way of perineal colostomy.

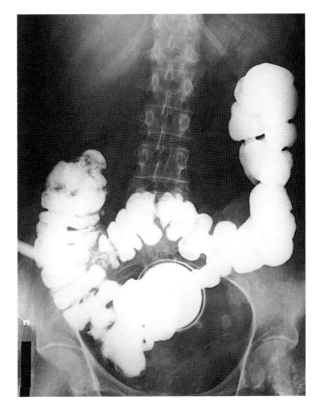

Fig. 17-130 Opaque colon by way of abdominal colostomy.

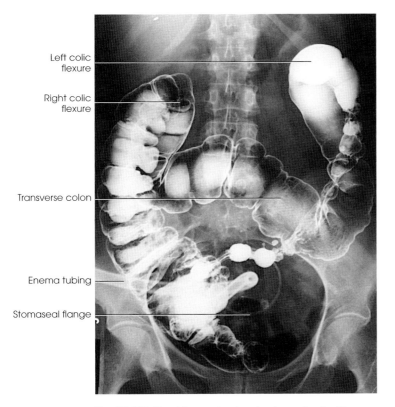

Left colic flexure

Right colic flexure

Transverse colon

Enema tubing

Stomaseal flange

Fig. 17-131 Double-contrast colon in patient with abdominal colostomy.

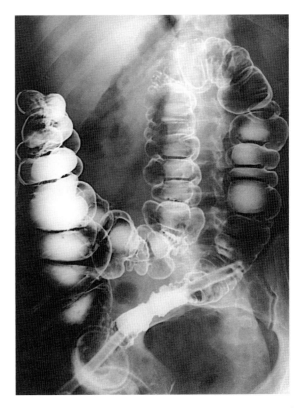

Fig. 17-132 Double-contrast AP oblique colon by way of abdominal colostomy.

Digestive system

DEFECOGRAPHY

Defecography, evacuation proctography, or *dynamic rectal examination* is a relatively new radiologic procedure performed on patients with defecational dysfunction. No preparation of the patient is necessary, and cleansing enemas are not recommended because water remaining in the rectum dilutes the contrast medium.

Early investigators[1] mixed a diluted suspension of barium sulfate, heated it, and added potato starch to form a smooth barium paste that was semisolid and malleable.[2,3] Barium manufacturers now package prepared barium products (≈100% weight/volume barium sulfate paste) with a special injector mechanism to instill the barium directly into the rectum. In addition, viscous barium may be introduced into the vagina and the bladder filled with aqueous iodinated contrast media.

[1]Burhenne HJ: Intestinal evacuation study: a new roentgenologic technique, *Radiol Clin (Basel)* 33:79, 1964.
[2]Mahieu P, Pringot J, Bodart P: Defecography. I. Description of a new procedure and results in normal patients, *Gastrointest Radiol* 9:247, 1984.
[3]Mahieu P, Pringot J, Bodart P: Defecography. II. Contribution to the diagnosis of defecation disorders, *Gastrointest Radiol* 9:253, 1984.

After the contrast media is instilled, the patient is usually seated in the lateral position on a commercially available radiolucent commode in front of a fluoroscopic unit. A special commode chair is recommended so that the anorectal junction and the zone of interest on the radiograph are not overexposed. Lateral projections are obtained during defecation by spot filming at the approximate rate of 1 to 2 frames per second. Video recording of the defecation process may be used, but the special equipment necessary to interpret the images is not always available and a hard copy of the images is not available.[1] The resulting images are then evaluated (Figs. 17-133). This evaluation includes measurements of the anorectal angle and the angle between the long axes of the anal canal and rectum. These measurements are then compared with normal values. In addition, changes in proximity of the rectum to the vagina and bladder during defecation are assessed when these structures have been filled with contrast media (Fig. 17-134).

[1]Mahieu PHG: Defecography. In Margulis AR, Burhenne H: *Alimentary tract radiology,* vol 1, ed 4, St Louis, 1989, Mosby.

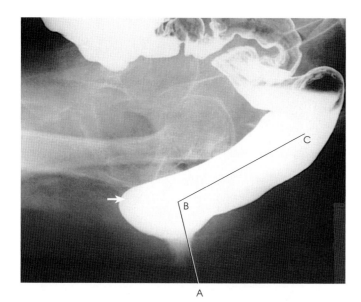

Fig. 17-133 Defecography: lateral anus and rectum spot image showing long axis of anal canal *(line A-B)* and long axis of rectal canal *(line B-C)* in a patient with an anorectal angle of 114 degrees. Also demonstrated is an anterior rectocele *(arrow).*

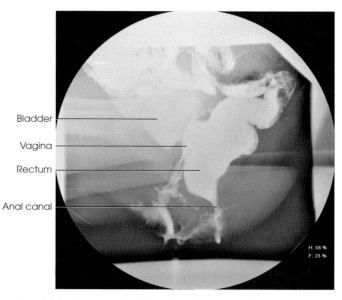

Bladder

Vagina

Rectum

Anal canal

Fig. 17-134 Defecography: lateral anal canal and rectum, vagina, and urinary bladder demonstrated during patient straining.

(Courtesy Michelle Alting, AS, RT(R).)

18

URINARY SYSTEM AND VENIPUNCTURE

VENIPUNCTURE CONTRIBUTED BY STEVEN C. JENSEN AND ERIC P. MATTHEWS

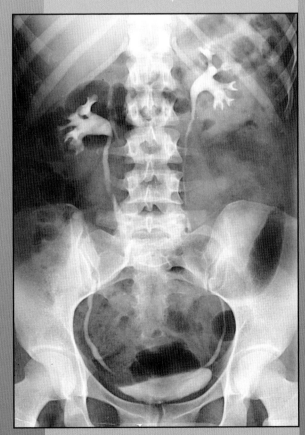

Excretory urogram.

SUMMARY OF PROJECTIONS

PROJECTIONS, POSITIONS, AND METHODS

Page	Essential	Anatomy	Projection	Position	Method
218	⚘	Urinary system	AP		
220	⚘	Urinary system	AP oblique	RPO and LPO	
221	⚘	Urinary system	Lateral	R or L	
222	⚘	Urinary system	Lateral	Dorsal decubitus	
223		Renal parenchymal	AP		
228	⚘	Pelvicaliceal system and ureters: *retrograde urography*	AP		
232	⚘	Urinary bladder	AP axial or PA axial		
234	⚘	Urinary bladder	AP oblique	RPO or LPO	
236	⚘	Urinary bladder	Lateral	R or L	
237	⚘	Male cystourethrography	AP oblique	RPO or LPO	
238		Female cystourethrography	AP		INJECTION

Icons in the Essential column indicate projections frequently performed in the United States and Canada. Students should be competent in these projections.

Urinary System

The *urinary system* includes the two *kidneys*, two *ureters*, one *urinary bladder*, and one *urethra* (Figs. 18-1 and 18-2). The functions of the kidneys include removing waste products from the blood, maintaining fluid and electrolyte balance, and secreting substances that affect blood pressure and other important body functions. The kidneys normally excrete 1 to 2 L of urine per day. This urine is expelled from the body via the *excretory system,* as the urinary system is often called. The excretory system consists of the following:

- A variable number of urine-draining branches in the kidney called the *calyces* and an expanded portion called the *renal pelvis,* which together are known as the *pelvicaliceal system*
- Two long tubes called *ureters,* with one ureter extending from the pelvis of each kidney
- A saclike portion, the *urinary bladder,* which receives the distal portion of the ureters and serves as a reservoir
- A third and smaller tubular portion, the *urethra,* which conveys the urine to the exterior of the body

Suprarenal Glands

Closely associated with the urinary system are the two *suprarenal,* or *adrenal, glands.* These ductless endocrine glands have no functional relationship with the urinary system but are included in this chapter because of their anatomic relationship with the kidneys. Each suprarenal gland consists of a small, flattened body composed of an internal *medullary portion* and an outer *cortical portion.* Each gland is enclosed in a fibrous sheath and is situated in the retroperitoneal tissue in close contact with the fatty capsule overlying the medial and superior aspects of the upper pole of the kidney. The suprarenal glands furnish two important substances: (1) epinephrine, which is secreted by the medulla, and (2) the cortical hormones, which are secreted by the cortex. These glands are subject to malfunction and a number of diseases. They are not usually demonstrated on preliminary radiographs but are delineated when computed tomography (CT) is used. The suprarenal circulation may be demonstrated by selective catheterization of a suprarenal artery or vein in angiographic procedures.

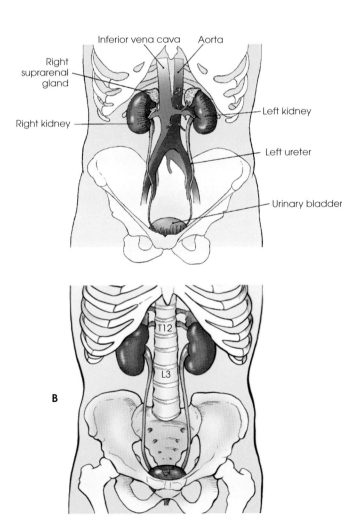

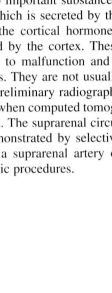

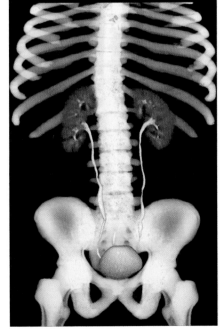

Fig. 18-1 Anterior aspect of urinary system in relation to surrounding structures. **A,** Abdominal structures. **B,** Bony structures. **C,** Three-dimensional CT image of urinary system in relation to bony structures.

Kidneys

The *kidneys* are bean-shaped bodies. The lateral border of each organ is convex, and the medial border is concave. They have slightly convex anterior and posterior surfaces, and they are arbitrarily divided into upper and lower poles. The kidneys measure approximately 4½ inches (11.5 cm) in length, 2 to 3 inches (5 to 7.6 cm) in width, and about 1¼ inches (3 cm) in thickness. The left kidney usually is slightly longer and narrower than the right kidney.

The kidneys are situated behind the peritoneum (retroperitoneal) and are in contact with the posterior wall of the abdominal cavity, one kidney lying on each side of and in the same coronal plane with L3. The superior aspect of the kidney lies more posterior than the inferior aspect (see Fig. 18-2). Each kidney lies in an oblique plane and is rotated about 30 degrees anteriorly toward the aorta, which lies on top of the vertebral body (Fig. 18-3). When the body is rotated 30 degrees for the AP oblique projection (LPO or RPO position), the lower kidney lies perpendicular and the upper kidney lies parallel to the IR. The kidneys normally extend from the level of the superior border of T12 to the level of transverse processes of L3 in persons of sthenic build; they are somewhat higher in individuals of hypersthenic habitus and somewhat lower in those of asthenic habitus. Because of the large space occupied by the liver, the right kidney is slightly lower in position than the left kidney.

The outer covering of the kidney is called the *renal capsule.* The capsule is a semitransparent membrane that is continuous with the outer coat of the ureter. Each kidney is embedded in a mass of fatty tissue called the adipose capsule. The capsule and kidney are enveloped in a sheath of superficial fascia, the renal fascia, which is attached to the diaphragm, lumbar vertebrae, peritoneum, and other adjacent structures. The kidneys are supported in a fairly fixed position, partially through the fascial attachments and partially by the surrounding organs. They have a respiratory movement of approximately 1 inch (2.5 cm) and normally drop no more than 2 inches (5 cm) in the change from supine to upright position.

The concave medial border of each kidney has a longitudinal slit, or *hilum,* for transmission of the blood and lymphatic vessels, nerves, and ureter (Fig. 18-4). The hilum expands into the body of the kidney to form a central cavity called the *renal sinus.* The renal sinus is a fat-filled space surrounding the renal pelvis and vessels.

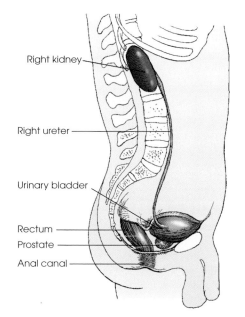

Fig. 18-2 Lateral aspect of male urinary system in relation to surrounding structures.

Right kidney
Right ureter
Urinary bladder
Rectum
Prostate
Anal canal

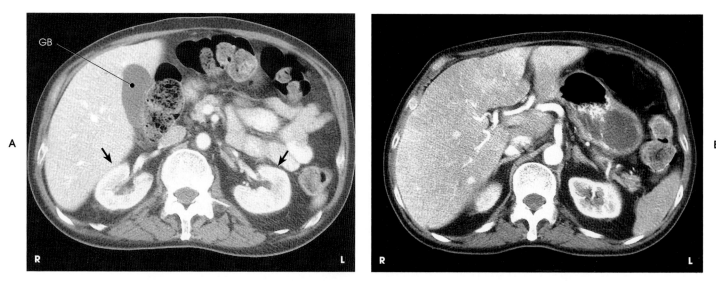

Fig. 18-3 A, Axial CT image through the center of the kidney. Note the 30-degree anterior angulation of the kidneys *(arrows). GB,* Gallbladder. **B,** Axial CT image of the upper abdomen. Note superior aspect of the right kidney and midportion of the left kidney demonstrating a lower-placed left kidney.

(From Kelley LL, Petersen CM: *Sectional anatomy for imaging professionals,* St Louis, 1997, Mosby.)

Each kidney has an outer renal cortex and an inner *renal medulla.* The renal medulla, composed mainly of the collecting tubules that give it a striated appearance, consists of 8 to 15 cone-shaped segments called the *renal pyramids.* The apices of the segments converge toward the renal sinus to drain into the pelvicaliceal system. The more compact renal cortex lies between the periphery of the organ and the bases of the medullary segments and extends medially between the pyramids to the renal sinus. These extensions of the cortex are called *renal columns.*

The essential microscopic components of the parenchyma of the kidney are called *nephrons* (Fig. 18-5). Each kidney contains approximately 1 million of these tubular structures. The individual nephron is composed of a *renal corpuscle* and a *renal tubule.* The renal corpuscle consists of a double-walled membranous cup called the *glomerular capsule* (Bowman's capsule) and a cluster of blood capillaries called the *glomerulus.* The glomerulus is formed by a minute branch of the renal artery entering the capsule and dividing

into capillaries. The capillaries then turn back and, as they ascend, unite to form a single vessel leaving the capsule.

The vessel entering the capsule is called the *afferent arteriole,* and the one leaving the capsule is termed the *efferent arteriole.* After exiting the glomerular capsules, the efferent arterioles form the capillary network surrounding the straight and convoluted tubules, and these capillaries reunite and continue on to communicate with the renal veins.

The thin inner wall of the capsule closely adheres to the capillary coils and is separated by a comparatively wide space from the outer layer, which is continuous with the beginning of a renal tubule. The glomerulus serves as a filter for the blood, permitting water and finely dissolved substances to pass through the walls of the capillaries into the capsule. The change from filtrate to urine is caused in part by the water and the usable dissolved substances being absorbed through the epithelial lining of the tubules into the surrounding capillary network.

Each *renal tubule* continues from a glomerular capsule in the cortex of the

kidney and then travels a circuitous path through the cortical and medullary substances, becoming the *proximal convoluted tubule,* the *nephron loop* (loop of Henle), and the *distal convoluted tubule.* The distal convoluted tubule opens into the collecting ducts that begin in the cortex. The *collecting ducts* converge toward the renal pelvis and unite along their course so that each group within the pyramid forms a central tubule that opens at a *renal papilla* and drains its tributaries into the minor calyx.

The *calyces* are cup-shaped stems arising at the sides of the papilla of each renal pyramid. Each calyx encloses one or more papillae, so that there are usually fewer calyces than pyramids. The beginning branches are called the *minor calyces* (numbering from 4 to 13), and they unite to form two or three larger tubes called the *major calyces.* The major calyces unite to form the expanded, funnel-shaped renal pelvis. The wide, upper portion of the *renal pelvis* lies within the hilum, and its tapering lower part passes through the hilum to become continuous with the ureter.

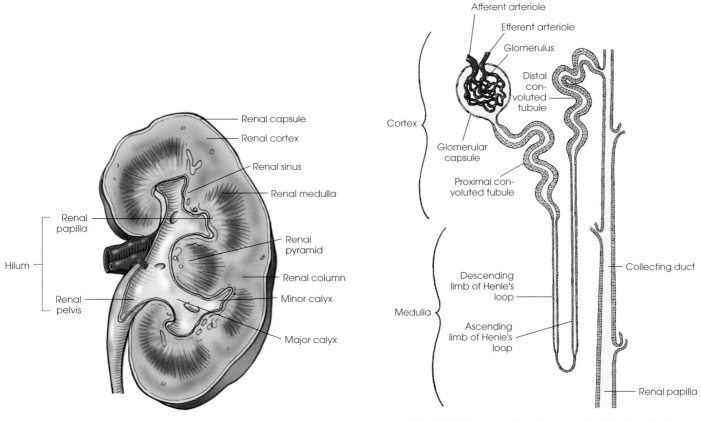

Fig. 18-4 Midcoronal section of kidney.

Fig. 18-5 Diagram of nephron and collecting duct.

Ureters

Each *ureter* is 10 to 12 inches (25 to 30 cm) long. They descend behind the peritoneum and in front of the psoas muscle and the transverse processes of the lumbar vertebrae, pass inferiorly and posteriorly in front of the sacral wing, and then curve anteriorly and medially to enter the posterolateral surface of the urinary bladder at approximately the level of the ischial spine. The ureters convey the urine from the renal pelves to the bladder by slow, rhythmic peristaltic contractions.

Urinary Bladder

The *urinary bladder* is a musculomembranous sac that serves as a reservoir for urine. The bladder is situated immediately posterior and superior to the pubic symphysis and is directly anterior to the rectum in the male and anterior to the vaginal canal in the female. The *apex* of the bladder is at the anterosuperior aspect and is adjacent to the superior aspect of the pubic symphysis. The most fixed part of the bladder is the neck, which rests on the prostate in the male and on the pelvic diaphragm in the female.

The bladder varies in size, shape, and position according to its content. It is freely movable and is held in position by folds of the peritoneum. When empty, the bladder is located in the pelvic cavity. As the bladder fills, it gradually assumes an oval shape while expanding superiorly and anteriorly into the abdominal cavity. The adult bladder can hold approximately 500 mL of fluid when completely full. The desire for *micturition* (urination) occurs when about 250 mL of urine is in the bladder.

The ureters enter the posterior wall of the bladder at the lateral margins of the superior part of its *base* and pass obliquely through the wall to their respective internal orifices (Fig. 18-6). These two openings are about 1 inch (2.5 cm) apart when the bladder is empty and about 2 inches (5 cm) apart when the bladder is distended. The openings are equidistant from the internal urethral orifice, which is situated at the neck (lowest part) of the bladder. The triangular area between the three orifices is called the *trigone*. The mucosa over the trigone is always smooth, whereas the remainder of the lining contains folds, called *rugae*, when the bladder is empty.

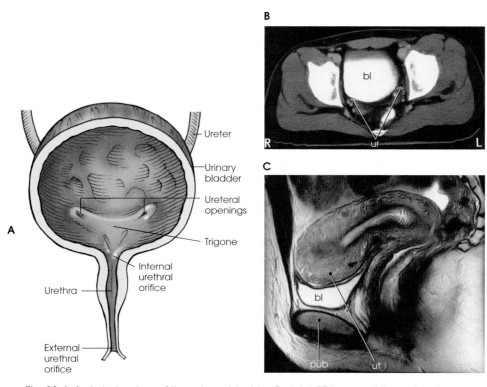

Fig. 18-6 A, Anterior view of the urinary bladder. **B,** Axial CT image of the pelvis demonstrating a contrast filled bladder *(bl)* and ureters *(ur)*. **C,** Sagittal MRI image of female pelvis showing contrast filled bladder *(bl)* and relationship to uterus *(ut)* and pubis *(pub)*.

(**B** and **C,** From Kelley LL, Petersen CM: *Sectional anatomy for imaging professionals,* St Louis, 1997, Mosby.)

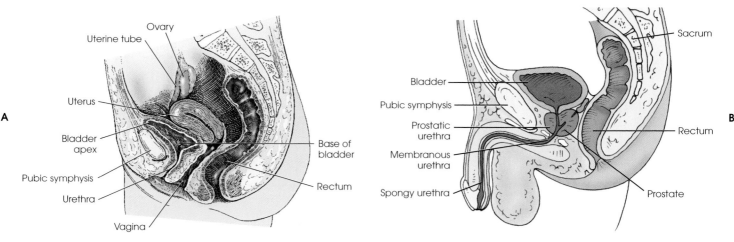

Fig. 18-7 A, Midsagittal section through female pelvis. **B,** Male pelvis.

Urethra

The *urethra,* which conveys the urine out of the body, is a narrow, musculomembranous tube with a sphincter type of muscle at the neck of the bladder. The urethra arises at the internal urethral orifice in the urinary bladder and extends about 1½ inches (3.8 cm) in the female and 7 to 8 inches (17.8 to 20 cm) in the male.

The female urethra passes along the thick anterior wall of the vagina to the external urethral orifice, which is located in the vestibule about 1 inch (2.5 cm) anterior to the vaginal opening (see Fig. 18-6). The male urethra extends from the bladder to the end of the penis and is divided into *prostatic, membranous,* and *spongy* portions (Fig. 18-7). The prostatic portion is about 1 inch (2.5 cm) in length, reaches from the bladder to the floor of the pelvis, and is completely surrounded by the prostate. The membranous portion of the canal passes through the urogenital diaphragm; it is slightly constricted and about ½ inch (1.3 cm) long. The spongy portion passes through the shaft of the penis, extending from the floor of the pelvis to the external urethral orifice. The distal prostatic, membranous, and spongy parts of the male urethra also serve as the excretory canal of the reproductive system.

Prostate

The *prostate* is a small glandular body surrounding the proximal part of the male urethra and is situated just posterior to the inferior portion of the pubic symphysis. The prostate is considered part of the male reproductive system but, because of its close proximity to the bladder, is commonly described with the urinary system. The conical base of the prostate is attached to the inferior surface of the urinary bladder, and its apex is in contact with the pelvic diaphragm. The prostate measures about 1½ inches (3.8 cm) transversely and ¾ inch (1.9 cm) anteroposteriorly at its base; vertically the prostate is approximately 1 inch (2.5 cm) long. The prostate gland secretes a milky fluid that combines with semen from the seminal vesicles and vas deferens. These secretions enter the urethra via ducts in the prostatic urethra.

SUMMARY OF ANATOMY

Urinary system (excretory system)	Kidneys	Urinary bladder
kidneys (2)	adipose capsule	apex
ureters (2)	renal fascia	base
urinary bladder	hilum	neck
urethra	renal capsule	trigone
	renal sinus	rugae
Suprarenal glands (adrenal glands)	renal cortex	
	renal columns	**Urethra**
medullary portion	renal medulla	male urethra
cortical portion	renal pyramids	prostatic
	nephrons	membranous
	renal corpuscle	spongy
	glomerular capsule (Bowman's capsule)	**Prostate**
	glomerulus	
	afferent arteriole	
	efferent arteriole	
	renal tubule	
	proximal convoluted tubule	
	nephron loop (loop of Henle)	
	distal convoluted tubule	
	collecting ducts	
	renal papilla	
	calyces	
	minor calyces	
	major calyces	
	renal pelvis	

SUMMARY OF PATHOLOGY

Condition	Definition
Benign Prostatic Hyperplasia (BPH)	Enlargement of the prostate
Calculus	Abnormal concretion of mineral salts, often called a stone
Carcinoma	Malignant new growth composed of epithelial cells
Bladder	Carcinoma located in the bladder
Renal Cell	Carcinoma located in the kidney
Congenital Anomaly	Abnormality present since birth
Duplicate Collecting System	Two renal pelvi and/or ureters from the same kidney
Horseshoe Kidney	Fusion of the kidneys, usually at the lower poles
Pelvic Kidney	Kidney that fails to ascend and remains in the pelvis
Cystitis	Inflammation of the bladder
Fistula	Abnormal connection between two internal organs or between an organ and the body surface
Glomerulonephritis	Inflammation of the capillary loops in the glomeruli of the kidney
Hydronephrosis	Distension of the renal pelvis and calyces with urine
Polycystic Kidney	Massive enlargement of the kidney with the formation of many cysts
Pyelonephritis	Inflammation of the kidney and renal pelvis
Renal Hypertension	Increased blood pressure to the kidneys
Renal Obstruction	Condition preventing the normal flow of urine through the urinary system
Stenosis	Narrowing or contraction of a passage
Tumor	New tissue growth where cell proliferation is uncontrolled
Wilms'	Most common childhood abdominal neoplasm affecting the kidney
Ureterocele	Ballooning of the lower end of the ureter into the bladder
Vesicoureteral Reflux	Backward flow of urine from the bladder into the ureters

EXPOSURE TECHNIQUE CHART ESSENTIAL PROJECTIONS

URINARY SYSTEM

Part	cm	kVp*	tm	mA	mAs	AEC	SID	IR	Dose† (mrad)
Urinary System (Urography)‡									
AP	21	75	0.08	200s	16		48"	35 × 43 cm	185
AP Oblique	24	75	0.09	200s	18		48"	35 × 43 cm	222
Lateral	27	90	0.11	200s	22		48"	35 × 43 cm	916
Lateral (decubitus)	30	95	0.11	200s	22		48"	35 × 43 cm	1040
Retrograde Urography‡									
AP	21	75	0.08	200s	16		48"	35 × 43 cm	185
Urinary Bladder‡									
AP and PA Axial	18	75	0.06	200s	12		48"	24 × 30 cm	148
AP Oblique	21	75	0.08	200s	16		48"	24 × 30 cm	185
Lateral	31	75	0.24	200s	48		48"	24 × 30 cm	1269
Male Cystourethrogram‡									
AP Oblique	21	75	0.08	200s	16		48"	24 × 30 cm	185

s, Small focal spot.
*kVp values are for a three-phase, 12-pulse generator.
†Relative doses for comparison use. All doses are skin entrance for average adult at cm indicated.
‡Bucky, 16:1 grid. Screen/film speed 300.

NEW ABBREVIATIONS USED IN CHAPTER 18

ACR	American College of Radiology
ASRT	American Society of Radiologic Technologists
BPH	Benign prostatic hyperplasia
BUN	Blood urea nitrogen
CDC	Centers for Disease Control and Prevention
IV	Intravenous
IVP	Intravenous pyelogram
VCUG	Voiding cystourethrogram

See Addendum B for a summary of all abbreviations used in Volume 2.

Overview

Radiography of the urinary system comprises numerous specialized procedures, each of which requires the use of an iodinated contrast medium and each of which was evolved to serve a specific purpose.

The specialized procedures are preceded by a plain, or scout, radiograph of the abdominopelvic areas for the detection of abnormalities demonstrable by this means. The preliminary examination may consist of no more than an AP projection of the abdomen. When indicated, oblique and/or lateral projections are taken to localize calcium and tumor masses, and an upright position may be used to demonstrate the mobility of the kidneys.

Preliminary radiography can usually demonstrate the position and mobility of the kidneys and usually their size and shape. This is possible because of the contrast furnished by the radiolucent fatty capsule surrounding the kidneys. In addition, properly selected CT soft-tissue windows can demonstrate the renal parenchyma without contrast media (Fig. 18-8). Visualization of the thin-walled drainage, or collecting, system (calyces and pelves, ureters, urinary bladder, and urethra) requires that the canals be filled with a contrast medium. The urinary bladder is outlined when it is filled with urine, but it is not adequately demonstrated. The ureters and the urethra cannot be distinguished on preliminary radiographs. However, a noncontrast media CT "stone protocol" can clearly demonstrate calcified renal stones (Fig. 18-9).

CONTRAST STUDIES

For the delineation and differentiation of cysts and tumor masses situated within the kidney, the renal parenchyma is opacified by an intravenously introduced organic, iodinated contrast medium and then radiographed by tomography (Fig. 8-10) or CT (Fig. 8-11). The contrast solution may be introduced into the vein by rapid injection or by infusion.

Angiographic procedures are used to investigate the blood vessels of the kidneys and the suprarenal glands (see Chapter 25). An example of the direct injection of contrast medium into the renal artery is shown in Fig. 18-12.

Radiologic investigations of the renal drainage, or collecting, system are performed by various procedures classified under the general term *urography*. This term embraces two regularly used techniques for filling the urinary canals with a contrast medium. Imaging of cutaneous urinary diversions has been described by Long.[1]

[1]Long BW: Radiography of cutaneous urinary diversions, *Radiol Technol* 60:109, 1988.

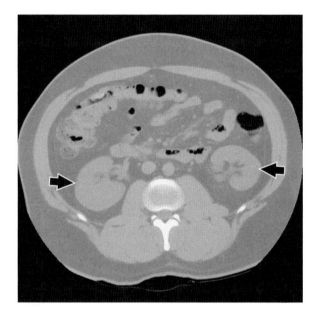

Fig. 18-8 Non–contrast media CT of the abdomen demonstrating the parenchyma and renal pelvis of both kidneys *(arrows).*

(Courtesy Karl Mockler, RT(R).)

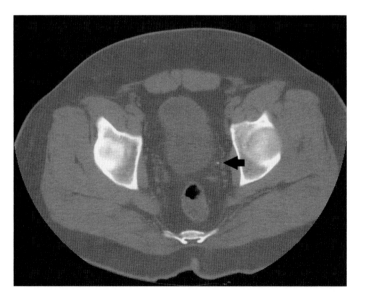

Fig. 18-9 Non–contrast media CT "stone protocol" demonstrating renal calculus in left distal ureter *(arrow).*

(Courtesy Karl Mockler, RT(R).)

Antegrade filling

Antegrade filling techniques allow the contrast medium to enter the kidney in the normal direction of blood flow. In selective patients this is done by introducing the contrast material directly into the kidney through a percutaneous puncture of the renal pelvis—a technique called percutaneous antegrade urography. Much more commonly used is the physiologic technique, in which the contrast agent is generally administered intravenously. This technique is called excretory or *intravenous urography* (IVU) and is shown in Fig. 18-13.

The excretory technique of urography is used in examinations of the upper urinary tract in infants and children and is generally considered to be the preferred technique in adults unless use of the retrograde technique is definitely indicated. Because the contrast medium is administered intravenously and all parts of the urinary system are normally demonstrated, the excretory technique is correctly referred to as intravenous urography. The term *pyelography* refers to the radiographic demonstration of the renal pelves and calyces. For years the examination has been erroneously called an intravenous pyelogram (IVP).

Once the opaque contrast medium enters the bloodstream, it is conveyed to the renal glomeruli and is discharged into the capsules with the glomerular filtrate, which is excreted as urine. With the reabsorption of water the contrast material becomes sufficiently concentrated to render the urinary canals radiopaque. The urinary bladder is well outlined by this technique, and satisfactory voiding urethrograms may be obtained.

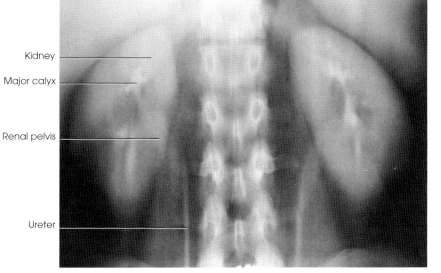

Kidney

Major calyx

Renal pelvis

Ureter

Fig. 18-10 Nephrotomogram.

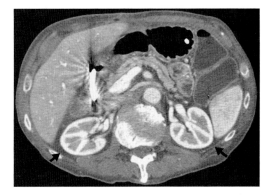

Fig. 18-11 CT image of the abdomen with contrast media demonstrating early filling of both kidneys *(arrows)*.

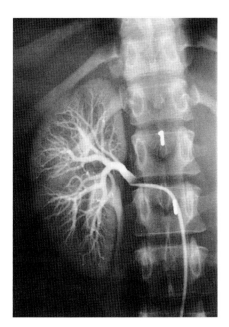

Fig. 18-12 Selective right renal arteriogram.

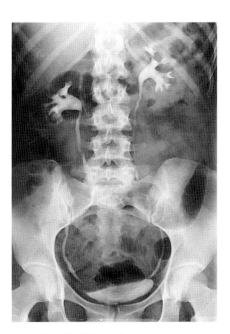

Fig. 18-13 Excretory urogram.

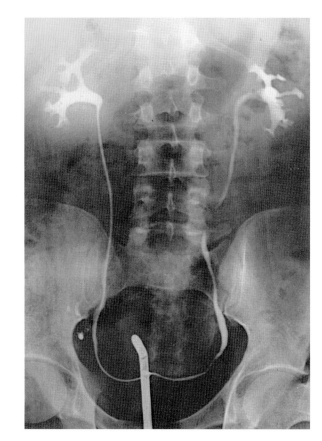

Fig. 18-14 Retrograde urogram.

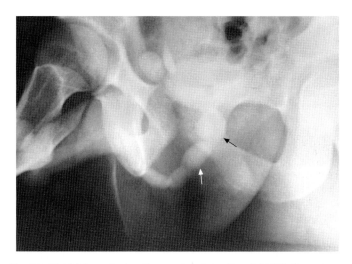

Fig. 18-15 Voiding study after routine injection IVU. Dilation of proximal urethra *(arrows)* is the result of urethral stricture.

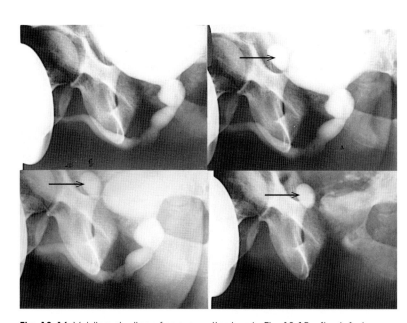

Fig. 18-16 Voiding studies of same patient as in Fig. 18-15 after infusion nephrourography. Note the increase in opacification of contrast-filled cavities by this method and the bladder diverticulum *(arrows)*.

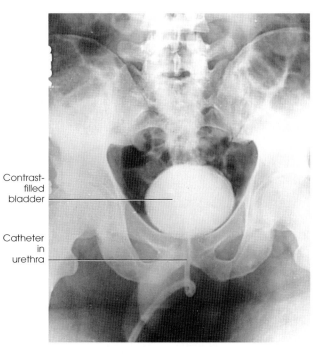

Contrast-filled bladder

Catheter in urethra

Fig. 18-17 Cystogram.

Retrograde filling

In some procedures involving the urinary system, the contrast material is introduced against the normal flow. This is called *retrograde* urography (Fig. 18-14). The contrast medium is injected directly into the canals by means of ureteral catheterization for contrast filling of the upper urinary tract and by means of urethral catheterization for contrast filling of the lower part of the urinary tract. Cystoscopy is required to localize the vesicoureteral orifices for the passage of ureteral catheters.

Retrograde urographic examination of the proximal urinary tract is primarily a urologic procedure. Catheterization and contrast filling of the urinary canals are performed by the attending urologist in conjunction with a physical or endoscopic examination. This technique enables the urologist to obtain catheterized specimens of urine directly from each renal pelvis. Because the canals can be fully distended by direct injection of the contrast agent, the retrograde urographic examination sometimes provides more information about the anatomy of the different parts of the collecting system than can be obtained by the excretory technique. For the retrograde procedure, an evaluation of kidney function depends on an intravenously administered dye substance to stain the color of the urine that subsequently trickles through the respective ureteral catheters. Both the antegrade and retrograde techniques of examination are occasionally required for a complete urologic study.

Investigations of the lower urinary tract—the bladder, lower ureters, and urethra—are usually made by the retrograde technique, which requires no instrumentation beyond passage of a urethral catheter. However, investigations may also be made by the physiologic technique (Figs. 18-15 and 18-16). Bladder examinations are usually denoted by the general term *cystography* (Fig. 18-17). A procedure understood to include inspection of the lower ureters is *cystoureterography* (Fig. 18-18), and a procedure understood to include inspection of the urethra is *cystourethrography* (Fig. 18-19).

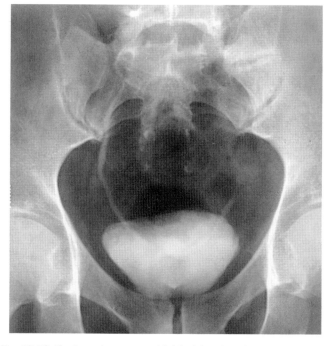

Fig. 18-18 Cystoureterogram: AP bladder showing distal ureters.

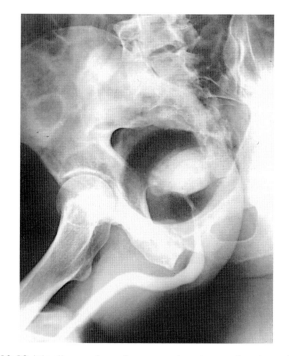

Fig. 18-19 Injection cystourethrogram showing urethra in male patient.

Contrast media

Retrograde urography (Figs. 18-20 and 18-21) was first performed in 1904 with the introduction of air into the urinary bladder. In 1906, retrograde urography and cystography were performed with the first opaque medium, a colloidal silver preparation that is no longer used. Silver iodide, which is a nontoxic inorganic compound, was introduced in 1911. Sodium iodide and sodium bromide, also inorganic compounds, were first used for retrograde urography in 1918. The bromides and iodides are no longer widely used for examinations of the renal pelves and ureters because they irritate the mucosa and commonly cause considerable patient discomfort.

Because a large quantity of solution is required to fill the urinary bladder, iodinated salts in concentrations of 30% or less are used in cystography. A large selection of commercially available contrast media may be used for all types of radiographic examinations of the urinary system. It is important to review the product insert packaged with every contrast agent.

Excretory urography (Figs. 18-22 and 18-23) was first reported by Rowntree et al. in 1923.[1] These investigators used a 10% solution of chemically pure sodium iodide as the contrast medium. However, this agent was excreted too slowly to give a satisfactory demonstration of the renal pelves and ureters, and it also proved too toxic for functional distribution. Early in 1929, Roseno and Jepkins[2] introduced a compound containing sodium iodide and urea. The latter constituent, which is one of the nitrogenous substances removed from the blood and eliminated by the kidneys, served to accelerate excretion and thus to quickly fill the renal pelves with opacified urine. Although satisfactory renal images were obtained with this compound, patients experienced considerable distress as a result of its toxicity.

[1]Rowntree LG et al: Roentgenography of the urinary tract during excretion of sodium iodide, *JAMA* 8:368, 1923.
[2]Roseno A, Jepkins H: Intravenous pyelography, *Fortschr Roentgenstr* 39:859, 1929. Abstract: *Am J Roentgenol* 22:685, 1929.

In 1929, Swick developed the organic compound Uroselectan, which had an iodine content of 42%. The present-day ionic contrast media for excretory urography are the result of extensive research by many investigators. These media are available under various trade names in concentrations ranging from approximately 50% to 70%. Sterile solutions of the media are supplied in dose-size ampules or vials.

In the early 1970s, research was initiated to develop nonionic contrast media. Development progressed, and several nonionic contrast agents are currently available for urographic, vascular, and intrathecal injection. Although nonionic contrast media are generally less likely to cause a reaction in the patient, they are twice as expensive as ionic agents.

Many institutions have developed criteria to determine which patient receives which contrast medium. The choice of whether to use an ionic or nonionic contrast medium depends on patient risk and economics.

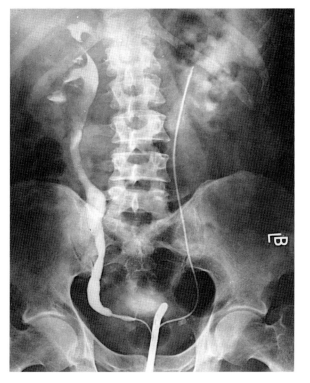

Fig. 18-20 Retrograde urogram with contrast medium–filled right renal pelvis and catheter in left renal pelvis.

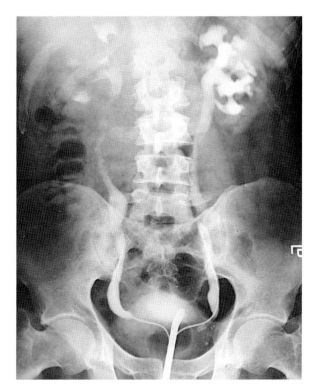

Fig. 18-21 Retrograde urogram.

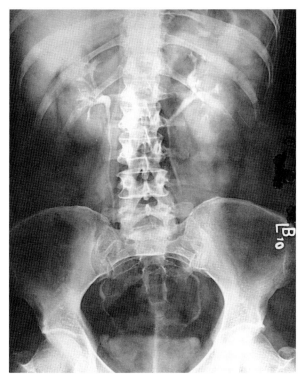

Fig. 18-22 Excretory urogram, 10 minutes after contrast medium injection.

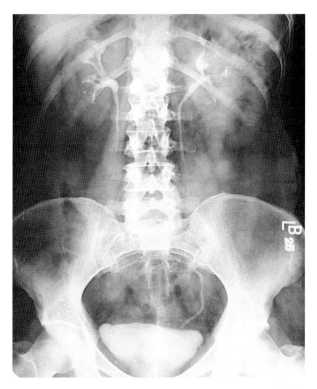

Fig. 18-23 Excretory urogram on same patient as in Fig. 18-22, 25 minutes after contrast medium injection.

Adverse reactions to iodinated media

The iodinated organic preparations that are compounded for urologic examinations are of low toxicity. Consequently, adverse reactions are usually mild and of short duration. The characteristic reactions are a feeling of warmth, flushing, and sometimes a few hives. Occasionally, nausea, vomiting, and edema of the respiratory mucous membrane result. Severe and serious reactions occur only rarely but are always a possibility. Therefore the clinical history of each patient must be carefully checked, and the patient must be kept under careful observation for any sign of systemic reactions. Most reactions to contrast media occur within the first 5 minutes after administration. Therefore the patient should not be left unattended during this time period. Emergency equipment and medication (Benadryl, epinephrine) to treat adverse reactions must be readily available.

Preparation of intestinal tract

Although unobstructed visualization of the urinary tracts requires that the intestinal tract be free of gas and solid fecal material (Fig. 18-24), bowel preparation is not attempted in infants and children. Furthermore, the use of cleansing measures in adults depends on the condition of the patient. Gas (particularly swallowed air, which is quickly dispersed through the small bowel) rather than fecal material usually interferes with the examination.

Hope and Campoy[1] recommended that infants and children be given a carbonated soft drink to distend the stomach with gas. By this maneuver, the gas-containing intestinal loops are usually pushed inferiorly and the upper urinary tracts, particularly those on the left side of the body, are then clearly visualized through the outline of the gas-filled stomach. Hope and Campoy stated that the aerated drink should be given in an amount adequate to fully inflate the stomach: at least 2 ounces are required for a newborn infant, and a full 12 ounces are required for a child 7 or 8 years old. In conjunction with the carbonated drink, Hope and Campoy recommended using a highly concentrated contrast medium. A gas-distended stomach is shown in Fig. 18-25.

[1]Hope JW, Campoy F: The use of carbonated beverages in pediatric excretory urography, *Radiology* 64:66, 1955.

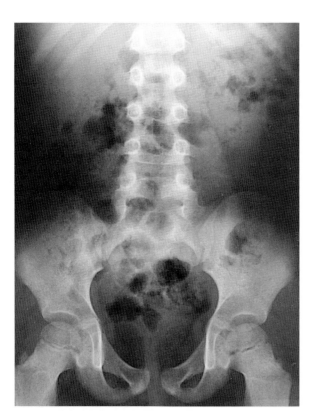

Fig. 18-24 Preliminary AP abdomen for urogram.

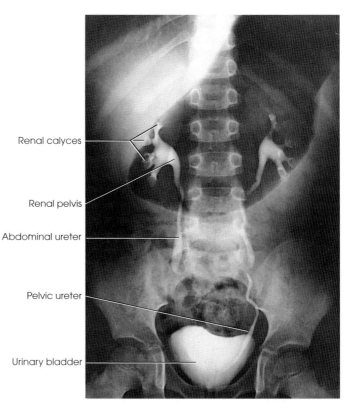

Renal calyces

Renal pelvis

Abdominal ureter

Pelvic ureter

Urinary bladder

Fig. 18-25 Supine urogram at 15-minute interval with gas-filled stomach.

Berdon, Baker, and Leonidas[2] stated that the prone position resolves the problem of obscuring gas in a majority of patients (Figs. 18-26 and 18-27). Therefore it is not necessary to inflate the stomach with air alone or with air as part of an aerated drink. By exerting pressure on the abdomen, the prone position moves the gas laterally away from the pelvicaliceal structures. Gas in the antral portion of the stomach is displaced into its fundic portion, gas in the transverse colon shifts into the ascending and descending segments, and gas in the sigmoid colon shifts into the descending colon and rectum. These investigators noted, however, that the prone position occasionally fails to produce the desired result in small infants when the small intestine is dilated. Gastric inflation also fails in these patients because the dilated small intestine merely elevates the gas-filled stomach and thus does not improve visualization. They recommended examination of such infants *after* the intestinal gas has passed.

[2]Berdon WE, Baker DH, Leonidas J: Prone radiography in intravenous pyelography in infants and children, *Am J Roentgenol* 103:444, 1968.

Preparation of patient

Medical opinion concerning preparative measures varies widely. However, with modifications as required, the following procedure seems to be in general use:

- When time permits, have the patient follow a low-residue diet for 1 to 2 days to prevent gas formation caused by excessive fermentation of the intestinal contents.
- Have the patient eat a light evening meal on the day before the examination.
- When indicated by costive bowel action, administer a non–gas-forming laxative the evening before the examination.
- Have the patient take nothing by mouth after midnight on the day of the examination. However, the patient should not be dehydrated. Patients with multiple myeloma, high uric acid levels, or diabetes must be well hydrated before IVU is performed; these patients are at increased risk for contrast medium–induced renal failure if they are dehydrated.

- In preparation for *retrograde urography,* have the patient drink a large amount of water (4 or 5 cups) several hours before the examination to ensure excretion of urine in an amount sufficient for bilateral catheterized specimens and renal function tests.
- Note that no patient preparation is usually necessary for examinations of the lower urinary tract.

Outpatients should be given explicit directions regarding any order from the physician pertaining to diet, fluid intake, and laxatives or other medication. The patient should also be given a suitable explanation for each preparative measure to ensure cooperation.

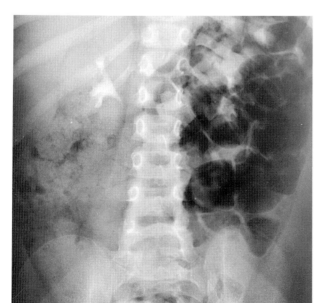

Fig. 18-26 Urogram: supine position. Intestinal gas obscuring the left kidney.

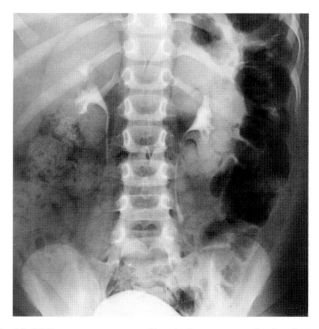

Fig. 18-27 Urogram: prone position, in the same patient as in Fig. 18-26. Visualization of the left kidney and ureter is markedly improved.

EQUIPMENT

A combination cystoscopic-radiographic unit facilitates retrograde urographic procedures requiring cystoscopy. Any standard radiographic table is suitable for the performance of preliminary excretory urography, as well as most retrograde studies of the bladder and urethra. The cystoscopic unit is also used for these procedures; however, for the patient's comfort, the table should have an extensible leg rest.

Infusion nephrourography requires a table equipped with tomographic apparatus. Tomography should be performed when intestinal gas obscures some of the underlying structures or when hypersthenic patients are being examined (Figs. 18-28 to 18-30).

For the patient's comfort and to prevent delays during the examination, all preparations for the examination should be completed before the patient is placed on the table. In addition to an identification and side marker, excretory urographic studies require a time-interval marker for each postinjection study. Body-position markers (supine, prone, upright or semiupright, Trendelenburg, decubitus) should also be used.

Some institutions perform excretory urograms (proximal urinary tract studies) using 24- × 30-cm or 30- × 35-cm IRs placed crosswise, but these studies can also be made on 35- × 43-cm IRs placed lengthwise. The upright study is made on a 35- × 43-cm IR because it is taken to demonstrate the mobility of the kidneys and to outline the lower ureters and bladder. Studies of the bladder before and after voiding are usually taken on 24- × 30-cm (10- × 12-inch) IRs.

The following guidelines are observed in preparing additional equipment for the examination:

- Have an emergency cart fully equipped and conveniently placed.
- Arrange the instruments for injection of the contrast agent on a small, movable table or on a tray.
- Have frequently used sterile items readily available. Disposable syringes and needles are available in standard sizes and are widely used in this procedure.
- Have required nonsterile items available: a tourniquet, a small waste basin, an emesis basin, general disposable wipes, one or two bottles of contrast medium, and a small prepared dressing for application to the puncture site.
- Have iodine or alcohol wipes available.
- Provide a folded towel or a small pillow that can be placed under the patient's elbow to relieve pressure during the injection.

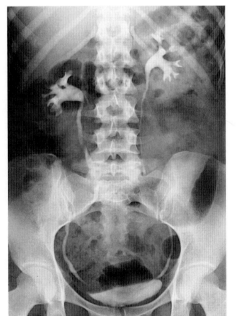

Fig. 18-28 Urogram: AP projection.

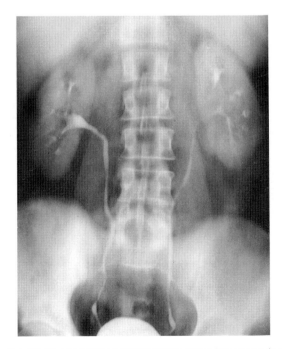

Fig. 18-29 Urogram: AP projection using tomography.

PROCEDURE

Image quality and exposure technique

Urograms should have the same contrast, density, and degree of soft tissue density as do abdominal radiographs. The radiographs must show a sharply defined outline of the kidneys, lower border of the liver, and lateral margin of the psoas muscles. The amount of bone detail visible in these studies varies according to the thickness of the abdomen (Fig. 18-31).

Motion control

An immobilization band usually is not applied over the upper abdomen in urographic examinations because the resultant pressure may interfere with the passage of fluid through the ureters and may also cause distortion of the canals. Thus the elimination of motion in urographic examinations depends on the exposure time and on securing the full cooperation of the patient.

The examination procedure should be explained so that the adult patient is prepared for any transitory distress caused by the injection of contrast solution or by the cystoscopic procedure. The patient should be assured that everything possible will be done for the patient's comfort. The success of the examinations depends in large part on the ability of the radiographer to gain the confidence of the patient.

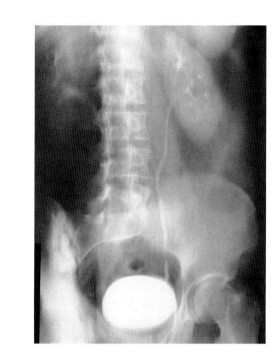

Fig. 18-30 Urogram: AP oblique projection, LPO position, using tomography. Note that the left kidney is perpendicular to IR.

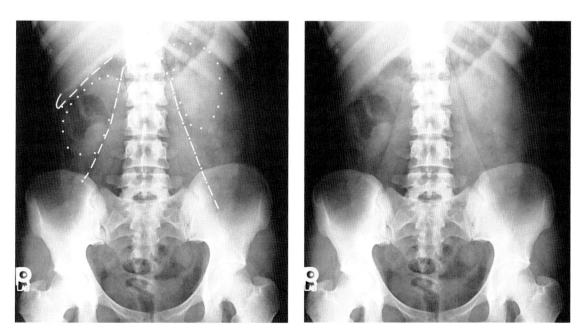

Fig. 18-31 AP abdomen showing margins of the kidney *(dots)*, liver *(dashes)*, and psoas muscles *(dot-dash lines)*.

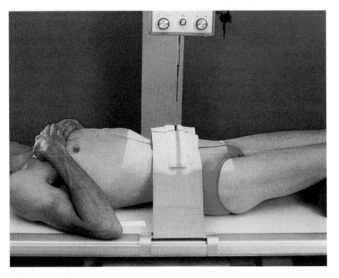

Fig. 18-32 Ureteral compression device in place for urogram.

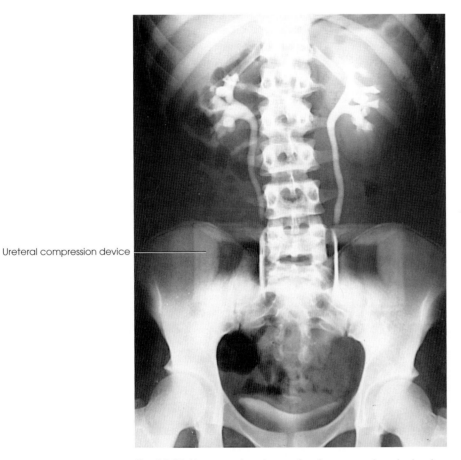

Ureteral compression device

Fig. 18-33 Urogram showing ureteral compression device in proper position over distal ureters.

Ureteral compression

In excretory urography, compression is sometimes applied over the distal ends of the ureters. This is done to retard flow of the opacified urine into the bladder and thus ensure adequate filling of the renal pelves and calyces. If compression is used, it must be placed so that the pressure over the distal ends of the ureters is centered at the level of the anterior superior iliac spine (ASIS). As much pressure as the patient can comfortably tolerate is then applied with the immobilization band (Figs. 18-32 and 18-33). The pressure should be released slowly when the compression device is removed to reduce pain caused by rapid change in intraabdominal pressure. Compression is generally contraindicated if a patient has urinary stones, an abdominal mass or aneurysm, a colostomy, a suprapubic catheter, or traumatic injury.

As a result of improvements in contrast agents, ureteral compression is not routinely used in most health care facilities. With the increased doses of contrast medium now employed, most of the ureteral area is usually demonstrated over a series of radiographs.

Respiration

For the purpose of comparison, all exposures are made at the end of the same phase of breathing—at the *end of expiration* unless otherwise requested. Because the normal respiratory excursion of the kidneys varies from ½ to 1½ inches (1.3 to 3.8 cm), it is occasionally possible to differentiate renal shadows from other shadows by making an exposure at a different phase of arrested respiration. When an exposure is made at a respiratory phase different from what is usually used, the image should be so marked.

PRELIMINARY EXAMINATION

A preliminary examination of the abdomen is made before a specialized investigation of the urinary tract is conducted. This examination sometimes reveals extrarenal lesions that are responsible for the symptoms attributed to the urinary tract and thereby renders the urographic procedure unnecessary. An upright AP projection may also be required to demonstrate the mobility of the kidneys. An oblique and/or lateral projection in the dorsal decubitus position may be required to localize a tumor mass or to differentiate renal stones from gallstones or calcified mesenteric nodes.

The scout radiograph—an AP projection with the patient recumbent—demonstrates the contour of the kidneys, their location in the supine position, and the presence of renal or other calculi (see Fig. 18-29). This radiograph also serves to check the preparation of the gastrointestinal tract and to enable the radiographer to make any necessary alteration in the exposure factors.

Radiation Protection

It is the responsibility of the radiographer to observe the following guidelines concerning radiation protection:

- Apply a gonadal shield if it does not overlap the area under investigation.
- Restrict radiation to the area of interest by close collimation.
- Work carefully so that repeat exposures are not necessary.

- Shield males for all examinations, except those of the urethra, by using a shadow shield or by placing a piece of lead just below the pubic symphysis.
- When excretory urography IRs are centered to the kidneys, place lead over the female pelvis for shielding. Unless the procedure is considered an emergency, perform radiography of the abdomen and pelvis only if there is no chance of patient pregnancy. For most projections in this chapter, females generally cannot be shielded without obscuring a portion of the urinary system. (Gonad shielding is not shown on the patient radiographs in this atlas for illustrative purposes.) Carefully follow department guidelines regarding gonad shielding.

Intravenous Urography

IVU demonstrates both the function and structure of the urinary system. *Function* is demonstrated by the ability of the kidneys to filter contrast medium from the blood and concentrate it with the urine. Anatomic *structures* are usually visualized as the contrast material follows the excretion route of the urine.

Indications for IVU include the following:

- Evaluation of abdominal masses, renal cysts, and renal tumors
- Urolithiasis—calculi or stones of the kidneys or urinary tract
- Pyelonephritis— infection of the upper urinary tract, which can be acute or chronic

- Hydronephrosis—abnormal dilation of the pelvicaliceal system (Urography is used to help determine the cause of the dilation.)
- Evaluation of the effects of trauma
- Preoperative evaluation of the function, location, size, and shape of the kidneys and ureters
- Renal hypertension (Urography is commonly performed to evaluate functional symmetry of the renal collecting systems.)

The most common contraindications for IVU relate to (1) the ability of the kidneys to filter contrast medium from the blood and (2) the patient's allergic history. Some contraindications can be overcome by the use of nonionic contrast agents. Patients with conditions in which the kidneys are unable to filter waste or excrete urine (renal failure, anuria) should have their kidneys evaluated by some technique other than excretory urography. Older patients or patients with any of the following risk factors are strong candidates to receive a nonionic contrast medium or should be examined using another modality: asthma, previous contrast media reaction, circulatory or cardiovascular disease, elevated creatinine level, sickle cell disease, diabetes mellitus, or multiple myeloma.

RADIOGRAPHIC PROCEDURE

Before the procedure begins, the patient should be instructed to empty the bladder and change into an appropriate radiolucent gown. Emptying the bladder prevents dilution of the contrast medium with urine. The patient's clinical history, allergic history, and blood chemistry levels should be reviewed. The normal creatinine level is 0.6 to 1.5 mg/100 mL, and the normal *blood urea nitrogen* (BUN) level is 8 to 25 mg/100 mL. Any significant elevation of these levels suggests renal dysfunction and should be reviewed by a physician before the procedure is continued. The radiographer then observes the following steps:

- Place the patient on the table in the supine position, and adjust the patient to center the midsagittal plane of the body to the midline of the grid.
- Place a support under the patient's knees to reduce the lordotic curvature of the lumbar spine and to provide more comfort for the patient (Fig. 18-34).

- Attach the footboard in preparation for a possible upright or semiupright position.
- If the head of the table is to be lowered farther to enhance pelvicaliceal filling, attach the shoulder support and adjust it to the patient's height.
- When ureteric compression is to be used, place the compression device so that it is ready for immediate application at the specified time.
- Obtain a preliminary, or scout, radiograph of the abdomen. Then prepare for the first postinjection exposure before the contrast medium is injected.
- Place the IR in the Bucky tray; position the identification, side, and time-interval markers; and then make any change in centering or exposure technique as indicated by the scout radiograph.
- Have ready a folded towel or other suitable support and the tourniquet for placement under the selected elbow.
- Prepare the contrast medium for injection using aseptic technique.
- According to the preference of the examining physician, administer 30 to 100 mL of the contrast medium to the

adult patient of average size. The dosage administered to infants and children is regulated according to age and weight.

- Produce radiographs at specified intervals from the time of the *completion of the injection* of contrast medium. (This may actually depend on the protocol of the department.) Depending on the patient's hydration status and the speed of the injection, the contrast agent normally begins to appear in the pelvicaliceal system within 2 to 8 minutes.

The uptake of contrast medium is seen in the nephrons of the kidney if a radiograph is exposed as the kidneys start to filter the contrast medium from the blood. The initial contrast "blush" of the kidney is termed the *nephrogram phase*. As the kidneys continue to filter and concentrate the contrast medium, it is directed to the pelvicaliceal system. The greatest concentration of contrast medium in the kidneys normally occurs 15 to 20 minutes after injection. Immediately after each IR is exposed, it is processed and reviewed to determine, according to the kidney function of the individual patient, the time intervals at which the most intense kidney image can be obtained.

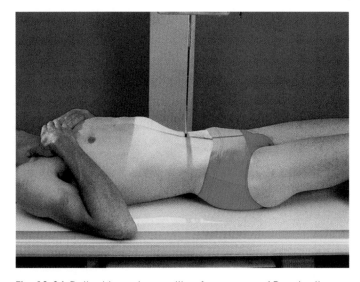

Fig. 18-34 Patient in supine position for urogram, AP projection. Note support under knees.

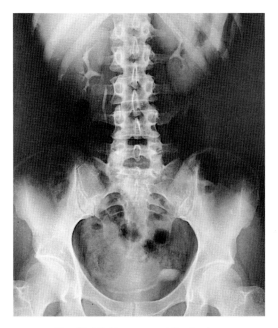

Fig. 18-35 Urogram at 3 minutes.

The most commonly recommended radiographs for IVU are AP projections at time intervals ranging from 3 to 20 minutes (Figs. 18-35 to 18-37). Some physicians prefer bolus injection of the contrast medium followed by a 30-second image to obtain a nephrogram. Thirty-degree AP oblique projections may be taken at 5- to 10-minute intervals. In some patients, supplemental radiographs are required to better demonstrate all parts of the urinary system and to differentiate normal anatomy from pathologic conditions. These may include an AP projection with the patient in the Trendelenburg or upright position, oblique or lateral projections, or a lateral projection with the patient in the dorsal or ventral decubitus position.

Unless further study of the bladder is indicated or voiding urethrograms are to be made, the patient is sent to the lavatory to void. A postvoid radiograph of the bladder (Figs. 18-38 and 18-39) may be taken to detect, by the presence of residual urine, conditions such as small tumor masses or, in male patients, enlargement of the prostate gland. When all the necessary radiographs have been obtained, the patient is released from the imaging department. Any contrast medium remaining in the body will be filtered from the blood by the kidneys and eventually excreted in the urine. Some physicians suggest having the patient drink extra fluids for a few days to help flush out the contrast medium.

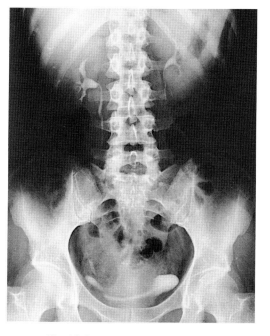

Fig. 18-36 Urogram at 6 minutes.

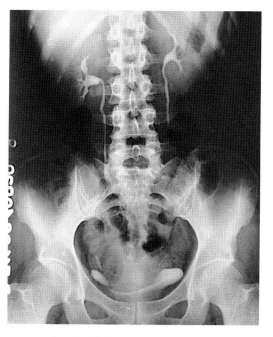

Fig. 18-37 Urogram at 9 minutes.

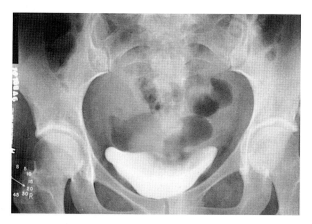

Fig. 18-38 Prevoiding filled bladder.

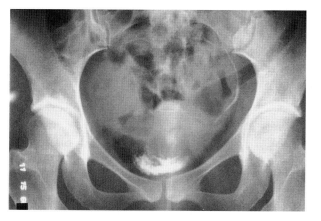

Fig. 18-39 Postvoiding emptied bladder.

⚕ AP PROJECTION

Image receptor: 35 × 43 cm lengthwise

Position of patient

- Place the patient supine on the radiographic table for the AP projection of the urinary system. Preliminary (scout) and postinjection radiographs are most commonly obtained with the patient supine (Fig. 18-40).
- Place a support under the patient's knees to relieve strain on the back.
- Place the patient in an upright or a semiupright position for an AP projection to demonstrate the opacified bladder and the mobility of the kidneys (Fig. 18-41).

- To demonstrate the lower ends of the ureters, it may be helpful to use the Trendelenburg position and an AP projection with the head of the table lowered 15 to 20 degrees and the central ray directed perpendicular to the IR. In this angled position, the weight of the contained fluid stretches the bladder fundus superiorly, providing an unobstructed image of the lower ureters and the vesicoureteral orifice areas.
- If needed, apply ureteral compression (see p. 214).

Position of part

- Center the midsagittal plane of the patient's body to the midline of the grid device.
- Place the patient's arms where they will not cast shadows on the IR.
- Center the IR at the level of the iliac crests. If the patient is too tall to include the entire urinary system, take a second exposure on a 24- × 30-cm IR centered to the bladder. The 24- × 30-cm IR is placed crosswise and centered 2 to 3 inches (5 to 7.6 cm) above the upper border of the pubic symphysis.
- *Shield gonads.*
- *Respiration:* Suspend at the end of expiration.

Central ray

- Perpendicular to the IR at the level of the iliac crests

Structures shown

An AP projection of the urinary system demonstrates the kidneys, ureters, and bladder filled with the contrast medium (Figs. 18-42 to 18-44).

NOTE: The prone position may be recommended for demonstration of the ureteropelvic region and for filling the obstructed ureter in the presence of hydronephrosis. The ureters fill better in the prone position, which reverses the curve of their inferior course. The kidneys are situated obliquely, slanting anteriorly in the transverse plane, so the opacified urine tends to collect in and distend the dependent part of the pelvicaliceal system. The supine position allows the more posteriorly placed upper calyces to fill more readily, and the anterior and inferior parts of the pelvicaliceal system fill more easily in the prone position.

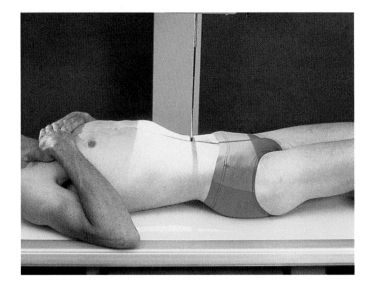

Fig. 18-40 Supine urogram: AP projection.

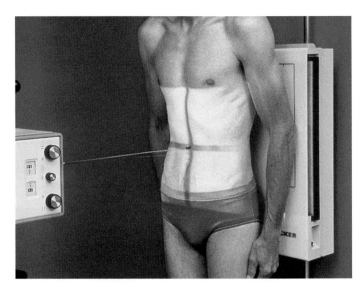

Fig. 18-41 Upright urogram: AP projection.

Urinary System

The following should be clearly demonstrated:

AP and PA projections

- Entire renal outlines
- Bladder and pubic symphysis (A separate radiograph of the bladder area is needed if the bladder was not included.)
- No motion
- Short scale of radiographic contrast clearly demonstrating contrast medium in the renal area, ureters, and bladder
- Compression devices, if used, centered over the upper sacrum and resulting in good renal filling
- Vertebral column centered on the radiograph
- No artifacts from elastic in the patient's underclothing
- Prostatic region inferior to the pubic symphysis on older male patients
- Time marker
- PA projection demonstrating the lower kidneys and entire ureters (bladder included if patient size permits)
- Superimposing intestinal gas in the AP projection moved for the PA projection

AP bladder

- Bladder
- No rotation of the pelvis
- Prostate area in male patients
- Postvoid radiographs clearly labeled and demonstrating only residual contrast medium

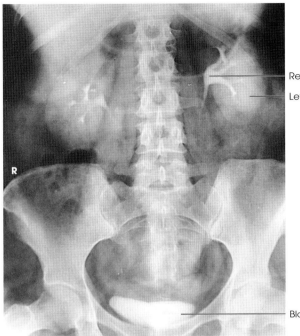

Fig. 18-42 Semiupright urogram: AP projection. Note mobility of kidneys.

Labels: Renal pelvis, Left kidney, Bladder

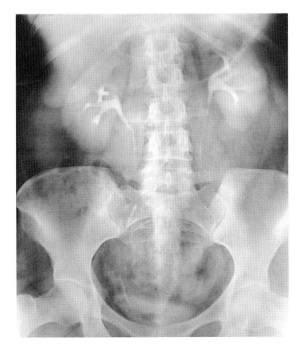

Fig. 18-43 Supine urogram: AP projection.

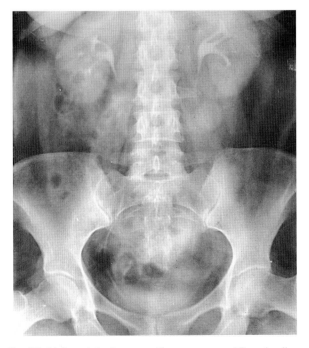

Fig. 18-44 Trendelenburg position urogram: AP projection.

♠ AP OBLIQUE PROJECTION
RPO and LPO positions

Image receptor: 35 × 43 cm lengthwise

Position of patient
- Place the patient supine on the radiographic table for oblique projections of the urinary system. The kidneys are situated obliquely, slanting anteriorly in the transverse plane.
- When performing AP oblique projections, remember that the kidney closer to the IR will be *perpendicular* to the plane of the IR and the kidney farther from the IR will be *parallel* with this plane.

Position of part
- Turn the patient so that the midcoronal plane forms an angle of 30 degrees from the IR plane.
- Adjust the patient's shoulders and hips so that they are in the same plane, and place suitable supports under the elevated side as needed.
- Place the arms so that they will not be superimposed on the urinary system.
- Center the spine to the grid (Fig. 18-45).
- Center the IR at the level of the iliac crests.
- *Shield gonads.*
- *Respiration:* Suspend at the end of expiration.

Central ray
- Perpendicular to the center of the IR at the level of the iliac crests, entering approximately 2 inches lateral to the midline on the elevated side

Structures shown
An AP oblique projection of the urinary system demonstrates the kidneys, ureters, and bladder filled with the contrast medium. The elevated kidney will be parallel with the IR, and the downside kidney will be perpendicular with the IR (Fig. 18-46).

The following should be clearly demonstrated:
- Patient rotated approximately 30 degrees
- No superimposition of the kidney remote from the IR on the vertebrae
- Entire down-side kidney
- Bladder and lower ureters on 35- × 43-cm IRs if the patient's size permits
- Time marker

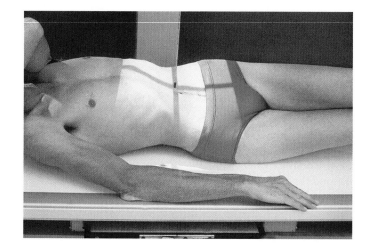

Fig. 18-45 Urogram: AP oblique projection, 30-degree RPO position.

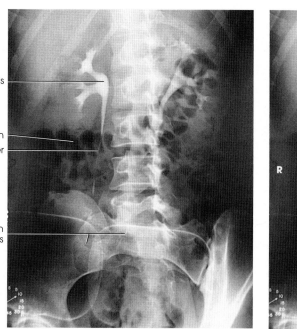
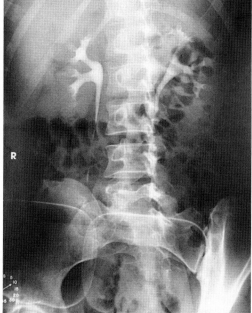

Renal pelvis

Gas in colon
Ureter

Ureteral compression devices

Fig. 18-46 Urogram at 10 minutes: AP oblique projection, RPO position.

⚘ LATERAL PROJECTION
R or L position

Image receptor: 35 × 43 cm lengthwise

Position of patient
- Turn the patient to a lateral recumbent position on the right or left side, as indicated.

Position of part
- Flex the patient's knees to a comfortable position, and adjust the body so that the midcoronal plane is centered to the midline of the grid.
- Place supports between the patient's knees and the ankles.
- Flex the patient's elbows, and place the hands under the patient's head (Fig. 18-47).
- Center the IR at the level of the iliac crests.
- *Shield gonads.*
- *Respiration:* Suspend at the end of expiration.

Central ray
- Perpendicular to the IR, entering the midcoronal plane at the level of the iliac crest

Structures shown
A lateral projection of the abdomen demonstrates the kidneys, ureters, and bladder filled with contrast material. Lateral projections are used to demonstrate conditions such as rotation or pressure displacement of a kidney and to localize calcareous areas and tumor masses (Fig. 18-48).

EVALUATION CRITERIA
The following should be clearly demonstrated:
- Entire urinary system
- Bladder and pubic symphysis
- Short scale of contrast clearly demonstrating contrast medium in the renal area, ureters, and bladder
- No rotation of the patient (Check pelvis and lumbar vertebrae.)
- Time marker

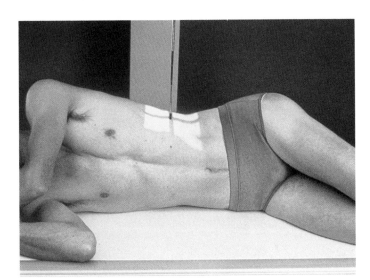

Fig. 18-47 Urogram: lateral projection.

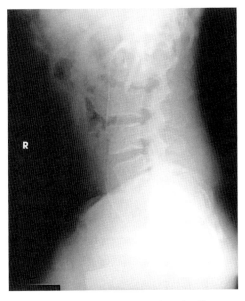

Fig. 18-48 Urogram: lateral projection.

⚜ LATERAL PROJECTION
Dorsal decubitus position

Image receptor: 35 × 43 cm

Position of patient
- Place the patient in the supine position on a radiographic cart with the side in question in contact with the vertical grid device. Ensure that the wheels are *locked.*
- Place the patient's arms across the upper chest to ensure that they are not projected over any abdominal contents, or place them behind the head.
- Flex the patient's knees slightly to relieve strain on the back.

Position of part
- Adjust the height of the vertical grid device so that the long axis of the IR is centered to the midcoronal plane of the patient's body.
- Position the patient so that a point approximately at the level of the iliac crests is centered to the IR (Fig. 18-49).
- Adjust the patient to ensure no rotation from the supine or prone position is present.
- *Shield gonads.*
- *Respiration:* Suspend at the end of expiration.

Central ray
- *Horizontal* and perpendicular to the center of the IR, entering the midcoronal plane at the level of the iliac crests

Structures shown
Rolleston and Reay[1] recommended the ventral decubitus position for demonstration of the ureteropelvic junction in the presence of hydronephrosis. Cook, Keats, and Seale[2] advocated this position to determine whether an extrarenal mass in the flank is intraperitoneal or extraperitoneal, and they stated that the position makes it easy to screen both kidneys and ureters for abnormal anterior displacement (Fig. 18-50).

---

[1]Rolleston GL, Reay ER: The pelvi-ureteric junction, *Br J Radiol* 30:617, 1957.
[2]Cook IK, Keats TE, Seale DL: Determination of the normal position of the upper urinary tract in the lateral abdominal urogram, *Radiology* 99:499, 1971.

The following should be clearly demonstrated:
- Entire urinary system
- Bladder and pubic symphysis
- Short scale of contrast clearly demonstrating contrast medium in the renal area, ureters, and bladder
- No rotation of the patient (Check pelvis and lumbar vertebrae.)
- Time marker
- Patient elevated so that entire abdomen is visible

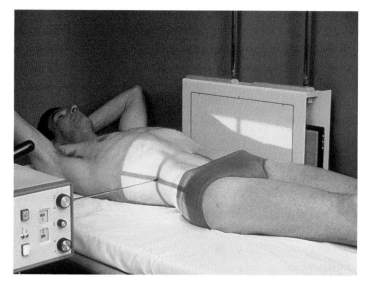

Fig. 18-49 Urogram: lateral projection, dorsal decubitus position.

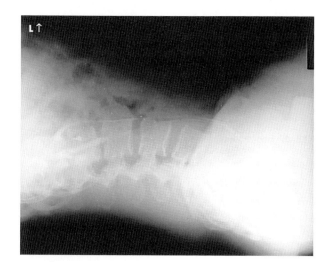

Fig. 18-50 Urogram: lateral projection, dorsal decubitus position.

Nephrotomography and Nephrourography

AP PROJECTION

The renal parenchyma, or the nephrons and collecting tubes, are best visualized by performing tomography immediately after the introduction of contrast medium. Evans et al.,[1,2] who introduced nephrotomography, found that by using tomography rather than stationary projections, they could eliminate intestinal-content superimpositions and more clearly define small intrarenal lesions.

Indications and contraindications

Nephrotomography is primarily performed to evaluate renal hypertension. It is also useful in delineating renal cysts and renal tumors.

Contraindications are mainly related to renal failure and contrast media sensitivity, as noted for IVU.

[1]Evans JA, Dubilier WJ, Monteith JC: Nephro–tomography, Am J Roentgenol 71:213, 1954.
[2]Evans JA: Nephrotomography in the investigation of renal masses, Radiology 69:684, 1957.

Contrast media

Many different contrast agents in various organic, iodinated concentrations are available for nephrography. These preparations are packaged in individual bottles with the IV tubing included. The actual dose may vary from patient to patient because renal failure induced by contrast media appears to be dose related.

A contrast medium can be administered rapidly by bolus injection or more slowly by IV infusion. Bolus injection nephrotomography was introduced by Weens et al.[1]

Bolus injection nephrotomography is performed by injecting a large amount of highly concentrated, iodinated contrast medium into the venous bloodstream by way of a large-bore needle inserted into an antecubital vein. With this rapid-injection technique, the renal blood vessels and corticomedullary structures are opacified only during the brief passage of the jet of contrast material. This short period requires that the imaging procedure be carried out as quickly as possible.

[1]Weens HS et al: Intravenous nephrography: a method of roentgen visualization of the kidney, Am J Roentgenol 65:411, 1951.

Infusion nephrotomography and nephrourography were first introduced by Schencker.[1] This method of administering a contrast medium provides opacification of both the renal parenchyma and drainage canals; thus it embraces both nephrography and urography. The examination is performed by a procedure somewhat similar to that used for preliminary IVU. The infusion procedure differs from the preliminary procedure in that (1) the contrast medium is introduced into the venous bloodstream by infusion rather than injection* and (2) both nephrotomographic and nephrourographic studies are made.

The infusion is made through an 18-gauge needle inserted into an antecubital vein, just as for preliminary IVU. The infusion bottle is hung on an IV stand, and the contrast solution is allowed to flow through the needle without restraint. The infusion requires several minutes for completion.

Preparation of patient

When preparation of the intestinal tract is possible, the patient may be given a low-residue diet for 1 to 2 days, and a non–gas-forming laxative may be given on the evening preceding the examination.

[1]Schencker B: Drip infusion pyelography: indications and applications in urologic roentgen diagnosis, Radiology 83:12, 1964.
*An injection is forced into a vessel or an organ, whereas an infusion flows in by gravity.

Examination procedure

The patient is placed in the supine position on a tomographic table. A scout radiograph of the abdomen is made to establish the exposure technique and determine the tomographic level for the nephrotomograms.

Before the examination is started, the procedure is explained to the patient. If the patient knows what sensations to expect, he or she will be better able to cooperate for the procedure.

After contrast medium has been injected, one AP projection of the abdomen is performed during the arterial phase of opacification (Fig. 18-51) and multiple tomograms of the upper abdomen are obtained during the nephrographic phase after the renal parenchyma becomes opacified—hence the term *nephrotomography* (Figs. 18-52 to 18-55). The nephrotic phase normally occurs within 5 minutes after completion of the injection or infusion.

Infusion studies of the urinary canals are usually made at intervals of 10, 20, and 30 minutes. Delayed urograms are taken as required. Urinary bladder studies and voiding urethrograms may be made. In addition to the AP projection, tomograms can also be made in the oblique and lateral projections as indicated (Fig. 18-56).

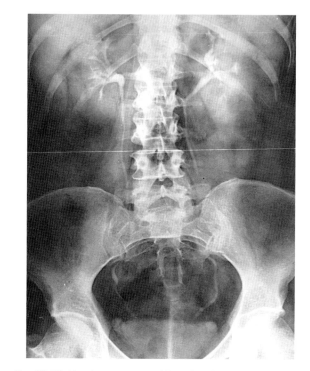

Fig. 18-51 Nephrourogram: AP projection, arterial phase.

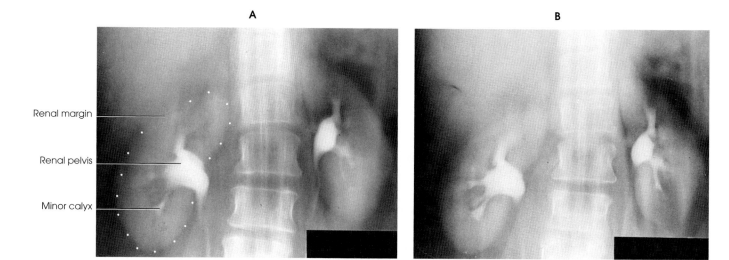

Renal margin

Renal pelvis

Minor calyx

Fig. 18-52 Nephrotomogram: AP projection at level of 9 cm **(A)** and 10 cm **(B)** in the same patient as in Fig. 18-51.

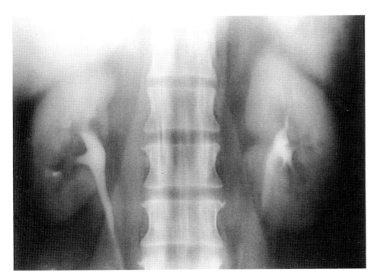

Fig. 18-53 Infusion nephrotomogram: AP projection at 9-cm level.

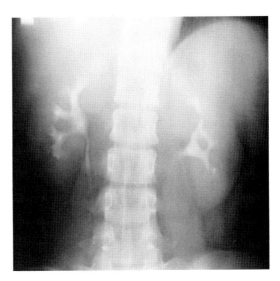

Fig. 18-54 Infusion nephrotomogram: AP projection at 5-cm level.

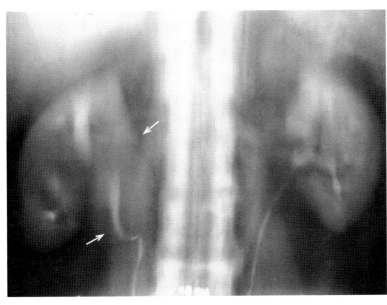

Fig. 18-55 Infusion nephrotomogram: AP projection demonstrating parapelvic cyst on right kidney *(arrows)*.

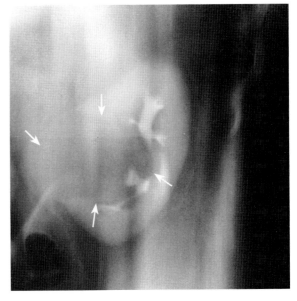

Fig. 18-56 Infusion nephrotomogram: lateral projection demonstrating parapelvic cyst *(arrows)*.

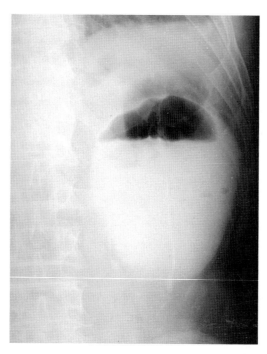

Fig. 18-57 Upright AP left kidney: percutaneous injection of iodinated contrast material and gas into renal cyst.

PERCUTANEOUS RENAL PUNCTURE

Percutaneous renal puncture, introduced by Lindblom,[1,2] is a radiologic procedure for the investigation of renal masses. Specifically, it is used to differentiate cysts and tumors of the renal parenchyma. This procedure is performed by direct injection of a contrast medium into the cyst under fluoroscopic control (Figs. 18-57 and 18-58). Ultrasonography of the kidney has practically eliminated the need for percutaneous renal puncture. Most masses that are clearly diagnosed as cystic by ultrasound examination are not surgically managed.

[1]Lindblom K: Percutaneous puncture of renal cysts and tumors, *Acta Radiol* 27:66, 1946.
[2]Lindblom K: Diagnostic kidney puncture in cysts and tumors, *Am J Roentgenol* 68:209, 1952.

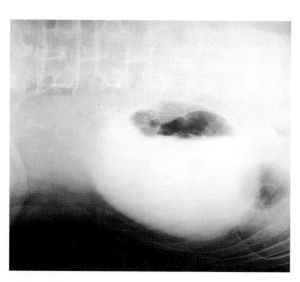

Fig. 18-58 AP projection left kidney, left lateral decubitus position, in the same patient as in Fig. 18-57.

In a similar procedure the renal pelvis is entered percutaneously for direct contrast filling of the pelvicaliceal system in selected patients with hydronephrosis.[1-3] This procedure, called *percutaneous antegrade pyelography*[3] to distinguish it from the retrograde technique of direct pelvicaliceal filling, is usually restricted to the investigation of patients with marked hydronephrosis and patients with suspected hydronephrosis for which conclusive information is not gained by excretory or retrograde urography (Fig. 18-59). Normally, AP abdominal radiographs are obtained for this procedure, although other projections may be requested.

[1]Wickbom I: Pyelography after direct puncture of the renal pelvis, *Acta Radiol* 41:505, 1954.
[2]Weens HS, Florence TJ: The diagnosis of hydronephrosis by percutaneous renal puncture, *J Urol* 72:589, 1954.
[3]Casey WC, Goodwin WE: Percutaneous antegrade pyelography and hydronephrosis, *J Urol* 74:164, 1955.

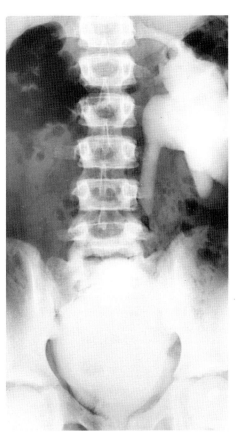

Fig. 18-59 AP projection left kidney, left lateral decubitus position, in the same patient as in Fig. 18-57.

Retrograde Urography

⚜ AP PROJECTION

Retrograde urography requires that the ureters be catheterized so that a contrast agent can be injected directly into the pelvicaliceal system. This technique provides improved opacification of the renal collecting system but little physiologic information about the urinary system.

Indications and contraindications

The retrograde urogram is indicated for evaluation of the collecting system in patients who have renal insufficiency or who are allergic to iodinated contrast media. Because the contrast medium is not introduced into the circulatory system, the incidence of reactions is reduced.

Examination procedure

Like all examinations requiring instrumentation, retrograde urography is classified as an operative procedure. This combined urologic-radiologic examination is carried out under careful aseptic conditions by the attending urologist with the assistance of a nurse and radiographer. The procedure is performed in a specially equipped cystoscopic-radiographic examining room that, because of its collaborative nature, may be located in the urology department or the radiology department. A nurse is responsible for the preparation of the instruments and the care and draping of the patient. One of the radiographer's responsibilities is to ensure that the overhead parts of the radiographic equipment are free of dust for the protection of the operative field and the sterile layout.

The radiographer positions the patient on the cystoscopic table with knees flexed over the stirrups of the adjustable leg supports (Fig. 18-60). This is a modified lithotomy position; the true lithotomy position requires acute flexion of the hips and knees.

If a general anesthetic is not used, the radiographer explains the breathing procedure to the patient and checks the patient's position on the table. The kidneys and the full extent of the ureters in patients of average height are included on a 35- × 43-cm IR when the third lumbar vertebra is centered to the grid.

If elevation of the thighs does not reduce the lumbar curve, a pillow is adjusted under the patient's head and shoulders so that the back is in contact with the table. Most cystoscopic-radiographic tables are equipped with an adjustable leg rest to permit extension of the patient's legs for certain radiographic studies.

The urologist then performs catheterization of the ureters through a ureterocystoscope, which is a cystoscope with an arrangement that aids insertion of the catheters into the vesicoureteral orifices. After the endoscopic examination, the urologist passes a ureteral catheter well into one or both ureters (Fig. 18-61) and, leaving the catheters in position, usually withdraws the cystoscope.

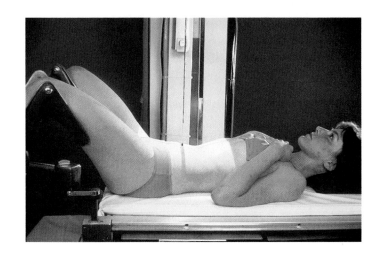

Fig. 18-60 Patient positioned on table for retrograde urography, modified lithotomy position.

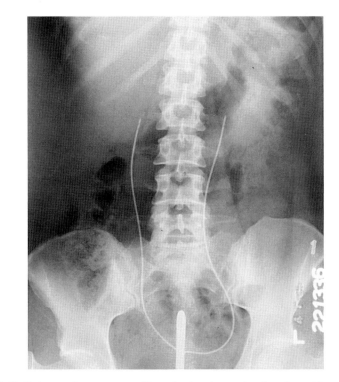

Fig. 18-61 Retrograde urogram with catheters in proximal ureters: AP projection.

After taking two catheterized specimens of urine from each kidney for laboratory tests—one specimen for culture and one for microscopic examination—the urologist tests kidney function. For this test, a color dye is injected intravenously, and the function of each kidney is determined by the specified time required for the dye substance to appear in the urine as it trickles through the respective catheters.

Immediately after the kidney function test, the radiographer rechecks the position of the patient and exposes the preliminary IR (if this has not been done previously) so that the radiographs will be ready for inspection by the time the kidney function test has been completed.

After reviewing the image, the urologist injects the contrast medium and proceeds with the urographic examination. When a bilateral examination is to be performed, both sides are filled simultaneously to avoid subjecting the patient to unnecessary radiation exposure. Additional studies in which only one side is refilled may then be made as indicated.

The most commonly used retrograde urographic series usually consists of three AP projections: the preliminary radiograph showing the ureteral catheters in position (see Fig. 18-61), the pyelogram, and the ureterogram. Some urologists recommend that the head of the table be lowered 10 to 15 degrees for the pyelogram to prevent the contrast solution from escaping into the ureters. Other urologists recommend that pressure be maintained on the syringe during the pyelographic exposure to ensure complete filling of the pelvicaliceal system. The head of the table may be elevated 35 to 40 degrees for the ureterogram to demonstrate any tortuosity of the ureters and the mobility of the kidneys.

Filling of the average normal renal pelvis requires 3 to 5 mL of contrast solution; however, a larger quantity is required when the structure is dilated. The best index of complete filling, and the one most commonly used, is an indication from the patient as soon as a sense of fullness is felt in the back.

When both sides are to be filled, the urologist injects the contrast solution through the catheters in an amount sufficient to fill the renal pelves and calyces. When signaled by the physician, the patient suspends respiration at the end of expiration, and the exposure for the pyelogram is then made (Fig. 18-62).

After the pyelographic exposure, the IR is quickly changed and the head of the table may be elevated in preparation for the ureterogram. For this exposure the patient is instructed to inspire deeply and then suspend respiration at the end of full expiration. Simultaneously with the breathing procedure, the catheters are slowly withdrawn to the lower ends of the ureters as the contrast solution is injected into the canals. At a signal from the urologist, the ureterographic exposure is made (Fig. 18-63).

Additional projections are sometimes required. RPO or LPO (AP oblique) projections are often necessary. Occasionally a lateral projection, with the patient turned onto the affected side, is performed to demonstrate anterior displacement of a kidney or ureter and to delineate a perinephric abscess. Lateral projections with the patient in the ventral or dorsal decubitus position (as required) are also useful, demonstrating the ureteropelvic region in patients with hydronephrosis.

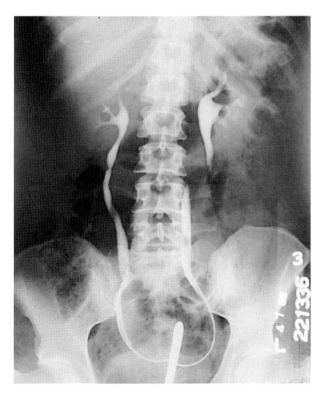

Fig. 18-62 Retrograde urogram with renal pelves filled: AP projection.

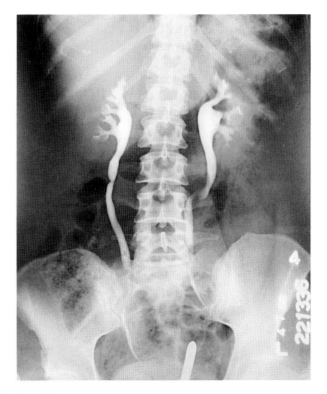

Fig. 18-63 Retrograde urogram showing renal pelves and contrast-filled ureters: AP projection.

Urinary Bladder, Lower Ureters, Urethra, and Prostate

With few exceptions, radiologic examinations of the lower urinary tract are performed with the retrograde technique of introducing contrast material. These examinations are identified, according to the specific purpose of the investigation, by the terms *cystography, cystoureterography, cystourethrography,* and *prostatography.* Most often they are denoted by the general term *cystography.* Cystoscopy is not required before retrograde contrast filling of the lower urinary canals, but when both examinations are indicated, they are usually performed in a single-stage procedure to spare the patient preparation and instrumentation for separate examinations. When cystoscopy is not indicated, these examinations are best carried out on an all-purpose radiographic table unless the combination table is equipped with an extensible leg rest.

Indications and contraindications

Retrograde studies of the lower urinary tract are indicated for vesicoureteral reflux, recurrent lower urinary tract infection, neurogenic bladder, bladder trauma, lower urinary tract fistulae, urethral stricture, and posterior urethral valves. Contraindications to lower urinary tract studies are related to catheterization of the urethra.

Contrast media

The contrast agents used for contrast studies of the lower urinary tracts are ionic solutions of either sodium or meglumine diatrizoates or the newer nonionic contrast media mentioned previously. These are the same organic compounds used for IVU, but their concentration is reduced for retrograde urography.

Injection equipment

The examinations are performed under careful aseptic conditions. Infants, children, and, usually, adults may be catheterized before they are brought to the radiology department. When the patient is to be catheterized in the radiology department, a sterile catheterization tray must be set up to specifications. Because of the danger of contamination in transferring a sterile liquid from one container to another, the use of commercially available premixed contrast solutions is recommended.

Preliminary preparations

The following guidelines are observed in preparing the patient for the examination:

- Protect the examination table from urine soilage with radiolucent plastic sheeting and disposable underpadding. Correctly arranged disposable padding does much to reduce soilage during voiding studies and consequently eliminates the need for extensive cleaning between patients. A suitable disposal receptacle should be available.
- A few minutes before the examination, accompany the patient to a lavatory. Give the patient supplies for perineal care, and instruct the patient to empty the bladder.
- Once the patient is prepared, place the patient on the examination table for the catheterization procedure.

Patients are usually tense, primarily because of embarrassment. It is important that they be given as much privacy as possible. Only the required personnel should be present during the examination, and patients should be properly draped and covered according to room temperature.

Contrast injection

For retrograde cystography (Figs. 18-64 and 18-65), cystourethrography, and voiding cystourethrography, the contrast material is introduced into the bladder by injection or infusion through a catheter passed into position by way of the urethral canal. A small, disposable Foley catheter is used to occlude the vesicourethral orifice in the examination of infants and children, and this catheter may be used in the examination of adults when interval studies are to be made for the detection of delayed ureteral reflux.

Studies are made during voiding for the delineation of the urethral canal and for the detection of ureteral reflux, which may occur only during urination (Fig. 18-66). When urethral studies are to be made during injection of contrast material, a soft-rubber urethral-orifice acorn is fitted directly onto a contrast-loaded syringe for female patients and is usually filled onto a cannula attached to a clamp device for male patients.

RETROGRADE CYSTOGRAPHY
Contrast injection technique

In preparing for this examination, the following steps are observed:

- With the urethral catheter in place, adjust the patient in the supine position for a preliminary radiograph and the first cystogram.
- Usually, take cystograms of adult patients on 24- × 30-cm IRs placed lengthwise.
- Center the IR at the level of the soft tissue depression just above the most prominent point of the greater trochanters. This centering coincides with the middle area of a filled bladder of average size. Therefore the 30-cm IR will include the region of the distal end of the ureters for demonstration of ureteral reflux, and it will also include the prostate and proximal part of the male urethra.
- Have large IRs nearby for use when ureteral reflux is shown. Some radiologists request studies during contrast filling of the bladder, as well as during voiding.

After the preliminary radiograph is taken, the physician removes the catheter clamp and the bladder is drained in preparation for the introduction of the contrast material. After introducing the contrast agent, the physician clamps the catheter and tapes it to the thigh to keep it from being displaced during position changes.

The initial cystographic images generally consist of four projections: one AP, two AP obliques, and one lateral. Additional studies, including voiding cystourethrograms, are obtained as indicated. The Chassard-Lapiné method (see Chapter 7), often called the "squat shot," is sometimes used to obtain an axial projection of the posterior surface of the bladder and the lower end of the ureters when they are opacified. These projections of the bladder are also made when it is opacified by the excretory technique of urography.

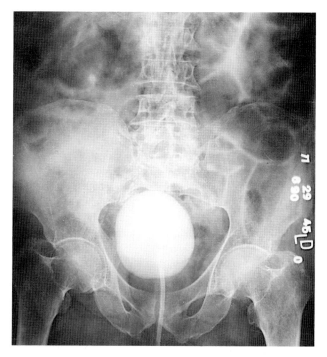

Fig. 18-64 Retrograde cystogram after introduction of contrast media: AP projection.

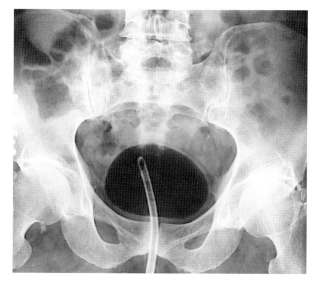

Fig. 18-65 Retrograde cystogram after introduction of air: AP projection.

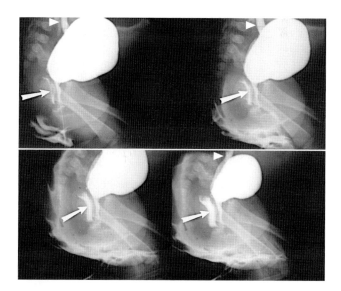

Fig. 18-66 Serial (polygraphic) voiding cystourethrograms in an infant girl with bilateral ureteral reflux *(arrowheads)*. Urethra is normal. Vaginal reflux *(arrows)* is a normal finding.

♠ AP AXIAL OR PA AXIAL PROJECTION

Image receptor: 24 × 30 cm lengthwise

Position of patient

- Place the patient supine on the radiographic table for the AP projection of the urinary bladder.

NOTE: Preliminary (scout) and postinjection radiographs are most commonly obtained with the patient supine. The prone position is sometimes used to image areas of the bladder not clearly seen on the AP axial projection. An AP axial projection using the Trendelenburg position at 15 to 20 degrees and with the central ray directed vertically is sometimes used to demonstrate the distal ends of the ureters. In this angled position, the weight of the contained fluid stretches the bladder fundus superiorly, giving an unobstructed projection of the lower ureters and the vesicoureteral orifice areas.

Position of part

- Center the midsagittal plane of the patient's body to the midline of the grid device.
- Adjust the patient's shoulders and hips so that they are equidistant from the IR.
- Place the patient's arms where they will not cast shadows on the IR.
- If the patient is positioned for a supine radiograph, have the patient's legs extended so that the lumbosacral area of the spine is arched enough to tilt the anterior pelvic bones inferiorly. In this position the pubic bones can more easily be projected below the bladder neck and proximal urethra (Fig. 18-67).
- Center the IR 2 inches (5 cm) above the upper border of the pubic symphysis (or at the pubic symphysis for voiding studies).
- *Respiration:* Suspend at the end of expiration.

Central ray

AP

- Angled 10 to 15 degrees caudal to the center of the IR. The central ray should enter 2 inches (5 cm) above the upper border of the pubic symphysis. When the bladder neck and proximal urethra are the main areas of interest, a 5-degree caudal angulation of the central ray is usually sufficient to project the pubic bones below them. More or less angulation may be necessary, depending on the amount of lordosis of the lumbar spine. With greater lordosis, less angulation may be needed (see Fig. 18-67).

PA

- When performing PA axial projections of the bladder, direct the central ray through the region of the bladder neck at an angle of 10 to 15 degrees cephalad, entering about 1 inch (2.5 cm) distal to the tip of the coccyx and exiting a little above the superior border of the pubic symphysis. If the prostate is the area of interest, the central ray is directed 20 to 25 degrees cephalad to project it above the pubic bones. For PA axial projections, the IR is centered to the central ray.
- Perpendicular to the pubic symphysis for voiding studies

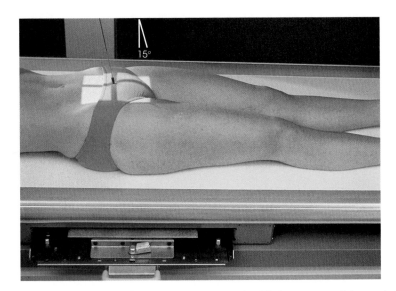

Fig. 18-67 Retrograde cystogram. AP axial bladder with 15-degree caudal angulation of central ray.

Structures shown

AP axial and PA axial projections demonstrate the bladder filled with contrast medium (Figs. 18-68 and 18-69). If reflux is present, the distal ureters are also visualized.

EVALUATION CRITERIA

The following should be clearly demonstrated:

- Regions of the distal end of the ureters, bladder, and proximal portion of the urethra
- Pubic bones projected below the bladder neck and proximal urethra
- Short scale of contrast clearly demonstrating contrast medium in the bladder, distal ureters, and proximal urethra

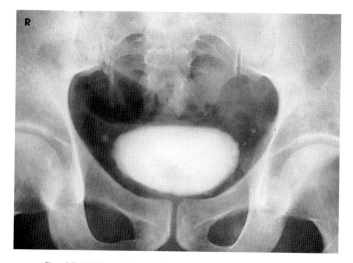

Fig. 18-68 Excretory cystogram: AP axial projection.

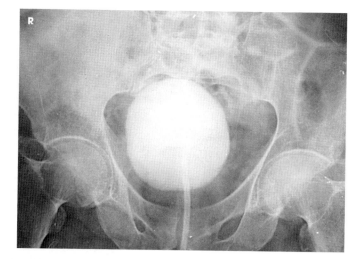

Fig. 18-69 Retrograde cystogram: AP axial projection. Note catheter in bladder.

▲ AP OBLIQUE PROJECTION
RPO or LPO position

Image receptor: 24 × 30 cm lengthwise

Position of patient
- Place the patient in the supine position on the radiographic table.

Position of part
- Rotate the patient 40 to 60 degrees RPO or LPO, according to the preference of the examining physician (Fig. 18-70).

- Adjust the patient so that the pubic arch closest to the table is aligned over the midline of the grid.
- Extend and abduct the uppermost thigh enough to prevent its superimposition on the bladder area.
- Center the IR 2 inches (5 cm) above the upper border of the pubic symphysis and approximately 2 inches (5 cm) medial to the upper ASIS (or at the pubic symphysis for voiding studies).
- *Respiration:* Suspend at the end of expiration.

Central ray
- Perpendicular to the center of the IR. The central ray will fall 2 inches (5 cm) above the upper border of the pubic symphysis and 2 inches (5 cm) medial to the upper ASIS. When the bladder neck and proximal urethra are the main areas of interest, a 10-degree caudal angulation of the central ray is usually sufficient to project the pubic bones below them.
- Perpendicular at the level of the pubic symphysis for voiding studies

Structures shown
Oblique projections demonstrate the bladder filled with the contrast medium. If reflux is present, the distal ureters are also visualized (Figs. 18-71 and 18-72).

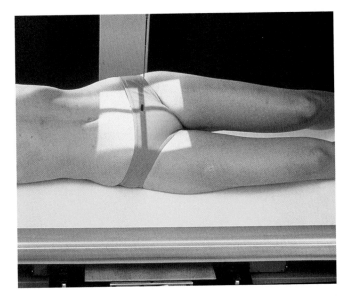

Fig. 18-70 Retrograde cystogram: AP oblique bladder, RPO position.

Urinary Bladder

EVALUATION CRITERIA

The following should be clearly demonstrated:

- Regions of the distal end of the ureters, bladder, and proximal portion of the urethra
- Pubic bones projected below the bladder neck and proximal urethra
- Short scale of contrast clearly demonstrating the contrast medium in the bladder, distal ureters, and proximal urethra
- No superimposition of the bladder by the uppermost thigh

Voiding studies

- Entire urethra visible and filled with the contrast medium
- Urethra overlapping the thigh on oblique projections for improved visibility
- Urethra lying posterior to the superimposed pubic and ischial rami on the side down in oblique projections

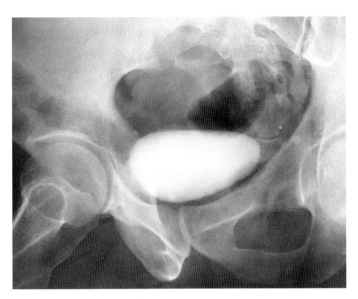

Fig. 18-71 Excretory cystogram: AP oblique bladder, RPO position.

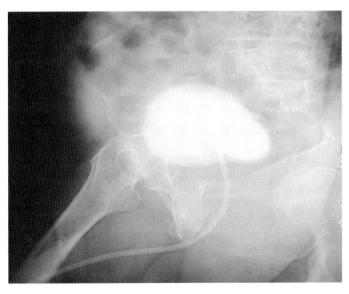

Fig. 18-72 Retrograde cystogram with catheter in bladder.

♠ LATERAL PROJECTION
R or L position

Image receptor: 24 × 30 cm lengthwise

Position of patient
- Place the patient in the lateral recumbent position on either the right or left side, as indicated.

Position of part
- Slightly flex the patient's knees to a comfortable position, and adjust the body so that the midcoronal plane is centered to the midline of the grid.
- Flex the patient's elbows, and place the hands under the head (Fig. 18-73).
- Center the IR 2 inches (5 cm) above the upper border of the pubic symphysis at the midcoronal plane.
- *Respiration:* Suspend at the end of expiration.

Central ray
- Perpendicular to the IR and 2 inches (5 cm) above the upper border of the pubic symphysis at the midcoronal plane

Structures shown
A lateral image demonstrates the bladder filled with the contrast medium. If reflux is present, the distal ureters are also visualized. Lateral projections demonstrate the anterior and posterior bladder walls and the base of the bladder (Fig. 18-74).

The following should be clearly demonstrated:
- Regions of the distal end of the ureters, bladder, and proximal portion of the urethra
- Short scale of contrast clearly demonstrating the contrast medium in the bladder, distal ureters, and proximal urethra
- Bladder and distal ureters visible through the pelvis
- Superimposed hips and femur

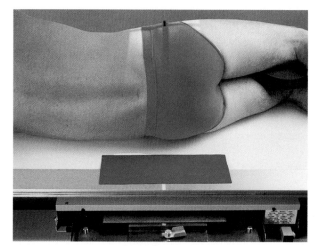

Fig. 18-73 Cystogram: lateral projection.

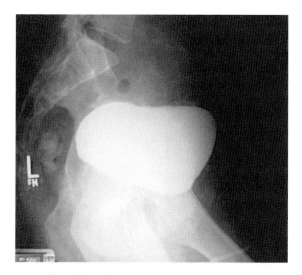

Fig. 18-74 Cystogram: lateral projection.

Urinary system and venipuncture

♣ AP OBLIQUE PROJECTION
RPO or LPO position

Male cystourethrography may be preceded by an endoscopic examination, after which the bladder is catheterized so that it can be drained just before contrast material is injected.

The following steps are observed:

- Use 24- × 30-cm IRs placed lengthwise for cystourethrograms in adult male patients.
- The patient is adjusted on the combination table so that the IR can be centered at the level of the superior border of the pubic symphysis. This centering coincides with the root of the penis, and a 30-cm (12-inch) IR will include both the bladder and the external urethral orifice.
- After inspecting the preliminary radiograph, the physician drains the bladder and withdraws the catheter.
- The supine patient is adjusted in an oblique position so that the bladder neck and the entire urethra are delineated as free of bony superimposition as possible. Rotate the patient's body 35 to 40 degrees, and adjust it so that the elevated pubis is centered to the midline of the grid. The superimposed pubic and ischial rami of the down side and the body of the elevated pubis usually are projected anterior to the bladder neck, proximal urethra, and prostate (Fig. 18-75).

- The patient's lower knee is flexed only slightly to keep the soft tissues on the medial side of the thigh as near to the center of the IR as possible.
- The elevated thigh is extended and retracted enough to prevent overlapping.
- With the patient in the correct position, the physician inserts the contrast-loaded urethral syringe or the nozzle of a device such as the Brodney clamp into the urethral orifice. The physician then extends the penis along the soft tissues of the medial side of the lower thigh to obtain a uniform density of both the deep and the cavernous portions of the urethral canal.

- At a signal from the physician, instruct the patient to hold still; make the exposure while the injection of the contrast material is continued to ensure filling of the entire urethra (Fig. 18-76).
- The bladder may then be filled with a contrast material so that a voiding study can be performed (Fig. 18-77). This is usually done without changing the patient's position. When a standing-upright voiding study is required, the patient is adjusted before a vertical grid device and is supplied with a urinal. (Further information on positioning is provided on pp. 232-236 of this volume.)

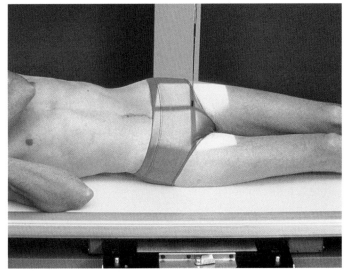

Fig. 18-75 Cystourethrogram: AP oblique projection, RPO position.

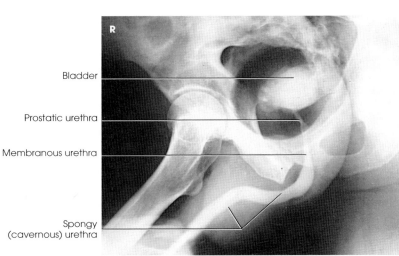

Bladder

Prostatic urethra

Membranous urethra

Spongy (cavernous) urethra

Fig. 18-76 Injection cystourethrogram: AP oblique urethra, RPO position.

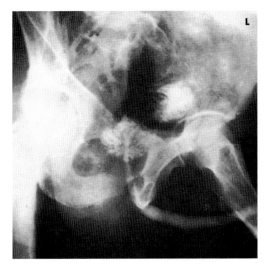

Fig. 18-77 Voiding cystourethrogram: AP oblique urethra, LPO position.

Urinary system and venipuncture

AP PROJECTION

INJECTION METHOD

The female urethra averages 3.5 cm in length. Its opening into the bladder is situated at the level of the superior border of the pubic symphysis. From this point the vessel slants obliquely inferiorly and anteriorly to its termination in the vestibule of the vulva, about 1 inch anterior to the vaginal orifice. The female urethra is subject to conditions such as tumors, abscesses, diverticula, dilation, and strictures. It is also subject to urinary incontinence during the stress of increased intraabdominal pressure, such as occurs during sneezing or coughing. In the investigation of abnormalities other than stress incontinence, contrast studies are made during the injection of contrast medium or during voiding.

Cystourethrography is usually preceded by an endoscopic examination. For this reason, it may be performed by the attending urologist or gynecologist with the assistance of a nurse and a radiographer.

The following steps are observed:

- After the physical examination, the cystoscope is removed and a catheter is inserted into the bladder so that the bladder can be drained just before injection of the contrast solution.

- The patient is adjusted in the supine position on the table.
- An 8- × 10-inch (18- × 24-cm) or 24- × 30-cm IR is placed lengthwise and centered at the level of the superior border of the pubic symphysis.
- A 5-degree caudal angulation of the central ray is usually sufficient to free the bladder neck of superimposition.
- After inspecting the preliminary radiograph, the physician drains the bladder and withdraws the catheter. The physician uses a syringe fitted with a blunt-nosed, soft-rubber acorn, which is held firmly against the urethral orifice to prevent reflux as the contrast solution is injected during the exposure.
- In addition to the AP projection, oblique projections may also be required. For the oblique projections, the patient is rotated 35 to 40 degrees so that the urethra is posterior to the pubic symphysis. The uppermost thigh is then extended and abducted enough to prevent overlapping.
- Further information on positioning is provided on pp. 232-236 of this volume.
- The physician fills the bladder for each voiding study to be made.

- For an AP projection (Figs. 18-78 and 18-79), the patient is maintained in the supine position, or the head of the table is elevated enough to place the patient in a semiseated position.
- A lateral voiding study of the female vesicourethral canal is performed with the patient recumbent or upright. In either case, the IR is centered at the level of the superior border of the pubic symphysis.

Metallic bead chain cystourethrography

The metallic bead chain technique of investigating anatomic abnormalities responsible for stress incontinence in women was described by Stevens and Smith[1] in 1937 and by Barnes[2] in 1940. This technique is used to delineate anatomic changes that occur in the shape and position of the bladder floor, in the poste-

---

[1]Stevens WE, Smith SP: Roentgenological examination of the female urethra, *J Urol* 37:194, 1937.
[2]Barnes AC: A method for evaluating the stress of urinary incontinence, *Am J Obstet Gynecol* 40:381, 1940.

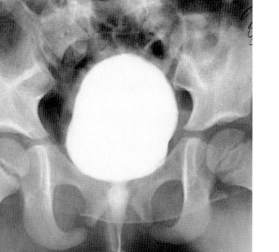

Fig. 18-78 Voiding cystourethrogram: AP projection.

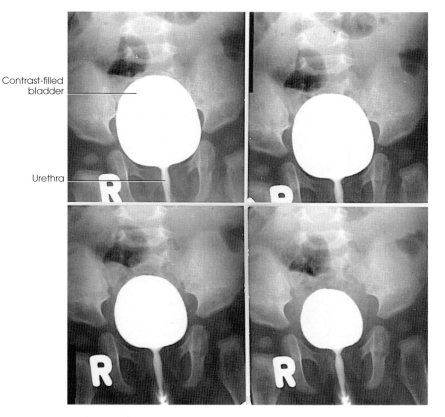

Contrast-filled bladder

Urethra

Fig. 18-79 Serial voiding images showing four stages of bladder emptying.

rior urethrovesical angle, in the position of the proximal urethral orifice, and in the angle of inclination of the urethral axis under the stress of increased intraabdominal pressure as exerted by the Valsalva maneuver.

Comparison AP and lateral projections are made with the patient standing at rest (Figs. 18-80 and 18-81) and straining (Figs. 18-82 and 18-83).

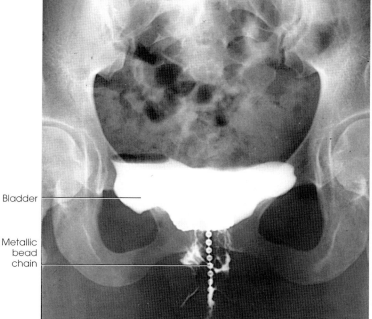

Bladder

Metallic
bead
chain

Fig. 18-80 Upright cystourethrogram: resting AP projection.

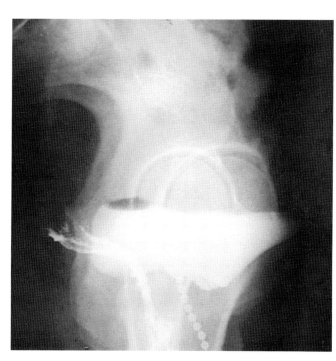

Fig. 18-81 Upright cystourethrogram: resting lateral projection.

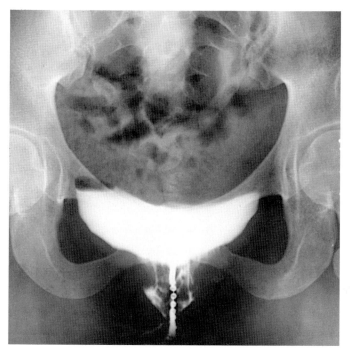

Fig. 18-82 Upright cystourethrogram: stress AP projection in the same patient as in Fig. 18-80.

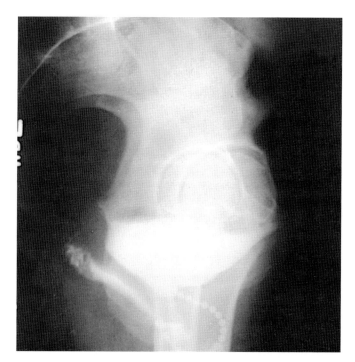

Fig. 18-83 Upright cystourethrogram: stress lateral projection.

For this examination the physician extends a flexible metallic bead chain through the urethral canal. The proximal portion of the chain rests within the bladder, and the distal end is taped to the thigh. For demonstration of the length of the urethra, a small, metal marker is attached with a piece of tape to the vaginal mucosa just lateral to the urethral orifice. After instillation of the metallic chain, a catheter is passed into the bladder, the contents of the bladder are drained, and an opaque contrast solution is injected. The catheter is removed for the imaging procedure.

Hodgkinson, Doub, and Kelly[1] recommended the upright position, which uses gravity and thus simulates normal body activity. Two sets of images (AP and lateral projections) are obtained, and the rest of the studies *must* be exposed before the stress studies are made because the bladder does not immediately return to its normal resting position after straining.

[1]Hodgkinson CP, Doub HP, Kelly WT: Urethrocystograms: metallic bead chain technique, *Clin Obstet Gynecol* 1:668, 1958.

After the metallic chain and contrast solution are instilled, the patient is usually prepared for upright radiographs. The examining room should be readied in advance so that the patient, who will be uncomfortable, can be given immediate attention. The patient must be given kind reassurance and must be examined in privacy. Klawon[1] found that the fear of involuntary voiding can be relieved by placing a folded towel or disposable pad between the patient's thighs before the stress radiographs are taken. Thus protected, the patient willingly applies full pressure during the stress studies.

The IR size and centering point are the same as for other female cystourethrograms. (Further information on positioning of the lower urinary tract is provided on pp. 232-236 of this volume.)

[1]Klawon Sister MM: Urethrocystography and urinary stress incontinence in women, *Radiol Techn* 39:353, 1968.

Advances in medical science and modern technology are creating tremendous changes and improvements in IV therapy, especially for those who perform diagnostic imaging. As IV therapy has evolved over the years, radiologic technologists are being assigned roles in the patient-focused, cost-effective collaborative team concept of modern health care. An estimated 80% of patients in acute-care settings require some type of IV medication. Administering medications accurately and safely is an important responsibility that must not be taken lightly.[1]

The principles of IV therapy include restoring and maintaining fluid and electrolyte balance, administering medication, transfusing blood, and delivering parenteral nutrition solutions. The radiologic technologist may initiate venipuncture and administer medications by physician order for specific indications in certain types of IV therapy related to radiographic procedures.[2]

Professional and Legal Considerations

Because of patient risk and legal liabilities, the radiologic technologist must follow professional recommendations, state regulations, and institutional policies for the administration of medications. The information presented in this section is meant to be an introduction to IV therapy. Competency in this area requires the completion of a formal course of instruction with supervised clinical practice and evaluation.

[1]Kowalczyk N, Donnett K: *Integrated patient care for the imaging professional,* St Louis, 1996, Mosby.
[2]Tortorici M: *Administration of imaging pharmaceuticals,* Philadelphia, 1996, Saunders.

The American Society of Radiologic Technologists (ASRT) includes venipuncture and IV medication administration in the curriculum guidelines for the educational opportunities offered to technologists. Additional support for the administration of medications and venipuncture as part of the technologist's scope of practice is found in the 1987 Resolution No. 27 from the American College of Radiology (ACR).[1] This resolution supports the injection of contrast materials and diagnostic levels of radiopharmaceuticals within specific established guidelines by certified and/or licensed radiologic technologists. The ASRT Standards of Practice for Radiography also support the administration of medication by technologists.

Technologists who perform venipuncture and contrast media administration must be knowledgeable about the specific state regulations and facility policies that govern these activities. Technologists also are responsible for professional decisions and actions in their practice. Competency in the skills of venipuncture and contrast media administration are based on cognitive knowledge, proficiency in psychomotor skills, positive affective values, and validation in a clinical setting.

Medications

Medications for a specific procedure are prescribed by a physician, who is also responsible for obtaining informed consent for the procedure. A technologist may administer medications for radiographic procedures, which can require medications for sedation, pain management, contrast media administration, and emergencies.[2] The technologist must have an extensive knowledge of all medications used in the radiology department. IV medications are administered into the body via the vascular system; once administered, they cannot be retrieved. Therefore before administering any medication, the technologist must know the medication's name, dosages, indications, contraindications, and possible adverse reactions (Table 18-1).

[1]Tortorici M: *Administration of imaging pharmaceuticals,* Philadelphia, 1996, Saunders.
[2]Kowalczyk N, Donnett K: *Integrated patient care for the imaging professional,* St Louis, 1996, Mosby.

Patient Education

The manner in which the technologist approaches the patient can have a direct influence on the patient's response to the procedure. Although the technologist may consider the procedure routine, the patient may be totally unfamiliar with its specifics. Apprehension experienced by the patient can cause vasoconstriction, making the venipuncture more difficult and more painful.[1] Careful explanation and a confident, sympathetic attitude can help the patient relax.

The technologist must provide information about the procedure in terms of the patient's understanding. The patient's questions must be answered in "layman's" language. By explaining the details of the procedure, the technologist can help alleviate fears and solicit cooperation from the patient. It is important to explain the steps in the procedure, its expected duration, and any limitations or restrictions associated with its performance. The patient may have heard an inaccurate "horror" story about the procedure from a neighbor or friend. Therefore the technologist may need to correct misconceptions and provide accurate information.

For simple procedures the patient must be reassured that the procedure is relatively straightforward and causes only slight discomfort. For more complex and longer procedures, the technologist must gain the patient's cooperation by providing appropriate, factual information and offering support. *The patient should never be told that insertion of the needle used in venipuncture does not hurt.* After all, a foreign object is going to be inserted through the patient's skin, which has a myriad of nerves that will be aggravated by insertion of a needle. The technologist must tell the truth and explain that the amount of pain experienced varies with each patient.[2]

[1]*IV therapy: skillbuilders,* Springhouse, Pa, 1991, Springhouse.
[2]Hoeltke L: *The complete textbook of phlebotomy,* ed 3, Albany, NY, 2006, Delmar.

Patient education

TABLE 18-1

Common medications used in an imaging department

Brand name	Generic name	Indications	Action	Adverse reactions
Atropine How supplied: Injection, tablets	atropine sulfate	Symptomatic brady-cardia, brad-yarrhythmia	Inhibits acetylcholine at the parasympathetic neuroef-fector junction, thereby enhancing/increasing heart rate	Bradycardia, headache, dry mouth, nausea, vom-iting
Benadryl How supplied: Tablets, capsules, elixir, syrup, injection	diphenhydramine hydrochloride	Allergic reactions, sedation	Competes with histamine for special receptors on effec-tor cells; prevents but does not reverse histamine-medi-ated responses	Seizures, sleepiness, insom-nia, incoordination, rest-lessness, nausea, vomit-ing, diarrhea
Demerol How supplied: Tablets, syrup, injection	meperidine hydrochloride	Mild to moderate pain Adjunct to anesthesia	Binds with opiate receptors of the CNS	Seizures, cardiac arrest, shock, respiratory depres-sion
Dopamine How supplied: Injection	dopamine hydrochloride	Shock, increase car-diac output, cor-rect hypotension	Stimulates dopaminergic and alpha and beta receptors of the sympathetic nervous system	Tachycardia, hypotension, nausea, vomiting, ana-phylactic reactions
Epinephrine How supplied: Injection, inhaler	adrenaline	Restore cardiac rhythm in cardiac arrest Bronchospasm Anaphylaxis	Relaxes bronchial smooth muscle by stimulating $beta_2$ receptors and alpha and beta receptors in the sym-pathetic nervous system	Palpations, ventricular fibril-lation, shock, nervousness
Glucagon How supplied: Injection	glucagon	Hypoglycemia	Raises blood glucose level by promoting catalytic depo-lymerization of hepatic gly-cogen to glucose	Bronchospasm, hypoten-sion, nausea, vomiting
Morphine How supplied: Tablets, syrup, oral suspension, injection	morphine sulfate	Severe pain	Binds with opiate receptors of the CNS	Bradycardia, shock, car-diac arrest, apnea, respi-ratory depression, respira-tory arrest
Noctec How supplied: Capsules, syrup, suppositories	chloral hydrate	Sedation	Unknown, sedative effects may be caused by its pri-mary metabolite	Drowsiness, nightmares, hallucinations, nausea, vomiting, diarrhea
Phenegran How supplied: Tablets, syrup, injection, supposi-tories	promethazine hydrochloride	Nausea, sedation	Competes with histamine for special receptors on effec-tor cells; prevents but does not reverse histamine-medi-ated responses	Dry mouth
Valium How supplied: Tablets, capsules, oral solutions, injections	diazepam	Anxiety	Unknown; probably depresses the CNS at the limbic and subcortical levels	Cardiovascular collapse, bradycardia, respiratory depression, acute with-drawal syndrome
Versed How supplied: Injection	midazolam hydrochloride	Preoperative seda-tion (to induce sleepiness or drows-iness and relieve apprehension)	Unknown; thought to depress CNS at the limbic and sub-cortical levels	Apnea, depressed respira-tory rate, nausea, vomit-ing, hiccups, pain at injection site
Vistaril How supplied: Tablets, syrup, cap-sules, injection	hydroxyzine hydrochloride	Nausea and vomit-ing, anxiety, pre-operative and postoperative adjunctive therapy	Unknown; actions may be due to a suppression of activity in key regions of the subcortical area of the CNS	Dry mouth, dyspnea, wheezing, chest tightness

Data from *Nursing 2006 drug handbook,* Ambler, Pa, 2006, Lippincott Williams & Wilkins.

Interactions	Effects on diagnostic imaging procedures	Contraindications	Patient care considerations
May increase anticholinergic drug effects; use together cautiously	None known	Patients with obstructive disease of the GI tract, paralytic ileus, toxic megacolon, tachycardia, myocardia/ischemia, or asthma	Watch for tachycardia in cardiac patients; may lead to ventricular fibrillation
Increased effects when used with other CNS depressants	None known	Hypersensitivity to drug, during acute asthmatic attacks, and in newborns or premature neonates and breastfeeding women	Use with extreme caution in patients with angle-closure glaucoma, asthma, COPD
May be incompatible when mixed in the same IV container	None known	Patients with hypersensitivity to drug and in those who have received MAO inhibitors within past 14 days	Give slowly by direct IV injection; oral dose is less than half as effective as parental dose Compatible with most IV solutions
Alpha and/or beta blockers may antagonize effects	None known	Patients with uncorrected tachycardias, pheochromocytoma, or ventricular fibrillation	During infusion, frequently monitor ECG, blood pressure, cardiac output, central venous pressure, pulse rate, urine output, and color and temperature of limbs
Avoid using with alpha blockers (may cause hypotension)	None known	Patients with shock, organic brain damage, cardiac dilation, arrhythmias, coronary insufficiency, or cerebral arteriosclerosis	Drug of choice in emergency treatment of acute anaphylactic reactions; avoid IM use of parenteral suspension into buttocks
Inhibits glucagon-induced insulin release	None known	Patients with hypersensitivity to drug or with pheochromocytoma	Arouse patient from coma as quickly as possible and give additional carbohydrates orally to prevent secondary hypoglycemic reactions
In combination with other depressants and narcotics, use with extreme caution	None known	Patients with hypersensitivity to drug or conditions that would preclude administration of IV opioids	Use with extreme caution in patients with head injuries or increased intracranial pressure and in the elderly
Alkaline solutions incompatible with aqueous solutions of chloral hydrate	None known	Patients with hepatic or renal impairment, severe cardiac disease, or hypersensitivity to drug	Note two strengths of oral liquid form; double-check dose, especially when administering to children
Increased effects when used with other CNS depressants	Discontinue drug 48 hours before a myelogram because of high risk of seizures	Patients with hypersensitivity to drug; intestinal obstruction, prostatic hyperplasias	Do not administer subcutaneously
Other CNS depressants	May cause minor changes in ECG patterns	Patients with hypersensitivity to drug or soy protein, shock, coma, or acute alcohol intoxication	Monitor respirations and have emergency resuscitation equipment available before administering
CNS depressants may increase risk of apnea	None known	Patients with hypersensitivity to drug, acute angle-closure glaucoma, shock, coma, or acute alcohol intoxication	Use cautiously in patients with uncompensated acute illness and in the elderly; have emergency resuscitation equipment available before administering
Can increase CNS depression	None known	Hypersensitivity to drug, during pregnancy, and in breastfeeding women	If used in conjunction with other CNS medication, observe for oversedation

Patient Assessment

The patient must be assessed before any medication is administered. A history of allergy must be obtained and documented. It is essential to determine whether the patient has any known allergies to foods, medications, environmental agents, or other substances. Before venipuncture is performed, the technologist needs to be aware of the potential for an allergic reaction to the iodine tincture used in puncture site preparation or an adverse reaction to the medication being injected.

Other assessment criteria include the patient's current medications. Knowledge of some common medication actions can help the radiologic technologist evaluate changes in a patient's condition during a procedure. Certain diabetic medications interact adversely with contrast media. Therefore assessment of the interaction of medications must be evaluated prior to the performance of the procedure.

During the physical evaluation, it is important to determine whether the patient has previously undergone surgical procedures that might affect site selection for venipuncture; for example, a mastectomy with resultant compromised lymph nodes and vascular abnormalities, such as arterioventricular (AV) shunts. To determine the appropriate type and amount of medication to be administered, the physician requires information about the patient's past and current disease processes, such as hypertension and renal disease. Evaluation of the BUN level (average range: 10 to 20 mg/dL) and the creatinine level (average range: 0.05 to 1.2 mg/dL) should be included as assessment criteria.

Infection Control

Each time the body system is entered, the potential for contamination exists.[1] Strict aseptic techniques and universal precautions must always be used when medications are administered with a needle.[2] If a medication is injected incorrectly, a microorganism may enter the body and cause an infection or other complications. The Centers for Disease Control and Prevention (CDC) have developed specific guidelines to prevent the transmission of infections during the preparation and administration of medications. These guidelines are part of the Standard Precautions used by every health care facility, and strict adherence to the guidelines must be followed by the technologist during the performance of radiologic procedures.

Studies using IV filters have shown a significant reduction in infusion phlebitis. Filters are devices located within the tubing used for IV administration. Filters prevent the injection of particulate and microbial matter into the circulatory system. The use of a filter for a bolus injection reduces the rate at which the medication can be injected. In addition, the viscosity of a medication may determine whether a filter is used and the rate of injection. Although a filter helps in reducing the possibility of bacteria being introduced into the blood, its use creates additional factors of risks versus benefits. The physician or health care facility should have policies to address these issues.

[1]Smith S et al: *Clinical nursing skills: basic to advanced skills,* ed 6, Stamford, Conn, 2003, Appleton and Lange.
[2]Adler AM, Carlton RR: *Introduction to radiography and patient care,* ed 3, Philadelphia, 2003, Saunders.

Venipuncture Supplies and Equipment

NEEDLES AND SYRINGES

The technologist assembles the proper syringe and needle for the planned injection. The syringe may be glass or plastic. Plastic syringes are disposed of after only one use; glass syringes may be cleaned and must be sterilized before they are used again. The syringe has three parts: the *tip,* where the needle attaches to the syringe; the *barrel,* which includes the calibration markings; and the *plunger,* which fits snugly inside the barrel and allows the user to instill the medication (Fig. 18-84). The tip of the syringe for an IV injection has a locking device to hold the needle securely. The size of the syringe depends on the volume of material to be injected. The technologist should select the next-larger size of syringe than the volume desired. This larger syringe assists in the accuracy of the dose by allowing the total amount of medication to be drawn into one syringe.

All needles used in venipuncture are disposable and are used only once. During the preparation and administration of contrast media, the technologist may use several types of needles, including a hypodermic needle, a butterfly set, and an over-the-needle cannula (Fig. 18-85).

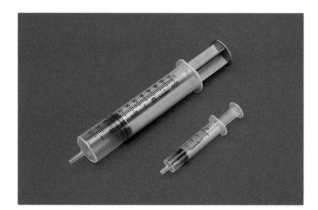

Fig. 18-84 Plastic disposable syringes.

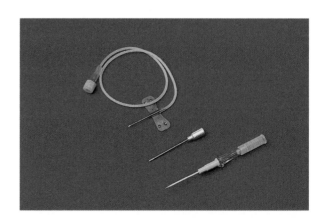

Fig. 18-85 Types of needles: over-the-cannula needle, or angio-catheter *(bottom),* a hypodermic needle *(center),* and metal butterfly needle *(top).*

Hypodermic needles vary in both gauge and length (see Fig. 18-83). Needle *gauge* refers to the *diameter* of the needle bore, with the gauge increasing as the diameter of the bore decreases. An 18-gauge needle is larger than a 22-gauge needle. As the bore of the needle increases, a given volume of fluid may be administered more rapidly. If bore size is reduced and fluid volume and rate of administration remain constant, the pressure (force) of the injection increases. The *length* of a needle is measured in inches and may vary from ½ inch (used for intradermal injections) to 4½ inches (used for intrathecal [spinal] injections). As a general rule, needles 1 to 1½ inches long are most commonly used for IV injections. The needle has three parts: the *hub,* which is the part that attaches to the syringe; the *cannula* or *shaft,* which is the length of the needle; and the *bevel,* which is the slanted portion of the needle tip. Needles should be visually examined before and after use to determine whether any structural defects, such as nonbeveled points or bent shafts, are present.[1]

Butterfly sets or *angiocatheters* are preferable to a conventional hypodermic needle for most radiographic IV therapies. The butterfly set consists of a stainless-steel needle with plastic appendages on either side and approximately 6 inches of plastic tubing that ends with a connector. The plastic appendages, often called wings, aid in inserting the needle and stabilization of the needle once venous patency has been confirmed.

The *over-the-needle cannula* is a device in which, once the venipuncture is made, the catheter is slipped off the needle into the vein and the steel needle is removed. This type of needle is recommended for long-term therapy or for rapid infusions. The choice of needle should be based on the assessment of the patient, institutional policy, and the technologist's preference.

MEDICATION PREPARATION

Although IV offers the most immediate results in terms of effect, certain safety precautions must be followed. The technologist must identify the correct patient before medication is administered. During preparation and again before administration, the medication in the container also must be verified.

[1]Strasinger S, DiLorenzo M: *Phlebotomy workbook for the multiskilled healthcare professional,* ed 2, Philadelphia, 2003, FA Davis.

If the medication is supplied in a bottle or vial, the preparation procedure has several variations. First, the solution must be evaluated for contamination. Then the protective cap is removed, with care taken not to contaminate the underlying surface. Containers have rubber stoppers through which a hypodermic needle can be inserted. If a single-dose vial is being used, and no contamination has occurred, the rubber stopper requires no additional cleansing. Multiple-dose vial stoppers must be cleaned with an alcohol wipe.

For a closed system to be maintained, and to reduce the chance of possible infection, a volume of air equal to the amount of desired fluid must be injected into the bottle. The plunger of the syringe is pulled back to the level of the desired amount of medication. The shaft of the plunger must not be contaminated at any time during preparation of the medica-

tion. The needle on the syringe is inserted into the rubber stopper, all the way to the hub of the needle. Then the vial is inverted by placing the end of the needle above the fluid level in the bottle (Fig. 18-86). Next, a small amount of air is *slowly* injected into the vial *above* the level of the fluid. This technique helps decrease air bubbles in the solution. After the air has been injected, the vial and syringe are held inverted and perpendicular to a horizontal plane, and the tip of the needle is pulled *below* the fluid level. The desired amount of medication is aspirated into the syringe by pulling down on the plunger of the syringe. The above procedure may have to be repeated several times to expel all of the medication. If air bubbles cling to the syringe casing, the syringe may be lightly tapped to release them. A one-handed method is used to recap the syringe (Fig. 18-87).

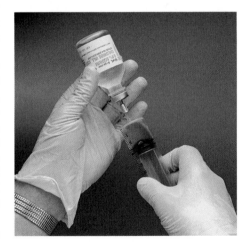

Fig. 18-86 Place the tip of the needle above the level of fluid before injection of air to decrease air bubbles in the solution.

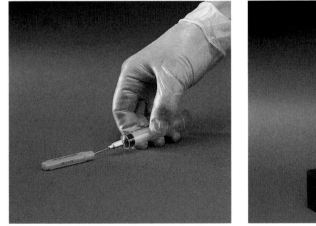 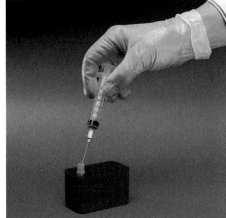

Fig. 18-87 When recapping a syringe, use a one-handed method.

Preparation of an infusion from a glass bottle or plastic bag begins with the identification and verification of the solution and its expiration date (Fig. 18-88). The solution should not contain any visible particles. The tubing used for the infusion is determined by the method of injection and the type of container. Electronic infusion devices require different tubing than gravity infusion devices. A glass container necessitates a vented tubing (Fig. 18-89), whereas a plastic container requires a nonvented tubing (Fig. 18-90).

To prepare for drip infusion of a medication, the technologist removes the tubing from the sterile package and closes the clamp (Fig. 18-91). Failure to close the clamp may result in loss of the vacuum in the solution container. The protective coverings are removed from the port of the solution and the tubing spike. Then the fill chamber of the tubing is squeezed, and the spike is inserted into the solution. The solution is then inverted and the chamber is released. The solution should fill the chamber to the measurement line. The tubing is primed by opening the clamp, which allows the solution to travel the length of the tubing, expelling any air. The tube is filled with solution, the clamp is closed, and the protective covering is secured. The solution is then ready for administration.

Procedure
SITE SELECTION

Selection of an appropriate vein for venipuncture is critical. Finding the vein is sometimes difficult, and the most visible veins are not always the best choice.[1] Technologists administer IV medication and contrast media via the venous system. Therefore if a pulse is palpated during assessment for a puncture site, that vessel must not be used *because* it is an *artery!* The prime factors to consider in selecting a vein are (1) suitability of location, (2) condition of the vein, (3) purpose of the infusion, and (4) duration of therapy. The veins most often used in establishing IV access are found on the anterior forearm, posterior hand, radial aspect of the wrist, and antecubital space on the anterior surface of the elbow (Fig. 18-92).

A general rule is to select the most distal site that can accept the desired-size needle and tolerate the injection rate and solution. Although the veins located at the antecubital space may be the most accessible, largest, and easiest to puncture, they may not be the best choice. Because of their convenient location, these sites may be overused and can become scarred or sclerotic. Antecubital accesses are located over an area of joint flexion; therefore any motion can dislodge the cannula and cause infiltration or result in mechanical phlebitis. A flexible IV catheter is the needle of choice for placement of a venous access in the antecubital space. The patient's arm should be immobilized to inhibit the ability to flex the elbow.

[1]Steele J: *Practical IV therapy,* Springhouse, Pa, 1988, Springhouse.

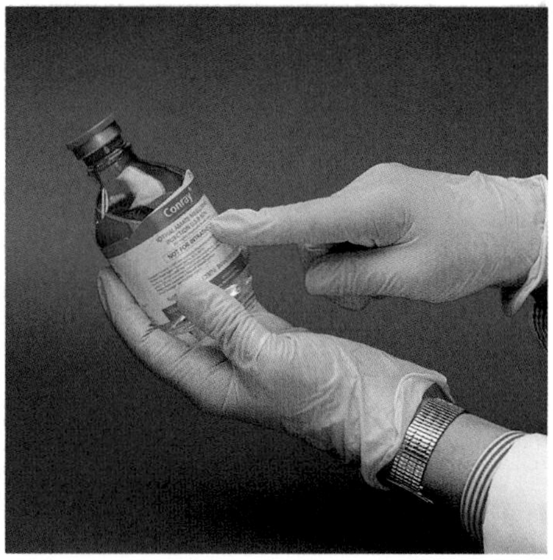

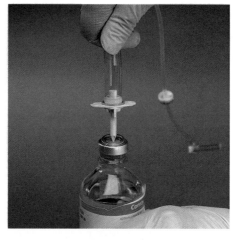

Fig. 18-88 Identify the correct solution and expiration date.

Fig. 18-89 A vented tubing is required for glass bottle containers.

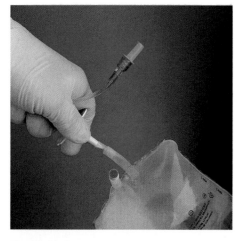

Fig. 18-90 Solutions in plastic bags require a nonvented tubing.

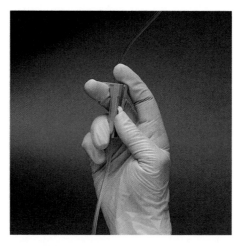

Fig. 18-91 Close the tubing clamp before inserting the spike into a container of solution.

The condition of the vein must also be considered in the selection of an appropriate puncture site. The selected vein must be able to tolerate the needed or desired cannula size. The vein should have resilience qualities and be anchored by surrounding supportive tissues to prevent rolling.

Another consideration in vein selection is the rate of flow required for the procedure and the viscosity and amount of medication to be administered. Because the purpose of the infusion determines the rate of flow, the solution to be infused should be evaluated during the site selection process. Larger veins should be selected for infusions of large quantities or for rapid infusions. Large veins are also used for the infusion of highly viscous solutions or those that are irritating to vessels.[1]

The expected duration of the therapy and the patient's comfort are other factors that must be considered in selecting a venipuncture site. If a prolonged course of therapy is anticipated, areas over flexion joints should be avoided, and the dorsal surfaces of the upper limbs should be carefully examined. Venous access in these locations will provide more freedom and comfort to the patient.

[1]Adler AM, Carlton RR: *Introduction to radiography and patient care,* ed 3, Philadelphia, 2003, Saunders.

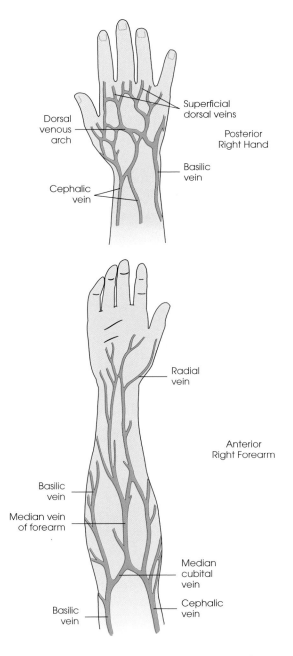

Fig. 18-92 Veins easily accessible for venipuncture.

SITE PREPARATION

The skin's surface must be prepared and cleaned. If the area selected for venipuncture is hairy, the hair should be clipped to permit better cleansing of the skin and visualization of the vein. This will also make removal of the cannula less painful when the infusion is terminated. Shaving is not recommended. The skin is cleansed with an antiseptic, which should remain in contact with the skin for at least 30 seconds. The preferred solution is iodine tincture 1% to 2%. Isopropyl alcohol 70% is recommended if the patient is sensitive to iodine. The skin should be cleaned in a *circular motion from the center of the injection site* to approximately a 2-inch circle. Once the swab has been placed on the skin, it should not be lifted from the surface until the cleansing process is complete (Fig. 18-93).

Many facilities have a policy that provides the patient an opportunity to request a local anesthetic for IV infusion catheter placement. This technique reduces the pain felt by the patient during insertion of an angiocatheter or needle. The local anesthetic can be administered topically or by injection.

A facility's procedure for local anesthetic determines the specific criteria for that institution. Commonly accepted guidelines are as follows: First, 0.1 to 0.2 mL of 1% lidocaine without epinephrine or sterile saline is prepared in a tuberculin or insulin syringe with a 23- to 25-gauge needle. The site for injection is selected and prepared. Then the anesthetic is injected subcutaneously (beneath the skin, into the soft tissue) or intradermally (immediately under the skin in the dermal layer) at the venipuncture site. Topical anesthesia is achieved by applying 5 g of eutectic mixture of local anesthetic cream and covering the area with an occlusive dressing. Maximum effects are achieved in 45 to 60 minutes.

The medication to be injected should already be prepared, and any tubing should be primed with the solution to prevent injection of any air into the vascular system.

VENIPUNCTURE

After the solution has been prepared, the site selected, and the type of syringe and needle to be used has been determined, the technologist is ready to perform the venipuncture.

Techniques for venipuncture follow one of two courses: (1) the *direct,* or *one-step,* entry method or (2) the *indirect* method. The *direct,* or *one-step,* method is performed by thrusting the cannula through the skin and into the vein in one quick motion. The needle and cannula enter the skin directly over the vein. This technique is excellent as long as large veins are available.[1] The *indirect* method is a two-step technique. First, the over-the-needle cannula is inserted through the skin adjacent to or below the point where the vein is visible. The cannula is then advanced and maneuvered to pierce the vein. For the actual venipuncture procedure, the technologist washes the hands. The patient is identified. Next the technologist instructs the patient about the procedure. The technologist performs the following steps:

1. The technologist puts on gloves and cleans the area in accordance with facility protocol (Fig. 18-94).

---

[1]Weinstein SM: *Plumer's principles and practice of intravenous therapy,* ed 8, Boston, 2006, Little, Brown.

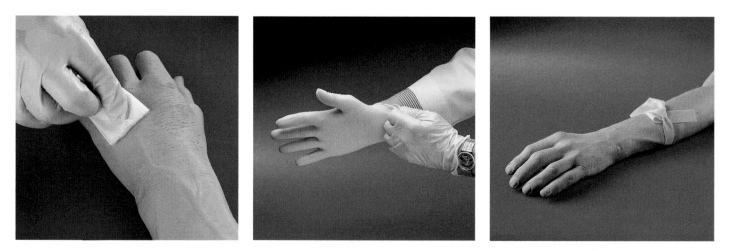

Fig. 18-93 Prepare the site for venipuncture.

Fig. 18-94 Put on clean gloves.

Fig. 18-95 Apply the tourniquet 6 to 8 inches above the intended venipuncture site, with its free end directed superiorly.

2. A local anesthetic is administered according to facility policy (optional).

3. A tourniquet is placed 6 to 8 inches *above* the intended site of puncture. The tourniquet should be tight enough to distend the vessels but not occlude them. The loose ends of the tourniquet should be placed away from the injection site to prevent contamination of the aseptic area (Fig. 18-95).

4. The technologist holds the patient's limb with the nondominant hand, using that thumb to stabilize and anchor the selected vein. The best method of accessing the vein—direct or indirect technique—is then determined.

5. Using the dominant hand, the technologist places the needle bevel up at a 45-degree angle to the skin's surface. The bevel-up position produces less trauma to the skin and vein (Fig. 18-96).

6. The technologist uses a quick, sharp darting motion to enter the skin with the needle. Upon entering the skin, the technologist decreases the angle of the needle to 15 degrees from the long axis of the vessel. Using an indirect method, the technologist slowly proceeds with a downward motion on the hub or wings of the needle; raising the point of the needle, the technologist advances the needle parallel and then punctures the vein. The needle may have to be maneuvered slightly to facilitate actual venous puncture. If the direct method of access is used, the needle is placed on the skin directly over the vein, and entry into the vein is accomplished in one movement of the needle through the skin and vein. Once the vein is entered, a backflow of blood may occur—this indicates a successful venipuncture.

7. Once the vein is punctured and a blood return is noted, the cannula is advanced cautiously up the lumen of the vessel for approximately ¾ inch.

8. Release the tourniquet (Fig. 18-97).

9. If a backflow of blood does not occur, verify venous access before injecting the medication. Aspiration of blood directly into the syringe of medication verifies placement before injecting. Another method of placement verification is to attach a syringe of normal saline to the hub of the needle before aspirating for blood. The advantage of this method is that only saline, an isotonic solution, is injected if the needle is not in place and extravasation occurs. A successful venipuncture does not guarantee a successful injection. If a bolus injection is desired, the tourniquet may not be released until the injection has been completed. If this technique is used, the protocol must be included in the facility's policies and procedures.

10. Anchor the needle with tape and a dressing, as required by policy (Fig. 18-98). Then administer the medication (Fig. 18-99).

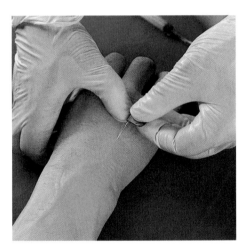

Fig. 18-96 Stabilize the vein and enter the skin with the needle at a 45-degree angle.

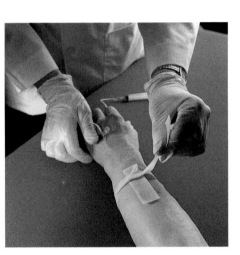

Fig. 18-97 Release the tourniquet after the venous access has been obtained. Do not permit the tourniquet to touch the needle.

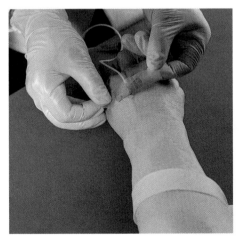

Fig. 18-98 Anchor the needle with tape to secure placement.

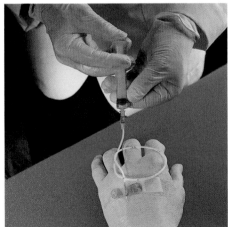

Fig. 18-99 Administer the medication.

With experience, a technologist's fingers become sensitive to the sensation of the needle entering the vein—the resistance encountered as the needle penetrates the wall of the vein and the "pop" felt at the loss of resistance as the cannula enters the lumen. If both walls of the vein are punctured with a needle, the vessel develops a hematoma. The cannula should be removed immediately, and direct pressure should be applied to the puncture site. If a venipuncture attempt is unsuccessful with an over-the-needle cannula and the needle has been removed from the cannula, the needle should not be reinserted into the catheter. Reinserting the needle into the cannula can shear a portion of the catheter.

ADMINISTRATION

The technologist should administer the medication and/or contrast medium at the established rate. During the injection process, the injection site should be observed and palpated proximal to the puncture for signs of infiltration. An infiltration, or extravasation, is a process whereby a fluid passes into the tissue instead of the vein.

A patient may have a venous access that was established before the radiologic procedure. A careful assessment of site and medication compatibility must be performed before the existing IV line can be used. (Compatibility is the ability of one medication to mix with another.) Special precautions should be taken with a patient who is currently receiving cardiac, blood pressure, heparin, or diabetes medications. The physician, nurse, or pharmacist should be consulted before medication is administered to such a patient. Verification must be obtained to ensure that the medication being infused through the established IV line is compatible with the *contrast medium* to be administered. Before the contrast medium is injected, the infusion should be stopped and the line should be flushed with normal saline through the port nearest the insertion site. The contrast *medium* is then administered, and the line is flushed again with normal saline. The amount of normal saline used depends on the facility's policies and procedures. Once the contrast medium has been administered, the IV infusion solution is restarted.

Heparin or saline locks allow intermittent injections through a port. The port is a small adapter with an access that is attached to an IV catheter when more than one injection is anticipated.[1] As determined by procedure criteria, the cannula is flushed with heparin and saline to maintain patency during dormant periods.

The patency (open, unobstructed flow) of the intermittent device is verified by aspirating blood and injecting normal saline without infiltration. Then the medication is administered. Finally, the medication is flushed through the device with saline. Depending on protocols, the device may then be flushed with heparin or normal saline.

After the medication has been administered and the radiologic procedure has been completed, the venous access may be discontinued. The radiologic technologist should carefully remove any tape or protective dressing covering the puncture site. Using a 2- × 2-inch gauze pad at the injection site, the technologist then removes the needle by pulling it straight from the vein. Direct pressure on the site is applied with the gauze only after the needle has been removed (Fig. 18-100). The technologist then puts the contaminated gloves, needles, and gauze in appropriate disposal containers (Fig. 18-101).

[1]Ehrlich R, McCloskey ED, Daly J: *Patient care in radiography,* ed 6, St Louis, 2004, Mosby.

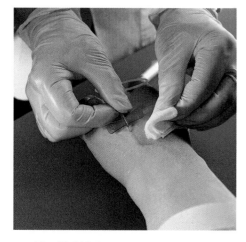

Fig. 18-100 Remove the IV access.

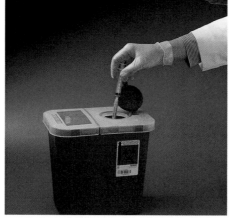

Fig. 18-101 Discard needles in puncture-resistant containers.

Reactions and Complications

Any *medication* has the potential to be harmful if it is not administered properly.[1] Technologists must be aware of possible untoward medication reactions and be able to recognize and report signs and symptoms of side effects as they occur.[2] The technologist who prepares a medication should also perform the administration.

Reactions can be mild, moderate, or severe. Mild reactions can include a sensation of warmth, a metallic taste, or sneezing. Moderate reactions can manifest as nausea, vomiting, or itching. Finally, a severe, or *anaphylactic*, reaction can cause a respiratory or cardiac crisis. The treatment for each category of reaction should be established in the procedures of each facility or department. The role of the radiologic technologist in the case of a reaction should also be defined in these documents. Competent professional standards of practice for the technologist include monitoring the patient's vital signs before, during, and after the injection of a contrast medium or certain types of medications. The specific monitoring criteria should be established by institutional policy. Therefore if an untoward event should occur, responding personnel will have access to important information about the patient's condition before the event occurred.

Every health care provider should be familiar with emergency procedures in the work environment. Emergency crash carts contain many medications and pieces of equipment that require regular review. Proficiency in the operation of equipment and the administration of medications must be maintained. The technologist must have the knowledge, proficiency, and confidence to manage crisis situations.

---

[1]Kowalczyk N, Donnett K: *Integrated patient care for the imaging professional,* St Louis, 1996, Mosby.
[2]Adler AM, Carlton RR: *Introduction to radiography and patient care,* ed 3, Philadelphia, 2003, Saunders.

Infiltration is another complication associated with the administration of contrast media or medications. This complication occurs when the medication or contrast material enters the soft tissue instead of the vein.[1] Signs of infiltration are swelling, redness, burning, and pain. The most common cause of extravasation is needle displacement. If infiltration occurs, the procedure should be stopped immediately and the venous access discontinued. The physician must be notified, and specific treatment instructions must be requested. Common therapies for infiltration are (1) the application of ice if less than 30 minutes have passed since the infiltration occurred or (2) the application of warm, wet compresses if the infiltration occurred more than 30 minutes previously.[1]

Documentation

In the administration of any medication, the radiologic technologist should always observe five "rights of medication administration":

- The right patient
- The right medication
- The right route
- The right amount
- The right time

The *right patient* must receive the medication. The identity of the patient must be confirmed before the medication is administered. Methods of patient identification include checking the patient's wristband and asking the patient to restate his or her name. If the patient is unable to speak, seek assistance in identifying the patient from a family member or significant other. Ensuring that the *right medication* is administered requires that the name of the medication be verified at least three times: during the selection process, during the preparation, and immediately before the administration. The amount of medication is determined by the physician or by departmental protocols. The *right route, right amount,* and *right time* are determined by the physician, the type of medication, and the procedure.

---

[1]Tortorici M: *Administration of imaging pharmaceuticals,* Philadelphia, 1996, Saunders.

Documentation of the five rights of medication administration is to be included in every patient's permanent medical record. In addition to these five rights, the documentation should include the size, type, and location of the needle; the number of venipuncture attempts; and the identity of the health care personnel who performed the procedure. Information about how the patient responded to the procedure should also be documented. The following is an example of correct documentation techniques for a technologist performing venipuncture and administering a medication:

4-15-99 at 0900 a venous access on Mr. John Q Public was performed using an 18-gauge angiocatheter. The access was established in the dorsum of the left hand after one attempt. Then 100 mL of [the specific name of the medication] was administered by IV push via the access. The patient tolerated the injection procedure and medication without complaints of pain or discomfort and with no unexpected side effects. (Sandy R. Ray, RT)

The objective of medication therapy and administration is to provide the maximum benefit to the patient with the minimum harm. Medications are intended to help maintain health, treat or prevent disease, relieve symptoms, alter body processes, and diagnose disease. Unfortunately, all medications are not ideal in their effects on the human body. It is important that health care providers understand their role and responsibilities in the administration of medications. Because the medications used by the radiologic technologist are less than perfect, caution for the patient's well-being and skill in the administration of the medications is a priority. Patients have the right to expect that the personnel who administer medications are informed about dosages, actions, indications, adverse reactions, interactions, contraindications, and special considerations. Education, training, licensing, and experience are critical in establishing competency in this area of practice.

19

REPRODUCTIVE SYSTEM

Vesiculogram demonstrating beginning (budding) metastasis of crista urethralis *(arrow)* discovered 2 years after prostatectomy for cancer of prostate.

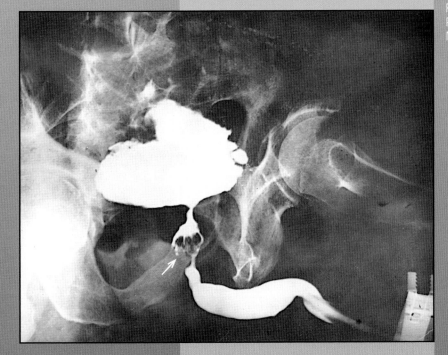

SUMMARY OF PROJECTIONS

PROJECTIONS, POSITIONS, AND METHODS

Page	Essential	Anatomy	Projection	Position	Method
262		Hysterosalpingography	AP, lateral, axial, oblique		
269		Pelvimetry	AP		COLCHER-SUSSMAN
270		Pelvimetry	Lateral	R or L	COLCHER-SUSSMAN
272		Seminal ducts	AP or AP oblique		

Female Reproductive System

The female reproductive system consists of an internal and an external group of organs, with the two groups connected by the vaginal canal. This chapter does not address the anatomy of the external genitalia because those structures do not require radiographic demonstration. The internal genital organs consist of the female gonads, or *ovaries,* which are two glandular bodies homologous to the male testes, and a system of canals made up of the *uterine tubes, uterus,* and *vagina.*

OVARIES

The two ovaries are small, glandular organs with an internal secretion that controls the menstrual cycle and an external secretion containing the *ova,* or female reproductive cells (Fig. 19-1). Each ovary is shaped approximately like an almond. The ovaries lie one on each side, inferior and posterior to the uterine tube and near the lateral wall of the pelvis. They are attached to the posterior surface of the broad ligament of the uterus by the *mesovarium.*

The ovary has a core of vascular tissue, the *medulla,* and an outer portion of glandular tissue termed the *cortex.* The cortex contains *ovarian follicles* in all stages of development, and each follicle contains one ovum. A fully developed ovarian follicle is referred to as a *graafian follicle.* As the minute ovum matures, the size of the follicle and its fluid content increase so that the wall of the follicle's sac approaches the surface of the ovary and in time ruptures, liberating the ovum and follicular fluid into the peritoneal cavity. Extrusion of an ovum by the rupture of a follicle is called *ovulation* and usually occurs one time during the menstrual cycle. Once the ovum is in the pelvic cavity, it is drawn toward the uterine tube.

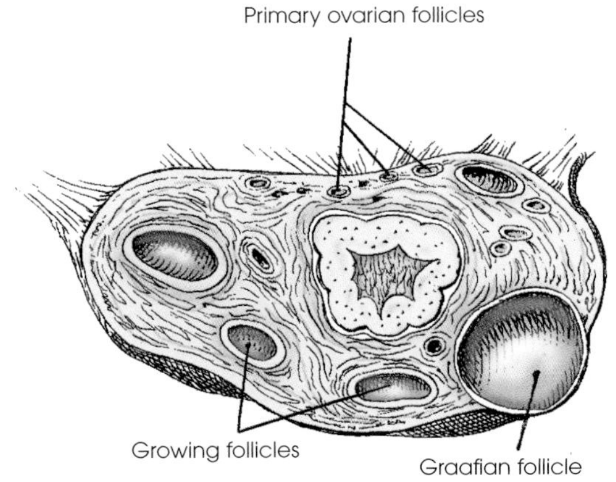

UTERINE TUBES

The two *uterine tubes,* or fallopian tubes, arise from the lateral angle of the uterus, pass laterally above the ovaries, and open into the peritoneal cavity. These tubes collect ova released by the ovaries and convey the cells to the uterine cavity. Each tube is 3 to 5 inches (7.6 to 13 cm) in length (Fig. 19-2) and has a small diameter at its uterine end, which opens into the cavity of the uterus by a minute orifice. The tube itself is divided into three parts: the isthmus, the ampulla, and the infundibulum. The *isthmus* is a short segment near the uterus. The *ampulla* comprises most of the tube and is wider than the isthmus. The terminal and lateral portion of the tube is the *infundibulum* and is flared in appearance. The infundibulum ends in a series of irregular prolonged processes called *fimbriae.* One of the fimbriae is attached either to or near the ovary.

The mucosal lining of the uterine tube contains hairlike projections called *cilia.* The lining is arranged in folds that increase in number and complexity as they approach the fimbriated extremity of the tube. The cilia draw the ovum into the tube, which then conveys it to the uterine cavity by peristaltic movements. The passage of the ovum through the tube requires several days. Fertilization of the cell occurs in the outer part of the tube, and the fertilized ovum then migrates to the uterus for implantation.

Primary ovarian follicles

Growing follicles

Graafian follicle

Fig. 19-1 Section of an ovary.

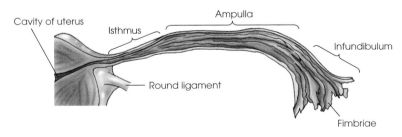

Cavity of uterus

Isthmus

Ampulla

Infundibulum

Round ligament

Fimbriae

Fig. 19-2 Section of left uterine tube.

UTERUS

The *uterus* is a pear-shaped, muscular organ (Figs. 19-3 and 19-4). Its primary functions are to receive and retain the fertilized ovum until development of the fetus is complete and, when the fetus is mature, to expel it during birth.

The uterus consists of four parts: the fundus, body, isthmus, and cervix. The *fundus* is the bluntly rounded, superior-most portion of the uterus. The *body* narrows from the fundus to the isthmus and is the point of attachment for the ligaments that secure the uterus within the pelvis. The *isthmus* (superior part of the cervix), a constricted area between the body and the cervix, is approximately ½ inch (1.3 cm) long. The *cervix* is the cylindric vaginal end of the uterus and is approximately 1 inch (2.5 cm) long. The vagina is attached around the circumference of the cervix.

The *nulliparous* uterus (i.e., the uterus of a woman who has not given birth) is approximately 3 inches (7.6 cm) in length, almost half of which represents the length of the cervix. The cervix is approximately ¾ inch (1.9 cm) in diameter. During pregnancy the body of the uterus gradually expands into the abdominal cavity, reaching the epigastric region in the eighth month. Following parturition, the organ shrinks to almost its original size but undergoes characteristic changes in shape.

The uterus is situated in the central part of the pelvic cavity, where it lies posterior and superior to the urinary bladder and anterior to the rectal ampulla. The long axis, which is slightly concave anteriorly, is directed inferiorly and posteriorly at a near right angle to the axis of the vaginal canal into which the lower end of the cervix projects.

The cavity of the body of the uterus, or the uterine cavity proper, is triangular in shape when viewed in the frontal plane. The canal of the cervix is dilated in the center and constricted at each extremity. The proximal end of the canal is continuous with the canal of the isthmus. The distal orifice is called the *uterine ostium.*

The mucosal lining of the uterine cavity is called the *endometrium.* This lining undergoes cyclic changes, called the *menstrual cycle,* at about 4-week intervals from puberty to menopause. During each premenstrual period the endometrium is prepared for the implantation and nutrition of the fertilized ovum. If fertilization has not occurred, the menstrual flow of blood and necrosed particles of uterine mucosa ensues.

VAGINA

The *vagina* is a muscular structure with walls and a canal lying posterior to the urinary bladder and urethra and anterior to the rectum. Averaging about 3 inches (7.6 cm) in length, the vagina extends inferiorly and anteriorly from the uterus to the exterior. The *mucosa* of the vagina is continuous with that of the uterus. The space between the labia minora is known as the *vaginal vestibule* and contains the *vaginal orifice* and the *urethral orifice.*

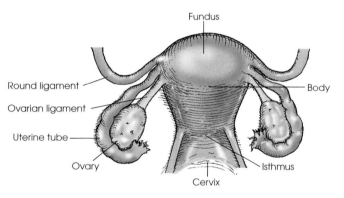

Fig. 19-3 Superoposterior view of uterus, ovaries, and uterine tubes.

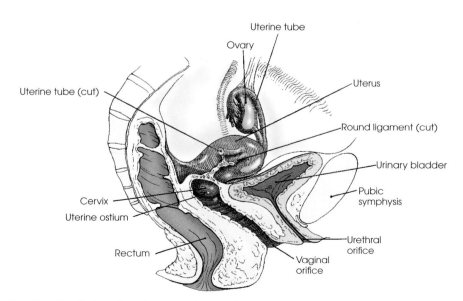

Fig. 19-4 Sagittal section showing relation of internal genitalia to surrounding structures.

FETAL DEVELOPMENT

During the *implantation* process, the fertilized ovum, called a *zygote,* is passed from the uterine tube into the uterine cavity, where it adheres to and becomes embedded in the uterine lining. About 2 weeks after fertilization of the ovum, the *embryo* begins to appear. Nine weeks after fertilization the embryo becomes a fetus and assumes a human appearance (Fig. 19-5).

During the first 2 weeks of embryonic development, the growing fertilized ovum is primarily concerned with the establishment of its nutritive and protective covering, the *chorion* and the *amnion.* As the chorion develops, it forms (1) the outer layer of the protective membranes enclosing the embryo and (2) the embryonic portion of the *placenta,* by which the umbilical cord is attached to the mother's uterus and through which food is supplied to and waste is removed from the fetus. The amnion, often referred to as the "bag of water" by the laity, forms the inner layer of the fetal membranes and contains amniotic fluid in which the fetus floats. Following the birth, the uterine lining is expelled with the fetal membranes and the placenta, constituting the afterbirth. A new endometrium is then regenerated.

The fertilized ovum usually becomes embedded near the fundus of the uterine cavity, most frequently on the anterior or posterior wall. Implantation occasionally occurs so low, however, that the fully developed placenta encroaches on or obstructs the cervical canal. This condition results in premature separation of the placenta, termed *placenta previa* (Fig. 19-6).

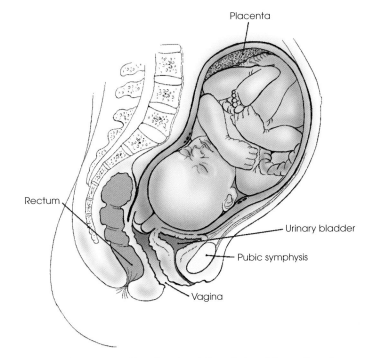

Fig. 19-5 Sagittal section showing fetus of about 7 months of age.

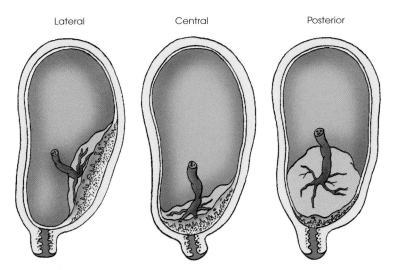

Fig. 19-6 Schematic drawings of several placental sites in low implantation.

Male Reproductive System

The male genital system consists of the following: a pair of male *gonads,* the *testes,* which produce spermatozoa; two excretory channels, the *ductus deferens,* or vas deferens; the *prostate;* the ejaculatory ducts; the *seminal vesicles;* and a pair of *bulbourethral glands,* which produce secretions that are added to the secretions of the testes and ductal mucosa to constitute the final product of seminal fluid. The *penis,* the *scrotum,* and the structures enclosed by the scrotal sac (testes, epididymides, spermatic cords, and part of the ductus deferens) are the external genital organs.

TESTES

The *testes* are ovoid bodies averaging 1½ inches (3.8 cm) in length and about 1 inch (2.5 cm) in both width and depth (Fig. 19-7). Each testis is divided into 200 to 300 partial compartments that constitute the glandular substance of the testis. Each compartment houses one or more convoluted, germ cell–producing tubules. These tubules in turn converge and unite to form 15 to 20 ductules that emerge from the testis to enter the head of the epididymis.

The *epididymis* is an oblong structure that is attached to the superior and lateroposterior aspects of the testis. The ductules leading out of the testis enter the head of the epididymis to become continuous with the coiled and convoluted ductules that comprise this structure. As the ductules pass inferiorly, they progressively unite to form the main duct, which is continuous with the ductus deferens.

DUCTUS DEFERENS

The *ductus deferens* is 16 to 18 inches (40 to 45 cm) long and extends from the tail of the epididymis to the posteroinferior surface of the urinary bladder. Only its first part is convoluted. From its beginning the ductus deferens ascends along the medial side of the epididymis on the posterior surface of the testis to join the other constituents of the spermatic cord, with which it emerges from the scrotal sac and passes into the pelvic cavity through the inguinal canal (Fig. 19-8). Near its termination the duct expands into an *ampulla* for the storage of seminal fluid and then ends by uniting with the duct of the seminal vesicle.

SEMINAL VESICLES

The two *seminal vesicles* are sacculated structures about 2 inches (5 cm) in length (Fig. 19-9). They are situated obliquely on the lateroposterior surface of the bladder, where, from the level of the ureterocystic junction, each slants inferiorly and medially to the base of the prostate. Each ampulla of the ductus deferens lies along the medial border of the seminal vesicle to form the ejaculatory duct.

EJACULATORY DUCTS

The *ejaculatory ducts* are formed by the union of the ductus deferens and the duct of the seminal vesicle. The ejaculatory ducts average about ½ inch (1.3 cm) in length and originate behind the neck of the bladder. The two ducts enter the base of the prostate and, passing obliquely inferiorly through the substance of the gland, open into the prostatic urethra at the lateral margins of the prostatic utricle. These ducts eject sperm into the urethra before ejaculation.

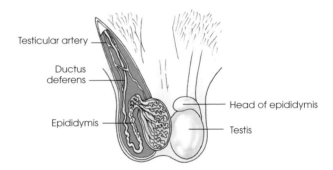

Fig. 19-7 Frontal section of testes and ductus deferens.

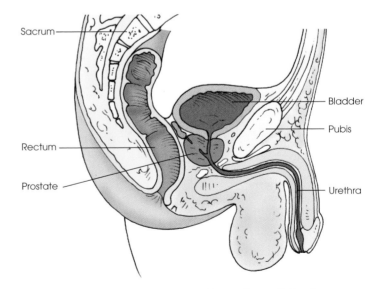

Fig. 19-8 Sagittal section showing male genital system.

PROSTATE

The *prostate,* an accessory genital organ, is a somewhat cone-shaped organ and averages 1¼ inches (3.2 cm) in length. The prostate encircles the proximal portion of the male urethra and, extending from the bladder neck to the pelvic floor, lies in front of the rectal ampulla approximately 1 inch (2.5 cm) posterior to the lower two thirds of the pubic symphysis (see Fig. 19-9). The prostate is composed of muscular and glandular tissue. The ducts of the prostate open into the prostatic portion of the urethra.

Because of advances in diagnostic ultrasound imaging, radiographic examinations of the male reproductive system are performed less often than in the past. The prostate can be ultrasonically imaged through the urine-filled bladder or using a special rectal transducer. The seminal ducts can be imaged when the rectum is filled with an ultrasound gel and a special rectal transducer is used. Testicular ultrasonic scans are performed to evaluate a palpable mass or an enlarged testis and to check for metastasis. The vast majority of the testicular scans are performed because of a palpable mass or an enlarged testis.

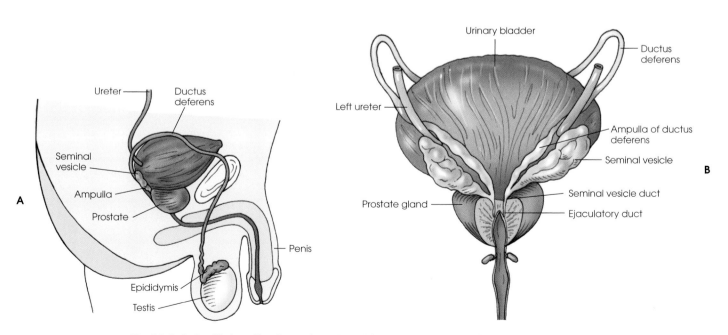

Fig. 19-9 A, Sagittal section through male pelvis. **B,** Posterior view of male reproductive organs.

SUMMARY OF ANATOMY

Female reproductive system
ovaries
uterine tubes
uterus
vagina

Ovaries
ova
mesovarium
medulla
cortex
  ovarian follicles
  graafian follicle
ovulation

Uterine tubes (fallopian tubes)
isthmus
ampulla
infundibulum
  fimbriae
cilia

Uterus
fundus
body
isthmus
cervix
uterine ostium
endometrium

Vagina
mucosa
vaginal vestibule
vaginal orifice
urethral orifice

Fetal development
zygote
embryo
fetus
placenta

Male reproductive system
testes
ductus deferens
  (vas deferens)
prostate
ejaculatory ducts
seminal vesicles
bulbourethral glands
penis
scrotum

Testes
epididymis

Ductus deferens
ampulla

SUMMARY OF PATHOLOGY

Condition	Definition
Adhesion	Union of two surfaces that are normally separate
Endometrial Polyp	Growth or mass protruding from the endometrium
Fallopian Tube Obstruction	Condition preventing normal flow through the fallopian tube
Fistula	Abnormal connection between two internal organs or between an organ and the body surface
Tumor	New tissue growth where cell proliferation is uncontrolled
Dermoid Cyst	Tumor of the ovary filled with sebaceous material and hair
Uterine Fibroid	Smooth-muscle tumor of the uterus

NEW ABBREVIATIONS USED IN CHAPTER 19

HSG	Hysterosalpingography
IUD	Intrauterine device

See Addendum B for a summary of all abbreviations used in Volume 2.

Male reproductive system

Female Radiography
NONPREGNANT PATIENT

Radiologic investigations of the non-pregnant uterus, accessory organs, and vagina are denoted by the terms *hysterosalpingography* (HSG), *pelvic pneumography,* and *vaginography.* Each procedure requires the use of a contrast medium and should be carried out under aseptic conditions. *HSG* involves the introduction of a radiopaque contrast medium through a uterine cannula. The procedure is performed to determine the size, shape, and position of the uterus and uterine tubes; to delineate lesions such as polyps, submucous tumor masses, or fistulous tracts; and to investigate the patency of the uterine tubes in patients who have been unable to conceive (Fig. 19-10).

Pelvic pneumography, which requires the introduction of a gaseous contrast medium directly into the peritoneal cavity, is now rarely performed because of the development of ultrasonic techniques for evaluating the pelvic cavity. *Vaginography* is performed to investigate congenital abnormalities, vaginal fistulae, and other pathologic conditions involving the vagina.

Contrast media

Various opaque media are used in examinations of the female genital passages. The water-soluble contrast media employed for intravenous urography are widely used for HSG and vaginography.

Preparation of intestinal tract

Preparation of the intestinal tract for any of these examinations usually consists of the following:

1. A non–gas-forming laxative is administered on the preceding evening if the patient is constipated.
2. Before reporting for the examination, the patient receives cleansing enemas until the return flow is clear.
3. The meal preceding the examination is withheld.

Appointment date and care of patient

Gynecologic examinations should be scheduled approximately 10 days after the onset of menstruation. This is the interval during which the endometrium is least congested. More importantly, because this time interval is a few days before ovulation normally occurs, there is little danger of irradiating a recently fertilized ovum.

The relatively minor instrumentation required for the introduction of contrast medium in these examinations normally necessitates neither hospitalization nor premedication. Some patients experience unpleasant but transitory aftereffects. Therefore the radiology department should have facilities for an outpatient to rest in the recumbent position before returning home.

The patient is requested to completely empty her bladder immediately before the examination. This procedure prevents pressure displacement of and superimposition of the bladder on the pelvic genitalia. In addition, the patient's vagina is irrigated just before the examination. At this time the patient should be given the necessary supplies and instructed to cleanse the perineal region.

Radiation protection

To deliver the least possible amount of radiation to the gonads, the radiologist restricts fluoroscopy and imaging to the minimum required for a satisfactory examination.

Hysterosalpingography

HSG is performed by a physician, with spot radiographs made while the patient is in the supine position on a fluoroscopic table. The examination may also be performed by the physician with conventional radiographs obtained using an overhead tube. When fluoroscopy is used, spot radiographs may be the only images obtained. Preparing the patient for the examination involves the following steps:

- After irrigation of the vaginal canal, complete emptying of the bladder, and perineal cleansing, place the patient on the examining table.
- Adjust the patient in the lithotomy position, with the knees flexed over leg rests.
- When a combination table is used, adjust the patient's position to permit the IRs to be centered to a point 2 inches (5 cm) proximal to the pubic symphysis; 24- × 30-cm IRs are used for all studies and are placed lengthwise.

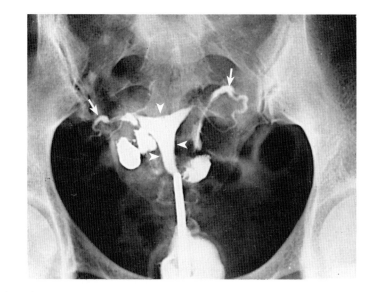

Fig. 19-10 HSG reveals bilateral hydrosalpinx of uterine tubes *(arrows)*. The contrast-filled uterine cavity is normal *(arrowheads)*.

After inspection of the preliminary radiograph and with a vaginal speculum in position, the physician inserts a uterine cannula through the cervical canal, fits the attached rubber plug, or acorn, firmly against the external cervical os, applies counterpressure with a tenaculum to prevent reflux of the contrast medium, and withdraws the speculum unless it is radiolucent. An opaque or a gaseous contrast medium may then be injected via the cannula into the uterine cavity. The contrast material flows through patent uterine tubes and "spills" into the peritoneal cavity (Figs. 19-11 to 19-13). Patency of the uterine tubes can be determined by transuterine gas insufflation (Rubin test), but the length, position, and course of the ducts can be demonstrated only by opacifying the lumina.

The free-flowing, iodinated organic contrast agents are usually injected at room temperature. These agents pass through patent uterine tubes quickly, and the resultant peritoneal spill is absorbed and eliminated by way of the urinary system, usually within 2 hours or less.

The contrast medium may be injected with a pressometer or a syringe. Intrauterine pressure is maintained for the radiographic studies by closing the cannular valve. In the absence of fluoroscopy the contrast medium is introduced in two to four fractional doses so that excessive peritoneal spillage does not occur. Each fractional dose is followed by a radiographic study to determine whether the filling is adequate as shown by the peritoneal spill.

The radiographs may consist of no more than a single AP projection taken at the end of each fractional injection. Other projections (oblique, axial, and lateral) are taken as indicated.

EVALUATION CRITERIA

The following should be clearly demonstrated:

- The pelvic region 2 inches (5 cm) above the pubic symphysis centered on the radiograph
- All contrast media visible, including any "spill" areas
- A short scale of contrast on radiographs

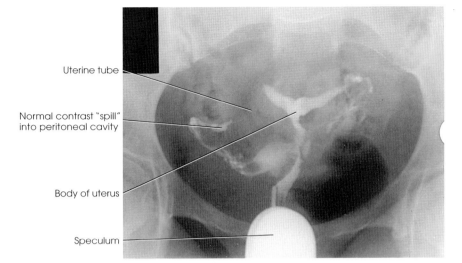

Uterine tube

Normal contrast "spill" into peritoneal cavity

Body of uterus

Speculum

Fig. 19-11 Hysterosalpingogram, AP projection, showing normal uterus and uterine tubes.

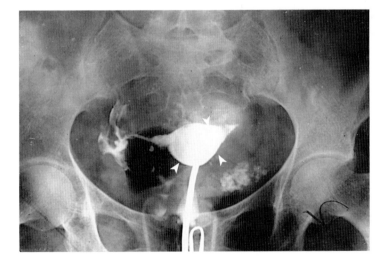

Fig. 19-12 Hysterosalpingogram, AP projection, showing submucous fibroid occupying entire uterine cavity *(arrowheads)*.

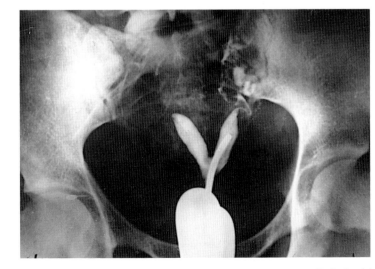

Fig. 19-13 Hysterosalpingogram, AP projection, revealing uterine cavity to be bicornate in outline.

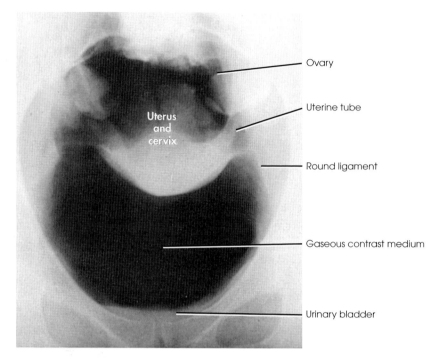

Ovary

Uterine tube

Uterus and cervix

Round ligament

Gaseous contrast medium

Urinary bladder

Fig. 19-14 Normal pelvic pneumogram. (See Fig. 19-3 for correlation with radiograph.)

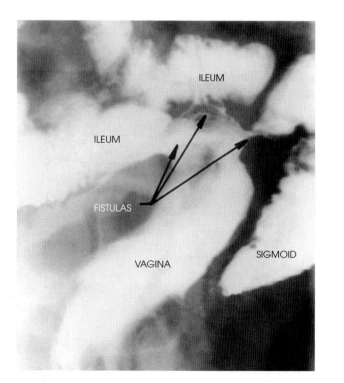

ILEUM

ILEUM

FISTULAS

VAGINA

SIGMOID

Fig. 19-15 Vaginogram, spot radiograph, PA oblique projection, LAO position. Sigmoid fistula and two ileum fistulas are shown.

Pelvic pneumography

Pelvic pneumography, gynecography, and *pangynecography* are the terms used to denote radiologic examinations of the female pelvic organs by means of intraperitoneal gas insufflation (Fig. 19-14). These procedures have essentially been replaced by ultrasonography and other diagnostic techniques. (Pelvic pneumography is described in Volume 3 of the fourth edition of this atlas.)

Vaginography

Vaginography is used in the investigation of congenital malformations and pathologic conditions such as vesicovaginal and enterovaginal fistulas. The examination is performed by introducing a contrast medium into the vaginal canal. Lambie, Rubin, and Dann[1] recommended the use of a thin barium sulfate mixture for the investigation of fistulous communications with the intestine. At the end of the examination the patient is instructed to expel as much of the barium mixture as possible, and the canal is then cleansed by vaginal irrigation. For the investigation of other conditions, Coe[2] advocated the use of an iodinated organic compound.

A rectal retention tube is employed for the introduction of the contrast medium so that the moderately inflated balloon can be used to prevent reflux. In one technique, the physician inserts only the tip of the tube into the vaginal orifice. The patient is then requested to extend the thighs and to hold them in close approximation to keep the inflated balloon pressed firmly against the vaginal entrance. In another technique, the tube is inserted far enough to place the deflated balloon within the distal end of the vagina, and the balloon is then inflated under fluoroscopic observation. The barium mixture is introduced with the usual enema equipment. The water-soluble medium is injected with a syringe.

Vaginography is performed on a combination fluoroscopic-radiographic table. The contrast medium is injected under fluoroscopic control, and spot radiographs are exposed as indicated during the filling (Fig. 19-15).

[1]Lambie RW, Rubin S, Dann DS: Demonstration of fistulas by vaginography, *AJR* 90:717, 1963.
[2]Coe FO: Vaginography, *AJR* 90:721, 1963.

The radiographs in Figs. 19-16 to 19-18 were taken with the central ray directed perpendicular to the midpoint of the IR. For localized studies, the central ray is centered at the level of the superior border of the pubic symphysis.

In each examination the radiographic projections required are determined by the radiologist according to the fluoroscopic findings. Low rectovaginal fistulas are best shown in the lateral projection, and fistulous communications with the sigmoid and/or ileum are best shown in oblique projections.

EVALUATION CRITERIA

The following should be clearly demonstrated:

- Superior border of the pubic symphysis centered on the radiograph
- Any fistulas in their entirety
- Optimal density and contrast to visualize the vagina and any fistula
- Pelvis on oblique projections not superimposed by the proximal thigh
- Superimposed hips and femora in the lateral image

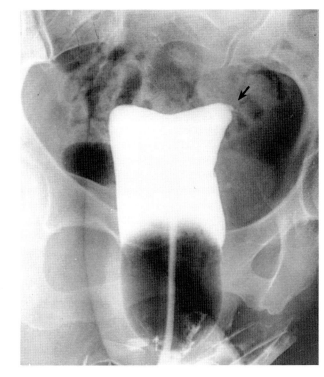

Fig. 19-16 Vaginogram, AP projection, showing small fistulous tract *(arrow)* projecting laterally from apex of vagina and ending in abscess.

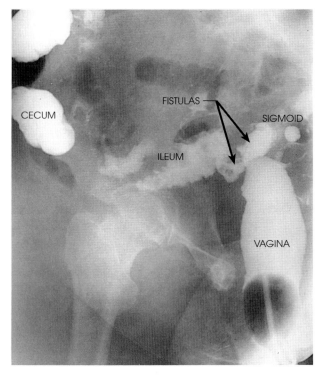

Fig. 19-17 Vaginogram, AP oblique projection, RPO position. Fistulas to ileum and sigmoid are shown.

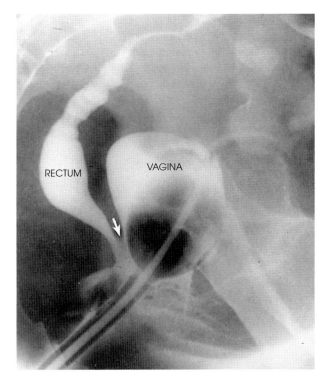

Fig. 19-18 Vaginogram, lateral projection, showing low rectovaginal fistula.

PREGNANT PATIENT

Because ultrasonography provides visualization of the fetus and placenta with no apparent risk to the patient or fetus, it has become the preferred diagnostic tool for examination of the pregnant female. In some situations, however, certain radiologic examinations are still indicated: *Fetography* is the demonstration of the fetus in utero. If possible, this examination technique is avoided until after the eighteenth week of gestation because of the danger of radiation-induced fetal malformations. Fetography is employed to detect suspected abnormalities of development, to confirm suspected fetal death, to determine the presentation and position of the fetus, and to determine whether the pregnancy is single or multiple.

Radiographic *pelvimetry* and *fetal cephalometry* are performed to demonstrate the architecture of the maternal pelvis and to compare the size of the fetal head with the size of the maternal bony pelvic outlet. This purpose of the procedure is to determine whether the pelvic diameters are adequate for normal parturition or whether cesarean section is necessary for the delivery. Although many techniques and combinations of techniques are employed in radiographic pelvimetry, only a few of the body positions and pertinent technical factors are included in this text.

Placentography is the radiographic examination in which the walls of the uterus are investigated to locate the placenta in cases of suspected placenta previa. At one time radiographs were the only means available to detect such conditions. With advances in technology and the concern about the dose of radiation received by the fetus, diagnostic ultrasound (see Chapter 34) has become a valuable diagnostic tool for placenta localization.

Radiation protection

Radiologic examinations of pregnant patients are performed only when required information can be obtained in no other way. In addition to the danger of genetic changes that may result from reproductive cell irradiation is the danger of radiation-induced malformations of the developing fetus. Whenever possible, radiation for any purpose is avoided during pregnancy, especially during the first trimester of gestation. If examination of the abdominopelvic region is necessary, it is restricted to the absolute minimum number of radiographs. The radiographer's responsibility is to carry out the work carefully and thoughtfully so that repeat exposures are not necessary.

Preparation of patient

Although it is desirable to clear the large bowel of gas and fecal material with a cleansing enema shortly before any radiologic examination, preliminary preparation depends on the condition of the patient. Under no circumstances is a cleansing enema administered without the express permission of the attending physician. The patient should completely empty the bladder immediately before the examination. This is particularly important when the upright position is used because the filled bladder prevents the fetus from descending to the most dependent portion of the uterine cavity.

Care of patient

The patient who is in labor or is bleeding because of a placental separation must be treated as an emergency and must be under constant observation by qualified personnel.

Respiration

A change in the oxygen content of the maternal blood causes the fetus to react quickly by movement. Just before suspension of respiration for the exposure, the mother's blood should be hyperaerated by having her inhale deeply several times and then suspend respiration during the inspiration phase.

Fetography

Fetography has generally been replaced by sonography and therefore is not fully described in this edition. A more complete description of this technique is provided in the seventh edition or even earlier editions of this atlas.

AP or PA and lateral projections are obtained to demonstrate the maternal pelvis and developing fetus (Figs. 19-19 to 19-21). The following steps are observed:
- Whenever possible, situate the patient in a prone position to place the fetus closer to the IR. To accomplish this, place supports under the chest, upper abdomen, and femora (Fig. 19-22).
- If the prone position cannot be used, place the patient supine on the radiographic table with a support under the knees to relieve back strain.
- For the lateral projection, have the patient lie on her side and support the abdomen to be parallel to the table if needed.
- Center the perpendicular central ray to the abdomen.

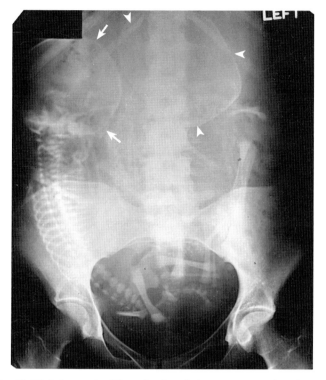

Fig. 19-19 Fetography, PA projection. Twin pregnancy showing two fetal heads *(arrows and arrowheads)*.

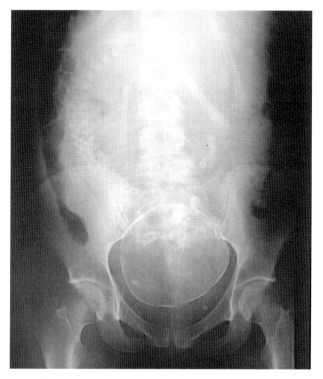

Fig. 19-20 Fetography, AP projection, showing one fetus.

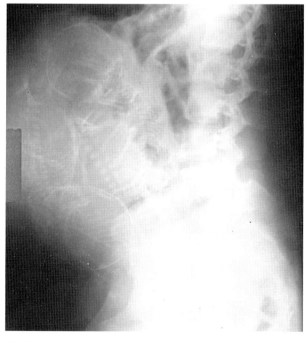

Fig. 19-21 Fetography, lateral projection, showing triplet pregnancy.

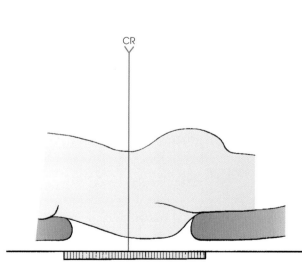

Fig. 19-22 Fetography, prone position, showing support under patient's legs and thorax.

Radiographic pelvimetry and cephalometry

Most pelvimetry techniques have been replaced by sonography. Thus the Ball and Thoms methods have been deleted from this edition. (See the seventh or earlier editions of this atlas for descriptions of these methods.) However, obtainable pelvic measurements and the Colcher-Sussman method of pelvimetry are described here.

The pelvimetry requires knowledge of pelvic anatomy. The entrance to the true pelvis, called the *superior strait* or *pelvic inlet,* is bounded by the sacral promontory, the linea terminalis, and the crests of the pubic bones and symphysis. The internal anteroposterior diameter of the inlet is measured from the center of the sacral promontory to the superoposterior margin of the pubic symphysis and is called the *internal conjugate diameter* or the *conjugata vera.* Other internal diameters of the pelvic cavity are shown in Figs. 19-23 and 19-24.

The *external conjugate diameter* extends from the space between the spinous process of L4-L5 to the top of the pubic symphysis. The posterior landmark—the interspinous space—can be palpated at the superior angle of the Michaelis rhomboid, which is the diamond-shaped depression overlying the lumbosacral region. This depression is bounded laterally by the dimples overlying the posterior superior iliac spines, superior to the L5 spinous process by the lines formed by the gluteus muscles, and inferior to the groove at the end of the vertebral column.

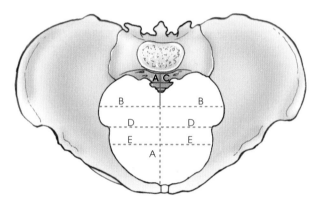

Fig. 19-23 Pelvis seen from above. *A,* Anteroposterior diameter of the inlet. *B,* Transverse diameter of inlet. *C,* Posterior sagittal diameter of inlet. *D,* Interspinous or transverse diameter of midplane. *E,* Widest transverse diameter of outlet.

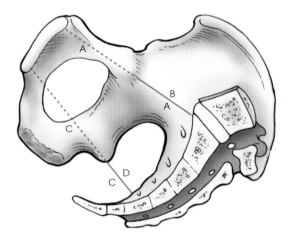

Fig. 19-24 Lateral aspect of pelvis. *A,* Anteroposterior diameter of inlet. *B,* Posterior sagittal diameter of inlet. *C,* Anteroposterior diameter of midplane. *D,* Posterior sagittal diameter of midplane.

Pelvimetry

AP PROJECTION

COLCHER-SUSSMAN METHOD

The two projections (AP and lateral) employed in this method of pelvimetry require the use of the Colcher-Sussman pelvimeter. This device consists of a metal ruler perforated at centimeter intervals and mounted on a small stand in such a way that it is always parallel to the plane of the IR. The ruler can be rotated in a complete circle and adjusted for height (Fig. 19-25).

> **Image receptor:** 35 × 43 cm for each exposure

Position of patient

- Place the patient in the supine position, and center the midsagittal plane of the body to the midline of the grid.

Position of part

- Flex the patient's knees to elevate the forepelvis, and separate the thighs enough to permit correct placement of the pelvimeter.
- Center the horizontal ruler to the gluteal fold at the level of the ischial tuberosities. The tuberosities are easily palpated through the median part of the buttocks. If preferred, localize the tuberosities by placing the ruler 10 cm below the superior border of the pubic symphysis (Fig. 19-26).
- Center the IR 1½ inches (3.8 cm) superior to the pubic symphysis (Fig. 19-27).
- *Respiration:* After determining that the fetus is quiet, instruct the patient to suspend respiration at the end of expiration.

Central ray

- Perpendicular to the midpoint of the IR and 1½ inches (3.8 cm) superior to the pubic symphysis

EVALUATION CRITERIA

The following should be clearly demonstrated:
- Entire pelvis
- Metal ruler with centimeter markings visible
- Density permitting visualization of all pelvic landmarks and intersecting diameters
- No rotation of the pelvis
- Entire fetal head

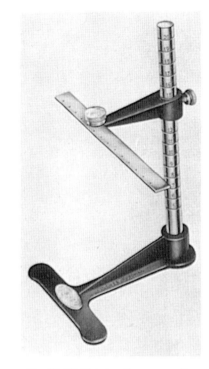

Fig. 19-25 Colcher-Sussman ruler.

Fig. 19-26 Pelvimetry, AP projection, with ruler in place.

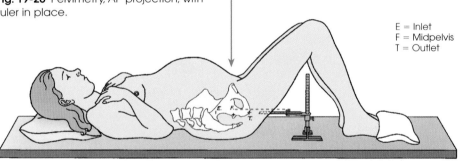

E = Inlet
F = Midpelvis
T = Outlet

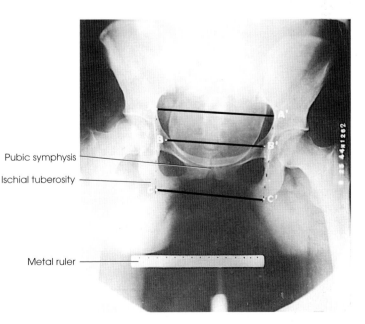

Pubic symphysis

Ischial tuberosity

Metal ruler

Fig. 19-27 Pelvimetry, AP projection.

Reproductive system

LATERAL PROJECTION
COLCHER-SUSSMAN METHOD
R or L position

Image receptor: 35 × 43 cm

Position of patient
- Ask the patient to turn to a lateral position, and center the midcoronal plane of the patient's body to the midline of the table.

Position of part
- Partially extend the patient's thighs so that they do not obscure the pubic bones.
- Place sandbags under and between the patient's knees and ankles to immobilize the legs.
- Place a folded sheet or other suitable support under the lower thorax, and adjust the support so that the long axis of the lumbar vertebrae is parallel with the tabletop.

- Adjust the patient's body in a true lateral position.
- Turn the ruler lengthwise, and adjust its height to coincide with the midsagittal plane of the patient's body.
- Place the pelvimeter so that the metal ruler lies within the upper part of the gluteal fold and against the midsacrum (Fig. 19-28).
- Center the IR at the level of the most prominent point of the greater trochanter (Fig. 19-29).
- *Respiration:* Suspend at the end of expiration.

Central ray
- Perpendicular to the most prominent point of the greater trochanter

EVALUATION CRITERIA

The following should be clearly demonstrated:
- Superimposed hips and femora
- No superimposition of the pubic symphysis by the femurs
- Entire pelvis, sacrum, and coccyx
- Metal ruler with centimeter markings visible
- Density permitting visualization of all pelvic landmarks and intersecting diameters
- Entire fetal head

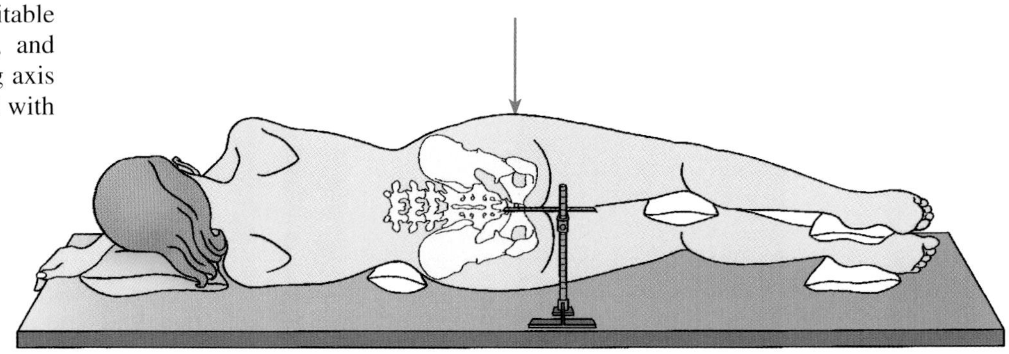

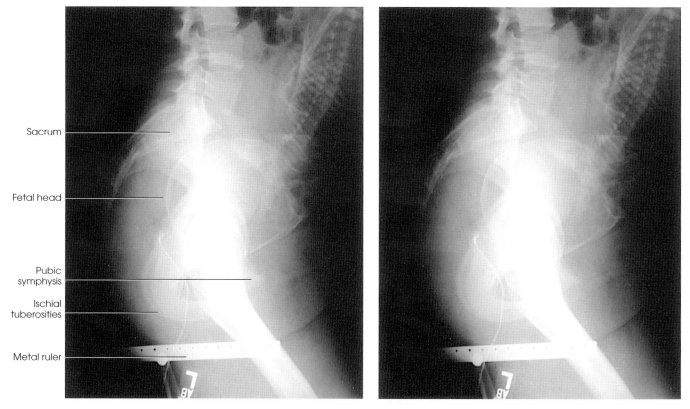

Fig. 19-28 Pelvimetry, lateral projection with ruler in place.

Sacrum

Fetal head

Pubic symphysis

Ischial tuberosities

Metal ruler

Fig. 19-29 Pelvimetry, lateral projection.

LOCALIZATION
OF INTRAUTERINE DEVICES

Intrauterine devices (IUDs) remain a contraceptive option. Occasionally an IUD becomes dislocated from the uterine cavity. If this occurs, the exact location of the device must be determined, in some cases by radiography. Therefore it is necessary to become acquainted with the radiographic appearance of IUDs.

The physician first performs a pelvic examination to determine the location of the IUD. If the IUD is not located, the physician passes a sterile probe into the uterine cavity and radiographs are taken.

AP and lateral projections of the abdomen are suggested for IUD localization. Occasionally, oblique projections are indicated. Most IUDs are radiopaque because of their inherent metallic density or because of barium impregnated in the plastic during their manufacture. It should be emphasized that radiography alone is *not* a reliable way to diagnose extrauterine localization of an IUD.

In the early 1980s, five types of IUDs were available for use. In the late 1980s, three IUDs were removed from the U.S. market by their manufacturers. At this time, only two IUDs are available for use in the United States: the Paragard and the Progestasert (Fig. 19-30).

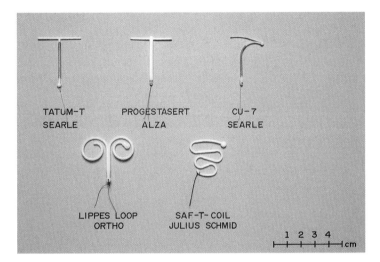

Fig. 19-30 Intrauterine contraceptive devices.

Male Radiography
SEMINAL DUCTS

Radiologic examinations of the seminal ducts[1-3] are performed in the investigation of selected genitourinary abnormalities such as cysts, abscesses, tumors, inflammation, and sterility. The regional terms applied to these examinations are *vesiculography, epididymography,* and, when combined, *epididymovesiculography.*

The contrast medium employed for these procedures is one of the water-soluble, iodinated compounds used for intravenous urography. A gaseous contrast medium can be injected into each scrotal sac to improve contrast in the examination of extrapelvic structures.

[1]Boreau J et al: Epididymography, *Med Radiogr Photogr* 29:63, 1953.
[2]Boreau J: *L'étude radiologique des voies séminales normales et pathologiques,* Paris, 1953, Masson and Cie.
[3]Vasselle B: *Etude radiologique des voies séminales de l'homme,* thesis, Paris, 1953.

The seminal vesicles are sometimes opacified directly by urethroscopic catheterization of the ejaculatory ducts. More frequently the entire duct system is inspected by introducing contrast solution into the canals by way of the ductus deferens. This requires small bilateral incisions in the upper part of the scrotum for the exposure and identification of these ducts. The needle that is used to inject the contrast medium is inserted into the duct in the direction of the portion of the tract under investigation—distally for study of the extrapelvic ducts and then proximally for study of the intrapelvic ducts.

A nongrid exposure technique is used for the delineation of extrapelvic structures (Figs. 19-31 to 19-33). The examining urologist places the IR and adjusts the position of the testes for the desired projections of the ducts. A grid technique is used to demonstrate the intrapelvic ducts (Figs. 19-34 to 19-36). AP and oblique projections are made on 8- × 10-inch (18- × 24-cm) or 24- × 30-cm IRs that are placed lengthwise and centered at the level of the superior border of the pubic symphysis.

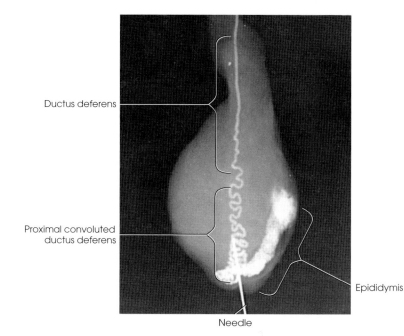

Ductus deferens

Proximal convoluted ductus deferens

Epididymis

Needle

Fig. 19-31 Epididymogram showing normal epididymis and origin of ductus deferens. The needle is at the epididymovasal kink, which can be palpated.

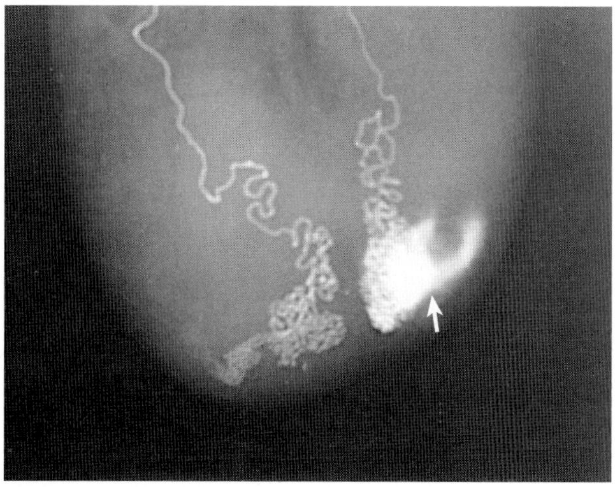

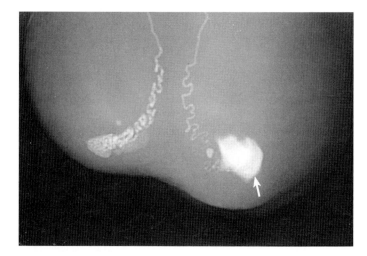

Fig. 19-32 Epididymogram demonstrating tuberculosis (cold abscess) of epididymis *(arrow).*

Fig. 19-33 Epididymogram showing epididymal abscess *(arrow)* observed during acute orchitis (third relapse). Epididymovasal kink is atrophic.

EVALUATION CRITERIA

The following should be clearly demonstrated:

AP projection

- IR centered at the level of the superior border of the pubic symphysis
- No rotation of the patient
- A short scale of contrast on radiograph

Oblique projection

- IR centered at the level of the superior border of the pubic symphysis
- No superimposition of the seminal ducts by the ilia
- No overlap of the region of the prostate or urethra by the uppermost thigh

PROSTATE

Prostatography is a term applied to the investigation of the prostate by radiographic, cystographic, or vesiculographic procedures. It is seldom performed today because of advancements in the diagnostic value of ultrasonography. Radiographic examination of the prostate gland was described in the eighth and earlier editions of this atlas.

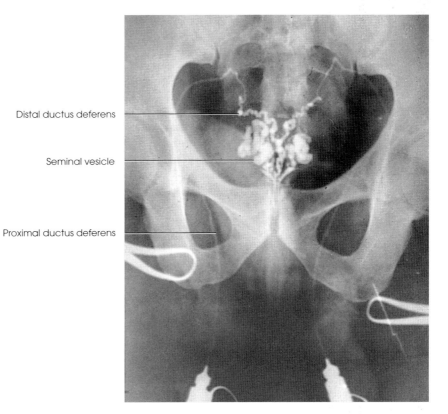

Distal ductus deferens

Seminal vesicle

Proximal ductus deferens

Fig. 19-34 Normal vesiculogram.

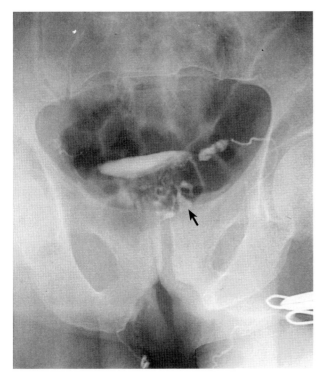

Fig. 19-35 Vesiculogram of tuberculous seminal vesicle associated with deferentitis, demonstrating small abscesses, ampullitis, and considerable vesiculitis on left *(arrow)*.

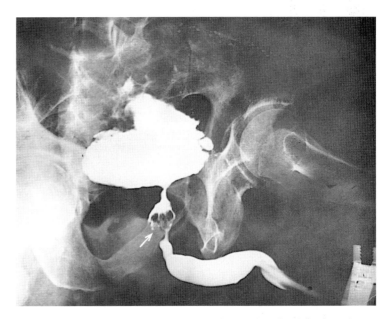

Fig. 19-36 Vesiculogram demonstrating beginning (budding) metastasis of crista urethralis *(arrow)* discovered 2 years after prostatectomy for cancer of prostate.

20

SKULL

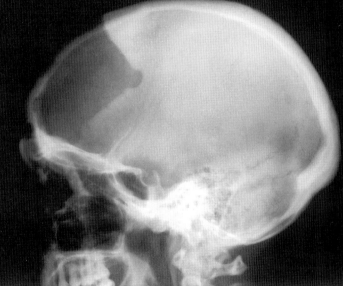

Lateral skull showing surgical removal of the frontal bone.

SUMMARY OF PROJECTIONS

PROJECTIONS, POSITIONS, AND METHODS

Page	Essential	Anatomy	Projection	Position	Method
306	♠	Cranium	Lateral	R or L	
308	♠	Cranium	Lateral	R or L dorsal decubitus	
308	♠	Cranium	Lateral	R or L supine lateral	
310	♠	Cranium	PA		
310	♠	Cranium	PA axial		CALDWELL
314	♠	Cranium	AP		
314	♠	Cranium	AP axial		
316	♠	Cranium	AP axial		TOWNE
322	♠	Cranium	PA axial		HAAS
324	♠	Cranial base	Submentovertical (SMV)		SCHÜLLER
328	♠	Petromastoid	Axiolateral oblique		MODIFIED LAW
330	♠	Petromastoid	Axiolateral oblique (posterior profile)		STENVERS
332	♠	Petromastoid	Axiolateral oblique (anterior profile)		ARCELIN
336	♠	Optic canal and foramen	Parietoorbital oblique		RHESE
341		Eye	Lateral	R or L	
342		Eye	PA axial		
343		Eye	Parietoacanthial		MODIFIED WATERS

Icons in the Essential column indicate projections frequently performed in the United States and Canada. Students should be competent in these projections.

Skull

The *skull* rests on the superior aspect of the vertebral column. It is composed of 22 separate bones divided into two distinct groups: 8 *cranial* bones and 14 *facial* bones. The cranial bones are further divided into the *calvaria* and *floor* (Box 20-1). The cranial bones form a protective housing for the brain. The facial bones provide structure, shape, and support for the face. They also form a protective housing for the upper ends of the respiratory and digestive tracts and, with several of the cranial bones, form the orbital sockets for protection of the organs of sight. The *hyoid bone* is commonly discussed with this group of bones.

The bones of the skull are identified in Figs. 20-1 to 20-3. The 22 primary bones of the skull should be located and recognized in the different views before they are studied in greater detail.

BOX 20-1
Skull bones

Cranial bones (8)		Facial bones (14)	
Calvaria		nasal	2
frontal	1	lacrimal	2
occipital	1	maxillary	2
right parietal	1	zygomatic	2
left parietal	1	palatine	2
		inferior nasal conchae	2
Floor		vomer	1
ethmoid	1	mandible	1
sphenoid	1		
right temporal	1		
left temporal	1		

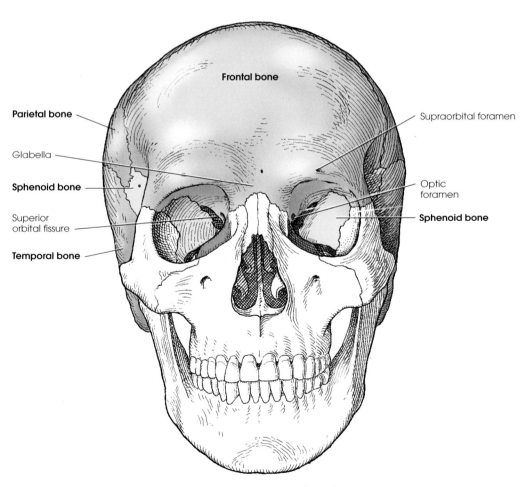

Fig. 20-1 Anterior aspect of cranium.

Labels: Frontal bone, Parietal bone, Glabella, Sphenoid bone, Superior orbital fissure, Temporal bone, Supraorbital foramen, Optic foramen, Sphenoid bone

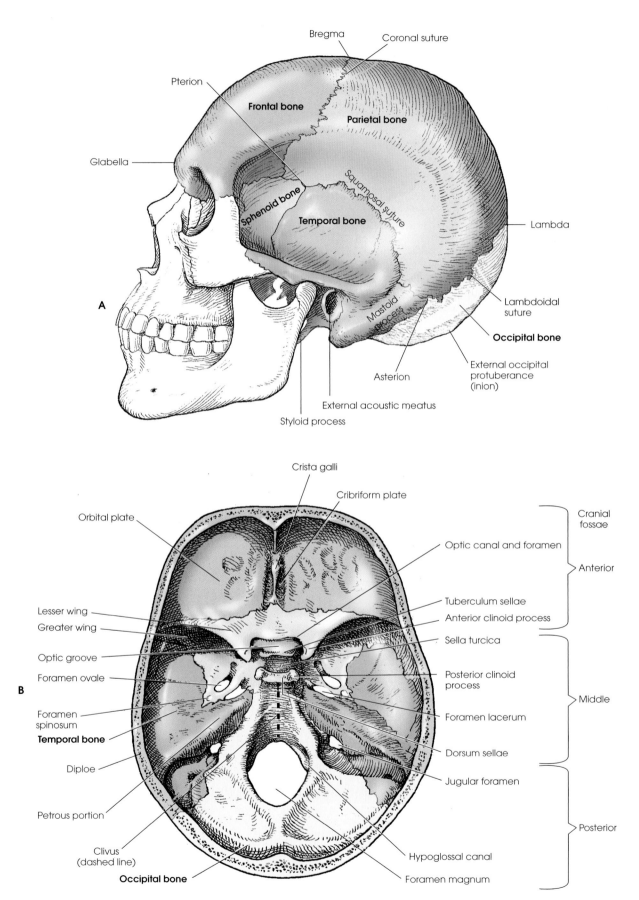

Bregma
Coronal suture
Pterion
Frontal bone
Parietal bone
Glabella
Sphenoid bone
Temporal bone
Squamosal suture
Lambda
Mastoid process
Lambdoidal suture
Occipital bone
Asterion
External occipital protuberance (inion)
External acoustic meatus
Styloid process

A

Crista galli
Cribriform plate
Orbital plate
Cranial fossae
Optic canal and foramen
Anterior
Lesser wing
Greater wing
Tuberculum sellae
Anterior clinoid process
Optic groove
Sella turcica
Foramen ovale
Posterior clinoid process
Foramen spinosum
Foramen lacerum
Temporal bone
Dorsum sellae
Middle
Diploe
Jugular foramen
Petrous portion
Clivus (dashed line)
Hypoglossal canal
Occipital bone
Foramen magnum
Posterior

B

Fig. 20-2 A, Lateral aspect of cranium. **B,** Superior aspect of cranial base.

The bones of the cranial vault are composed of two plates of compact tissue separated by an inner layer of spongy tissue called *diploë*. The outer plate, or table, is thicker than the inner table over most of the vault, and the thickness of the layer of spongy tissue varies considerably.

Except for the mandible, the bones of the cranium and face are joined by fibrous joints called *sutures*. The sutures are named *coronal, sagittal, squamosal,* and *lambdoidal* (see Figs. 20-1 and 20-2). The *coronal suture* is found between the frontal and parietal bones. The *sagittal suture* is located on the top of the head between the two parietal bones and just behind the coronal suture line (not visible in Figs. 20-1 and 20-2). The junction of the coronal and sagittal sutures is the *bregma.* Between the temporal bones and the parietal bones are the *squamosal sutures.* Between the occipital bone and the parietal bones is the *lambdoidal suture.* The *lambda* is the junction of the lambdoidal and sagittal sutures. On the lateral aspect of the skull, the junction of the parietal bone, squamosal suture, and greater wing of the sphenoid is the *pterion,* which overlies the middle meningeal artery. At the junction of the occipital bone, parietal bone, and mastoid portion of the temporal bone is the *asterion.*

In the newborn infant, the bones of the cranium are thin and not fully developed. They contain a small amount of calcium, are indistinctly marked, and present six

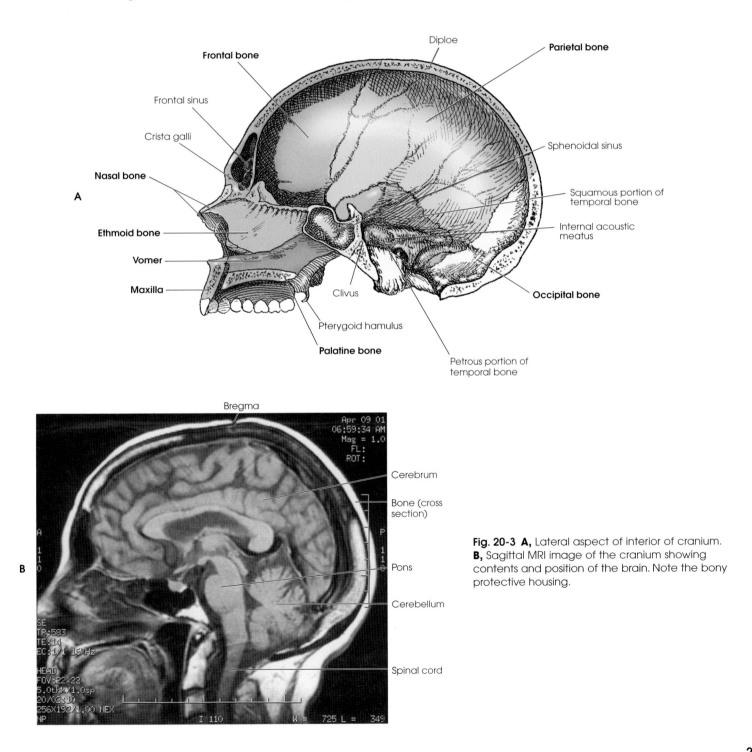

Fig. 20-3 **A,** Lateral aspect of interior of cranium. **B,** Sagittal MRI image of the cranium showing contents and position of the brain. Note the bony protective housing.

areas of incomplete ossification called *fontanels* (Fig. 20-4). Two of the fontanels are situated in the midsagittal plane at the superior and posterior angles of the parietal bones. The *anterior fontanel* is located at the junction of the two parietal bones and the one frontal bone at the bregma. Posteriorly and in the midsagittal plane is the *posterior fontanel,* located at the point labeled *lambda* in Fig. 20-2. Two fontanels are also on each side at the inferior angles of the parietal bones. Each *sphenoidal fontanel* is found at the site of the pterion; the *mastoid fontanels* are found at the asteria. The posterior and sphenoidal fontanels normally close in the first and third months after birth, respectively, and the anterior and mastoid fontanels close during the second year of life.

The cranium develops rapidly in size and density during the first 5 or 6 years, after which a gradual increase occurs until adult size and density are achieved, usually by the age of 12 years. The thickness and degree of mineralization in normal adult crania show comparatively little difference in radiopacity from person to person, and the atrophy of old age is less marked than in other regions of the body.

Internally, the cranial floor is divided into three regions: the anterior, middle, and posterior cranial fossae (see Fig. 20-2, *B*). The *anterior cranial fossa* extends from the anterior frontal bone to the lesser wings of the sphenoid. It is associated mainly with the frontal lobes of the cerebrum. The *middle cranial fossa* accommodates the temporal lobes and associated neurovascular structures and extends from the lesser wings of the sphenoid bone to the apices of the petrous portions of the temporal bones. The deep depression posterior to the petrous ridges is the *posterior cranial fossa,* which protects the cerebellum, pons, and medulla oblongata (see Fig. 20-3, *B*).

The average or so-called normal cranium is more or less oval in shape, being wider in back than in front. The average cranium measures approximately 6 inches (15 cm) at its widest point from side to side, 7 inches (17.8 cm) at its longest point from front to back, and 9 inches (22 cm) at its deepest point from the vertex to the submental region. Crania vary in size and shape, with resultant variation in the position and relationship of internal parts.

Internal deviations from the norm are usually indicated by external deviations and thus can be estimated with a reasonable degree of accuracy. The length and width of the normally shaped head vary by 1 inch (2.5 cm). Any deviation from this relationship indicates a comparable change in the position and relationship of the internal structures. If the deviation involves more than a 5-degree change, it must be compensated for by a change in either part rotation or central ray angulation. This "rule" applies to all images except direct lateral projections. A ½-inch (1.3 cm) change in the 1-inch (2.5-cm) width-to-length measurement indicates an approximately 5-degree change in the direction of the internal parts with reference to the midsagittal plane.

It is important for the radiographer to understand cranial anatomy from the standpoint of the size, shape, position, and relationship of the component parts of the cranium so that estimations and compensations can be made for deviations from the norm.

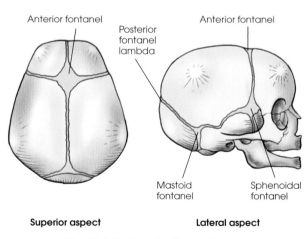

Superior aspect　　　　Lateral aspect

Fig. 20-4 Fontanels of a newborn.

Cranial Bones
FRONTAL BONE

The *frontal bone* has a vertical portion and horizontal portions. The vertical portion, called the *frontal squama,* forms the forehead and the anterior part of the vault. The horizontal portions form the orbital plates (roofs of the orbits), part of the roof of the nasal cavity, and the greater part of the anterior cranial fossa (Figs. 20-5 to 20-7).

On each side of the midsagittal plane of the superior portion of the squama is a rounded elevation called the *frontal emi-nence.* Below the frontal eminences, just above the *supraorbital margins,* are two arched ridges that correspond in position to the eyebrows. These ridges are called the *superciliary arches.* In the center of the supraorbital margin is an opening for nerves and blood vessels called the *supra-orbital foramen.* The smooth elevation between the superciliary arches is termed the *glabella.*

The *frontal sinuses* (see Chapter 22) are situated between the two tables of the squama on each side of the midsagittal plane. These irregularly shaped sinuses are separated by a bony wall, which may be incomplete and usually deviates from the midline.

The squama articulates with the parietal bones at the coronal suture, the greater wing of the sphenoid bone at the fronto-sphenoidal suture, and the nasal bones at the frontonasal suture. The midpoint of the frontonasal suture is termed the *nasion.*

The frontal bone articulates with the right and left parietals, the sphenoid, and the ethmoid bones of the cranium.

The *orbital plates* of the horizontal portion of the frontal bone are separated by a notch called the *ethmoidal notch.* This notch receives the cribriform plate of the ethmoid bone. At the anterior edge of the ethmoidal notch is a small inferior projection of bone, the *nasal spine,* which is the most superior component of the bony nasal septum. The posterior margins of the orbital plates articulate with the lesser wings of the sphenoid bone.

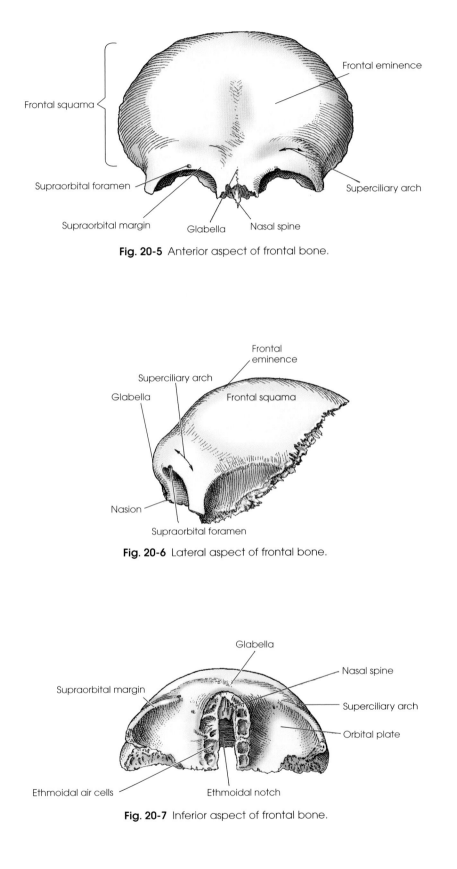

Fig. 20-5 Anterior aspect of frontal bone.

Fig. 20-6 Lateral aspect of frontal bone.

Fig. 20-7 Inferior aspect of frontal bone.

ETHMOID BONE

The *ethmoid bone* is a small, cube-shaped bone that consists of a horizontal plate, a vertical plate, and two light, spongy lateral masses called *labyrinths* (Figs. 20-8 to 20-11). Situated between the orbits, the ethmoid bone forms part of the anterior cranial fossa, the nasal cavity and orbital walls, and the bony nasal septum.

The horizontal portion of the ethmoid bone, called the *cribriform plate*, is received into the ethmoidal notch of the frontal bone. The cribriform plate is perforated by many foramina for the transmission of olfactory nerves. The plate also has a thick, conical process, the *crista galli*, which projects superiorly from its anterior midline and serves as the anterior attachment for the falx cerebri.

The vertical portion of the ethmoid bone is called the *perpendicular plate*. This plate is a thin, flat bone that projects inferiorly from the inferior surface of the cribriform plate and, with the nasal spine, forms the superior portion of the bony septum of the nose.

The *labyrinths* contain the *ethmoidal sinuses,* or air cells. The cells of each side are arbitrarily divided into three groups: the *anterior, middle,* and *posterior ethmoidal air cells.* The walls of the labyrinths form a part of the medial walls of the orbits and a part of the lateral walls of the nasal cavity. Projecting inferiorly from each medial wall of the labyrinths are two thin, scroll-shaped processes called the *superior* and *middle nasal conchae.*

The ethmoid bone articulates with the frontal and sphenoid bones of the cranium.

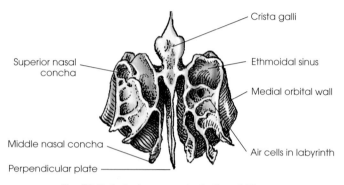

Fig. 20-8 Anterior aspect of ethmoid bone.

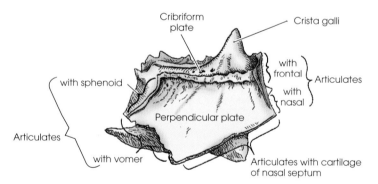

Fig. 20-9 Lateral aspect of ethmoid bone with labyrinth removed.

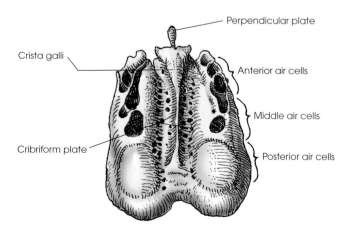

Fig. 20-10 Superior aspect of ethmoid bone.

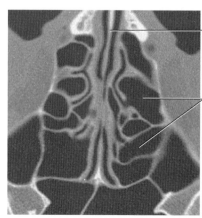

Fig. 20-11 Axial CT of ethmoidal sinus and perpendicular plate.

Skull

PARIETAL BONES

The two *parietal bones* are somewhat square and have a convex external surface and a concave internal surface (Figs. 20-12 and 20-13). The parietal bones form a large portion of the sides of the cranium. By their articulation with each other at the sagittal suture in the midsagittal plane, they also form the posterior portion of the cranial roof.

Each parietal bone presents a prominent bulge, called the *parietal eminence,* near the central portion of its external surface. In radiography, the width of the head should be measured at this point because it is the widest point of the head.

Each parietal bone articulates with the frontal, temporal, occipital, sphenoid, and opposite parietal bone of the cranium.

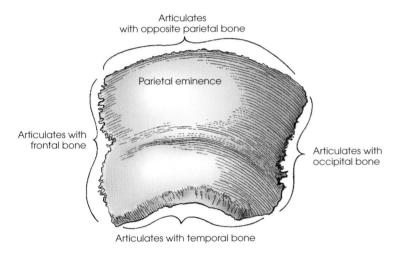

Fig. 20-12 External surface of parietal bone.

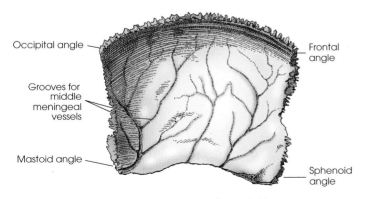

Fig. 20-13 Internal surface of parietal bone.

SPHENOID BONE

The *sphenoid bone* is an irregularly wedge-shaped bone that somewhat resembles a bat with its wings extended. It is situated in the base of the cranium anterior to the temporal bones and basilar part of the occipital bone (Figs. 20-14 to 20-16). The sphenoid bone consists of a body; two lesser wings and two greater wings, which project laterally from the sides of the body; and two pterygoid processes, which project inferiorly from each side of the inferior surface of the body.

The *body* of the sphenoid bone contains the two *sphenoidal sinuses,* which are incompletely separated by a median septum. The anterior surface of the body forms the posterior bony wall of the nasal cavity. The superior surface presents a deep depression called the *sella turcica* and contains a gland called the pituitary gland. The sella turcica lies in the midsagittal plane of the cranium at a point ¾ inch (1.9 cm) anterior to and ¾ inch (2 cm) superior to the level of the *external acoustic meatus* (EAM). The sella turcica

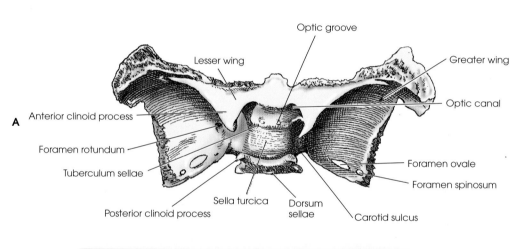

A, Lesser wing — Optic groove — Greater wing — Anterior clinoid process — Optic canal — Foramen rotundum — Tuberculum sellae — Foramen ovale — Foramen spinosum — Posterior clinoid process — Sella turcica — Dorsum sellae — Carotid sulcus

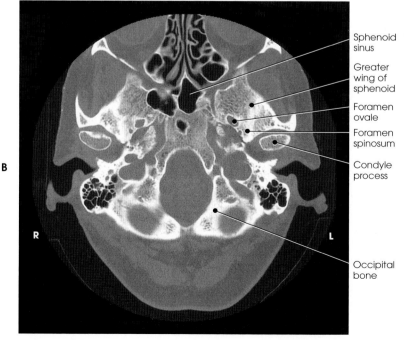

B, Sphenoid sinus — Greater wing of sphenoid — Foramen ovale — Foramen spinosum — Condyle process — Occipital bone

Fig. 20-14 A, Superior aspect of sphenoid bone. **B,** Axial CT of the sphenoid bone.

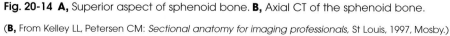

(**B,** From Kelley LL, Petersen CM: *Sectional anatomy for imaging professionals,* St Louis, 1997, Mosby.)

is bounded anteriorly by the *tuberculum sellae* and posteriorly by the *dorsum sellae,* which bears the *posterior clinoid processes.* The slanted area of bone posterior and inferior to the dorsum sellae is continuous with the basilar portion of the occipital bone and is called the *clivus.* The clivus supports the pons. On either side of the sella turcica is a groove, the *carotid sulcus,* in which the internal carotid artery and cavernous sinus lie.

The *optic groove* extends across the anterior portion of the tuberculum sellae. The groove ends on each side at the *optic canal.* The optic canal is the opening into the apex of the orbit for the transmission of the optic nerve and ophthalmic artery. The actual opening is called the *optic foramen.*

The *lesser wings* are triangular in shape and nearly horizontal in position. They arise, one on each side, from the antero-superior portion of the body of the sphenoid bone and project laterally, ending in sharp points. The lesser wings form the posteromedial portion of the roofs of the orbits, the posterior portion of the anterior cranial fossa, the upper margin of the *superior orbital fissures,* and the optic canals. The medial ends of their posterior borders form the *anterior clinoid processes.* Each process arises from two roots. The anterior (superior) root is thin and flat, and the posterior (inferior) root, referred to as the *sphenoid strut,* is thick and rounded. The circular opening between the two roots is the *optic canal.*

The *greater wings* arise from the sides of the body of the sphenoid bone and curve laterally, posteriorly, anteriorly, and superiorly. The greater wings form a part of the middle cranial fossa, the posterolateral walls of the orbits, the lower margin of the superior orbital sulci, and the greater part of the posterior margin of the inferior orbital sulci. The *foramina rotundum, ovale,* and *spinosum* are paired and are situated in the greater wings. Because these foramina transmit nerves and blood vessels, they are subject to radiologic investigation for the detection of erosive lesions of neurogenic or vascular origin.

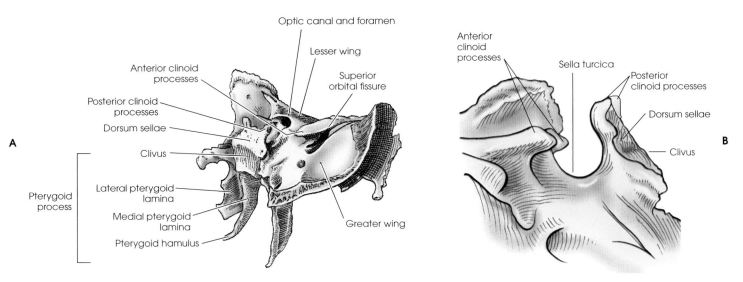

A

B

Fig. 20-15 A, Oblique aspect of upper and lateroposterior aspects of sphenoid bone (right lateral pterygoid lamina removed). **B,** Sella turcica of sphenoid bone, lateral view.

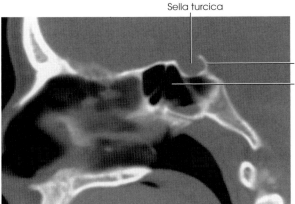

Fig. 20-16 Sagittal CT of sella turcica and sphenoid sinus.

The *pterygoid processes* arise from the lateral portions of the inferior surface of the body of the sphenoid bone and the medial portions of the inferior surfaces of the greater wings. These processes project inferiorly and curve laterally. Each pterygoid process consists of two plates of bone, the *medial* and *lateral pterygoid laminae,* which are fused at their superoanterior parts. The inferior extremity of the medial lamina possesses an elongated, hook-shaped process, the *pterygoid hamulus,* which makes it longer and narrower than the lateral lamina. The pterygoid processes articulate with the palatine bones anteriorly and with the wings of the vomer, where they enter into the formation of the nasal cavity.

The sphenoid bone articulates with each of the other seven bones of the cranium.

OCCIPITAL BONE

The *occipital bone* is situated at the posteroinferior part of the cranium. It forms the posterior half of the base of the cranium and the greater part of the posterior cranial fossa (Figs. 20-17 to 20-19). The occipital bone has four parts: the *squama,* which is saucer shaped, being convex externally; *two occipital condyles,* which extend anteriorly, one on each side of the foramen magnum; and the *basilar portion.* The occipital bone also has a large

aperture, the *foramen magnum,* through which the inferior portion of the medulla oblongata passes as it exits the cranial cavity and joins the spinal cord.

The *squama* curves posteriorly and superiorly from the foramen magnum and is also curved from side to side. It articulates with the parietal bones at the lambdoidal suture and with the mastoid portions of the temporal bones at the occipitomastoid sutures. On the external surface of the squama, midway between its summit and the foramen magnum, is a prominent process termed the *external occipital protuberance,* or *inion,* that corresponds in position with the *internal occipital protuberance.*

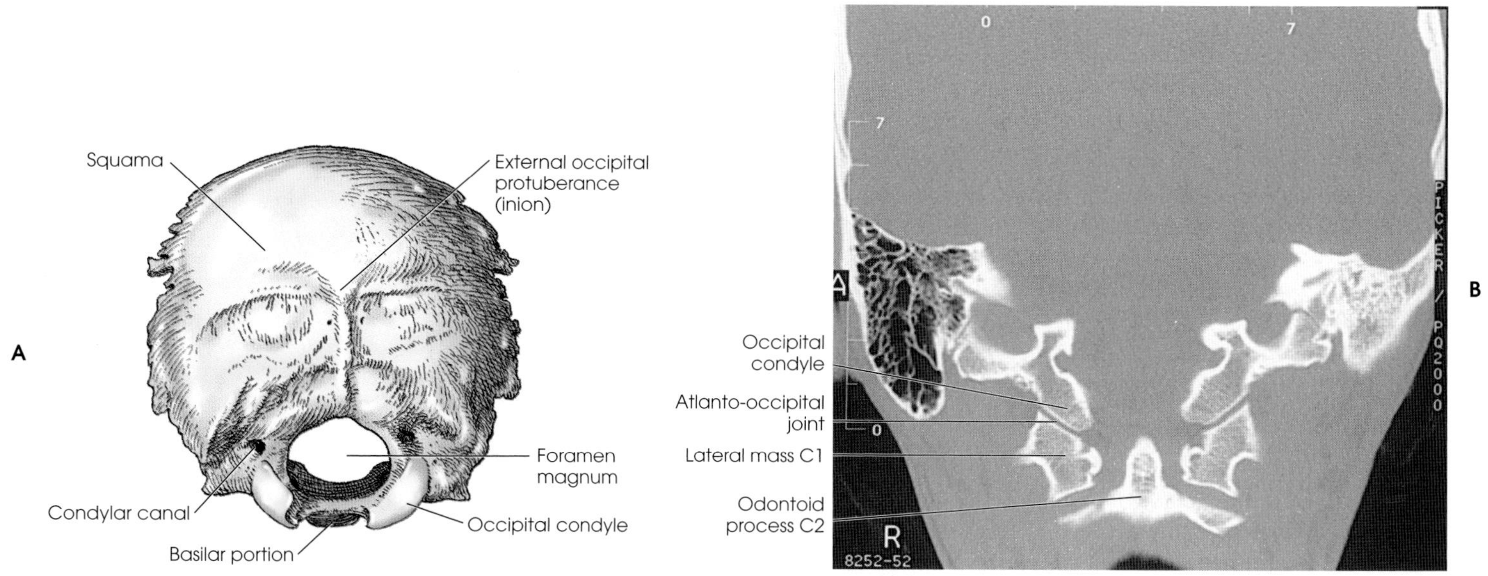

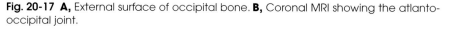

Fig. 20-17 A, External surface of occipital bone. **B,** Coronal MRI showing the atlanto-occipital joint.

(**B,** Courtesy Siemens Medical Systems, Iselin, NJ.)

The *occipital condyles* project anteriorly, one from each side of the squama, for articulation with the atlas of the cervical spine. Part of each lateral portion curves medially to fuse with the basilar portion and thus complete the foramen magnum, and part of it projects laterally to form the jugular process. On the inferior surface of the curved parts, extending from the level of the middle of the foramen magnum anteriorly to the level of its anterior margin, reciprocally shaped condyles articulate with the superior facets of the atlas. These articulations, known as the *occipitoatlantal joints,* are the only bony articulations between the skull and the neck. The *hypoglossal canals* are found at the anterior ends of the condyles and transmit the hypoglossal nerves. At the posterior end of the condyles are the *condylar canals,* through which the emissary veins pass. The anterior portion of the occipital bone contains a deep notch that forms a part of the *jugular foramen* (see Fig. 20-2, *B*). The jugular foramen is an important large opening in the skull for two reasons: it allows blood to drain from the brain via the internal jugular vein, and it lets three cranial nerves pass through it.

The *basilar portion* of the occipital bone curves anteriorly and superiorly to its junction with the body of the sphenoid. In the adult the basilar part of the occipital bone fuses with the body of the sphenoid bone, resulting in the formation of a continuous bone. The sloping surface of this junction between the dorsum sellae of the sphenoid bone and the basilar portion of the occipital bone is called the *clivus.*

The occipital bone articulates with the two parietals, the two temporals and the sphenoid of the cranium, and the first cervical vertebra.

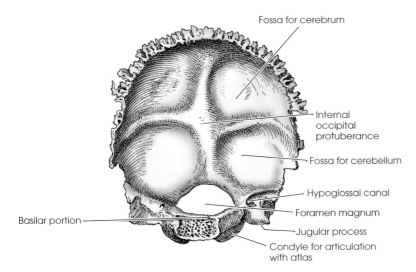

Fossa for cerebrum

Internal occipital protuberance

Fossa for cerebellum

Hypoglossal canal

Foramen magnum

Jugular process

Condyle for articulation with atlas

Basilar portion

Fig. 20-18 Internal surface of occipital bone.

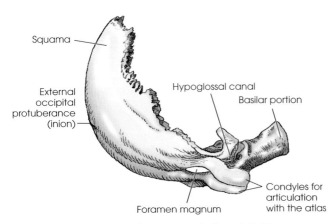

Squama

External occipital protuberance (inion)

Hypoglossal canal

Basilar portion

Condyles for articulation with the atlas

Foramen magnum

Fig. 20-19 Lateroinferior aspect of occipital bone.

TEMPORAL BONES

The temporal bones are irregular in shape and are situated on each side of the base of the cranium between the greater wings of the sphenoid bone and the occipital bone (Figs. 20-20 to 20-24). The temporal bones form a large part of the middle fossa of the cranium and a small part of the posterior fossa. Each temporal bone consists of a squamous portion, a tympanic portion, a styloid process, a zygomatic process, and a petromastoid portion (the mastoid and petrous portions) that contains the organs of hearing and balance.

The *squamous portion* is the thin upper portion of the temporal bone. It forms a part of the side wall of the cranium and has a prominent arched process, the *zygomatic process,* which projects anteriorly to articulate with the zygomatic bone of the face and thus complete the zygomatic arch. On the inferior border of the zygomatic process is a rounded eminence, the *articular tubercle,* which forms the anterior boundary of the *mandibular fossa.* The mandibular fossa receives the condyle of the mandible to form the *temporomandibular joint* (TMJ).

The *tympanic portion* is situated below the squama and in front of the mastoid and petrous portions of the temporal bone. This portion forms the anterior wall, inferior wall, and part of the posterior walls of the EAM. The EAM is approximately ½ inch (1.3 cm) in length and projects medially, anteriorly, and slightly superiorly.

The *styloid process,* a slender, pointed bone of variable length, projects inferiorly, anteriorly, and slightly medially from the inferior portion of the tympanic part of the temporal bone.

Petromastoid portion

The petrous and mastoid portions together are called the *petromastoid portion.* The mastoid portion, which forms the inferior, posterior part of the temporal bone is prolonged into the conical *mastoid process* (see Figs. 20-22 and 20-24).

The *mastoid portion* articulates with the parietal bone at its superior border through the parietomastoid suture and with the occipital bone at its posterior border through the occipitomastoid suture, which is contiguous with the lambdoidal suture. The *mastoid process* varies considerably in size, depending on its pneumatization, and is larger in males than in females.

The first of the *mastoid air cells* to develop is situated at the upper anterior part of the process and is termed the *mastoid antrum.* This air cell is quite large and communicates with the tympanic cavity. Shortly before or after birth, smaller air cells begin to develop around the mastoid antrum and continue to increase in number and size until around puberty. However, the air cells vary considerably in both size and number. Occasionally they are absent altogether, in which case the mastoid process is solid bone and is usually small.

The *petrous portion,* often called the *petrous pyramid,* is conical or pyramidal and is the thickest, densest bone in the cranium. This part of the temporal bone contains the organs of hearing and balance. From its base at the squamous and mastoid portions, the petrous portion projects medially and anteriorly between the greater wing of the sphenoid bone and the occipital bone to the body of the sphenoid bone, with which its apex articulates. The internal carotid artery in the *carotid canal* enters the inferior aspect of the petrous portion, passes superior to the cochlea, then passes medially to exit the *petrous apex.* Near the petrous apex is a ragged foramen called the *foramen lacerum.* The carotid canal opens into this foramen, which contains the internal carotid artery (see Fig. 20-2, *B*). At the center of the posterior aspect of the petrous portion is the *internal acoustic meatus* (IAM), which transmits the vestibulocochlear and facial nerves. The upper border of the petrous portion is commonly referred to as the *petrous ridge.* The top of the ridge lies approximately at the level of an external radiography landmark called the *top of ear attachment* (TEA).

The temporal bone articulates with the parietal, occipital, and sphenoid bones of the cranium.

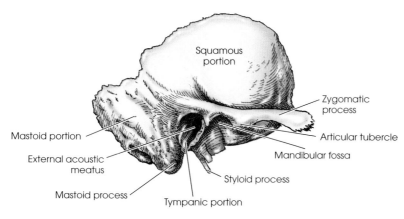

Fig. 20-20 Lateral aspect of temporal bone.

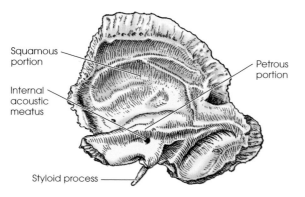

Fig. 20-21 Internal surface of temporal bone.

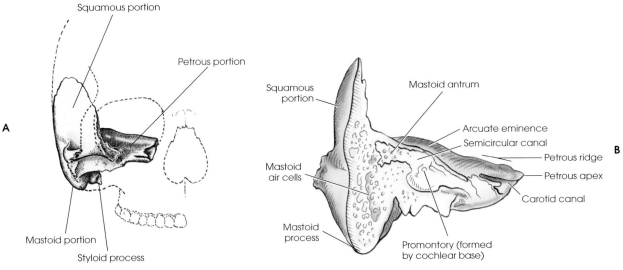

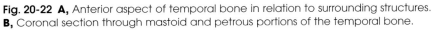

Fig. 20-22 A, Anterior aspect of temporal bone in relation to surrounding structures.
B, Coronal section through mastoid and petrous portions of the temporal bone.

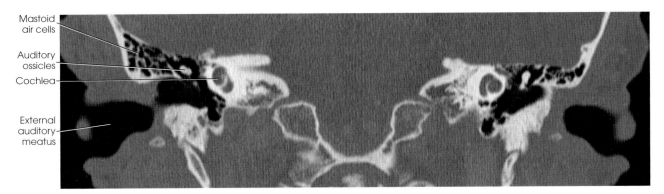

Fig. 20-23 Coronal CT through temporal bones.

(Courtesy Karl Mockler, RT(R).)

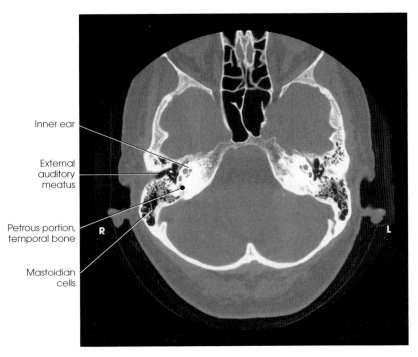

Fig. 20-24 Axial CT of the petrous portion at the level of the external auditory meatus.

(From Kelley LL, Petersen CM: *Sectional anatomy for imaging professionals,* St Louis, 1997, Mosby.)

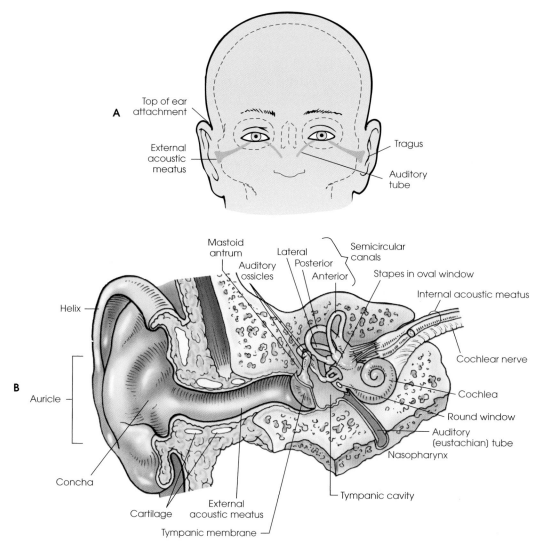

Fig. 20-25 A, Frontal view of the face, showing internal structures of ear *(shaded area)*. **B,** External, middle, and internal ear.

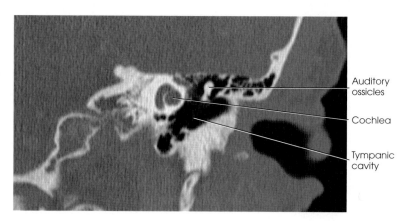

Fig. 20-26 Coronal CT through petrous portion of temporal bone, demonstrating middle and inner ear.

(Courtesy Karl Mockler, RT(R).)

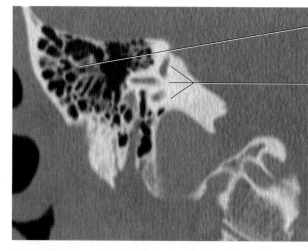

Fig. 20-27 Coronal CT of petromastoid portion of temporal bone, demonstrating semicircular canals and mastoid air cells.

(Courtesy Karl Mockler, RT(R).)

Ear

The ear is the organ of hearing and balance (Fig. 20-25). The essential parts of the ear are housed in the petrous portion of the temporal bone. The organs of hearing and equilibrium consist of three main divisions: the external ear, middle ear, and internal ear.

EXTERNAL EAR

The *external ear* consists of two parts: (1) the oval-shaped, fibrocartilaginous, sound-collecting organ situated on the side of the head known as the *auricle,* and (2) a sound-conducting canal, the *EAM.* The auricle has a deep central depression, the *concha,* the lower part of which leads into the EAM. At its anterior margin the auricle has a prominent cartilaginous lip, the *tragus,* which projects posteriorly over the entrance of the meatus. The outer rim of the ear is the *helix.* The EAM is about 1 inch (2.5 cm) in length. The outer third of the canal wall is cartilaginous, and the inner two thirds are osseous. From the meatal orifice the canal forms a slight curve as it passes medially and anteriorly in line with the axis of the IAM. The EAM ends at the tympanic membrane of the middle ear.

MIDDLE EAR

The *middle ear* is situated between the external and internal ear. The middle ear proper consists of (1) the *tympanic membrane* (or eardrum), (2) an irregularly shaped, air-containing compartment called the *tympanic cavity,* and (3) three small bones called the *auditory ossicles* (Fig. 20-26). The middle ear communicates with the mastoid antrum and auditory eustachian tube.

The *tympanic membrane* is a thin, concavoconvex, membranous disk with an elliptic shape. The disk, the convex surface of which is directed medially, is situated obliquely over the medial end of the EAM and serves as a partition between the external and middle ear. The function of the tympanic membrane is the transmission of sound vibrations.

The *tympanic cavity* is a narrow, irregularly shaped chamber that lies just posterior and medial to the mandibular fossa. The cavity is separated from the external ear by the tympanic membrane and from the internal ear by the bony labyrinth. The tympanic cavity communicates with the nasopharynx through the *auditory (eustachian) tube,* a passage by which air pressure in the middle ear is equalized with the pressure in the outside air passages. The auditory tube is about 1¼ inches (3 cm) long. From its entrance into the tympanic cavity, the auditory tube passes medially and inferiorly to its orifice on the lateral wall of the nasopharynx.

The mastoid antrum is the large air cavity situated in the temporal bone above the mastoid air cells and immediately behind the posterior wall of the middle ear.

The *auditory ossicles,* named for their shape, are the *malleus* (hammer), *incus* (anvil), and *stapes* (stirrup). These three delicate bones are articulated to permit vibratory motion. They bridge the middle ear cavity for the transmission of sound vibrations from the tympanic membrane to the internal ear. The handle of the malleus (the outermost ossicle) is attached to the tympanic membrane, and its head articulates with the icus (the central ossicle). The head of the stapes (the innermost ossicle) articulates with the incus, and its base is fitted into the oval window of the inner ear.

INTERNAL EAR

The *internal ear* contains the essential sensory apparatus of hearing and equilibrium and lies on the densest portion of the petrous portion immediately below the arcuate eminence. Composed of an irregularly shaped bony chamber called the *bony labyrinth,* the internal ear is housed within the bony chamber and is an intercommunicating system of ducts and sacs known as the *membranous labyrinth.* The bony labyrinth consists of three distinctly shaped parts: (1) a spiral-coiled, tubular part called the *cochlea,* which communicates with the middle ear through the membranous covering of the *round window* (see Fig. 20-26); (2) a small, ovoid central compartment behind the cochlea, known as the *vestibule,* which communicates with the middle ear by way of the *oval window;* and (3) three unequally sized *semicircular canals* that form right angles to one another and are called, according to their positions, the *anterior, posterior,* and *lateral semicircular canals* (Fig. 20-27). From its cranial orifice, the IAM passes inferiorly and laterally for a distance of about ½ inch (1.3 cm). It is through this canal that the cochlear and vestibular nerves pass from their fibers in the respective parts of the membranous labyrinth to the brain. The cochlea is used for hearing, and the vestibule and semicircular canals are involved with equilibrium.

Facial Bones

NASAL BONES

The two small, thin *nasal bones* vary in size and shape in different individuals (Figs. 20-28 and 20-29). They form the superior bony wall (called the *bridge* of the nose) of the nasal cavity. The nasal bones articulate in the midsagittal plane, where at their posterosuperior surface they also articulate with the perpendicular plate of the ethmoid bone. They articulate with the frontal bone above and with the maxillae at the sides.

LACRIMAL BONES

The two *lacrimal bones,* which are the smallest bones in the skull, are very thin and are situated at the anterior part of the medial wall of the orbits between the labyrinth of the ethmoid bone and the maxilla (see Figs. 20-28 and 20-29). Together with the maxillae, the lacrimal bones form the lacrimal fossae, which accommodate the lacrimal sacs. Each lacrimal bone contains a *lacrimal foramen* through which a tear duct passes. Each lacrimal bone articulates with the frontal and ethmoid cranial bones and the maxilla and inferior nasal concha facial bones. The lacrimal bones can be seen on PA and lateral projections of the skull.

MAXILLARY BONES

The two *maxillary bones* are the largest of the immovable bones of the face (see Figs. 20-28 and 20-29). Each articulates with all other facial bones except the mandible. Each also articulates with the frontal and ethmoid bones of the cranium. The maxillary bones form part of the lateral walls and most of the floor of the nasal cavity, part of the floor of the orbital cavities, and three fourths of the roof of the mouth. Their zygomatic processes articulate with the zygomatic bones and assist in the formation of the prominence of the cheeks. The body of each maxilla contains a large, pyramidal cavity called the *maxillary sinus,* which empties into the nasal cavity. An *infraorbital foramen* is located under each orbit and serves as a passage through which the infraorbital nerve and artery reach the nose.

At their inferior borders the maxillae possess a thick, spongy ridge called the *alveolar process,* which supports the roots of the teeth. In the anterior midsagittal plane at their junction with each other, the maxillary bones form a pointed, forward-projecting process called the *anterior nasal spine.* The midpoint of this prominence is called the *acanthion.*

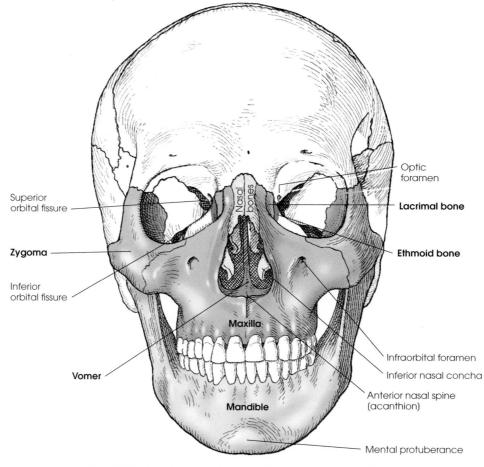

Fig. 20-28 Anterior aspect of skull demonstrating facial bones.

ZYGOMATIC BONES

The zygomatic bones form the prominence of the cheeks and a part of the side wall and floor of the orbital cavities (see Figs. 20-28 and 20-29). A posteriorly extending *temporal process* unites with the zygomatic process of the temporal bone to form the *zygomatic arch.* The zygomatic bones articulate with the frontal bone superiorly, with the zygomatic process of the temporal bone at the side, with the maxilla anteriorly, and with the sphenoid bone posteriorly.

PALATINE BONES

The two palatine bones are L-shaped bones composed of *vertical* and *horizontal plates.* The horizontal plates articulate with the maxillae to complete the posterior fourth of the bony palate, or roof of the mouth (see Fig. 20-3). The vertical portions of the palatine bones extend upward between the maxillae and the pterygoid processes of the sphenoid bone in the posterior nasal cavity. The superior tips of the vertical portions of the palatine bones assist in forming the posteromedial bony orbit.

INFERIOR NASAL CONCHAE

The inferior nasal conchae extend diagonally and inferiorly from the lateral walls of the nasal cavity at approximately its lower third (see Fig. 20-28). They are long, narrow, and extremely thin; they curl laterally, which gives them a scroll-like appearance.

The upper two nasal conchae are processes of the ethmoid bone. The three nasal conchae project into and divide the lateral portion of the respective sides of the nasal cavity into superior, middle, and inferior meatuses. They are covered with a mucous membrane to warm, moisten, and cleanse inhaled air.

VOMER

The *vomer* is a thin plate of bone situated in the midsagittal plane of the floor of the nasal cavity, where it forms the inferior part of the *nasal septum* (see Fig. 20-28). The anterior border of the vomer slants superiorly and posteriorly from the anterior nasal spine to the body of the sphenoid bone, with which its superior border articulates. The superior part of its anterior border articulates with the perpendicular plate of the ethmoid bone; its posterior border is free.

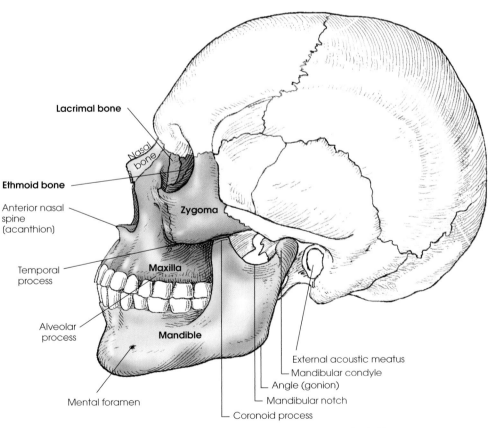

Fig. 20-29 Lateral aspect of skull demonstrating facial bones.

MANDIBLE

The *mandible,* the largest and densest bone of the face, consists of a curved horizontal portion, called the *body,* and two vertical portions, called the *rami,* which unite with the body at the *angle* of the mandible, or *gonion* (Fig. 20-30). At birth the mandible consists of bilateral pieces held together by a fibrous symphysis that ossifies during the first year of life. At the site of ossification is a slight ridge that ends below in a triangular prominence, the *mental protuberance.* The *symphysis* is the most anterior and central part of the mandible. This is where the left and right halves of the mandible have fused.

The superior border of the body of the mandible consists of spongy bone, called the *alveolar portion,* which supports the roots of the teeth. Below the second premolar tooth, approximately halfway between the superior and inferior borders of the bone, is a small opening on each side for the transmission of nerves and blood vessels. These two openings are called the *mental foramina.*

The rami project superiorly at an obtuse angle to the body of the mandible, and their broad surface forms an angle of approximately 110 to 120 degrees. Each ramus presents two processes at its upper extremity, one coronoid and one condylar, which are separated by a concave area called the *mandibular notch.* The anterior process, the *coronoid process,* is thin and tapered and projects to a higher level than the posterior process. The *condylar process* consists of a constricted area, the *neck,* above which is a broad, thick, almost transversely placed *condyle* that articulates with the mandibular fossa of the temporal bone (Fig. 20-31). This articulation, the TMJ, slants posteriorly approximately 15 degrees and inferiorly and medially approximately 15 degrees. Radiographic projections, produced from the opposite side, must reverse these directions. In other words, the central ray angulation must be superior and anterior to coincide with the long axis of the joint. The TMJ is situated immediately in front of the EAM.

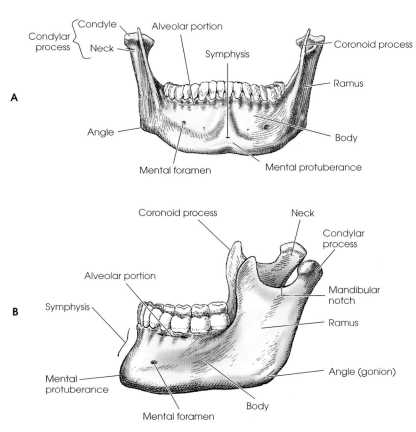

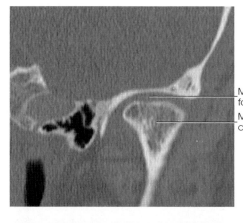

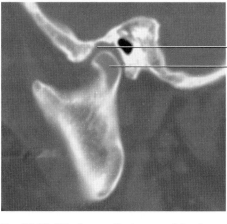

Fig. 20-30 A, Anterior aspect of mandible. **B,** Lateral aspect of mandible.

Fig. 20-31 CT of mandibular condyle situated in the mandibular fossa. **A,** Coronal. **B,** Sagittal.

(Courtesy Karl Mockler, RT(R).)

HYOID BONE

The *hyoid bone* is a small, U-shaped structure situated at the base of the tongue, where it is held in position in part by the stylohyoid ligaments extending from the styloid processes of the temporal bones (Fig. 20-32). Although the hyoid bone is an accessory bone of the axial skeleton, it is described in this chapter because of its connection with the temporal bones. The hyoid is the only bone in the body that does not articulate with any other bone.

The hyoid bone is divided into a *body,* two *greater cornua,* and two *lesser cornua.* The bone serves as an attachment for certain muscles of the larynx and tongue and is easily palpated just above the larynx.

ORBITS

Each orbit is composed of *seven* different bones (Fig. 20-33). Three of these are cranial bones: *frontal, sphenoid,* and *ethmoid.* The other four bones are the facial bones: *maxilla, zygoma, lacrimal,* and *palatine.* The circumference of the orbit, or outer rim area, is composed of three of the seven bones—the frontal, zygoma, and maxilla. The remaining four bones comprise most of the posterior aspect of the orbit.

Articulations of the Skull

The sutures of the skull are connected by toothlike projections of bone interlocked with a thin layer of fibrous tissue. These articulations allow for no movement and are classified as *fibrous* joints of the *suture* type. The articulations of the facial bones, including the joints between the roots of the teeth and the jawbones, are *fibrous gomphoses.* The exception is the point at which the rounded condyle of the mandible articulates with the mandibular fossa of the temporal bone to form the TMJ. The TMJ articulation is a *synovial* joint of both the *hinge* and *gliding* type. The atlanto-occipital joint is a *synovial ellipsoidal* joint that joins the base of the skull (occipital bone) with the atlas of the cervical spine. The seven joints of the skull are summarized in Table 20-1.

Text continued on p. 300

TABLE 20-1

Joints of the skull

Joint	Structural classification		Movement
	Tissue	Type	
Coronal suture	Fibrous	Suture	Immovable
Sagittal suture	Fibrous	Suture	Immovable
Lambdoidal suture	Fibrous	Suture	Immovable
Squamosal suture	Fibrous	Suture	Immovable
Temporomandibular	Synovial	Hinge and gliding	Freely movable
Alveolar sockets	Fibrous	Gomphosis	Immovable
Atlanto-occipital	Synovial	Ellipsoidal	Freely moveable

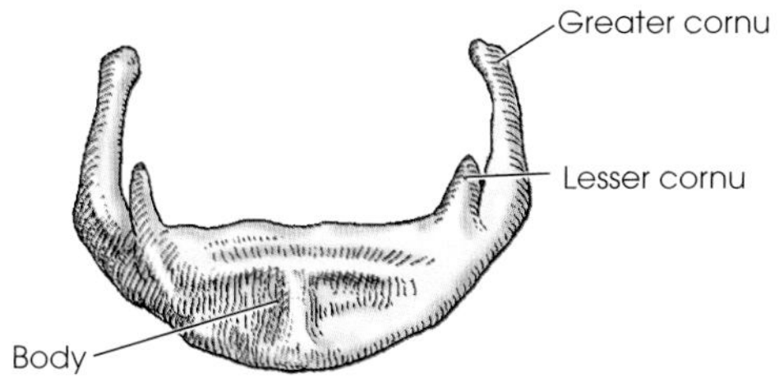

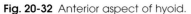

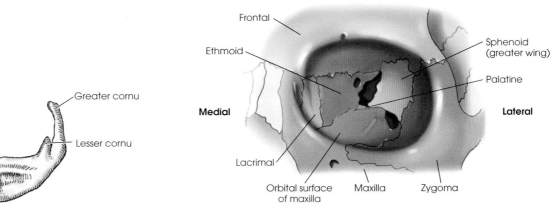

Fig. 20-32 Anterior aspect of hyoid.

Fig. 20-33 The orbit. The seven bones of the orbit are shown.

SUMMARY OF ANATOMY

Skull
cranial bones (8)
facial bones (14)

Cranial bones
calvaria
  frontal
  right parietal
  left parietal
  occipital
floor
  right temporal
  left temporal
  sphenoid
  ethmoid
diploë

Sutures
coronal suture
sagittal suture
squamosal sutures
lambdoidal suture
bregma
lambda
pterion
asterion

Fontanels
anterior fontanel
posterior fontanel
sphenoidal fontanels (2)
mastoid fontanels (2)

Fossae
anterior cranial fossa
middle cranial fossa
posterior cranial fossa

Frontal bone
frontal squama
frontal eminence
supraorbital margins
superciliary arches
supraorbital foramen
glabella
frontal sinuses
nasion
orbital plates
  ethmoidal notch
  nasal spine

Ethmoid bone
cribriform plate
  crista galli
perpendicular plate
labyrinths
  anterior air cells
  middle air cells
  posterior air cells
  ethmoidal sinuses
  superior nasal conchae
  middle nasal conchae

Parietal bones
parietal eminence

Sphenoid bone
body
  sphenoidal sinuses
  sella turcica
    tuberculum sellae
    dorsum sellae
    posterior clinoid
      processes
    clivus
carotid sulcus
optic groove
  optic canals
  optic foramen
lesser wings
  superior orbital fissures
  anterior clinoid
    processes
  sphenoid strut
greater wings
  foramen rotundum
  foramen ovale
  foramen spinosum
  pterygoid processes
    medial pterygoid
    lamina
    pterygoid hamulus
    lateral pterygoid
    lamina

Occipital bone
foramen magnum
squama
  external occipital
    protuberance (inion)
  internal occipital
    protuberance
  occipital condyles
    hypoglossal canals
    condylar canals
    jugular foramen
  basilar portion
    clivus

Temporal bones
squamous portions
  zygomatic process
  articular tubercle
  mandibular fossa
tympanic portions
  external acoustic meatus (EAM)
  styloid process
petromastoid portions
  mastoid portions
    mastoid process
    mastoid antrum
    mastoid air cells
  petrous portions (petrous pyramids)
    carotid canals
    petrous apex
    foramen lacerum
    internal acoustic meatus (IAM)
    petrous ridge
    top of ear attachment (TEA)

Ear
external ear
  auricle
    concha
    tragus
    helix
  EAM
middle ear
  tympanic membrane
  tympanic cavity
    auditory (eustachian)
    tube
auditory ossicles
  malleus
  incus
  stapes
internal ear
  arcuate eminence
  bony labyrinth
    cochlea
    round window
    vestibule
    oval window
    semicircular canals
      anterior
      posterior
      lateral
  membranous labyrinth

Facial bones (14)
nasal (2)
lacrimal (2)
maxillary (2)
zygomatic (2)
palatine (2)
inferior nasal conchae (2)
vomer (1)
mandible (1)
hyoid bone
diploë

Lacrimal bones (2)
lacrimal foramen

Maxillary bones (2)
maxillary sinus
infraorbital foramen
alveolar process
anterior nasal spine
acanthion

Zygomatic bones (2)
temporal process
zygomatic arch

Palatine bones (2)
vertical plates
horizontal plates

Inferior nasal conchae (2)

Vomer (1)
nasal septum

Mandible (1)
body
  alveolar portion
  mental foramina
angle (gonion)
rami
  coronoid process
  condylar process
    condyle
    neck
    temporomandibular
    joint (TMJ)
  mandibular notch
mental protuberance
(mentum)
symphysis

Hyoid bone
body
greater cornua
lesser cornua

Articulations
coronal suture
sagittal suture
lambdoidal sutures
squamosal sutures
temporomandibular
alveolar sockets
atlanto-occipital

Morphology
mesocephalic
brachycephalic
dolicocephalic

Orbit
base
apex
optic foramen
superior orbital fissures
inferior orbital fissures

Eye
eyeball
conjunctiva
sclera
cornea
retina
  rods
  cones

Articulations of the skull

SUMMARY OF PATHOLOGY

Condition	Definition
Fracture	Disruption in the continuity of bone
Basal	Fracture located at the base of the skull
Blowout	Fracture of the floor of the orbit
Contre-Coup	Fracture to one side of a structure caused by trauma to the other side
Depressed	Fracture causing a portion of the skull to be depressed into the cranial cavity
Le Fort	Bilateral horizontal fractures of the maxillae
Linear	Irregular or jagged fracture of the skull
Tripod	Fracture of the zygomatic arch and orbital floor or rim and dislocation of the frontozygomatic suture
Mastoiditis	Inflammation of the mastoid antrum and air cells
Metastases	Transfer of a cancerous lesion from one area to another
Osteomyelitis	Inflammation of bone due to a pyogenic infection
Osteopetrosis	Increased density of atypically soft bone
Osteoporosis	Loss of bone density
Paget's Disease	Thick, soft bone marked by bowing and fractures
Polyp	Growth or mass protruding from a mucous membrane
Sinusitis	Inflammation of one or more of the paranasal sinuses
TMJ Syndrome	Dysfunction of the temporomandibular joint (TMJ)
Tumor	New tissue growth where cell proliferation is uncontrolled
Acoustic Neuroma	Benign tumor arising from Schwann cells of the eighth cranial nerve
Multiple Myeloma	Malignant neoplasm of plasma cells involving the bone marrow and causing destruction of the bone
Osteoma	Tumor composed of bony tissue
Pituitary Adenoma	Tumor arising from the pituitary gland, usually in the anterior lobe

EXPOSURE TECHNIQUE CHART ESSENTIAL PROJECTIONS

SKULL

Part	cm	kVp*	tm	mA	mAs	AEC	SID	IR	Dose† (mrad)
Cranium‡									
Lateral	15	80		200s		⚆	48″	24 × 30 cm	98
PA	20	80		200s		⚆	48″	24 × 30 cm	211
PA Axial (Caldwell)	20	80		200s		⚆	48″	24 × 30 cm	211
AP	20	80		200s		⚆	48″	24 × 30 cm	211
AP Axial	20	80		200s		⚆	48″	24 × 30 cm	211
AP Axial (Towne)	22	80		200s		⚆	48″	24 × 30 cm	252
PA Axial (Haas)	21	80		200s		⚆	48″	24 × 30 cm	220
Cranial Base‡									
SMV	23	80		200s		⚆	48″	24 × 30 cm	329
Petromastoid Portion‡									
Modified Law	15	75	0.17	200s	14	⚆	48″	8 × 10 in	117
Stenvers	16	75	0.10	200s	20	⚆	48″	8 × 10 in	167
Arcelin	15	75	0.10	200s	20	⚆	48″	8 × 10 in	167
Optic Canal and Foramen‡									
Parietoorbital Oblique	21	80	0.09	200s	18		48″	8 × 10 in	220

s, Small focal spot.
*kVp values are for a three-phase, 12-pulse generator.
†Relative doses for comparison use. All doses are skin entrance for average adult at cm indicated.
‡Bucky, 16:1 grid. Screen/film speed 300.

NEW ABBREVIATIONS USED IN CHAPTER 20

AML	Acanthiomeatal line
GML	Glabellomeatal line
IAM	Internal acoustic meatus
IPL	Interpupillary line
OID	Object–to–image-receptor distance
TEA	Top of ear attachment

See Addendum B for a summary of all abbreviations used in Volume 2.

Skull

Skull Topography

The basic localization points and planes of the skull (all of which can be either seen or palpated) used in radiographic positioning are illustrated in Figs. 20-34 and 20-35.

Accurate positioning of the skull requires a full understanding of these landmarks, *which should be studied thoroughly before positioning of the skull is learned.* The planes, points, lines, and abbreviations most frequently used in skull positioning are as follows:

- Midsagittal plane
- Interpupillary line
- Acanthion
- Outer canthus
- Infraorbital margin
- External acoustic meatus (EAM)
- Orbitomeatal line (OML)
- Infraorbitomeatal line (IOML)
- Acanthiomeatal line (AML)
- Mentomeatal line (MML)

In the adult, an average 7-degree angle difference exists between the OML and IOML, and an average 8-degree angle difference exists between the OML and the glabellomeatal line. The degree difference between the cranial positioning lines must be recognized. Often the relationship of the patient, IR, and central ray is the same, but the angle that is described may vary depending on the cranial line of reference.

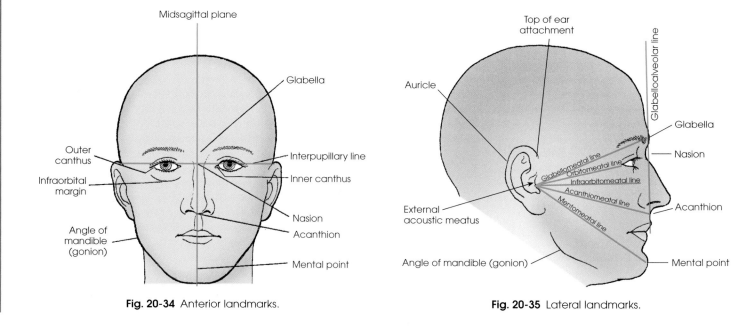

Fig. 20-34 Anterior landmarks.

Fig. 20-35 Lateral landmarks.

Skull Morphology

Radiographic images of the skull are all based on the normal size and shape of the cranium. Rules have been established for the centering and adjustment of localization points and planes and for the exact degree of central ray angulation for each projection. Although the heads of many patients fall within the limits of normality and can be radiographed satisfactorily using the established positions, a considerable number of skulls vary enough in shape that the standard procedure must be adjusted to obtain an undistorted image.

In the typically shaped head (Fig. 20-36), the petrous pyramids project anteriorly and medially at an angle of 47 degrees from the midsagittal plane of the skull. The superior borders of these structures are situated in the base of the cranium.

Depending on its shape, the atypical cranium requires more or less rotation of the head or an increase or decrease in the angulation of the central ray compared with the typical, or *mesocephalic,* skull (see Fig. 20-36). In the *brachycephalic* skull (Fig. 20-37), which is short from front to back, broad from side to side, and shallow from vertex to base, the internal structures are higher with reference to the IOML and their long axes are more frontal in position (i.e., the petrous pyramids form a wider angle with the midsagittal plane). The petrous pyramids lie at an average angle of 54 degrees. In the *dolichocephalic* skull (Fig. 20-38), which is long from front to back, narrow from side to side, and deep from vertex to base, the internal structures are lower with reference to the IOML and their long axes are

less frontal in position (i.e., the petrous pyramids form a narrower angle with the midsagittal plane). The petrous pyramids form an average angle of 40 degrees in the dolichocephalic skull.

Asymmetry must also be considered. For example, the orbits are not always symmetric in size and shape, the lower jaw is often asymmetric, and the nasal bones and cartilage are frequently deviated from the midsagittal plane. Many deviations are not as obvious as these, but if the radiographer adheres to the fundamental rules of positioning, relatively little difficulty will be encountered. Varying the position of the part or the degree of central ray angulation to compensate for structural variations becomes a simple procedure if care and precision are used initially.

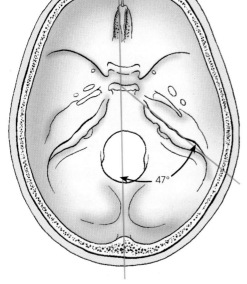

Fig. 20-36 Mesocephalic skull.

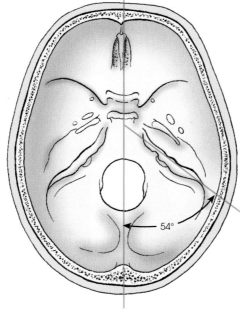

Fig. 20-37 Brachycephalic skull.

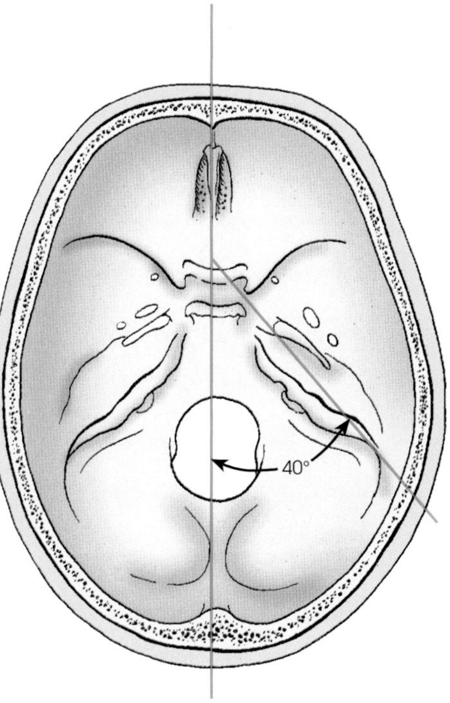

Fig. 20-38 Dolichocephalic skull.

If possible, the radiography student should obtain a dry skull specimen and radiograph it in the standard positions. This is the best technique for studying the anatomy of the different parts of the cranium from both actual and radiographic standpoints. It is important to compare the actual structure (its position in the head, its relationship to adjacent structures in each radiographic position, and its relationship to the IR and the central ray angulation) with the resultant image on the radiograph. In this way the radiographer can develop the ability to look at a head as though it were transparent—to visualize the location and direction of the internal parts according to the shape of the cranium. By studying the image cast by the part being examined with reference to its relationship to the images of the adjacent structures, the radiographer learns to detect quickly and accurately any error in the image and any deviation from the normal cranium that requires compensation.

It is also advisable to keep a complete set of radiographs of a normally shaped skull. These radiographs can be used for comparison with atypical skulls in determining the deviation and the correct adjustment to make in the degree and direction of part rotation or central ray angulation. Radiographic examples of correct and incorrect skull rotation are shown in Figs. 20-39 and 20-40.

The radiographic positions depicted in Chapters 20 to 22 show the patient either seated at the vertical grid device or lying on a radiographic table. Whether the radiographer elects to perform the examination with the patient in the recumbent or upright position depends on four variables: (1) the equipment available, (2) the age and condition of the patient, (3) the preference of the radiographer and/ or radiologist, and (4) whether upright images would increase diagnostic value, such as showing air-fluid levels in paranasal sinuses.

With the exception of paranasal sinuses, which should be radiographed upright, the remaining radiographic positions are shown with the patient *either* upright or recumbent. Comparable radiographs can usually be obtained with the patient either upright or recumbent. For example, a recumbent skull radiograph can also be obtained with the patient upright as long as the OML and central ray angulation remain constant. Therefore unless specifically noted in the text, the photographic illustration does *not* constitute a recommendation for performing the examination with the patient in either the upright or recumbent position. Line drawings illustrating both table and upright radiography are included for most radiographic positions in this chapter.

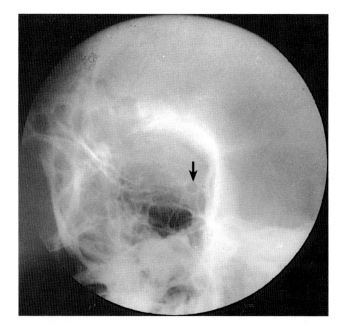

Fig. 20-39 Correct rotation clearly showing optic canal *(arrow)*.

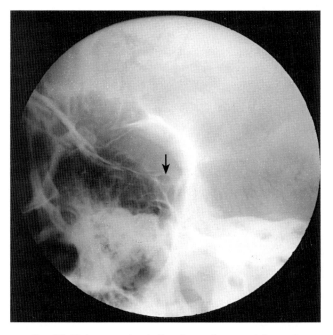

Fig. 20-40 Incorrect rotation for optic canal *(arrow)*.

Technical Considerations

GENERAL BODY POSITION

The position of the body is important in radiography of the skull. Uncomfortable body position resulting in rotation or other motion is responsible for the majority of repeat examinations. The radiographer, engrossed in adjusting the patient's head, may forget that the head is attached to a body. If the body is not correctly adjusted, it places so great a strain on the muscles that they cannot support the position. This is especially true when recumbent positions are used for skull radiography. Some guidelines to alleviate strain and facilitate accurate positioning are as follows:

- To prevent lateral rotation of the head, place the patient's body so that its long axis, depending on the image, either coincides with or is parallel to the midline of the radiographic table. To prevent superior or inferior pull on the head, resulting in longitudinal angulation or tilt, place the patient's body so that the long axis of the cervical vertebrae coincides with the level of the midpoint of the foramen magnum.
- Support any elevated part, such as the patient's shoulder or hip, on a pillow or sandbags to relieve strain.
- For examinations of hyposthenic or asthenic patients, elevate the patient's chest on a small pillow to raise the cervical vertebrae to the correct level for the lateral, PA, and oblique projections when the patient is recumbent.
- For examinations of obese or hypersthenic patients, elevate the patient's head on a radiolucent pad to obtain the correct part-IR relationship if needed. An advantage of a head unit is that it simplifies the handling of these patients.

- While adjusting the body, stand in a position that facilitates estimation of the approximate part position. For example, stand so that the longitudinal axis of the radiographic table is visible as the midsagittal plane of the body is being centered. This allows the anterior surface of the forehead to be viewed while the degree of body rotation for a lateral projection of the skull is adjusted. Therefore the body can be adjusted in such a way that it does not interfere with the final adjustment of the head, and the final position is comfortable for the patient.

When the body is correctly placed and adjusted so that the long axis of the cervical vertebrae is supported at the level of the foramen magnum, the final position of the head requires only minor adjustments. The average patient can maintain this relatively comfortable position without the aid of elaborate immobilization devices, although the following techniques may be helpful:

- If necessary, apply a head clamp with equal pressure on the two sides of the head.
- If such a clamp is not available, use a strip of adhesive tape where it will not be projected onto the image. The portion of the tape touching the hair should have the adhesive side covered with a second piece of tape so that the hairs are not pulled out when the tape is removed. Do not place adhesive tape directly on the patient's skin.
- When the area to be exposed is small, immobilize the head with sandbags placed against the sides or vertex.

Correct basic body positions and compensatory adjustments for recumbent radiography are illustrated in Figs. 20-41 to 20-48.

CLEANLINESS

The hair and face are naturally oily and leave a residue, even with the most hygienic patients. If the patient is sick, the residue is worse. During positioning of the skull, the patient's hair, mouth, nose, and eyes come in direct contact with the vertical grid device, tabletop, or IR. For medical asepsis, a paper towel or a cloth sheet may be placed between the imaging surface and the patient. As part of standard procedure the contacted area should be cleaned with a disinfectant before and after positioning.

Radiation Protection

Protection of the patient from unnecessary radiation is a professional responsibility of the radiographer (see Chapters 1 and 2 for specific guidelines). In this chapter, radiation shielding of the patient is not specified or illustrated. The federal government has reported that placing a lead shield over a patient's pelvis does not significantly reduce gonadal exposure during imaging of the skull.[1] However, lead shields should be used to reassure the patient.

Infants and children should receive radiation shielding of the thyroid and thymus glands and the gonads. The protective lead shielding used to cover the thyroid and thymus glands can also assist in immobilizing the pediatric patient.

The most effective way to protect the patient from unnecessary radiation is to restrict the radiation beam by using proper collimation. Taking care to ensure that the patient is properly instructed and immobilized also reduces the likelihood of having to repeat the procedure, thereby further limiting the radiation exposure received by the patient.

---

[1]HEW 76-8013 *Handbook of Selected Organ Doses.*

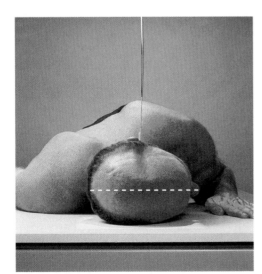

A

B

Fig. 20-41 Horizontal sagittal plane *(dashed lines).*

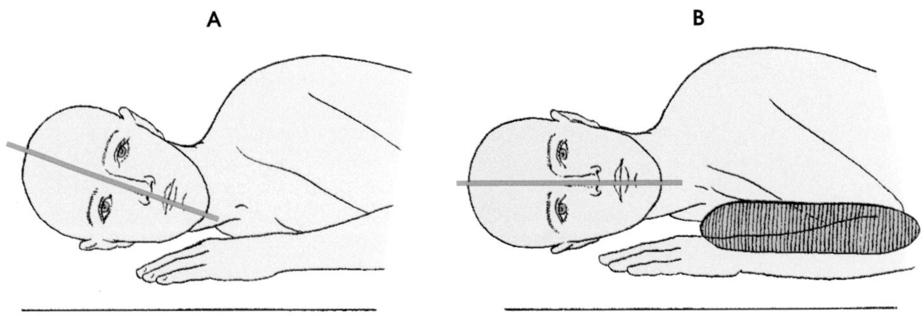

Fig. 20-42 Adjusting the sagittal planes to horizontal position. **A,** Asthenic or hyposthenic patient. **B,** Angulation corrected.

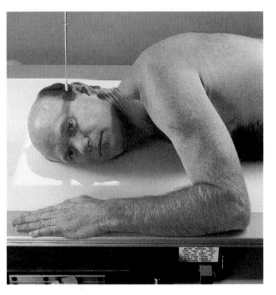

Fig. 20-43 Horizontal sagittal plane.

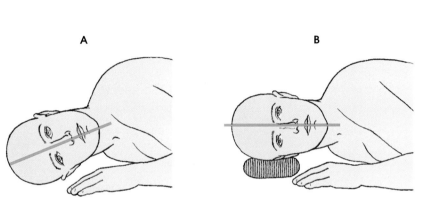

Fig. 20-44 Adjusting the sagittal plane to horizontal position. **A,** Hypersthenic patient. **B,** Angulation corrected.

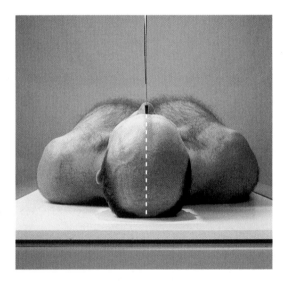

Fig. 20-45 Perpendicular sagittal plane *(dashed lines)*.

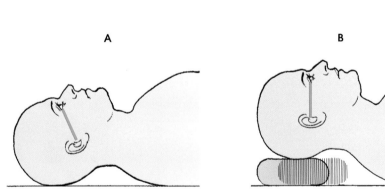

Fig. 20-46 Adjusting the OML to vertical position. **A,** Hypersthenic or round-shouldered patient. **B,** Angulation corrected.

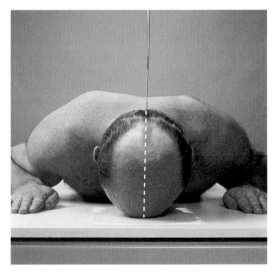

Fig. 20-47 Perpendicular sagittal plane *(dashed lines)*.

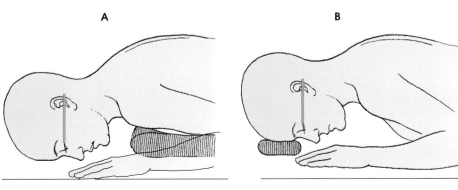

Fig. 20-48 Adjusting the OML to vertical position. **A,** Correction for hyposthenic patient. **B,** Correction for hypersthenic patient.

♠ LATERAL PROJECTION
R or L position

Image receptor: 24 × 30 cm crosswise

Position of patient
- Place the patient in the seated-upright or semiprone position.
- If a semiprone position is used, have the patient rest on the forearm and flexed knee of the elevated side.

Position of part
- With the side of interest closest to the IR, place one hand under the mandibular region and the opposite hand on the upper parietal region of the patient's head to help guide it into a true lateral position.
- Adjust the patient's head so that the midsagittal plane is parallel to the plane of the IR. If necessary, place a support under the side of the mandible to prevent it from sagging.
- Adjust the flexion of the patient's neck so that the IOML is perpendicular to the front edge of the IR. The IOML also should be parallel to the long axis of the IR.
- Check the head position so that the interpupillary line is perpendicular to the IR (Figs. 20-49 to 20-52).
- Immobilize the head.
- *Respiration:* Suspend.

Central ray
- Perpendicular, entering 2 inches (5 cm) superior to the EAM
- Center the IR to the central ray.

Structures shown
This lateral image of the superimposed halves of the cranium shows the detail of the side adjacent to the IR. The sella turcica, anterior clinoid processes, dorsum sellae, and posterior clinoid processes are well demonstrated in the lateral projection.

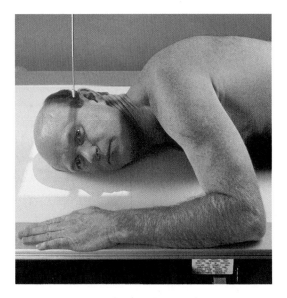

Fig. 20-49 Lateral skull.

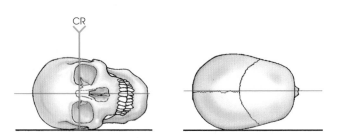

Fig. 20-50 Table radiography.

EVALUATION CRITERIA

The following should be clearly demonstrated:

- Entire cranium without rotation or tilt
- Superimposed orbital roofs and greater wings of sphenoid
- Superimposed mastoid regions and EAMs
- Superimposed TMJs
- Sella turcica seen in profile
- Radiographic penetration of parietal region
- No overlap of cervical spine by mandible

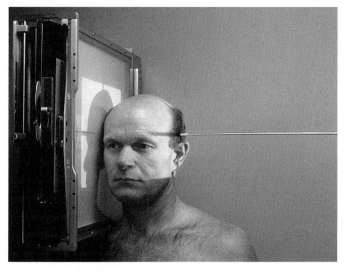

Fig. 20-51 Lateral skull centered over sella turcica.

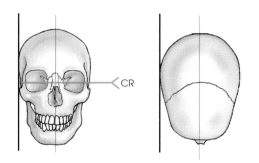

Fig. 20-52 Upright radiography.

Skull

☀ LATERAL PROJECTION
Dorsal decubitus or supine lateral position
R or L position

Dorsal decubitus

- With the patient supine, adjust the shoulders to lie in the same horizontal plane.
- After ruling out cervical injury, place the side of interest closest to the vertically placed grid IR. Elevate the patient's head enough to center it to the IR, and then support it on a radiolucent sponge.
- Adjust the patient's head so that the midsagittal plane is vertical and the interpupillary line is perpendicular to the IR (Fig. 20-53).
- Direct the central ray perpendicular to the IR and center it 2 inches (5 cm) superior to the EAM.
- Robinson, Meares, and Goree[1] recommended using the dorsal decubitus lateral projection for the demonstration of traumatic sphenoid sinus effusion (Fig. 20-54). They stated that this finding may be the only clue to the presence of a basal skull fracture.

[1]Robinson AE, Meares BM, Goree JA: Traumatic sphenoid sinus effusion, *AJR* 101:795, 1967.

Supine lateral

- Place the patient in a supine or semisupine position, and turn the head toward the side being examined.
- Elevate and support the opposite shoulder and hip enough that the midsagittal plane of the head is parallel and the interpupillary line is perpendicular to the IR.
- Support the patient's head with a radiolucent sponge.
- Direct the central ray perpendicular to enter 2 inches (5 cm) superior to the EAM (Fig. 20-55).
- Center the IR to the central ray.

Structures shown

This lateral image of the superimposed halves of the cranium shows the detail of the side adjacent to the IR. The sella turcica, anterior clinoid processes, dorsum sellae, and posterior clinoid processes are well demonstrated in the lateral projection (Fig. 20-56).

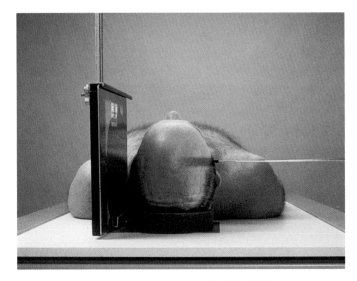

Fig. 20-53 Dorsal decubitus lateral skull.

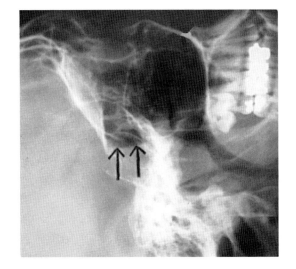

Fig. 20-54 Dorsal decubitus lateral skull showing sphenoid sinus effusion *(arrows)*.

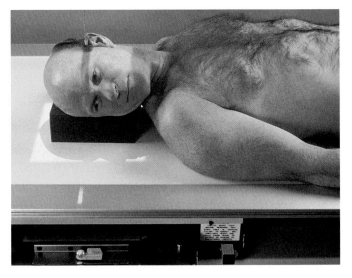

Fig. 20-55 Lateral skull with patient supine.

EVALUATION CRITERIA

The following should be clearly demonstrated:

- Entire cranium without rotation or tilt
- Superimposed orbital roofs and greater wings of sphenoid
- Superimposed mastoid regions and EAMs
- Superimposed TMJs
- Sella turcica seen in profile
- Radiographic penetration of parietal region
- No overlap of cervical spine by mandible

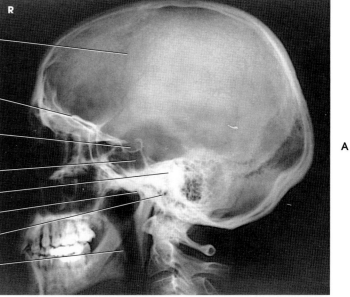

Coronal suture

Orbital roof

Sella turcica

Sphenoidal sinus

Petrous portion of temporal bone

Temporomandibular joint

External acoustic meatus

Mandibular rami

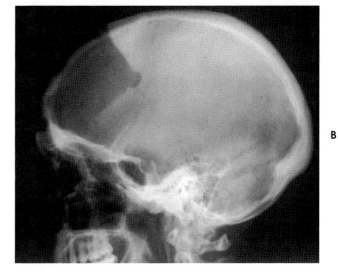

Fig. 20-56 A, Lateral skull. **B,** Lateral skull showing surgical removal of the frontal bone.

♠ PA PROJECTION
♠ PA AXIAL PROJECTION
CALDWELL METHOD

Image receptor: 24 × 30 cm lengthwise

Position of patient
- Place the patient in either a prone or seated position.
- Center the midsagittal plane of the patient's body to the midline of the grid.
- Rest the patient's forehead and nose on the table or against the upright Bucky.
- Flex the patient's elbows, place the arms in a comfortable position.

Position of part
- Adjust the flexion of the patient's neck so that the OML is perpendicular to the plane of the IR.
- If the patient is recumbent, support the chin on a radiolucent sponge if needed.
- If the patient is obese or hypersthenic, a small radiolucent sponge may need to be placed under (or in front of) the forehead.
- Align the midsagittal plane perpendicular to the IR. This is accomplished by adjusting the lateral margins of the orbits or the EAMs equidistant from the tabletop.
- Immobilize the patient's head, and center the IR to the nasion (Figs. 20-57 to 20-60).
- *Respiration:* Suspend.

Central ray
- For the PA projection, when the frontal bone is of primary interest, direct the central ray perpendicular to exit the nasion.
- For the Caldwell method, direct the central ray to exit the nasion at an angle of 15 degrees caudad.
- Center the IR to the central ray.
- For demonstration of the superior orbital fissures, direct the central ray through the midorbits at an angle of 20 to 25 degrees caudad.
- For demonstration of the rotundum foramina, direct the central ray to the nasion at an angle of 25 to 30 degrees caudad. (The Waters method is also used for demonstration of the rotundum foramina; see Chapter 22.)

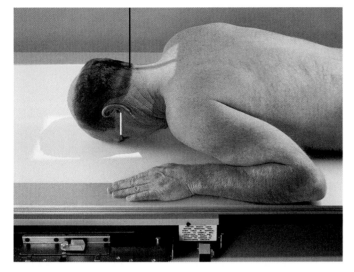

Fig. 20-57 PA skull: central ray angulation of 0 degrees for frontal bone.

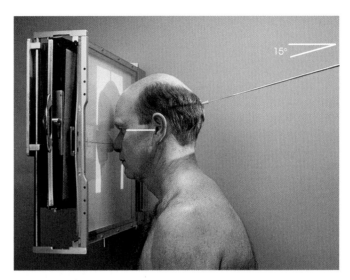

Fig. 20-58 PA axial skull: Caldwell method with central ray angulation of 15 degrees.

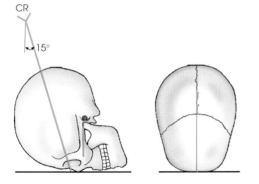

Fig. 20-59 Table radiography: Caldwell method.

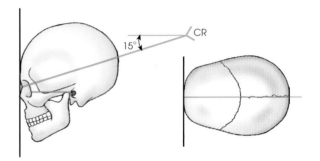

Fig. 20-60 Upright radiography: Caldwell method.

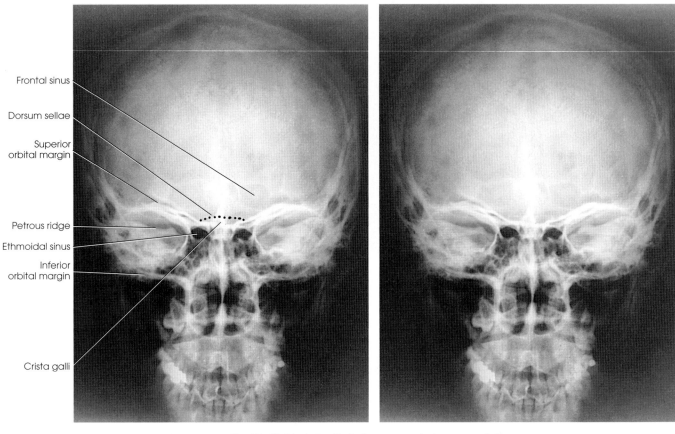

Frontal sinus

Dorsum sellae

Superior
orbital margin

Petrous ridge

Ethmoidal sinus

Inferior
orbital margin

Crista galli

Fig. 20-61 PA skull with 0-degree central ray angulation.

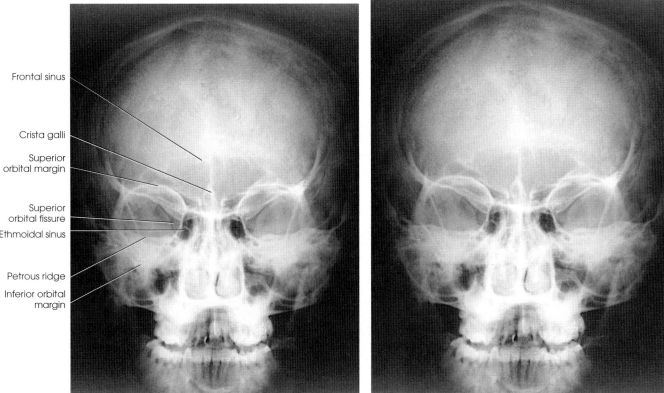

Frontal sinus

Crista galli

Superior
orbital margin

Superior
orbital fissure

Ethmoidal sinus

Petrous ridge

Inferior orbital
margin

Fig. 20-62 PA axial skull: Caldwell method with caudal central ray angulation of 15 degrees.

Structures shown

For the PA projection with a perpendicular central ray (Fig. 20-61), the orbits are filled by the margins of the petrous pyramids. Other structures demonstrated include the posterior ethmoidal air cells, crista galli, frontal bone, and frontal sinuses. The dorsum sellae is seen as a curved line extending between the orbits, just above the ethmoidal air cells.

When the central ray is angled 15 degrees caudad to the nasion for the Caldwell method, many of the same structures that appear in the direct PA projection are seen (Fig. 20-62). The petrous ridges, however, are projected into the lower third of the orbits. The Caldwell method also demonstrates the anterior ethmoidal air cells. Schüller,[1] who first described this positioning for the skull, recommended a caudal angle of 25 degrees.

---

[1]Schüller A: Die Schädelbasis im Rontgenbild, *Fortschr Roentgenstr* 11:215, 1905.

Stretcher and bedside examinations
Lateral decubitus position

- When the patient cannot be turned to the prone position for the PA Caldwell projection and cervical spinal injury has been ruled out, elevate one side enough to place the patient's head in a true lateral position and support the shoulder and hip on pillows or sandbags if needed.
- Elevate the patient's head on a suitable support, and adjust its height to center the midsagittal plane of the head to a vertically positioned grid.
- Adjust the patient's head so that the OML is perpendicular to the plane of the IR (Fig. 20-63).
- Direct the *horizontal* central ray perpendicular, or 15 degrees caudad, to exit the nasion.

The following should be clearly demonstrated:

- Entire cranial perimeter showing three distinct tables of squamous bone
- Equal distance from lateral border of skull to lateral border of orbit on both sides
- Symmetric petrous ridges
- Petrous pyramids lying in lower third of orbit with a caudal central ray angulation of 15 degrees and filling the orbits with 0-degree central ray angulation
- Penetration of frontal bone without excessive density at lateral borders of skull

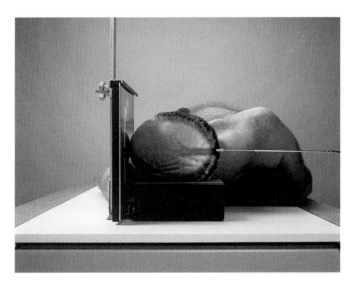

Fig. 20-63 PA skull with patient semisupine.

▲ AP PROJECTION
▲ AP AXIAL PROJECTION

Image receptor: 24 × 30 cm lengthwise

When the patient cannot be positioned for a PA or PA axial projection, a similar but somewhat magnified image can be obtained with an AP projection.

Position of patient and part
• Position the patient supine with the midsagittal plane of the body centered to the grid.
• Make certain that the midsagittal plane and the OML are perpendicular to the IR.

Central ray
• Perpendicular (Fig. 20-64) or directed to the nasion at an angle of 15 degrees cephalad (Fig. 20-65)
• Center the IR to the central ray.

Structures shown
The structures shown on the AP projection are the same as those demonstrated on the PA projection. On the AP projection (Fig. 20-66), the orbits are considerably magnified because of the increased object–to–image-receptor distance (OID). Similarly, because of the magnification, the distance from the lateral margin of the orbit to the lateral margin of the temporal bone measures less on the AP projection than on the PA projection.

EVALUATION CRITERIA
The following should be clearly demonstrated:
■ Entire cranial perimeter showing three distinct areas of squamous bone
■ Equal distance from lateral border of skull to lateral border of orbit on both sides
■ Symmetric petrous ridges
■ Petrous pyramids lying in lower third of orbit with a cephalad central ray angulation of 15 degrees and filling orbits with a 0-degree central ray angulation
■ Penetration of frontal bone without excessive density at lateral borders of skull

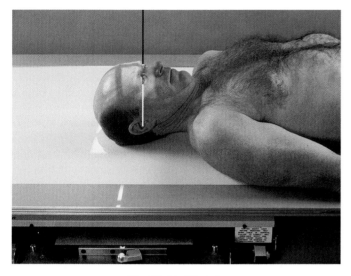

Fig. 20-64 AP skull.

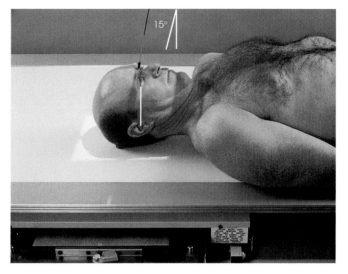

Fig. 20-65 AP axial skull with 15-degree cephalad central ray.

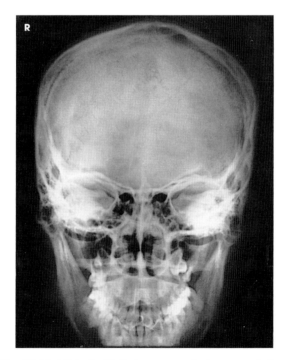

Fig. 20-66 AP skull with 0-degree central ray angulation.

⚘ AP AXIAL PROJECTION
TOWNE METHOD

Image receptor: 24 × 30 cm lengthwise

NOTE: Although this technique is most commonly referred to as the Towne method,[1] numerous authors have described slightly different variations. In 1912, Grashey[2] published the first description of the AP axial projection of the cranium. In 1926, Altschul[3] and Towne[1] described the position. Altschul recommended strong depression of the chin and direction of the central ray through the foramen magnum at a caudal angle of 40 degrees. Towne (citing Chamberlain) recommended that with the patient's chin depressed, the central ray should be directed through the midsagittal plane from a point about 3 inches (7.6 cm) above the eyebrows to the foramen magnum. Towne gave no specific central ray angulation, but the angulation would, of course, depend on the flexion of the neck.

[1]Towne EB: Erosion of the petrous bone by acoustic nerve tumor, *Arch Otolaryngol* 4:515, 1926.
[2]Grashey R: Atlas typischer Röntgenbilder vom normalen Menschen. In *Lehmann's medizinische Atlanten*, ed 2, vol 5, Munich, 1912, JF Lehmann.
[3]Altschul W: Beiträg zur Röntgenologie des Gehörorganes, *Z Hals Nas Ohr* 14:335, 1926.

Position of patient
- With the patient either supine or seated upright, center the midsagittal plane of the patient's body to the midline of the grid.
- Place the patient's arms in a comfortable position, and adjust the shoulders to lie in the same horizontal plane.
- To ensure the patient's comfort without increasing the IR distance, examine the hypersthenic or obese patient in the seated-upright position if possible.
- The skull can be brought closer to the IR by having the patient lean back lordotically and rest the shoulders against the vertical grid device. When this is not possible, the desired projection of the occipitobasal region may be obtained by using the PA axial projection described by Haas (p. 322). The Haas method is the reverse of the AP axial projection and produces a comparable result.

Position of part
- Adjust the patient's head so that the midsagittal plane is perpendicular to the midline of the IR.
- Flex the patient's neck enough to place the OML perpendicular to the plane of the IR.
- When the patient cannot flex the neck to this extent, adjust the neck so that the IOML is perpendicular and then increase the central ray angulation by 7 degrees (Figs. 20-67 to 20-70).
- Position the IR so that its upper margin is at the level of the highest point of the cranial vertex. This will place the center at or near the level of the foramen magnum.
- For a localized image of the dorsum sellae and petrous pyramids, adjust the IR so that its midpoint coincides with the central ray. This means that the IR is centered at or slightly below the level of the occlusal plane.
- Recheck the position and immobilize the head.
- *Respiration:* Suspend.

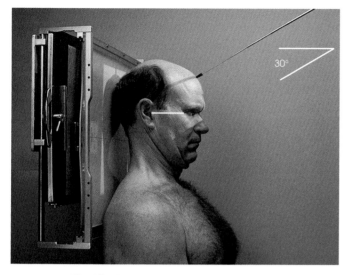

Fig. 20-67 AP axial skull: Towne method.

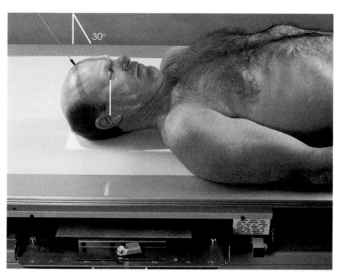

Fig. 20-68 AP axial skull: Towne method.

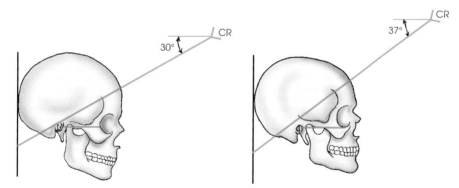

Fig. 20-69 Upright radiography. Same radiographic result with central ray directed 30 degrees to OML or 37 degrees to IOML.

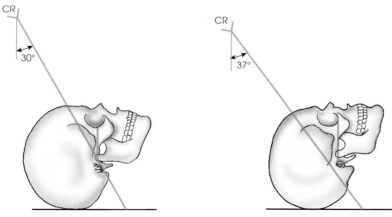

Fig. 20-70 Table radiography.

Central ray

- Directed through the foramen magnum at a caudal angle of 30 degrees to the OML or 37 degrees to the IOML. The central ray enters approximately 2½ inches (6.3 cm) above the glabella and passes through the level of the EAM.

Structures shown

The AP axial projection shows a symmetric image of the petrous pyramids, the posterior portion of the foramen magnum, the dorsum sellae and posterior clinoid processes projected within the foramen magnum, the occipital bone, and the posterior portion of the parietal bones (Fig. 20-71). This projection is also used for tomographic studies of the ears, facial canal, jugular foramina, and rotundum foramina.

EVALUATION CRITERIA

The following should be clearly demonstrated:

- Equal distance from lateral border of skull to lateral margin of foramen magnum on both sides, indicating no rotation
- Symmetric petrous pyramids
- Dorsum sellae and posterior clinoid processes visible within foramen magnum
- Penetration of occipital bone without excessive density at lateral borders of skull

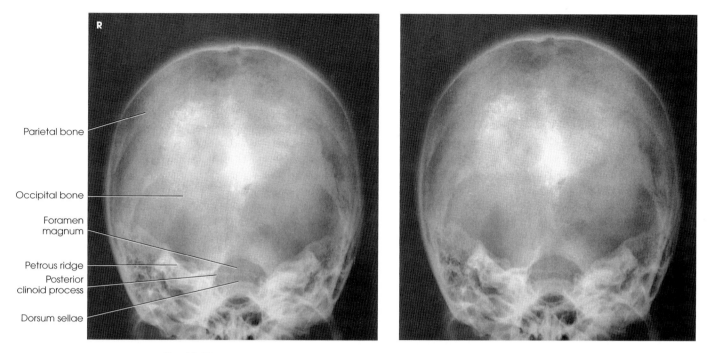

Parietal bone

Occipital bone

Foramen magnum

Petrous ridge

Posterior clinoid process

Dorsum sellae

Fig. 20-71 AP axial skull: Towne method with 30-degree central ray angulation to OML.

Pathologic condition or trauma

For demonstration of the entire foramen magnum, the caudal angulation of the central ray is increased from 40 to 60 degrees to the OML (Figs. 20-72 to 20-76).

Lateral decubitus position

For pathologic conditions, trauma, or a deformity such as a strongly accentuated dorsal kyphosis when the patient cannot be examined in a direct supine or prone position, the following steps should be observed:

- Adjust and support the body in a semi-recumbent position; this allows the head to be placed in a true lateral position.

- Immobilize the IR and grid in a vertical position behind the patient's occiput.
- Direct the *horizontal* central ray 30 degrees caudally to the OML (Fig. 20-77).

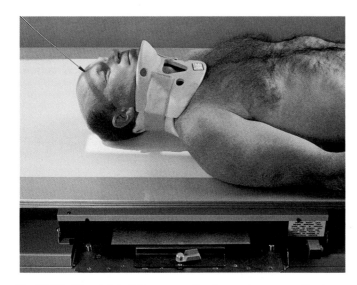

Fig. 20-72 AP axial skull, Towne method, on a trauma patient. Note that the OML and IOML lines are not perpendicular, which would require a central ray angulation greater than 37 degrees.

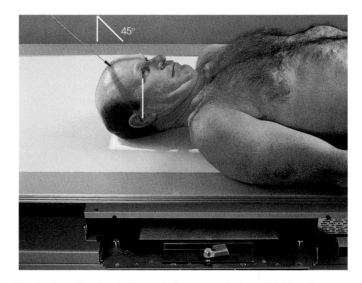

Fig. 20-73 AP axial skull: central ray angulation of 40 to 45 degrees.

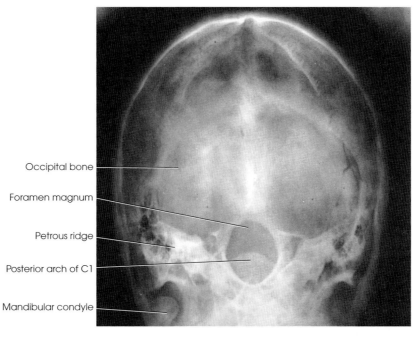

Occipital bone

Foramen magnum

Petrous ridge

Posterior arch of C1

Mandibular condyle

Fig. 20-74 AP axial skull: central ray angulation of 45 degrees.

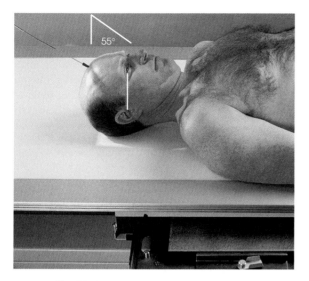

Fig. 20-75 AP axial foramen magnum.

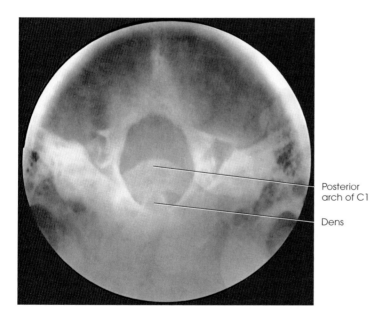

Posterior
arch of C1

Dens

Fig. 20-76 AP axial foramen magnum: central ray angulation of 55 degrees.

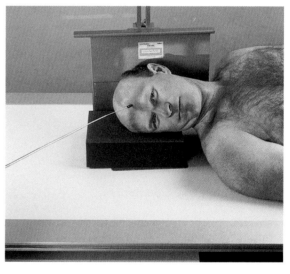

Fig. 20-77 AP axial skull, with the patient's head in lateral decubitus position and with the IR and grid vertical.

Skull

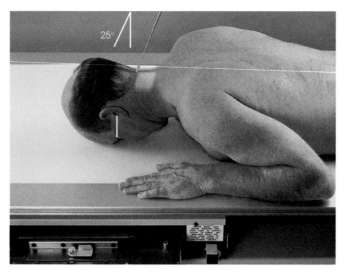

Fig. 20-78 PA axial skull: Haas method.

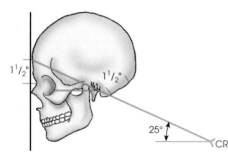

Fig. 20-79 Upright radiography.

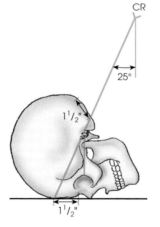

Fig. 20-80 Table radiography.

★ PA AXIAL PROJECTION
HAAS METHOD

Haas[1] devised this projection for obtaining an image of the sellar structures projected within the foramen magnum on hypersthenic, obese, or other patients who cannot be adjusted correctly for the AP axial (Towne) projection.

Image receptor: 24 × 30 cm lengthwise

Position of patient
- Adjust the patient in the prone or seated-upright position, and center the midsagittal plane of the body to the midline of the grid.
- Flex the patient's elbows, place the arms in a comfortable position, and adjust the shoulders to lie in the same horizontal plane.

Position of part
- Rest the patient's forehead and nose on the table, with the midsagittal plane perpendicular to the midline of the grid.
- Adjust the flexion of the neck so that the OML is perpendicular to the IR (Figs. 20-78 to 20-80).
- Immobilize the head.
- For a localized image of the sellar region and/or the petrous pyramids, adjust the position of the IR so that the midpoint will coincide with the central ray; shift the IR cephalad approximately 3 inches (7.6 cm) to include the vertex of the skull. An 18- × 24-cm (8- × 10-inch) IR is recommended.
- *Respiration:* Suspend.

---

[1]Haas L: Verfahren zur sagittalen Aufnahme der Sellagegend, *Fortschr Roentgenstr* 36:1198, 1927.

Central ray

- Directed at a cephalad angle of 25 degrees to the OML to enter a point 1½ inches (3.8 cm) below the external occipital protuberance (inion) and to exit approximately 1½ inches (3.8 cm) superior to the nasion. The central ray can be varied to demonstrate other cranial anatomy.

Structures shown

A PA axial projection demonstrates the occipital region of the cranium and shows a symmetric image of the petrous pyramids and the dorsum sellae and posterior clinoid processes within the foramen magnum (Figs. 20-81 and 20-82).

EVALUATION CRITERIA

The following should be clearly demonstrated:

- Projection of dorsum sellae and posterior clinoid processes within foramen magnum
- Equal distance from lateral border of skull to lateral margin of foramen magnum on both sides, indicating no rotation
- Symmetric petrous pyramids
- Entire cranium

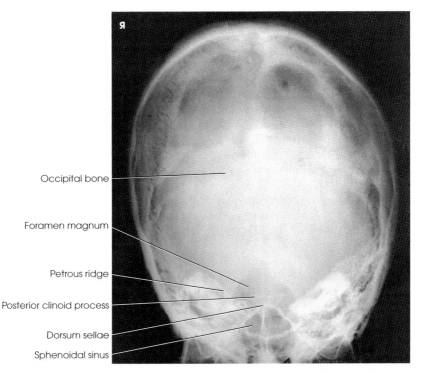

Occipital bone

Foramen magnum

Petrous ridge

Posterior clinoid process

Dorsum sellae

Sphenoidal sinus

Fig. 20-81 PA axial skull: Haas method, with central ray angulation of 25 degrees.

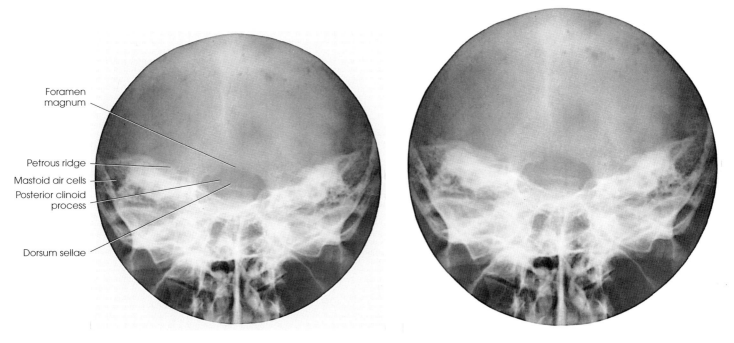

Foramen magnum

Petrous ridge

Mastoid air cells

Posterior clinoid process

Dorsum sellae

Fig. 20-82 PA axial sella turcica: Haas method, using a cylindric extension cone that restricts collimation to a small area. Beam restriction decreases scatter radiation and increases the visibility of detail of the sellar structures.

♠ SUBMENTOVERTICAL PROJECTION
SCHÜLLER METHOD

Image receptor: 24 × 30 cm lengthwise

Position of patient
The success of the submentovertical (SMV) projection of the cranial base depends on placing the IOML as nearly parallel with the plane of the IR as possible and directing the central ray perpendicular to the IOML. The following steps are observed:

- Place the patient in the supine or the seated-upright position; the latter is more comfortable. If a chair that supports the back is used, the upright position also allows greater freedom in positioning the patient's body to place the IOML parallel with the IR. If the patient is seated far enough away from the vertical grid device, the head can usually be adjusted without placing great pressure on the neck.
- When the patient is placed in the supine position, elevate the torso on firm pillows or a suitable pad to allow the head to rest on the vertex with the neck in hyperextension.

- Flex the patient's knees to relax the abdominal muscles.
- Place the patient's arms in a comfortable position, and adjust the shoulders to lie in the same horizontal plane.
- Do not keep the patient in the final adjustment longer than is absolutely necessary because the supine position places considerable strain on the neck.

Position of part
- With the midsagittal plane of the patient's body centered to the midline of the grid, extend the patient's neck to the greatest extent as can be achieved, placing the IOML as parallel as possible to the IR.
- Adjust the patient's head so that the midsagittal plane is perpendicular to the IR (Figs. 20-83 to 20-86).

NOTE: Patients placed in the supine position for the cranial base may have increased intracranial pressure. As a result, they may be dizzy or unstable for a few minutes after having been in this position. Use of the upright position may alleviate some of this pressure.

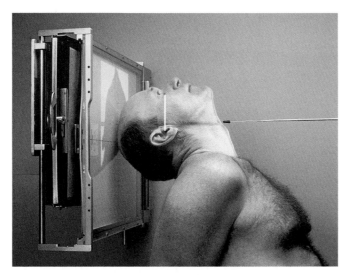

Fig. 20-83 SMV cranial base.

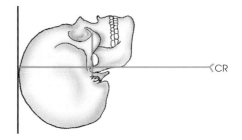

Fig. 20-84 Upright radiography.

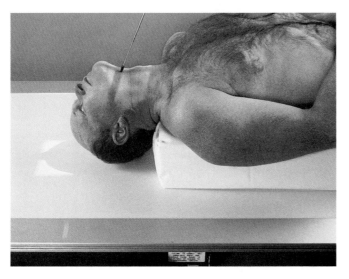

Fig. 20-85 SMV cranial base.

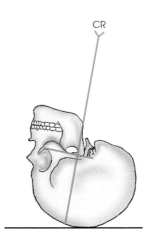

Fig. 20-86 Table radiography.

- Immobilize the patient's head. In the absence of a head clamp, place a suitably backed strip of adhesive tape across the tip of the chin and anchor it to the sides of the radiographic unit if needed. (The part of the tape touching the skin should be covered.)
- *Respiration:* Suspend.

Central ray

- Directed through the sella turcica perpendicular to the IOML. The central ray enters the midsagittal plane of the throat between the angles of the mandible and passes through a point ¾ inch (1.9 cm) anterior to the level of the EAMs.
- Center the IR to the central ray. The IR should be parallel to the IOML.

Structures shown

An SMV projection of the cranial base demonstrates symmetric images of the petrosae, the mastoid processes, the foramina ovale and spinosum (which are best shown in this projection), the carotid canals, the sphenoidal and ethmoidal sinuses, the mandible, the bony nasal septum, the dens of the axis, and the occipital bone. The maxillary sinuses are superimposed over the mandible (Fig. 20-87).

The SMV projection is also used for axial tomography of the orbits, optic canals, ethmoid bone, maxillary sinuses, and mastoid processes. With a decrease in the exposure factors, the zygomatic arches are also well demonstrated in this position (see Chapter 22).

EVALUATION CRITERIA

The following should be clearly demonstrated:

- Clearly visible structures of the cranial base, indicated by adequate penetration
- Equal distance from lateral border of skull to mandibular condyles on both sides, indicating no tilt.
- Superimposition of mental protuberance over anterior frontal bone, indicating full extension of neck
- Mandibular condyles anterior to petrous pyramids
- Symmetric petrosae

NOTE: Schüller[1] described and illustrated the basal projections—SMV and verticosubmental (VSM)—but Pfeiffer[2] gave specific directions for the central ray angulation.

---

[1]Schüller A: Die Schädelbasis im Rontgenbild, *Fortshr Reontgenstr* 11:215, 1905.
[2]Pfeiffer W: Beitrag zum Wert des axialen Schädelskiagrammes, *Arch Laryngol Rhinol* 30:1, 1916.

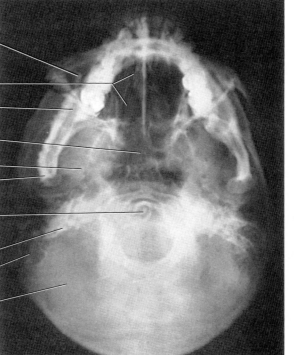
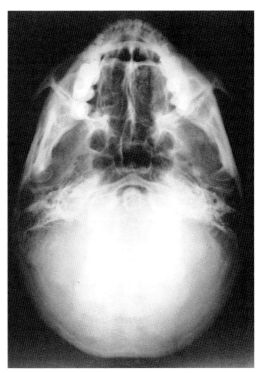

Maxillary sinus

Ethmoidal air cells

Mandible

Sphenoidal sinus

Foramen spinosum

Mandibular condyle

Dens (odontoid process)

Petrosa

Mastoid process

Occipital bone

Fig. 20-87 SMV cranial base.

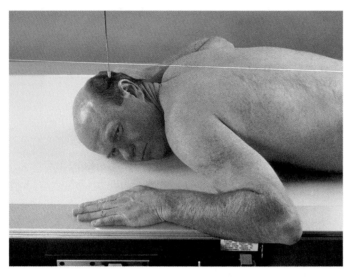

Fig. 20-88 Midsagittal rotation of 15 degrees for mastoid process.

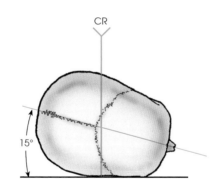

Fig. 20-89 Midsagittal rotation of 15 degrees.

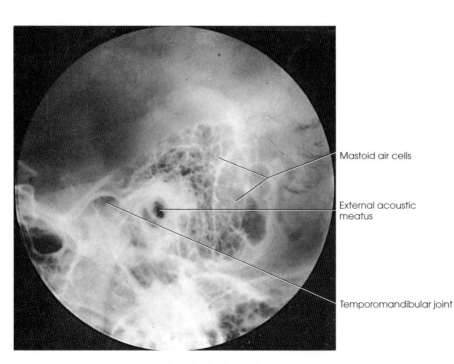

Mastoid air cells

External acoustic
meatus

Temporomandibular joint

Fig. 20-90 Mastoid process.

General Procedures

In an AP or lateral projection of the cranium, the mastoid process is obscured by superimposition of the dense petrous pyramids or the contralateral mastoid process. An unobstructed lateral projection of the mastoid process requires a slightly oblique orientation, which can be obtained by angling either the head or the central ray (Figs. 20-88 to 20-90). The degrees of angulation that are recommended for this purpose by various authors cover a considerable range. The 15-degree double-angle technique and the 15-degree and 25-degree single-angle techniques are most commonly used.

Both mastoid processes are always examined for comparison purposes. Therefore the radiographs must be exact duplicates in both part position and technical quality. Likewise, radiographs made in follow-up examinations must be exact duplicates of those made in preceding examinations. Every effort must be made to establish an exact procedure in centering and adjusting the part according to the specific localization points and planes used in the particular image. Errors in centering the part can be minimized by first adjusting the patient's head and then checking the position with a protractor.

The auricles of the ears may be folded forward to keep the relatively dense margins cast by the ear cartilages from obscuring the superimposed mastoid cells. Taping each auricle forward with a narrow strip of adhesive tape keeps them in place and at the same time minimizes discomfort to the patient by eliminating the necessity of repeated handling of a part that is often inflamed and tender. To prevent the adhesive strip from overlapping the mastoid cells, it should be placed so that it does not extend beyond the posterior junction of the auricle and the head. Figs. 20-91 and 20-92 demonstrate how the auricle can obscure the mastoid cells.

Visualization of the sharp outlines of the thin, fragile walls of the mastoid cells requires the following:

1. The effective focal spot of the x-ray tube must be no larger than 0.6 mm.
2. High-resolution imaging systems must be used to demonstrate the small mastoid structures.
3. Perfect film-screen contact and clean screens are essential.
4. The collimator must be adjusted to the smallest possible field size. Limiting the radiation area reduces the amount of secondary radiation that reaches the film.
5. During the exposure, complete head immobilization and cessation of respiration are necessary. The slightest movement, although not enough to cause visible blurring of the outlines of the comparatively gross surrounding structures, can diffuse the outlines of the thin cell walls. Unfortunately, when confined to the cellular structure, the diffusion cannot always be recognized as motion. For this reason the head must be rigidly immobilized.

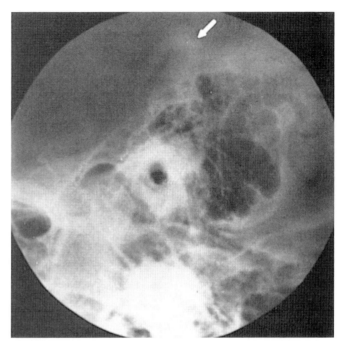

Fig. 20-91 Mastoid process: auricle folded forward (*arrow*).

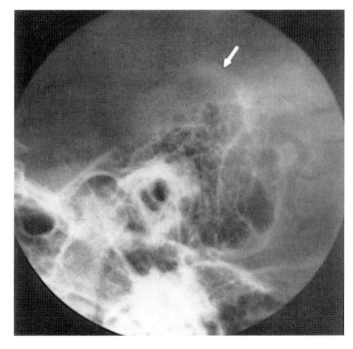

Fig. 20-92 Mastoid process: auricle not folded forward (*arrow*).

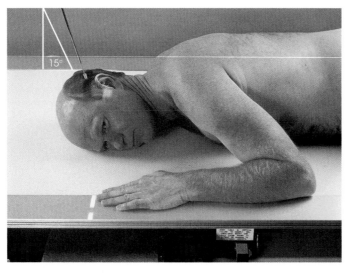

Fig. 20-93 Axiolateral petromastoid portion: modified Law method with single-tube angulation.

♠ AXIOLATERAL OBLIQUE PROJECTION
MODIFIED LAW METHOD
Single-tube angulation

Image receptor: 8 × 10 inch (18 × 24 cm)

Position of patient
- Place the patient on the table in the prone position, or seat the patient before a vertical grid device.
- Tape each auricle forward with a narrow strip of adhesive tape.

Position of part
- Position the patient's head in a lateral position with the affected side closest to the IR.
- Adjust the flexion of the patient's head so that the IOML is parallel with the IR and the interpupillary line is perpendicular to the IR.
- Rotate the patient's head toward the IR until the midsagittal plane is adjusted to an angle of 15 degrees (Figs. 20-93 and 20-94).
- Check the position of the head with a protractor.
- Immobilize the head.
- *Respiration*: Suspend.

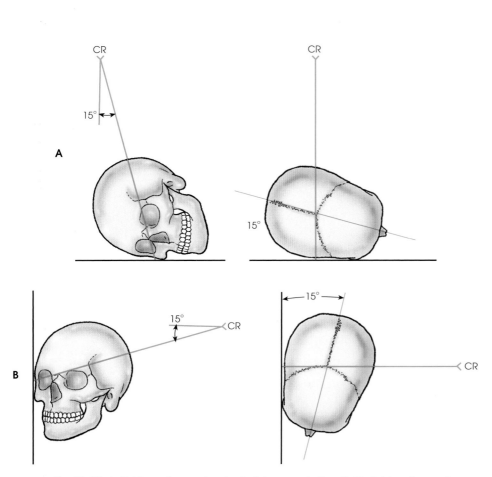

Fig. 20-94 A, Table radiography: single-tube angulation. **B,** Upright radiography.

Central ray

- Directed to the midpoint of the grid at an angle of 15 degrees caudad to exit the downside mastoid tip approximately 1 inch (2.5 cm) posterior to the EAM. The central ray enters approximately 2 inches (5 cm) posterior to and 2 inches (5 cm) superior to the uppermost EAM.
- Center the IR to the central ray.

Structures shown

The axiolateral oblique projection demonstrates the mastoid cells, the lateral portion of the petrous pyramid, the superimposed IAM and EAM, and, when present, the mastoid emissary vessel (Fig. 20-95).

The following should be clearly demonstrated:

- Mastoid process closest to IR, with air cells centered to IR
- Opposite mastoid process not superimposing but lying inferior and slightly anterior to mastoid process of interest
- Auricle of ear not superimposing mastoid process
- Superimposition of IAM and EAM
- TMJ visible anterior to mastoid process
- Close beam restriction to mastoid region

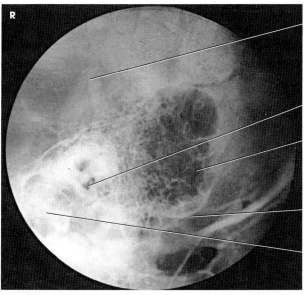

Auricle (taped forward)

Internal and external acoustic meatuses

Mastoid air cells

Mastoid process

Mandibular condyle

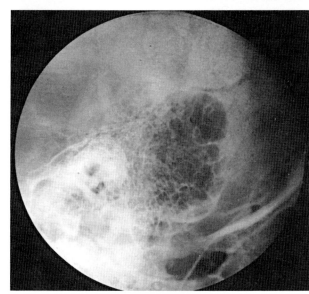

Fig. 20-95 Axiolateral petromastoid portion: modified Law method.

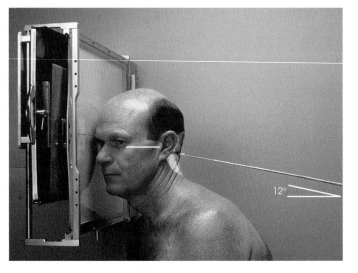

Fig. 20-96 Axiolateral oblique projection demonstrating right petromastoid portion: posterior profile, Stenvers method.

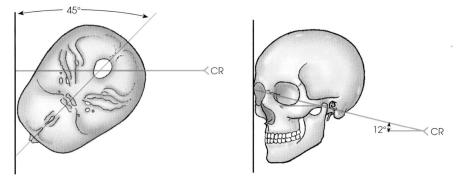

Fig. 20-97 Upright radiography.

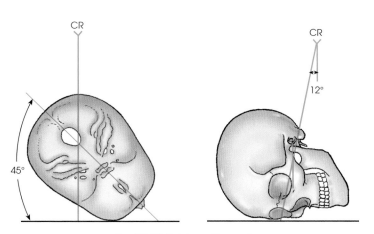

Fig. 20-98 Table radiography.

♠ AXIOLATERAL OBLIQUE PROJECTION

STENVERS METHOD
Posterior profile

Image receptor: 8 × 10 inch (18 × 24 cm)

Position of patient
- Place the patient in the prone position, or seat the patient before a vertical grid device.

Position of part
- Rest the patient's head on the forehead, nose, and cheek, with the side being examined closest to the IR.
- Adjust the flexion of the patient's neck so that the IOML is parallel with the transverse axis of the IR.
- Using a protractor as a guide, adjust the midsagittal plane of the head to form an angle of 45 degrees with the plane of the IR (Figs. 20-96 to 20-98).
- In patients with brachycephalic (short front-to-back) skulls, the petrous ridges form an angle of approximately 54 degrees with the midsagittal plane of the head. Patients with this skull type require less than normal rotation of the midsagittal plane to place the petrous ridge parallel with the IR. In patients with dolichocephalic (long front-to-back) skulls, the petrous ridges form an angle of approximately 40 degrees with the midsagittal plane. Patients with this skull type require more rotation of the midsagittal plane to place the petrous ridge parallel with the IR.
- Immobilize the head.
- *Respiration:* Suspend.

Central ray
- Directed 12 degrees cephalad. The central ray enters about 3 to 4 inches (7.6 to 10 cm) posterior and ½ inch (1.3 cm) inferior to the upside EAM and exits about 1 inch (2.5 cm) anterior to the downside EAM.
- Center the IR to the central ray.

Petromastoid Portion

Structures shown

The Stenvers method shows a profile image of the petromastoid portion closest to the IR. When the patient is correctly positioned, the petrous pyramid of interest is parallel with the plane of the IR (Fig. 20-99). The resultant image demonstrates the petrous ridge, the cellular structure of the mastoid process, the mastoid antrum, the area of the tympanic cavity, the bony labyrinth, the internal acoustic canal, and the cellular structure of the petrous apex.

EVALUATION CRITERIA

The following should be clearly demonstrated:

- Petromastoid portion in profile without distortion
- Lateral border of skull to lateral border of orbit
- Petrous ridge extended to a point approximately two thirds up the lateral border of orbit
- Mastoid process in profile below margin of cranium (Air cells are not well visualized when internal aspects of the petrosa are properly exposed.)
- Posterior margin of mandibular ramus superimposing lateral border of cervical column
- Mandibular condyle projecting over the atlas near the petrosa
- Close beam restriction to the petrous pyramid and mastoid region

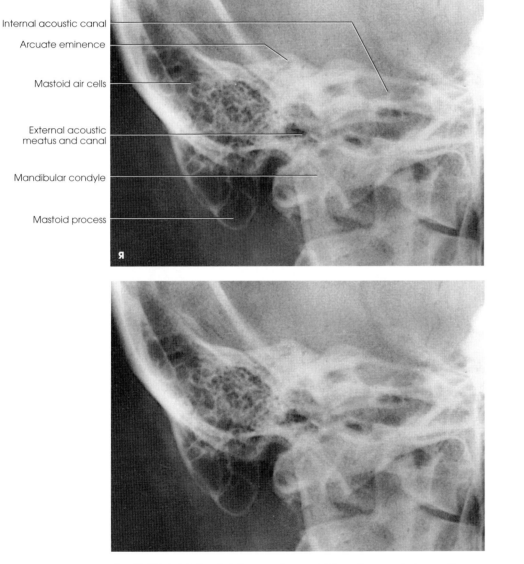

Internal acoustic canal
Arcuate eminence
Mastoid air cells
External acoustic meatus and canal
Mandibular condyle
Mastoid process

Fig. 20-99 Axiolateral oblique petromastoid portion: posterior profile, Stenvers method.

Petromastoid portion

331

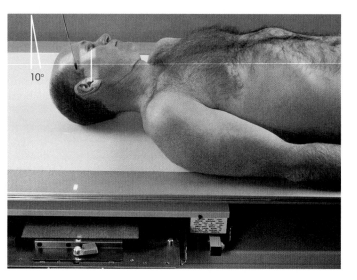

Fig. 20-100 Axiolateral oblique demonstrating right petromastoid portion: anterior profile, Arcelin method.

♠ AXIOLATERAL OBLIQUE PROJECTION
ARCELIN METHOD
Anterior profile

The Arcelin method is particularly useful in children and in adults who cannot be placed in the prone or seated-upright position for the Stenvers method. This projection is the exact opposite of the Stenvers method, and the petromastoid portion is more magnified.

Image receptor: 8 × 10 inch (18 × 24 cm)

Position of patient
- Place the patient in the supine position.
- Center the midsagittal plane of the patient's body to the midline of the radiographic table.

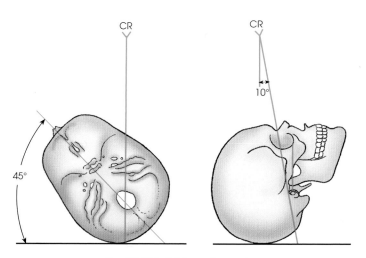

Fig. 20-101 Table radiography.

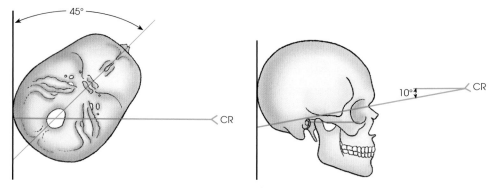

Fig. 20-102 Upright radiography.

Skull

Position of part

- Rotate the patient's face away from the side being examined so that the midsagittal plane forms an angle of 45 degrees with the plane of the IR.
- Adjust the flexion of the patient's neck so that the IOML is perpendicular to the plane of the IR (Figs. 20-100 to 20-102.
- In patients with brachycephalic (short front-to-back) skulls, the petrous ridges form an angle of approximately 54 degrees with the midsagittal plane. Patients with this skull type require less than normal rotation of the midsagittal plane to place the petrous ridges parallel with the IR. In patients with dolichocephalic (long front-to-back) skulls, the petrous ridges form an angle of approximately 40 degrees with the midsagittal plane. Patients with this skull type require more rotation of the midsagittal plane to place the petrous ridge parallel with the IR.
- Immobilize the head.
- *Respiration*: Suspend.

Central ray

- Directed at an angle of 10 degrees caudad. The central ray enters the temporal area at a point approximately 1 inch (2.5 cm) anterior to the EAM and ¾ inch (1.9 cm) above it.
- Center the IR to the central ray.

Structures shown

The anterior-profile Arcelin method (Fig. 20-103), the exact reverse of the Stenvers method, demonstrates the petrous portion of the temporal bone farthest from the IR.

The following should be clearly demonstrated:

- Petromastoid portion in profile
- Lateral border of skull to lateral border of orbit
- Petrous ridge lying horizontally and at a point approximately two thirds up the lateral border of orbit
- Mastoid process in profile below margin of cranium (Air cells are not well visualized when petrous pyramid is properly exposed.)
- Posterior surface of mandibular ramus parallel to lateral surface of cervical vertebrae
- Mandibular condyle projected over the atlas near the petrous pyramid
- Close beam restriction to petrous pyramid and mastoid region

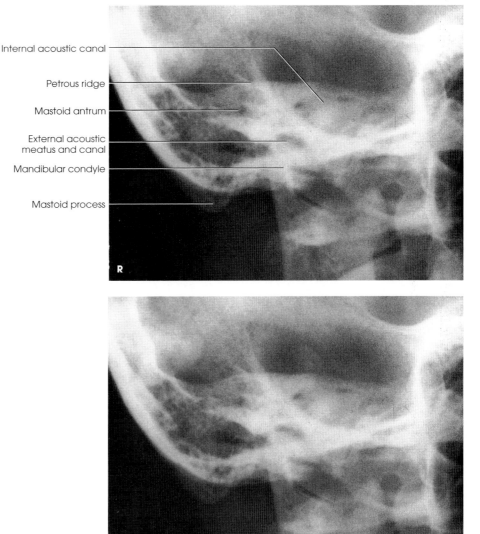

Internal acoustic canal
Petrous ridge
Mastoid antrum
External acoustic meatus and canal
Mandibular condyle
Mastoid process

R

Fig. 20-103 Axiolateral oblique petromastoid portion: anterior profile, Arcelin method.

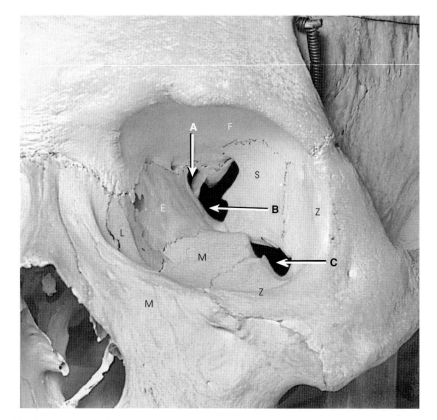

Orbit

The orbits are cone-shaped, bony-walled cavities situated on each side of the midsagittal plane of the head (Fig. 20-104). They are formed by the seven previously described and illustrated bones of the cranium (frontal, ethmoid, and sphenoid) and the face (lacrimal, palatine, maxillary, and zygomatic). Each orbit has a roof, a medial wall, a lateral wall, and a floor. The easily palpable, quadrilateral-shaped anterior circumference of the orbit is called its *base*. The *apex* of the orbit corresponds to the *optic foramen*. The long axis of each orbit is directed obliquely, posteriorly, and medially at an average angle of 37 degrees to the midsagittal plane of the head and also superiorly at an angle of about 30 degrees from the OML (Fig. 20-105).

Fig. 20-104 Bones of left orbit of dry specimen. **A,** Optic canal and foramen. **B,** Superior orbital fissure. **C,** Inferior orbital fissure. *E,* Ethmoid; *F,* frontal; *L,* lacrimal; *M,* maxilla; *S,* sphenoid; *Z,* zygomatic (palatine not shown).

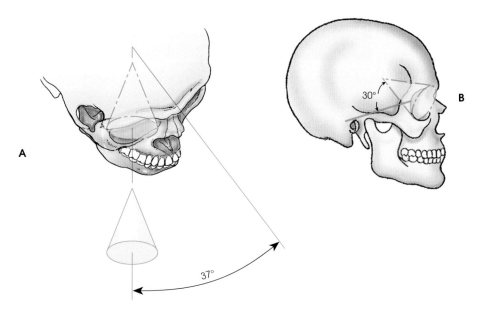

Fig. 20-105 Cone-shaped orbit. **A,** Average angle of 37 degrees from the midsagittal plane. **B,** Average angle of 30 degrees superior to the OML.

The orbits serve primarily as bony sockets for the eyeballs and the structures associated with them, but they also contain blood vessels and nerves that pass through openings in their walls to other regions. The major and frequently radiographed openings are the previously described optic foramina and the superior and inferior orbital sulci.

The *superior orbital fissure* is the cleft between the greater and lesser wings of the sphenoid bone. From the body of the sphenoid at a point near the orbital apex, this sulcus extends superiorly and laterally between the roof and the lateral wall of the orbit. The *inferior orbital fissure* is the narrow cleft extending from the lower anterolateral aspect of the sphenoid body anteriorly and laterally between the floor and lateral wall of the orbit. The anterior margin of the cleft is formed by the orbital plate of the maxilla, and its posterior margin is formed by the greater wing of the sphenoid bone and the zygomatic bone.

Because the walls of the orbits are thin, they are subject to fracture. For example, when a person is forcibly struck squarely on the eyeball (by a fist, a piece of sporting equipment, etc.), the resulting pressure directed to the eyeball forces the eyeball into the cone-shaped orbit and "blows out" the thin, delicate bony floor of the orbit (Figs. 20-106 and 20-107). The injury must be diagnosed and treated accurately so that the person's vision is not jeopardized. Blowout fractures may be demonstrated using any combination of radiographs obtained with the patient positioned for parietoacanthial projections (Waters method), radiographic tomography, and/or CT.

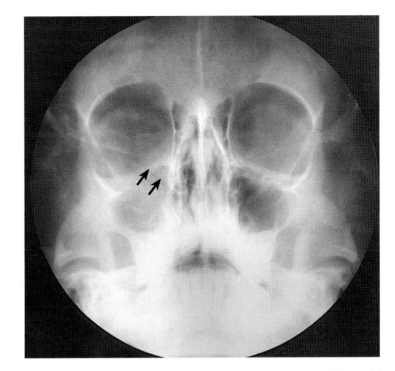

Fig. 20-106 Parietoacanthial orbits using Waters method and showing blowout fracture of orbit *(arrows)*.

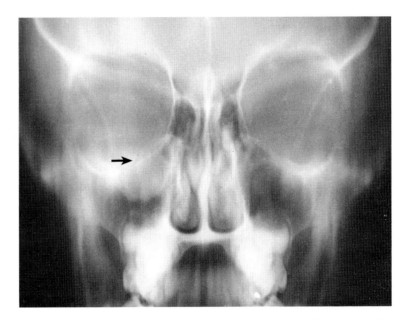

Fig. 20-107 Tomogram: AP projection showing fracture *(arrow)* in the same patient as in Fig. 20-106.

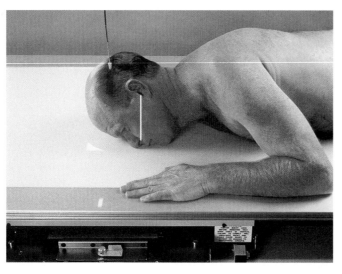

Fig. 20-108 Parietoorbital oblique projection: Rhese method.

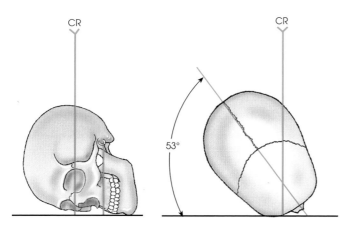

Fig. 20-109 Table radiography.

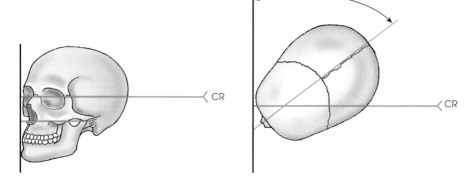

Fig. 20-110 Upright radiography.

▲ PARIETOORBITAL OBLIQUE PROJECTION

RHESE METHOD

Image receptor: 8 × 10 inch (18 × 24 cm)

Position of patient

- Place the patient in the semiprone or seated-upright position.
- Place the patient's arms in a comfortable position, and adjust the shoulders to lie in the same horizontal plane.

Position of part

- Center the affected orbit to the unmasked half of the IR, and rest the zygoma, nose, and chin on the radiographic table or against the upright Bucky.
- Adjust the flexion of the patient's neck to place the AML perpendicular to the plane of the IR.
- Adjust the rotation of the patient's head so that the midsagittal plane forms an angle of 53 degrees to the plane of the IR (Figs. 20-108 to 20-110). A protractor may be used to obtain an accurate 53-degree angle.
- Immobilize the patient's head.
- *Respiration:* Suspend.

Central ray

- Perpendicular, entering approximately 1 inch (2.5 cm) superior and posterior to the upside TEA. The central ray exits through the affected orbit *closest* to the IR.
- Collimate the beam closely to the orbit resting on table.
- Center the IR to the central ray.

Structures shown

This projection demonstrates the optic canal "on end" and the optic foramen lying in the inferior and lateral quadrant of the projected orbit (Fig. 20-111). Any lateral deviation of this location indicates incorrect rotation of the head. Any longitudinal deviation indicates incorrect angulation of the AML. Both sides are examined for comparison.

A parietoorbital projection of the ethmoidal, sphenoidal, and frontal sinuses is also demonstrated (Fig. 20-112).

EVALUATION CRITERIA

The following should be clearly demonstrated:

- Optic canal and foramen visible at end of sphenoid ridge in inferior and lateral quadrant of orbit
- Entire orbital rim
- Supraorbital margins lying in same horizontal line
- Close beam restriction to the orbital region

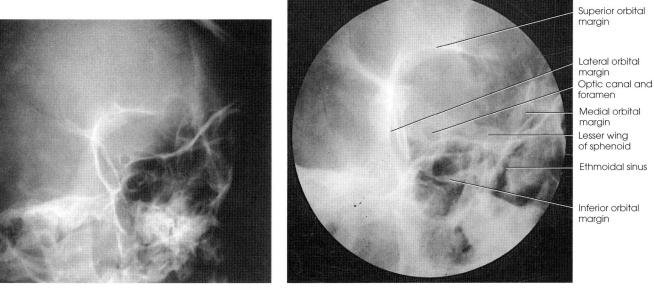

Superior orbital margin

Lateral orbital margin

Optic canal and foramen

Medial orbital margin

Lesser wing of sphenoid

Ethmoidal sinus

Inferior orbital margin

Fig. 20-111 Parietoorbital oblique projection: Rhese method.

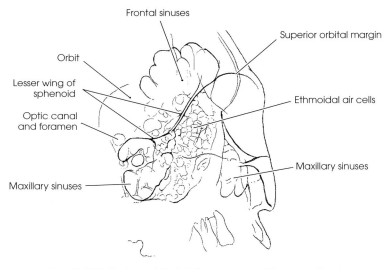

Frontal sinuses

Orbit

Lesser wing of sphenoid

Optic canal and foramen

Maxillary sinuses

Superior orbital margin

Ethmoidal air cells

Maxillary sinuses

Fig. 20-112 Parietoorbital oblique sinuses: Rhese method.

Eye

The organ of vision, or eye (Latin, *oculus;* Greek, *ophthalmos*), consists of the following: eyeball; the optic nerve, which connects the eyeball to the brain; the blood vessels; and accessory organs such as the extrinsic muscles, lacrimal apparatus, and eyelids (Figs. 20-113 and 20-114).

The *eyeball* is situated in the anterior part of the orbital cavity. Its posterior segment (about two thirds of the bulb) is adjacent to the soft parts that occupy the remainder of the orbital cavity (chiefly muscles, fat, and connective tissue). The anterior portion of the eyeball is exposed and projects somewhat beyond the base of the orbit. Therefore bone-free radiographic images of the anterior segment of the eye can be obtained. The exposed part of the eyeball is covered by a thin mucous membrane known as the *conjunctiva,* portions of which line the eyelids. The conjunctival membrane is kept moist by tear secretions from the lacrimal gland. These secretions prevent drying and friction irritation during movements of the eyeball and eyelids.

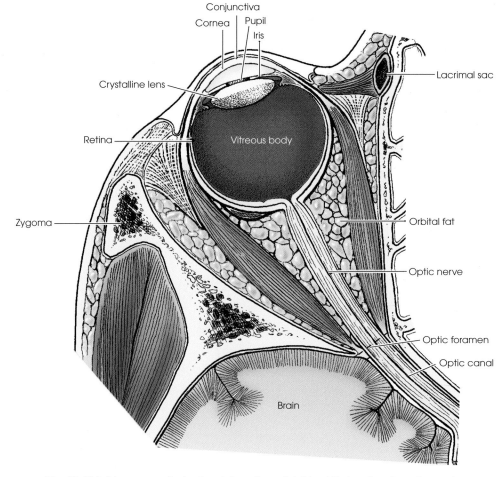

Fig. 20-113 Diagrammatic horizontal section of right orbital region: top-down view.

The outer, supporting coat of the eyeball is a firm, fibrous membrane consisting of a posterior segment called the *sclera* and an anterior segment called the *cornea.* The opaque, white sclera is commonly referred to as the "white of the eye." The cornea is situated in front of the *iris,* with its center point corresponding to the pupil. The corneal part of the membrane is transparent, allowing the passage of light into the eyeball, and it serves as one of the four refractive media of the eye.

The inner coat of the eyeball is called the *retina.* This delicate membrane is contiguous with the optic nerve. The retina is composed chiefly of nervous tissue and several million minute receptor organs, called *rods* and *cones,* which transmit light impulses to the brain. The rods and cones are important radiographically because they play a role in the ability of the radiologist or radiographer to see the fluoroscopic image. Their function is described in discussions of fluoroscopy in radiography physics and imaging textbooks.

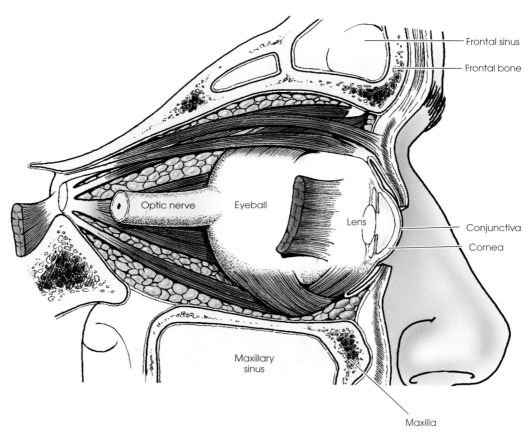

Fig. 20-114 Diagrammatic sagittal section of right orbital region.

LOCALIZATION OF FOREIGN BODIES WITHIN ORBIT OR EYE

Ultrasonography and CT (Fig. 20-115) have been increasingly used to locate foreign bodies in the eye. (Magnetic resonance imaging is not used for foreign body localization because movement of a metallic foreign object by the magnetic field could lead to hemorrhage or other serious complications.) Whether an ultrasound or a radiographic approach is used, accurate localization of foreign particles lodged within the orbit or eye requires the use of a precision localization technique.

Localization methods removed

The *Vogt method, Sweet method, Pfeiffer-Comberg method,* and parallax *motion method* are sometimes used to localize foreign bodies in the eye. These methods were described briefly in the eighth edition of this atlas. Complete descriptions appeared in the seventh and earlier editions.

Image quality

Ultrafine recorded detail is essential to the detection and localization of minute foreign particles within the orbit or eyeball. The following are required:

1. The geometric unsharpness must be reduced as much as possible by the use of a close OID and a small, undamaged focal spot at a source–to–image-receptor distance (SID) that is as long as is consistent with the exposure factors required.
2. Secondary radiation must be minimized by close collimation.
3. Motion must be eliminated by firmly immobilizing the patient's head and by having the patient gaze steadily at a fixed object, thereby immobilizing the eyeballs.

An artifact can cast an image that simulates the appearance of a foreign body located within the orbit or eye. Therefore IRs and screens must be impeccably clean before each examination. In institutions and clinics that often perform these examinations, an adequate number of IR holders are kept in reserve for eye studies only. This measure protects them from the wear of routine use in less-critical procedures.

PRELIMINARY EXAMINATION

Lateral projections, PA projections, and bone-free studies are taken to determine whether a radiographically demonstrable foreign body is present. For these radiographs, the patient may be placed in the recumbent position or may be seated upright before a vertical grid device.

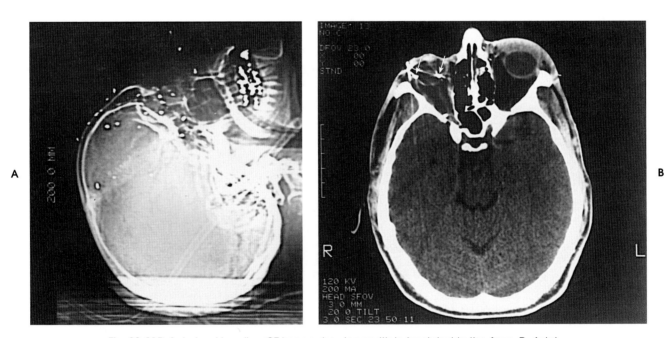

Fig. 20-115 A, Lateral localizer CT image showing multiple buckshot in the face. **B,** Axial CT image of same patient, showing shotgun pellets within the eye *(arrows)*.

LATERAL PROJECTION

R or L position

A nongrid (very high-resolution) technique is recommended to reduce magnification and eliminate possible artifacts in or on the radiographic table and grid. The following steps are observed:

- With the patient either semiprone or seated upright, place the outer canthus of the affected eye adjacent to and centered over the midpoint of the IR.
- Adjust the patient's head to place the midsagittal plane parallel with the plane of the IR and the interpupillary line perpendicular to the IR plane.
- *Respiration:* Suspend.

Central ray

- Perpendicular through the outer canthus
- Instruct the patient to look straight ahead for the exposure (Figs. 20-116 and 20-117).

EVALUATION CRITERIA

The following should be clearly demonstrated:

- ■ Density and contrast permitting optimal visibility of orbit and eye for localization of foreign bodies
- ■ Superimposed orbital roofs
- ■ Close beam restriction centered to orbital region

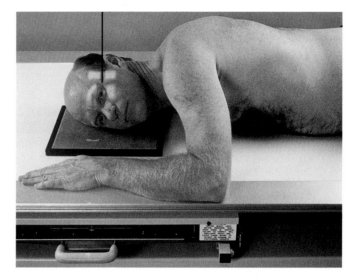

Fig. 20-116 Lateral projection for orbital foreign body localization.

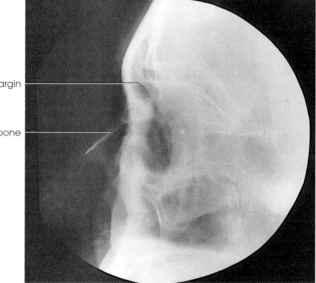

Superior orbital margin

Nasal bone

Fig. 20-117 Lateral projection showing foreign body (*white speck*).

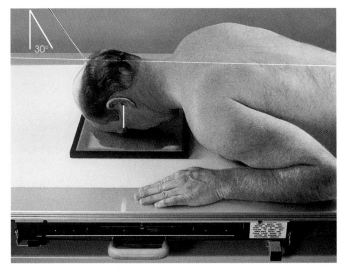

Fig. 20-118 PA axial projection for orbital foreign body localization.

PA AXIAL PROJECTION

A nongrid (very high-resolution) technique is recommended to reduce magnification and eliminate possible artifacts in or on the radiographic table and grid. The following steps are observed:

- Rest the patient's forehead and nose on the IR holder, and center the holder ¾ inch (1.9 cm) distal to the nasion.
- Adjust the patient's head so that the midsagittal plane and the OML are perpendicular to the plane of the IR.
- *Respiration:* Suspend.

Central ray

- Directed through the center of the orbits at a caudal angulation of 30 degrees. This angulation is used to project the petrous portions of the temporal bones below the inferior margin of the orbits (Figs. 20-118 and 20-119).
- Instruct the patient to close the eyes and to concentrate on holding them still for the exposure.

EVALUATION CRITERIA

The following should be clearly demonstrated:

- Petrous pyramids lying below orbital shadows
- No rotation of cranium
- Close beam restriction centered to orbital region

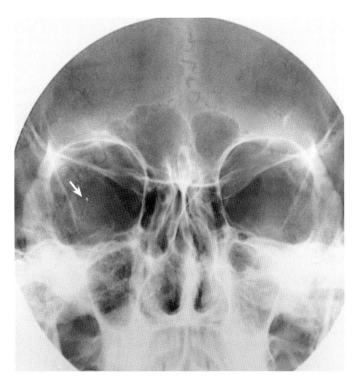

Fig. 20-119 PA axial projection demonstrating foreign body *(arrow)* in right eye.

PARIETOACANTHIAL PROJECTION
MODIFIED WATERS METHOD

Some physicians prefer to have the PA projection performed with the patient's head adjusted in a modified Waters position so that the petrous margins are displaced by part adjustment rather than by central ray angulation. The following steps are observed:
- With the IR centered at the level of the center of the orbits, rest the patient's chin on the IR holder.
- Adjust the patient's head so that the midsagittal plane is perpendicular to the plane of the IR.
- Adjust the flexion of the patient's neck so that the OML forms an angle of 50 degrees with the plane of the IR.
- *Respiration*: Suspend.

Central ray
- Perpendicular through the midorbits (Figs. 20-120 and 20-121)
- Instruct the patient to close the eyes and to concentrate on holding them still for the exposure.

EVALUATION CRITERIA

The following should be clearly demonstrated:
- Petrous pyramids lying well below orbital shadows
- Symmetric visualization of orbits, indicating no rotation of cranium
- Close beam restriction centered to the orbital region

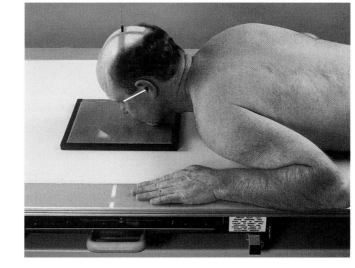

Fig. 20-120 Parietoacanthial projection, modified Waters method, for orbital foreign body localization.

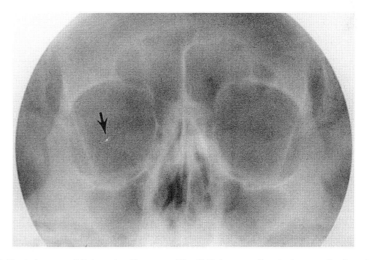

Fig. 20-121 Parietoacanthial projection, modified Waters method, demonstrating foreign body *(arrow)*.

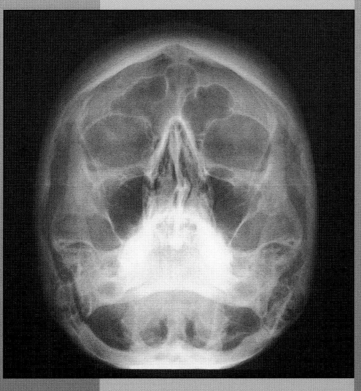

21

FACIAL BONES*

Parietoacanthial facial bones,
Waters method.

*For a complete description of the anatomy of the
facial bones, see Chapter 20.

SUMMARY OF PROJECTIONS

PROJECTIONS, POSITIONS, AND METHODS

Page	Essential	Anatomy	Projection	Position	Method
349	🌲	Facial bones	Lateral	R or L	
352	🌲	Facial bones	Parietoacanthial		WATERS
354		Facial bones	Modified parietoacanthial		MODIFIED WATERS
356	🌲	Facial bones	Acanthioparietal		REVERSE WATERS
358	🌲	Facial bones	PA axial		CALDWELL
360	🌲	Nasal bones	Lateral	R and L	
362	🌲	Zygomatic arches	Submentovertical		
364	🌲	Zygomatic arch	Tangential		
366	🌲	Zygomatic arches	AP axial		MODIFIED TOWNE
368	🌲	Mandibular rami	PA		
369	🌲	Mandibular rami	PA axial		
370		Mandibular body	PA		
371		Mandibular body	PA axial		
372	🌲	Mandible	Axiolateral oblique		
375		Mandible	Submentovertical		
376	🌲	Temporomandibular articulations	AP axial		
378		Temporomandibular articulations	Axiolateral	R and L	
380	🌲	Temporomandibular articulations	Axiolateral oblique	R and L	
382		Mandible	Panoramic		TOMOGRAPHY

Icons in the Essential column indicate projections frequently performed in the United States and Canada. Students should be competent in these projections.

Summary of Pathology

Please refer to Chapter 20 for a summary
of pathology for this chapter.

EXPOSURE TECHNIQUE CHART ESSENTIAL PROJECTIONS

FACIAL BONES

Part	cm	kVp*	tm	mA	mAs	AEC	SID	IR	Dose† (mrad)
Facial Bones‡									
Lateral	15	70		200s		●○○	48″	8 × 10 in	130
Waters Method	24	80		200s		●○○	48″	8 × 10 in	251
Reverse Waters	24	80		200s		●○○	48″	8 × 10 in	251
Caldwell Method	20	75		200s		●○○	48″	8 × 10 in	240
Nasal Bones‡									
Lateral	2	50		200s	3		48″	8 × 10 in	8
Zygomatic Arches‡									
SMV	23	65	0.03	200s	6		48″	8 × 10 in	43
Tangential	20	65	0.03	200s	6		48″	8 × 10 in	53
AP Axial	17	70	0.08	200s	16		48″	8 × 10 in	158
Mandibular Rami‡									
PA	17	75	0.06	200s	12		48″	8 × 10 in	109
PA Axial	17	75	0.06	200s	12		48″	8 × 10 in	109
Mandible‡									
Axiolateral Oblique	13	75	0.025	200s	5		48″	8 × 10 in	40
TMJ‡									
AP Axial	21	80	0.08	200s	16		48″	8 × 10 in	211
Axiolateral Oblique	15	75	0.07	200s	14		48″	8 × 10 in	120

s, Small focal spot.
*kVp values are for a three-phase, 12-pulse generator.
†Relative doses for comparison use. All doses are skin entrance for average adult at cm indicated.
‡Bucky, 16:1 grid. Screen/film speed 300.

Radiation Protection

Protection of the patient from unnecessary radiation is a professional responsibility of the radiographer (see Chapter 1 for specific guidelines). In this chapter *(with a few exceptions),* because of central ray angulations, radiation shielding of the patient is not specified or illustrated because the professional community and the federal government have reported that a lead shield over the patient's pelvis does not significantly reduce gonadal exposure during radiography of the facial bones. Nonetheless, shielding the abdomen of a pregnant woman is recommended by the authors of this atlas.

Infants and children, however, should be protected from radiation by shielding the thyroid and thymus glands and the gonads. The protective lead shielding used to cover the thyroid and thymus glands can also assist in immobilizing the pediatric patient.

The most effective way to protect patients from unnecessary radiation is to restrict the radiation beam by using proper collimation. Taking care to ensure that the patient is properly instructed and immobilized also reduces the chance of having to repeat the procedure and thereby expose the patient to more radiation.

PROJECTIONS REMOVED

The following projections have been removed from this edition of the atlas.

Facial profile
- Lateral projection

Nasal bones
- Tangential projection

Zygomatic arch
- Tangential projection: May method

Mandibular symphysis
- AP axial projection

Mandible
- Verticosubmental projection

♠ LATERAL PROJECTION
R or L position

Image receptor: 8 × 10 inch (18 × 24 cm) lengthwise

Position of patient
- Place the patient in a semiprone or obliquely seated position before a vertical grid device.

Position of part
- Adjust the patient's head so that the midsagittal plane is parallel with the IR and the interpupillary line is perpendicular to the IR.
- Adjust the flexion of the patient's neck so that the infraorbitomeatal line (IOML) is parallel with the transverse axis of the IR (Figs. 21-1 to 21-3).
- Immobilize the head.
- *Respiration:* Suspend.

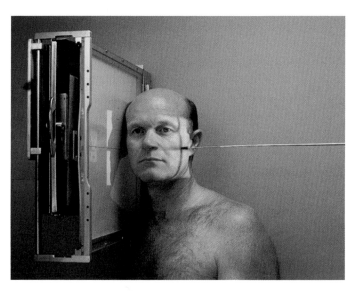

Fig. 21-1 Lateral facial bones.

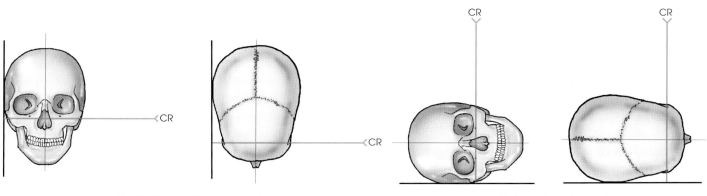

Fig. 21-2 Upright radiography.

Fig. 21-3 Table radiography.

Central ray

- Perpendicular and entering the lateral surface of the zygomatic bone halfway between the outer canthus and the external acoustic meatus (EAM)
- Center the IR to the central ray.

Structures shown

This projection demonstrates a lateral image of the bones of the face, with the right and left sides superimposed (Fig. 21-4).

EVALUATION CRITERIA

The following should be clearly demonstrated:

- ■ All facial bones in their entirety, with the zygomatic bone in the center
- ■ Almost perfectly superimposed mandibular rami
- ■ Superimposed orbital roofs
- ■ No rotation of sella turcica

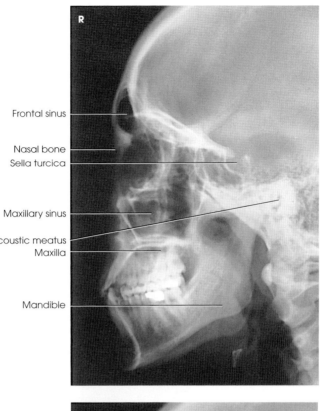

Frontal sinus

Nasal bone
Sella turcica

Maxillary sinus

External acoustic meatus
Maxilla

Mandible

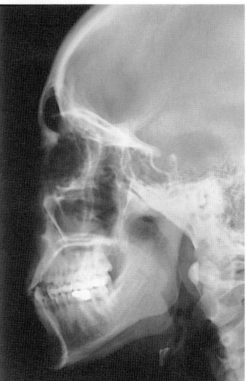

Fig. 21-4 Lateral facial bones.

✳ PARIETOACANTHIAL PROJECTION
WATERS METHOD[1]

Image receptor: 8 × 10 inch (18 × 24 cm) lengthwise

Position of patient
- Place the patient in the prone or seated-upright position.
- Center the midsagittal plane of the patient's body to the midline of the grid device.

[1]Waters CA: Modification of the occipito-frontal position in roentgenography of the accessory nasal sinuses, *Arch Radiol Electrotherapy* 20:15, 1915.

Position of part
- Rest the patient's head on the tip of the extended chin. Hyperextend the neck so that the orbitomeatal line (OML) forms a 37-degree angle with the plane of the IR.
- Note that the mentomeatal line (MML) will be approximately perpendicular to the plane of the IR; the average patient's nose will be about ¾ inch (1.9 cm) away from the grid device.
- Adjust the head so that the midsagittal plane is perpendicular to the plane of the IR (Figs. 21-5 to 21-7).
- Center the IR at the level of the acanthion.
- Immobilize the head.
- *Respiration:* Suspend.

Central ray
- Perpendicular to exit the acanthion

Structures shown
The Waters method demonstrates the orbits, maxillae, and zygomatic arches (Fig. 21-8).

EVALUATION CRITERIA

The following should be clearly demonstrated:
- Distance between the lateral border of the skull and the orbit equal on each side
- Petrous ridges projected immediately below maxillary sinuses

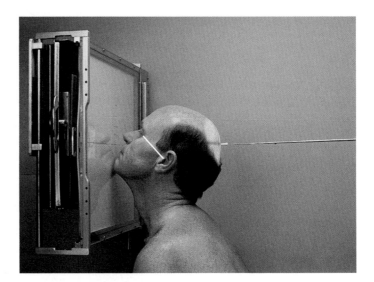

Fig. 21-5 Parietoacanthial facial bones: Waters method.

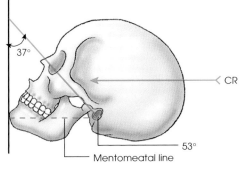

37°

53°

CR

Mentomeatal line

Fig. 21-6 Upright radiography.

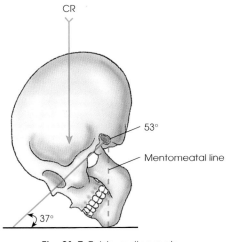

CR

53°

Mentomeatal line

37°

Fig. 21-7 Table radiography.

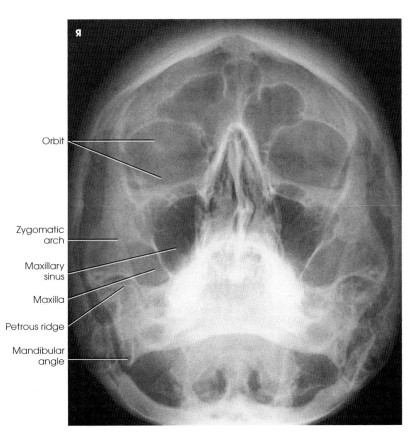

Orbit

Zygomatic arch

Maxillary sinus

Maxilla

Petrous ridge

Mandibular angle

Fig. 21-8 Parietoacanthial facial bones: Waters method.

MODIFIED PARIETOACANTHIAL PROJECTION

MODIFIED WATERS METHOD

Although the parietoacanthial projection (Waters method) is widely used, many institutions modify the projection by radiographing the patient using less extension of the patient's neck. This modification, although sometimes called a "shallow" Waters, actually increases the angulation of the OML by placing it more perpendicular to the plane of the IR. The patient's head is positioned as described using the Waters method, but the neck is extended a lesser amount. In the modification, the OML is adjusted to form an approximately 55-degree angle with the plane of the IR (Figs. 21-9 to 21-11). The resulting radiograph demonstrates the facial bones with less axial angulation than with the Waters method (see Fig. 21-8). With the modified Waters method, the petrous ridges are projected immediately below the inferior border of the orbits at a level midway through the maxillary sinuses (Fig. 21-12).

The modified Waters method is a good projection to demonstrate blowout fractures. This places the orbital floor perpendicular to the IR and parallel to the central ray, demonstrating inferior displacement of the orbital floor and the commonly associated opacified maxillary sinus.

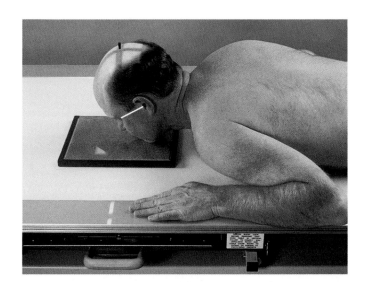

Fig. 21-9 Modified parietoacanthial facial bones: Waters method.

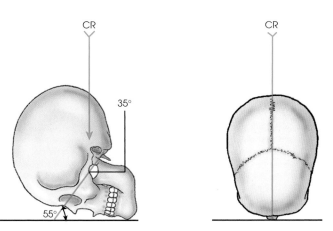

Fig. 21-10 Table radiography, modified parietoacanthial facial bones: Waters method with OML adjusted to 55 degrees.

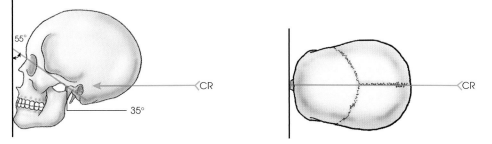

Fig. 21-11 Upright radiography, modified parietoacanthial facial bones: Waters method with OML adjusted to 55 degrees.

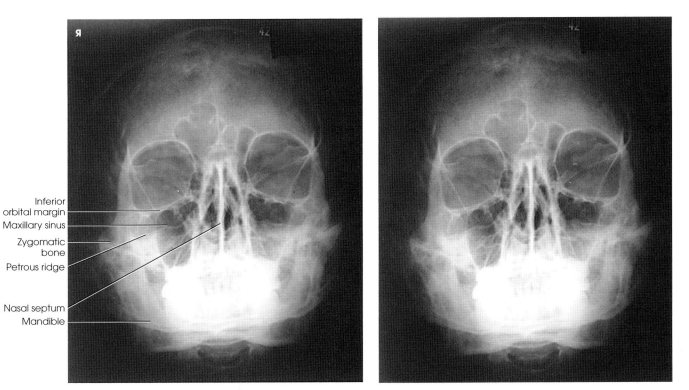

Inferior orbital margin
Maxillary sinus
Zygomatic bone
Petrous ridge

Nasal septum
Mandible

Fig. 21-12 Modified parietoacanthial facial bones: Waters method.

▲ ACANTHIOPARIETAL PROJECTION

REVERSE WATERS METHOD

Image receptor: 24 × 30 cm lengthwise

The *reverse* Waters method is used to demonstrate the facial bones when the patient cannot be placed in the prone position.

Position of patient

- With the patient in the supine position, center the midsagittal plane of the body to the midline of the grid.

Position of part

- Bringing the patient's chin up, adjust the extension of the neck so that the OML forms a 37-degree angle with the plane of the IR (Fig. 21-13). If necessary, place a support under the patient's shoulders to help extend the neck.
- Note that the MML is approximately perpendicular to the plane of the IR.
- Adjust the patient's head so that the midsagittal plane is perpendicular to the plane of the IR.
- Immobilize the head.
- *Respiration:* Suspend.

Central ray

- Perpendicular to enter the acanthion and centered to the IR

Structures shown

The *reverse* Waters method demonstrates the superior facial bones. The image is similar to that obtained with the Waters method, but the facial structures are considerably magnified (Fig. 21-14).

The following should be clearly demonstrated:

- Distance between lateral border of the skull and orbit equal on each side
- Petrous ridges projected below maxillary sinuses

ACANTHIOPARIETAL PROJECTION FOR TRAUMA

Trauma patients are often unable to hyperextend the neck far enough to place the OML 37 degrees to the IR and the MML perpendicular to the plane of the IR. In these patients, the acanthioparietal projection, or the reverse Waters projection, can be achieved by adjusting the central ray so that it enters the acanthion while remaining parallel with the MML (Fig. 21-15).

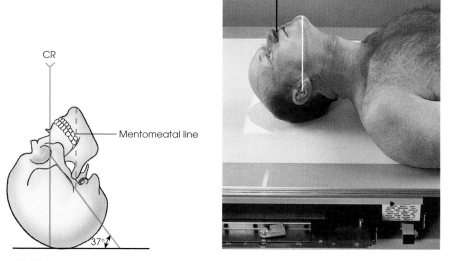

Fig. 21-13 Table radiography. Acanthioparietal facial bones: reverse Waters method with neck extended. Note that the MML is perpendicular to the IR.

CR

Mentomeatal line

37°

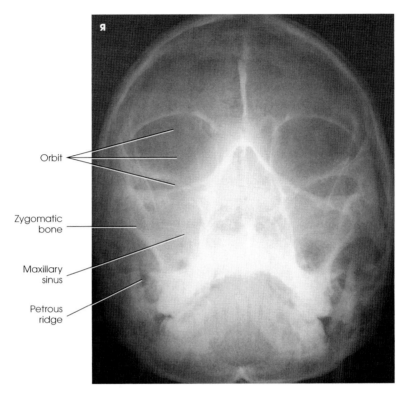

Orbit

Zygomatic bone

Maxillary sinus

Petrous ridge

Fig. 21-14 Acanthioparietal facial bones: reverse Waters method.

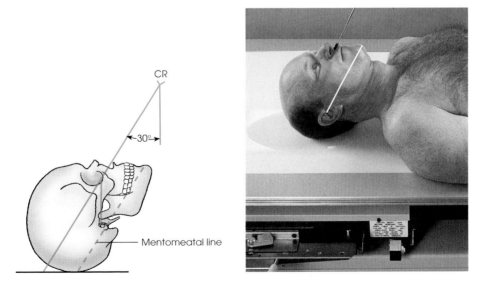

CR

30°

Mentomeatal line

Fig. 21-15 Table radiography. Acanthioparietal facial bones: reverse Waters method with central ray *(CR)* parallel to MML.

♠ PA AXIAL PROJECTION
CALDWELL METHOD

Image receptor: 24 × 30 cm lengthwise

Position of patient
- Place the patient in either a prone or seated position.
- Center the midsagittal plane of the patient's body to the midline of the grid.
- Rest the patient's forehead and nose on the table or against the upright Bucky.
- Flex the patient's elbows, and place the arms in a comfortable position.

Position of part
- Adjust the flexion of the patient's neck so that the OML is perpendicular to the plane of the IR.
- If the patient is obese or hypersthenic, a small radiolucent sponge may need to be placed in front of the forehead.
- Align the midsagittal plane perpendicular to the IR. This is accomplished by adjusting the lateral margins of the orbits or the EAMs equidistant from the tabletop.
- Immobilize the patient's head, and center the IR to the nasion (Figs. 21-16).
- *Respiration:* Suspend.

Central ray
- Direct the central ray to exit the nasion at an angle of 15 degrees caudad.
- For demonstration of the orbital rims, in particular the orbital floors, use a 30-degree caudal angle (sometimes referred to as the exaggerated Caldwell).
- Center the IR to the central ray.

Structures shown
The PA axial projection, Caldwell method, demonstrates the orbital rims, maxillae, nasal septum, zygomatic bones, and the anterior nasal spine. When the central ray is angled 15 degrees caudad to the nasion, the petrous ridges are projected into the lower third of the orbits (Fig. 21-17). When the central ray is angled 30 degrees caudad, the petrous ridges are projected below the inferior margins of the orbits.

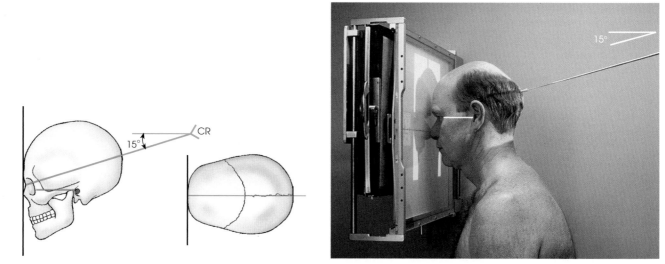

Fig. 21-16 Upright radiography, PA axial facial bones: Caldwell method.

EVALUATION CRITERIA

The following should be clearly demonstrated:

- Entire cranial perimeter showing three distinct tables of squamous bone
- Equal distance from lateral border of skull to lateral border of orbit on both sides
- Symmetric petrous ridges lying in lower third of orbit
- Penetration of frontal bone without excessive density at lateral borders of skull, which will then demonstrate the facial bones

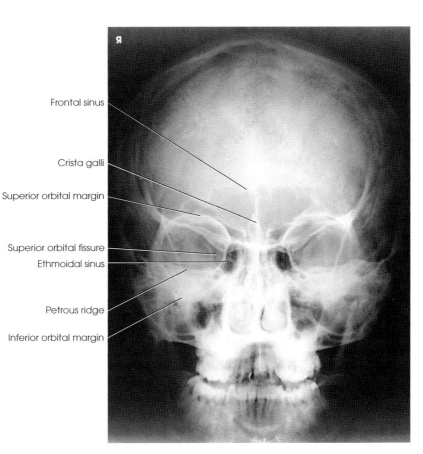

Frontal sinus

Crista galli

Superior orbital margin

Superior orbital fissure

Ethmoidal sinus

Petrous ridge

Inferior orbital margin

Fig. 21-17 PA axial facial bones: Caldwell method.

⚹ LATERAL PROJECTION
R and L positions

Image receptor: 8 × 10 inch (18 × 24 cm) crosswise for two exposures on one IR or a 2½- × 3-inch (57- × 76-mm) occlusal film for each

Position of patient
- With the patient in a semiprone position, adjust the rotation of the body so that the midsagittal plane of the head can be placed horizontally.

Position of part
- Adjust the head so that the midsagittal plane is parallel with the tabletop and the interpupillary line is perpendicular to the tabletop.
- Adjust the flexion of the patient's neck so that the IOML is parallel with the transverse axis of the IR (Figs. 21-18 and 21-19).
- Support the mandible to prevent rotation.
- *Respiration:* Suspend.

Placement of IR
- When using an 8- × 10-inch (18- × 24-cm) IR, slide the unmasked half of the IR under the frontonasal region and center it to the nasion (see Fig. 21-18). This centering allows space for the identification marker to be projected across the upper part of the IR. Tape the side marker (R or L) in position.

Placement of film
- When using occlusal film for the examination, tape the side marker onto the outer lower corner of the pebbled side of the film packet.
- Place a sandbag under the side of the nose, against the orbit and cheek, to support the film packet.
- Adjust the film packet so that the pebbled surface faces and is parallel with the midsagittal plane and so that its upper border projects approximately ½ inch (1.3 cm) above the supraorbital ridge.
- Press the film packet firmly against the maxilla and supraorbital ridge (Fig. 21-20).

Bridge of the nose, flat or concave
- Place the film packet at an angle under the supraorbital ridge.
- Turn the corner of the packet back enough to ease the sharp edge so that it can be placed without discomfort to the patient.
- Place the rounded corner just medial to the inner canthus, and press the upper border firmly against the inferior surface of the supraorbital ridge.
- Instruct the patient to hold the film packet in position so that its plane is parallel with the midsagittal plane of the head.

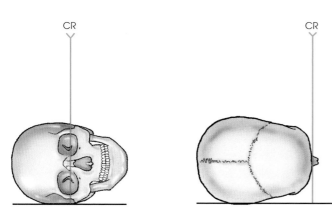

Fig. 21-18 Lateral nasal bones.

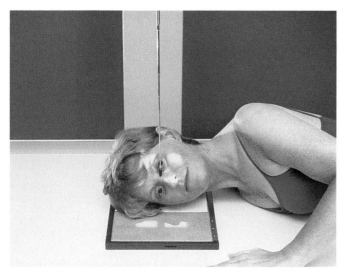

Fig. 21-19 Table radiography.

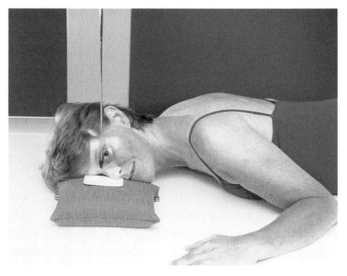

Fig. 21-20 Lateral nasal bones using occlusal film.

Central ray

- Perpendicular to the bridge of the nose at a point ½ inch (1.3 cm) distal to the nasion
- Use close collimation.

Structures shown

The lateral images of the nasal bones demonstrate the side nearer the film or IR and the soft structures of the nose (Figs. 21-21 and 21-22). Both sides are examined for comparison.

EVALUATION CRITERIA

The following should be clearly demonstrated:
- No rotation of nasal bone and soft tissue
- Anterior nasal spine and frontonasal suture

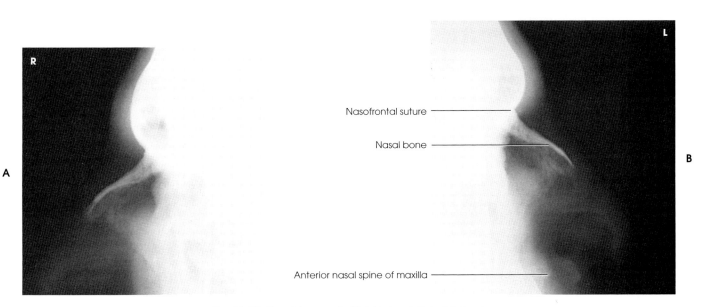

Nasofrontal suture

Nasal bone

Anterior nasal spine of maxilla

Fig. 21-21 Nasal bones. **A,** Right lateral. **B,** Left lateral.

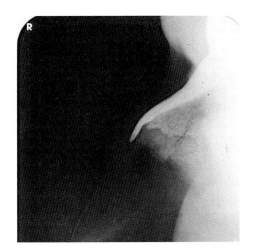

Fig. 21-22 Lateral nasal bones using occlusal film.

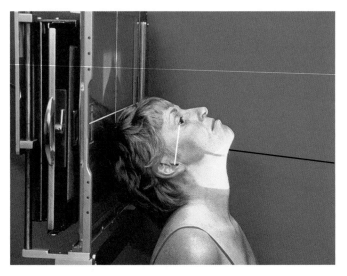

Fig. 21-23 SMV zygomatic arches.

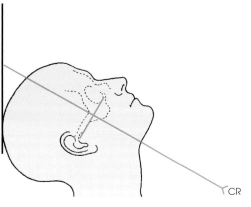

Fig. 21-24 Upright radiography.

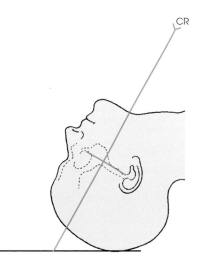

Fig. 21-25 Table radiography.

☀ SUBMENTOVERTICAL PROJECTION

This projection is similar to the submentovertical (SMV) projection described in Chapter 20.

> **Image receptor:** 8 × 10 inch (18 × 24 cm) crosswise

Position of patient

- Place the patient in a seated upright or supine position. A vertical head unit greatly assists the patient who is unable to hyperextend the neck.
- When the supine position is used, elevate the patient's trunk on several firm pillows or a suitable pad to allow complete extension of the neck. Flex the patient's knees to relax the abdominal muscles.
- Center the midsagittal plane of the patient's body to the midline of the grid device.

Position of part

- Hyperextend the patient's neck completely so that the IOML is as nearly parallel with the plane of the IR as possible.
- Rest the patient's head on its vertex, and adjust the head so that the midsagittal plane is perpendicular to the plane of the IR (Figs. 21-23 to 21-25).
- *Respiration:* Suspend.

Zygomatic Arches

Central ray

- Perpendicular to the IOML and entering the midsagittal plane of the throat at a level approximately 1 inch (2.5 cm) posterior to the outer canthi
- Center the IR to the central ray.

Structures shown

Bilateral symmetric SMV images of the zygomatic arches are shown, projected free of superimposed structures (Fig. 21-26). Unless very flat or traumatically depressed, the arches, being farther from the IR, are projected beyond the prominent parietal eminences by the divergent x-ray beam.

The following should be clearly demonstrated:
- Zygomatic arches free from overlying structures
- Zygomatic arches symmetric and without foreshortening
- No rotation of head

NOTE: The zygomatic arches are well demonstrated with a decrease in the exposure factors used for this projection of the cranial base.

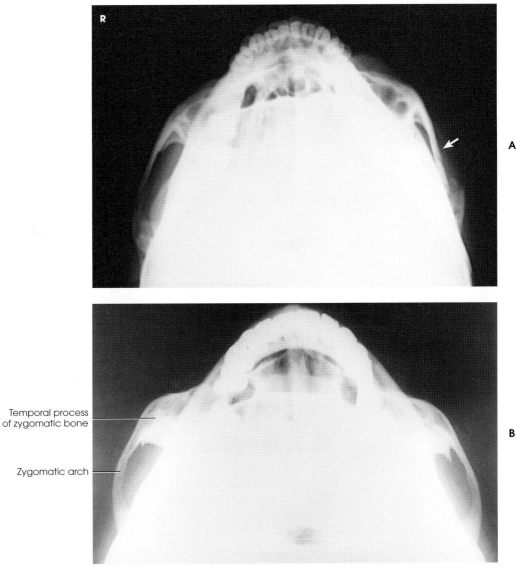

Fig. 21-26 A, SMV projection demonstrating normal zygomatic arch *(right)* and depressed fracture *(arrow)* of left zygomatic arch caused by patient being struck during a fistfight. **B,** Tangential zygomatic arches.

Temporal process of zygomatic bone

Zygomatic arch

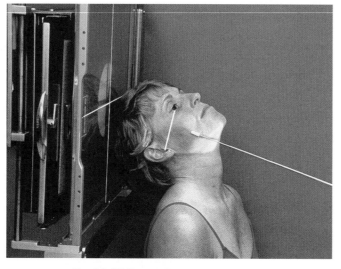

Fig. 21-27 Tangential zygomatic arch.

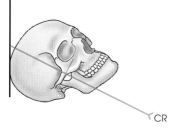 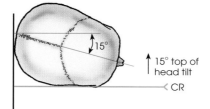

Fig. 21-28 Upright radiography.

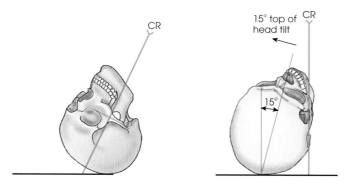

Fig. 21-29 Table radiography.

▲ TANGENTIAL PROJECTION

Image receptor: 8 × 10 inch (18 × 24 cm)

Position of patient
- Seat the patient with the back against a vertical grid device, or place the patient in the supine position with the trunk elevated on several firm pillows and the knees flexed to permit complete extension of the neck.

Position of part
Seated position
- Hyperextend the patient's neck, and rest the head on its vertex.
- Adjust the position of the patient's head so that the IOML is as parallel as possible with the plane of the IR.
- Rotate the midsagittal plane of the head approximately 15 degrees toward the side being examined.
- Tilt the top of the head approximately 15 degrees away from the side being examined. This rotation and tilt ensure that the central ray is tangent to the lateral surface of the skull. The central ray thus skims across the lateral portion of the mandibular angle and the parietal bone to project the zygomatic arch onto the IR.
- Center the zygomatic arch to the IR (Figs. 21-27 and 21-28).

Facial bones

Zygomatic Arch

Supine position

- Rest the patient's head on its vertex.
- Elevate the upper end of the IR on sandbags, or place it on an angled sponge of suitable size.
- Adjust the elevation of the IR and the extension of the patient's neck so that the IOML is placed as nearly parallel with the plane of the IR as possible.
- Rotate and tilt the midsagittal plane of the head approximately 15 degrees toward the side being examined (similar to the upright position).
- If the IOML is parallel with the plane of the IR, center the IR to the zygomatic arch; if not, displace the IR so that the midpoint of the IR coincides with the central ray (Fig. 21-29).
- Attach a strip of adhesive tape to the inferior surface of the chin; draw the tape upward, and anchor it to the edge of the table or IR stand. This usually affords sufficient support. Do not put the adhesive surface directly on the patient's skin.
- *Respiration:* Suspend.

Central ray

- Perpendicular to the IOML and centered to the zygomatic arch at a point approximately 1 inch (2.5 cm) posterior to the outer canthus
- Centered to the IR

Structures shown

A tangential image of one zygomatic arch is seen free of superimposition (Fig. 21-30). This projection is particularly useful in patients with depressed fractures or flat cheekbones.

The following should be clearly demonstrated:

- Zygomatic arch free from overlying structures
- Zygomatic arch not overexposed

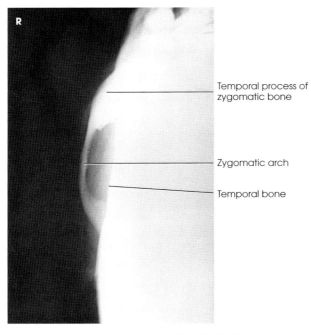 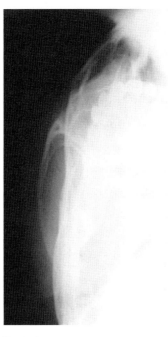

Temporal process of zygomatic bone

Zygomatic arch

Temporal bone

Fig. 21-30 Tangential zygomatic arch.

⚚ AP AXIAL PROJECTION
MODIFIED TOWNE METHOD

Image receptor: 8 × 10 inch (18 × 24 cm) crosswise

Position of patient
- Place the patient in the seated-upright or supine position.
- Center the midsagittal plane of the body to the midline of the grid.

Position of part
- Adjust the patient's head so that the midsagittal plane is perpendicular to the midline of the grid.
- Adjust the flexion of the neck so that the OML is perpendicular to the plane of the IR (Figs. 21-31 to 21-33).
- *Respiration*: Suspend.

Central ray
- Directed to enter the glabella approximately 1 inch (2.5 cm) above the nasion at an angle of 30 degrees caudad
- If the patient is unable to sufficiently flex the neck, adjust the IOML perpendicular with the IR and direct the central ray 37 degrees caudad.
- Center the IR to the central ray.

Structures shown
A symmetric AP axial projection of both zygomatic arches is demonstrated. The arches should be projected free of superimposition (Fig. 21-34).

The following should be clearly demonstrated:
- No overlap of zygomatic arches by mandible
- No rotation evident because arches are symmetric
- Zygomatic arches projected lateral to mandibular rami

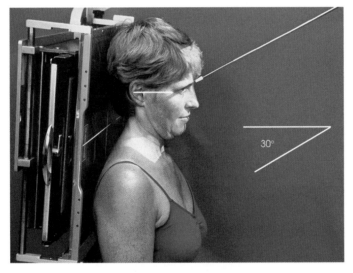

Fig. 21-31 AP axial zygomatic arches: modified Towne method.

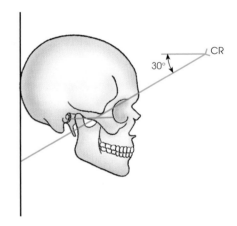

Fig. 21-32 Upright radiography: modified Towne method.

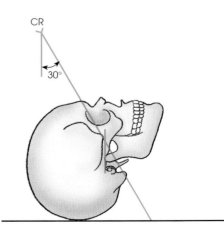

Fig. 21-33 Table radiography: modified Towne method.

Facial bones

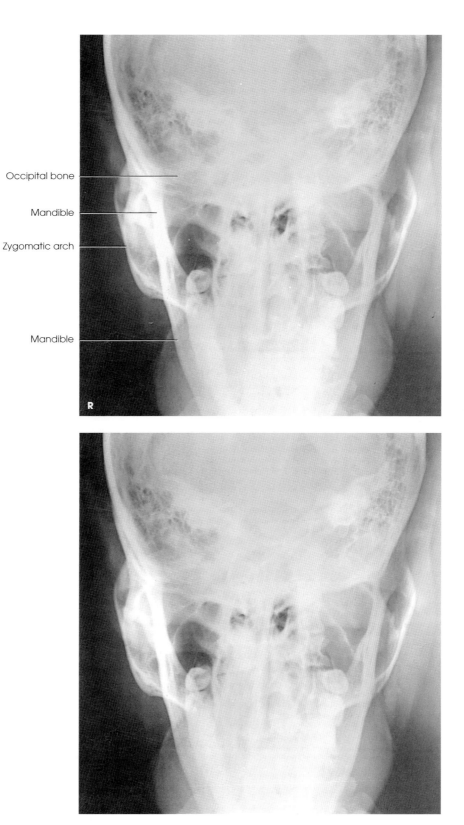

Occipital bone

Mandible

Zygomatic arch

Mandible

R

Fig. 21-34 AP axial zygomatic arches: modified Towne method.

☀ PA PROJECTION

Image receptor: 8 × 10 inch (18 × 24 cm) lengthwise

Position of patient
- Place the patient in the prone position, or seat the patient before a vertical grid device.

Position of part
- Rest the patient's forehead and nose on the IR. Adjust the OML to be perpendicular to the plane of the IR.
- Adjust the head so that its midsagittal plane is perpendicular to the plane of the IR (Fig. 21-35).
- Immobilize the head.
- *Respiration*: Suspend.

Central ray
- Perpendicular to exit the acanthion
- Center the IR to the central ray.

Structures shown
The PA projection shows the mandibular body and rami (Figs. 21-36 and 21-37). The central part of the body is not well shown because of the superimposed spine. This radiographic approach is usually employed to demonstrate medial or lateral displacement of fragments in fractures of the rami.

EVALUATION CRITERIA
The following should be clearly demonstrated:
- Mandibular body and rami symmetric on each side
- Entire mandible

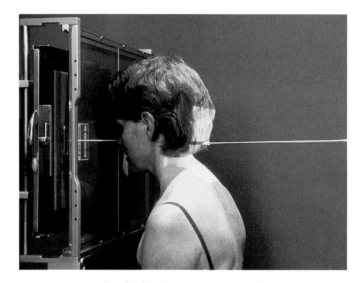

Fig. 21-35 PA mandibular rami.

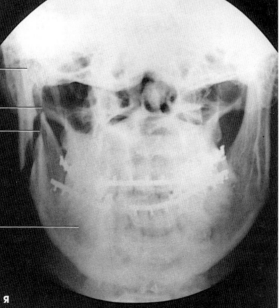

Fig. 21-36 PA mandibular rami showing fracture of right superior ramus.

Condyle

Mastoid process

Fracture

Body

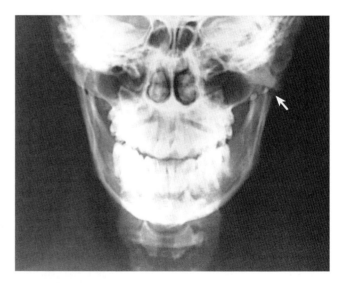

Fig. 21-37 Fracture of left mandibular ramus *(arrow)* incurred when the patient's chin struck the steering wheel during a motor vehicle accident.

⚛ PA AXIAL PROJECTION

Image receptor: 8 × 10 inch (18 × 24 cm) lengthwise

Position of patient
- Place the patient in the prone position, or seat the patient before a vertical grid device.

Position of part
- Rest the patient's forehead and nose on the IR holder.
- Adjust the OML to be perpendicular to the plane of the IR.
- Adjust the patient's head so that the midsagittal plane is perpendicular to the plane of the IR (Fig. 21-38).
- Immobilize the patient's head.
- *Respiration:* Suspend.

Central ray
- Directed 20 or 25 degrees cephalad to exit at the acanthion
- Center the IR to the central ray.

Structures shown
The PA axial projection shows the mandibular body and rami (Fig. 21-39). The central part of the body is not well shown because of the superimposed spine. This radiographic approach is usually employed to demonstrate medial or lateral displacement of fragments in fractures of the rami.

EVALUATION CRITERIA

The following should be clearly demonstrated:
- Mandibular body and rami symmetric on each side
- Condylar processes
- Entire mandible

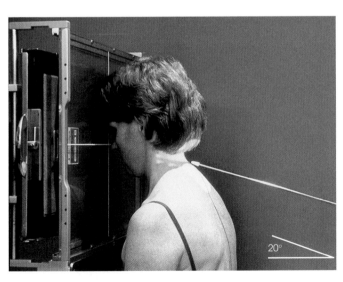

Fig. 21-38 PA axial mandibular rami.

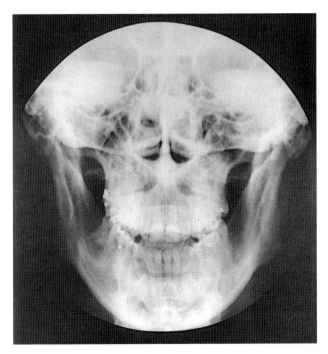

Fig. 21-39 PA axial mandibular body and rami.

PA PROJECTION

Image receptor: 8 × 10 inch (18 × 24 cm) lengthwise

Position of patient
- Place the patient in the prone position, or seat the patient before a vertical grid device.

Position of part
- With the midsagittal plane of the patient's head centered to the midline of the IR, rest the head on the nose and chin so that the anterior surface of the mandibular symphysis is parallel with the plane of the IR. This position places the acanthiomeatal line (AML) nearly perpendicular to the IR plane.
- Adjust the patient's head so that the midsagittal plane is perpendicular to the plane of the IR (Fig. 21-40).
- *Respiration:* Suspend.

Central ray
- Perpendicular to the level of the lips
- Center the IR to the central ray.

Structures shown
This image demonstrates the mandibular body (Fig. 21-41).

The following should be clearly demonstrated:
- ▪ Mandibular body symmetric on each side

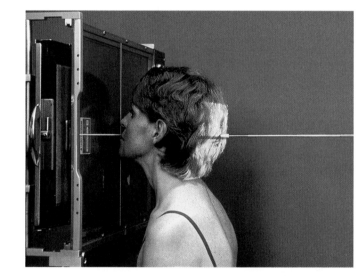

Fig. 21-40 PA mandibular body.

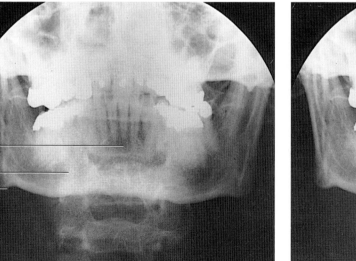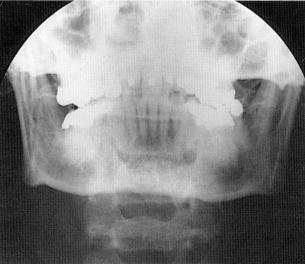

Ramus
Symphysis
Body
Angle

Fig. 21-41 PA mandibular body.

Facial bones

PA AXIAL PROJECTION

Image receptor: 8 × 10 inch (18 × 24 cm) lengthwise

Position of patient

- Place the patient in the prone position, or seat the patient before a vertical grid device.

Position of part

- With the midsagittal plane of the patient's head centered to the midline of the IR, rest the head on the nose and chin so that the anterior surface of the mandibular symphysis is parallel with the plane of the IR. This position places the AML nearly perpendicular to the plane of the IR.
- Adjust the patient's head so that the midsagittal plane is perpendicular to the plane of the IR (Fig. 21-42).
- *Respiration*: Suspend.

Central ray

- Directed midway between the temporomandibular joints (TMJs) at an angle of 30 degrees cephalad. Zanelli[1] recommended that better contrast around the TMJs could be obtained if the patient was instructed to fill the mouth with air for this projection.
- Center the IR to the central ray.

[1]Zanelli A: Le proiezioni radiografiche dell'articolazione temporomandibolare, *Radiol Med* 16:495, 1929.

Structures shown

This image shows the mandibular body and TMJs (Fig. 21-43).

EVALUATION CRITERIA

The following should be clearly demonstrated:

- TMJs just inferior to the mastoid process
- Symmetric rami

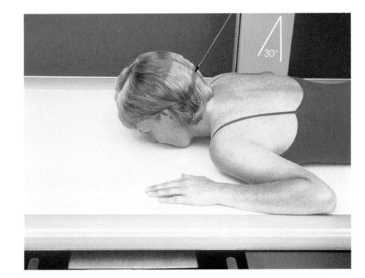

Fig. 21-42 PA axial mandibular body.

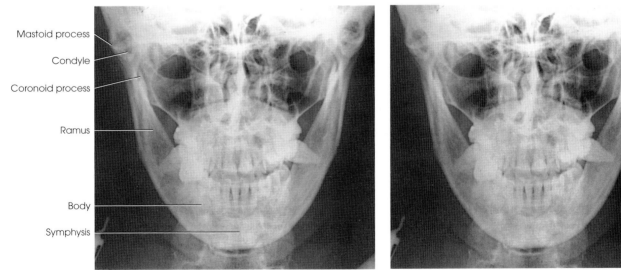

Mastoid process
Condyle
Coronoid process
Ramus
Body
Symphysis

Fig. 21-43 PA axial mandibular body.

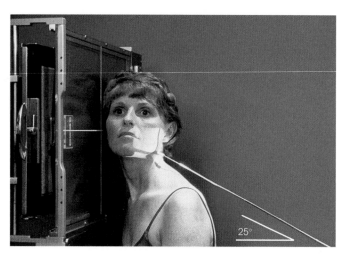

Fig. 21-44 Axiolateral oblique mandibular ramus.

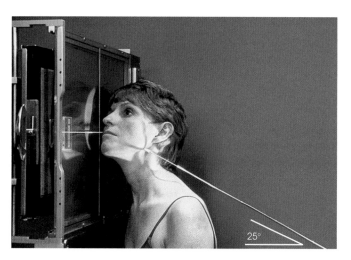

Fig. 21-45 Axiolateral oblique mandibular body.

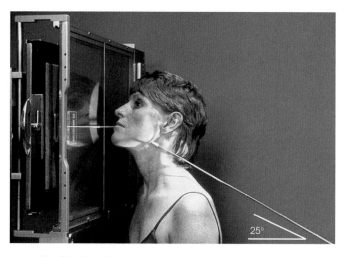

Fig. 21-46 Axiolateral oblique mandibular symphysis.

⚜ AXIOLATERAL OBLIQUE PROJECTION

The goal of this projection is to place the desired portion of the mandible parallel with the IR.

> **Image receptor:** 8- × 10-inch (18- × 24-cm) IR placed according to region

Position of patient
- Place the patient in the seated, semiprone, or semisupine position.

Position of part
- Place the patient's head in a lateral position with the interpupillary line perpendicular to the IR. The mouth should be closed with the teeth together.
- Extend the patient's neck enough that the long axis of the mandibular body is parallel with the transverse axis of the IR. This prevents superimposition of the cervical spine.
- If the projection is to be performed on the tabletop, position the IR so that the complete body of the mandible is on the IR.
- Adjust the rotation of the patient's head to place the area of interest parallel to the IR, as follows:
  Ramus
- Keep the patient's head in a true lateral position (Fig. 21-44).
  Body
- Rotate the patient's head 30 degrees toward the IR (Fig. 21-45).
  Symphysis
- Rotate the patient's head 45 degrees toward the IR (Fig. 21-46).

NOTE: When the patient is in the semisupine position, place the IR on a wedge device or wedge sponge (Fig. 21-47).

Central ray
- Directed 25 degrees cephalad to pass directly through the mandibular region of interest (See note on p. 374.)
- Center the IR to the central ray for projections done on upright grid units.

Structures shown
Each axiolateral oblique projection demonstrates the region of the mandible that was parallel with the IR (Figs. 21-48 to 21-50).

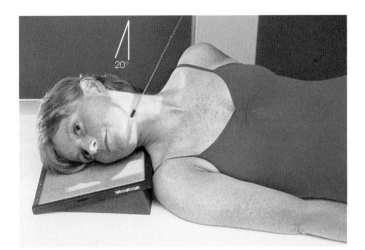

Fig. 21-47 Semisupine axiolateral oblique mandibular body and symphysis.

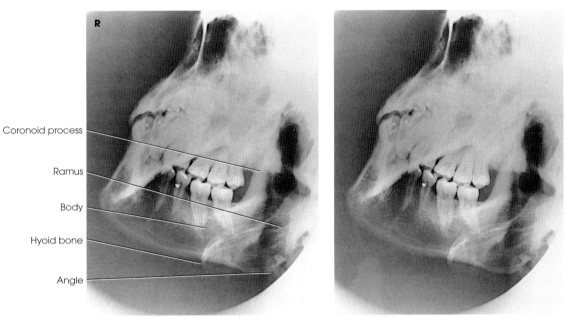

Coronoid process
Ramus
Body
Hyoid bone
Angle

R

Fig. 21-48 Axiolateral oblique mandibular body.

EVALUATION CRITERIA

The following should be clearly demonstrated:

Ramus and body

- No overlap of the ramus by the opposite side of the mandible
- No elongation or foreshortening of ramus or body

- No superimposition of the ramus by the cervical spine

Symphysis

- No overlap of the mentum region by the opposite side of the mandible
- No foreshortening of the mentum region

NOTE: To reduce the possibility of projecting the shoulder over the mandible when radiographing muscular or hypersthenic patients, adjust the midsagittal plane of the patient's skull with an approximately 15-degree angle, open inferiorly. The cephalad angulation of 10 degrees of the central ray maintains the optimal 25-degree central ray/part angle relationship.

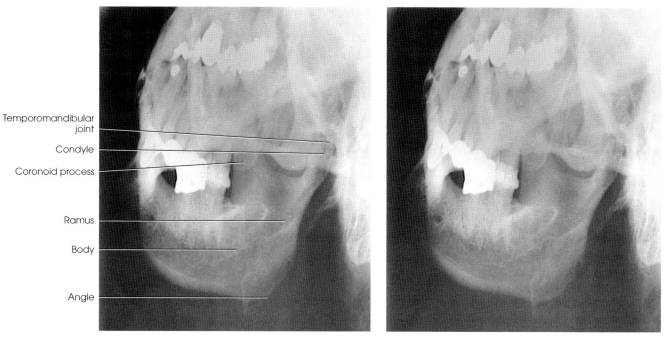

Temporomandibular joint
Condyle
Coronoid process
Ramus
Body
Angle

Fig. 21-49 Axiolateral oblique mandibular ramus.

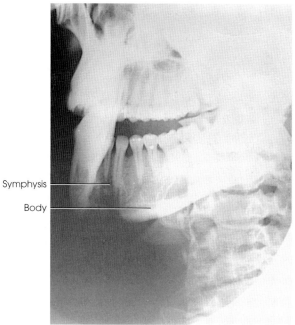

Symphysis
Body

Fig. 21-50 Axiolateral oblique mandibular symphysis.

SUBMENTOVERTICAL PROJECTION

Image receptor: 8 × 10 inch (18 × 24 cm) lengthwise

Position of patient

- Place the patient upright in front of a vertical grid device or in the supine position. When the patient is supine, elevate the shoulders on firm pillows to permit complete extension of the neck.
- Flex the patient's knees to relax the abdominal muscles and thus relieve strain on the neck muscles.
- Center the midsagittal plane of the body to the midline of the grid device.

Position of part

- With the neck fully extended, rest the head on its vertex and adjust the head so that the midsagittal plane is vertical.
- Adjust the IOML as parallel as possible with the plane of the IR (Fig. 21-51).
- When the neck cannot be extended enough so that the IOML is parallel with the IR plane, angle the *grid device* and place it parallel to the IOML.
- Immobilize the head.
- *Respiration:* Suspend.

Central ray

- Perpendicular to the IOML and centered midway between the angles of the mandible

Structures shown

The SMV projection of the mandibular body shows the coronoid and condyloid processes of the rami (Fig. 21-52).

EVALUATION CRITERIA

The following should be clearly demonstrated:

- Distance between the lateral border of the skull and the mandible equal on both sides
- Condyles of the mandible anterior to the pars petrosae
- Symphysis extending almost to the anterior border of the face so that the mandible is not foreshortened

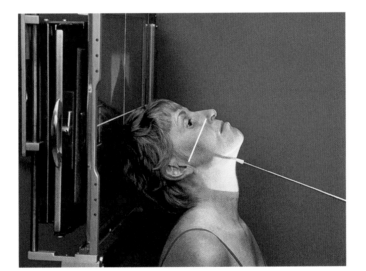

Fig. 21-51 SMV mandible.

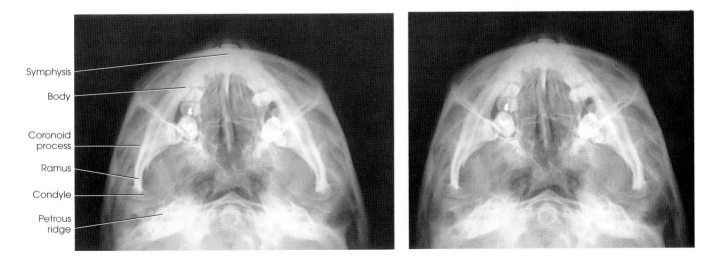

Symphysis
Body
Coronoid process
Ramus
Condyle
Petrous ridge

Fig. 21-52 SMV mandible.

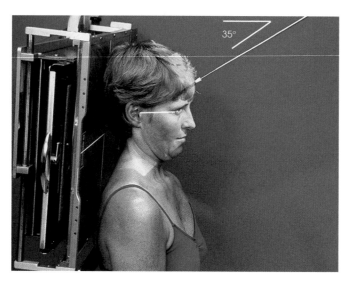

Fig. 21-53 AP axial TMJs.

♠ AP AXIAL PROJECTION

For radiography of the TMJs in the closed-mouth position, *the posterior teeth,* rather than the incisors, must be in contact. Occlusion of the incisors places the mandible in a position of protrusion, and the condyles are carried out of the mandibular fossae. In the open-mouth position, the mouth should be opened as wide as possible but not with the mandible protruded (jutted forward).

Because of the danger of fragment displacement, the open-mouth position should not be attempted in patients with recent injury. Trauma patients are examined without any stress movement of the mandible. Tomography is particularly useful when a fracture or dislocation is suspected.

Image receptor: 8×10 inch (18×24 cm) lengthwise

Position of patient
- Place the patient in a supine or seated-upright position with the posterior skull in contact with the upright Bucky.

Position of part
- Adjust the patient's head so that the midsagittal plane is perpendicular to the plane of the IR.
- Flex the patient's neck so that the OML is perpendicular to the plane of the IR (Figs. 21-53 to 21-55).
- *Respiration*: Suspend.

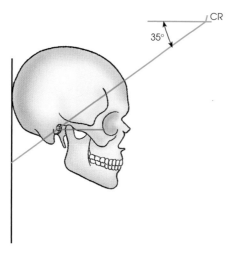

Fig. 21-54 Upright radiography.

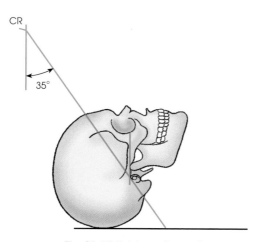

Fig. 21-55 Table radiography.

Central ray

- Directed 35 degrees caudad, centered midway between the TMJs, and entering at a point approximately 3 inches (7.6 cm) above the nasion
- Expose one image with the mouth closed; when not contraindicated, expose one image with the mouth open.
- Center the IR to the central ray.

Structures shown

The AP axial projection demonstrates the condyles of the mandible and the mandibular fossae of the temporal bones (Figs. 21-56 and 21-57).

EVALUATION CRITERIA

The following should be clearly demonstrated:

- No rotation of head
- Minimal superimposition of petrosa on the condyle in the closed-mouth examination
- Condyle and temporomandibular articulation below pars petrosa in the open-mouth position

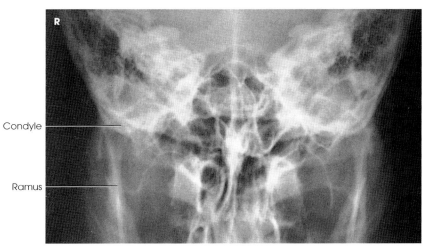

Fig. 21-56 AP axial TMJs: mouth closed.

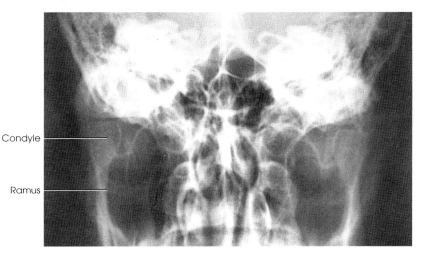

Fig. 21-57 AP axial TMJs: mouth open.

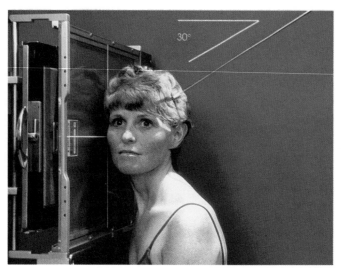

Fig. 21-58 Axiolateral TMJ: mouth closed.

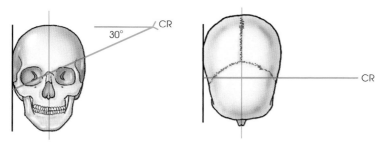

Fig. 21-59 Upright radiography.

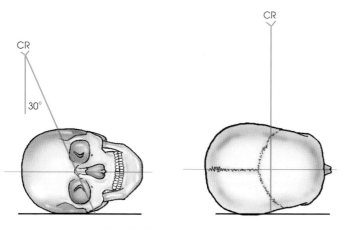

Fig. 21-60 Table radiography.

AXIOLATERAL PROJECTION
R and L positions

> **Image receptor:** 8 × 10 inch (18 × 24 cm) crosswise

Position of patient
- Put a mark on each cheek at a point ½ inch (1.3 cm) anterior to the EAM and 1 inch (2.5 cm) inferior to the EAM to localize the TMJ if needed.
- Place the patient in a semiprone position, or seat the patient before a vertical grid device.

Position of part
- Center a point ½ inch (1.3 cm) anterior to the EAM to the IR, and place the patient's head in the lateral position with the affected side closest to the IR.
- Adjust the patient's head so that the midsagittal plane is parallel with the plane of the IR and the interpupillary line is perpendicular to the IR plane (Figs. 21-58 to 21-60).
- Immobilize the head.
- *Respiration:* Suspend.
- After making the exposure with the patient's mouth closed, change the IR; then, unless contraindicated, have the patient open the mouth widely (Fig. 21-61).
- Recheck the patient's position, and make the second exposure.

Central ray

- Directed to the midpoint of the IR at an angle of 25 or 30 degrees caudad. The central ray enters about ½ inch (1.3 cm) anterior and 2 inches (5 cm) superior to the upside EAM.

Structures shown

These images show the TMJ when the mouth is open and closed (Figs. 21-62 and 21-63). Examine both sides for comparison.

EVALUATION CRITERIA

The following should be clearly demonstrated:

- Temporomandibular articulation lying anterior to the EAM
- Condyle lying in mandibular fossa in the closed-mouth examination
- Condyle lying inferior to articular tubercle in the open-mouth examination if the patient is normal and able to open the mouth widely

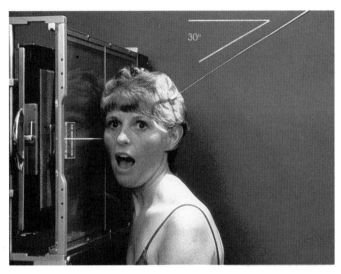

Fig. 21-61 Axiolateral TMJ with mouth open.

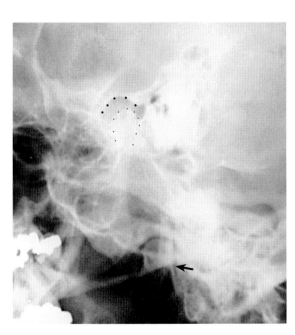

Fig. 21-62 Axiolateral TMJ, mouth closed. Mandibular condyle *(small dots)* and mandibular fossa *(large dots)* are demonstrated. Mandibular condyle of side away from film is also seen *(arrow)*.

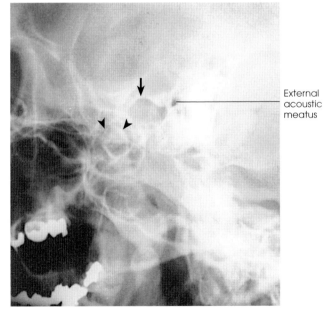

Fig. 21-63 Axiolateral TMJ, mouth open. Mandibular fossa *(arrow)* and mandibular condyle *(arrowheads)* are demonstrated.

External acoustic meatus

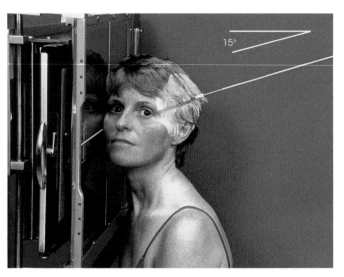

Fig. 21-64 Axiolateral oblique TMJ.

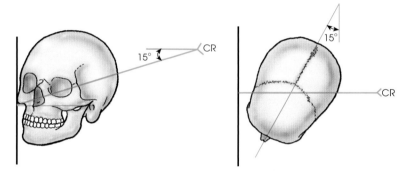

Fig. 21-65 Upright radiography.

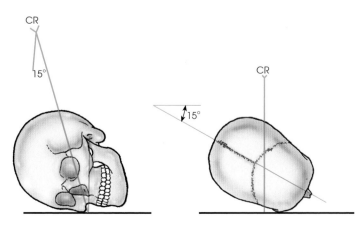

Fig. 21-66 Table radiography.

⚜ AXIOLATERAL OBLIQUE PROJECTION
R and L positions

Image receptor: 8 × 10 inch (18 × 24 cm) crosswise

Position of patient
- Place the patient in a semiprone position, or seat the patient before a vertical grid device.
- In TMJ examinations, make one exposure with the mouth closed and, when not contraindicated, make one exposure with the mouth open.
- Use an IR-changing tunnel or Bucky tray so that the patient's head does not have to be adjusted between the two exposures.
- Examine both sides for comparison.

Position of part
- Center a point ½ inch (1.3 cm) anterior to the EAM to the IR, and rest the patient's cheek on the grid device.
- Rotate the midsagittal plane of the head approximately 15 degrees toward the IR.
- Adjust the interpupillary line perpendicular to the plane of the IR.
- Adjust the flexion of the patient's neck so that the AML is parallel with the transverse axis of the IR (Figs. 21-64 to 21-66).
- Immobilize the head.
- *Respiration:* Suspend.
- After making the exposure with the mouth closed, change the IR and instruct the patient to open the mouth widely.
- Recheck the position of the AML, and make the second exposure.

Central ray
- Directed 15 degrees caudad and exiting through the TMJ closest to the IR. The central ray enters about 1½ inches (3.8 cm) superior to the upside EAM.

Structures shown

The images in the open-mouth and closed-mouth positions demonstrate the condyles and necks of the mandible. The images also show the relation between the mandibular fossa and the condyle. The open-mouth position demonstrates the mandibular fossa and the inferior and anterior excursion of the condyle. Both sides are examined for comparison (Fig. 21-67). The closed-mouth position demonstrates fractures of the neck and condyle of the ramus.

EVALUATION CRITERIA

The following should be clearly demonstrated:

■ Temporomandibular articulation
■ Condyle lying in mandibular fossa in the closed-mouth examination
■ Condyle lying inferior to articular tubercle in the open-mouth projection if the patient is normal and is able to open the mouth widely

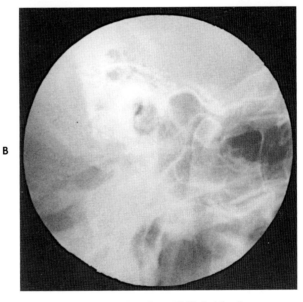

Mandibular fossa
Articular tubercle
External acoustic meatus
Condyle

A
B

Fig. 21-67 Axiolateral oblique TMJ. **A,** Mouth open, right side. **B,** Mouth open, left side (same patient), showing more movement on the left side.

Panoramic Tomography of the Mandible

Panoramic tomography, pantomography, and *rotational tomography* are terms used to designate the technique employed to produce tomograms of curved surfaces. This technique of body-section radiography provides a panoramic image of the entire mandible, including the TMJ, and of both dental arches on one long, narrow film curved to conform to the shape of the patient's jaw. Only the structures near the axis of rotation are sharply defined.

Two types of equipment are available for pantomography. In the first type, the patient and film are rotated before a stationary x-ray tube. This type of machine consists of (1) a specially designed chair mounted on a turntable and (2) a second turntable to support a 4- × 10-inch (10.2- × 25.4-cm) film enclosed in a flexible IR. The seated and immobilized patient and the film are electronically rotated in *opposite* directions at coordinated speeds. The x-ray tube remains stationary. In one machine the exposure is interrupted in the midline.

In the second type of unit, the x-ray tube and the IR rotate in the *same direction* around the seated and immobilized patient (Fig. 21-68). The x-ray tube and IR drum are attached to an overhead carriage that is supported by the vertical stand assembly. The chair of this unit is fixed to the base but can be removed to accommodate patients in wheelchairs. The attached head holder and radiolucent bite device center and immobilize the patient's head. A scale on the head holder indicates the jaw size. The film, 5 × 12 inches (12.7 × 30.5 cm) or 5 × 14 inches (12.7 × 35.6 cm) as indicated, is placed in a flexible IR that attaches firmly to the film drum.

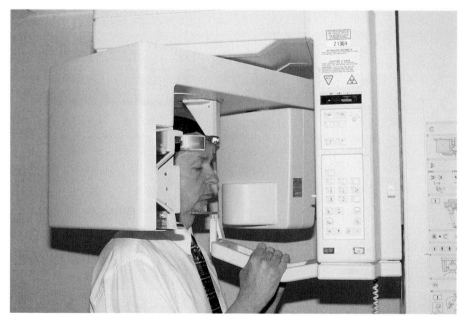

Fig. 21-68 Panograph radiographic unit.

(Courtesy Gendex.)

In both types of equipment the beam of radiation is sharply collimated at the tube aperture by a lead diaphragm with a narrow vertical slit. A corresponding slit diaphragm is fixed between the patient and the IR so that the patient and the IR (or the tube and the film) rotate. Each narrow area of the part is recorded on the film without overlap and without fogging from scattered and secondary radiation.

The rotation time varies from 10 to 20 seconds in different makes of equipment. This requires a long exposure time. Because of the slit diaphragm, however, radiation exposure to the patient at each fraction of a second is restricted to the skin surface that is passing before the narrow vertical slit aperture.

Panoramic tomography provides a distortion-free lateral image of the entire mandible (Fig. 21-69). It also affords the most comfortable way to position patients who have sustained severe mandibular or TMJ trauma, both before and after splint wiring of the teeth. It must, of course, be supplemented with an AP, PA, or a verticosubmental projection to establish fragment position.

This tomographic technique is useful for general survey studies of various dental and facial bone abnormalities. It is also used to supplement rather than replace conventional periapical radiographs.

NOTE: A more comprehensive discussion of basic tomographic principles is presented in Chapter 31.

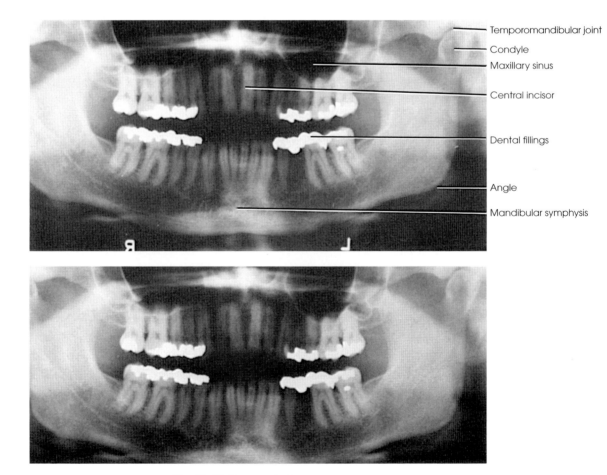

Temporomandibular joint
Condyle
Maxillary sinus
Central incisor
Dental fillings
Angle
Mandibular symphysis

Fig. 21-69 Panoramic tomogram.

22

PARANASAL SINUSES

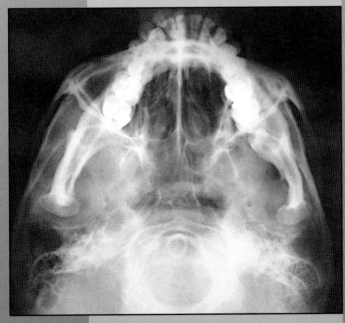

Submentovertical sinuses.

SUMMARY OF PROJECTIONS

PROJECTIONS, POSITIONS, AND METHODS

Page	Essential	Anatomy	Projection	Position	Method
394	♠	Paranasal sinuses	Lateral	R or L	
396	♠	Frontal and anterior ethmoidal sinuses	PA axial		CALDWELL
398	♠	Maxillary sinuses	Parietoacanthial		WATERS
400	♠	Maxillary and sphenoidal sinuses	Parietoacanthial	Open mouth	WATERS
402	♠	Ethmoidal and sphenoidal sinuses	Submentovertical		

Icons in the Essential column indicate projections frequently performed in the United States and Canada. Students should be competent in these projections.

Sinuses

The air-containing cavities situated in the frontal, ethmoidal, and sphenoidal bones of the cranium and the maxillary bones of the face are called the *paranasal sinuses* because of their formation from the nasal mucosa and their continued communication with the nasal fossae (Figs. 22-1 and 22-2). Although the functions of the sinuses are not agreed on by all anatomists, these cavities are believed to do the following:

- Serve as a resonating chamber for the voice
- Decrease the weight of the skull by containing air
- Help warm and moisten inhaled air
- Act as shock absorbers in trauma (as airbags do in automobiles)
- Possibly control the immune system

The sinuses begin to develop early in fetal life, at first appearing as small sacculations of the mucosa of the nasal meatus and recesses. As the pouches, or sacs, grow, they gradually invade the respective bones to form the air sinuses and cells. The maxillary sinuses are usually sufficiently well developed and aerated at birth to be demonstrated radiographically. The other groups of sinuses develop more slowly, so that by age 6 or 7 years the frontal and sphenoidal sinuses are distinguishable from the ethmoidal air cells, which they resemble in both size and position. The ethmoidal air cells develop during puberty, and the sinuses are not completely developed until the seventeenth or eighteenth year of life. When fully developed, each of the sinuses communicates with the others and with the nasal cavity.

An understanding of the actual size, shape, and position of the sinuses within the skull is made possible by studying the sinuses on computed tomography (CT) head images (see Fig. 22-2).

Maxillary Sinuses

The largest sinuses, the *maxillary sinuses,* are paired and are located in the body of each maxilla (see Figs. 22-1 and 22-2). Although the maxillary sinuses appear rectangular in the lateral image, they are approximately pyramidal in shape and have only three walls. The apices are directed inferiorly and laterally. The two maxillary sinuses vary considerably in size and shape but are usually symmetric. In adults, each maxillary sinus is approximately 3.5 cm high and 2.5 to 3 cm wide. The sinus is often divided into subcompartments by partial septa, and occasionally it is divided into two sinuses by a complete septum. The sinus floor presents several elevations that correspond to the roots of the subjacent teeth. The maxillary sinuses communicate with the middle nasal meatus at the superior aspect of the sinus.

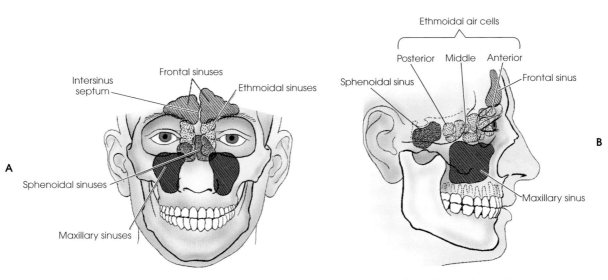

Fig. 22-1 A, Anterior aspect of paranasal sinuses, showing lateral relationship to each other and to surrounding parts. **B,** Schematic drawing of paranasal sinuses, showing AP relationship to each other and surrounding parts.

Maxillary sinuses

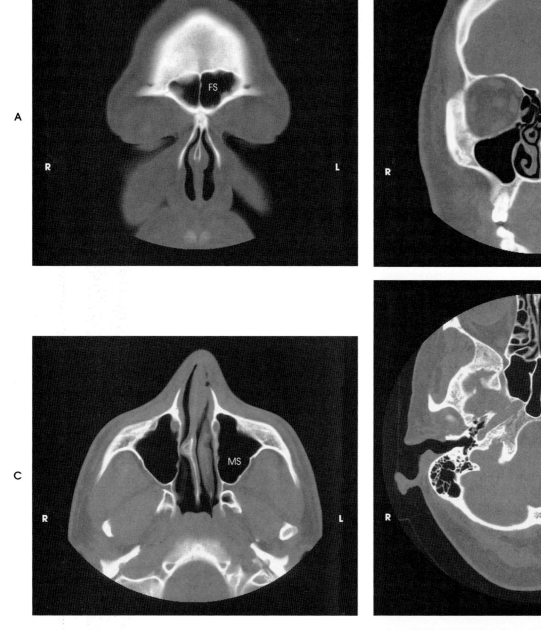

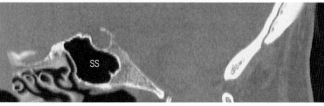

Fig. 22-2 A, Coronal CT image of the frontal sinuses *(FS)*.
B, Coronal CT scan of the maxillary sinuses *(MS)*. **C,** Axial CT image of the maxillary sinuses *(MS)*. **D,** Axial CT image of the sphenoid sinuses *(SS)*. **E,** Sagittal CT image of the sphenoidal sinus *(SS)*.

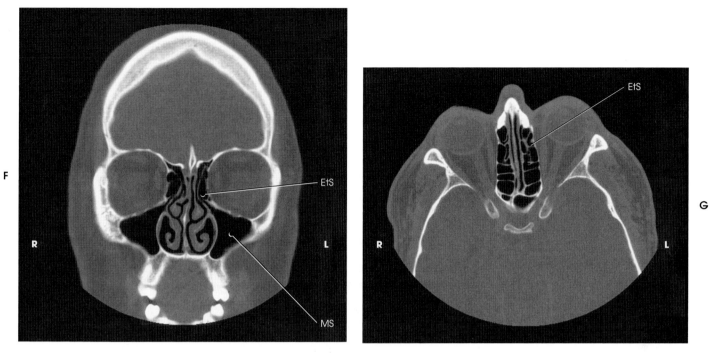

Fig. 22-2, cont'd F, Coronal CT image of the ethmoidal sinuses *(EtS)*. *MS,* Maxillary sinus. **G,** Axial CT image of the ethmoidal sinuses *(EtS)*.

(From Kelley LL, Petersen CM: *Sectional anatomy for imaging professionals,* St Louis, 1997, Mosby.)

Frontal Sinuses

The *frontal sinuses,* the second-largest sinuses, are paired and are normally located between the tables of the vertical plate of the frontal bone (see Figs. 22-1 and 22-2). The frontal sinuses vary greatly in size and form. Occasionally they are absent. One or both may be as large as approximately 2 to 2.5 cm in the vertical or lateral dimension. The sinuses often extend beyond the frontal region of the bone, most frequently into the orbital plates. The *intersinus septum* is usually deviated from the midline; for this reason the frontal sinuses are rarely symmetric. Multiple septa are sometimes present. Like maxillary sinuses, the frontal sinuses drain into the middle nasal meatus.

Ethmoidal Sinuses

The two *ethmoidal sinuses* are located within the lateral masses of the labyrinths of the ethmoid bone. They are composed of a varying number of air cells that are divided into three main groups: *anterior, middle,* and *posterior* (see Figs. 22-1 and 22-2). The anterior and middle ethmoidal cells vary in number from two to eight, and each group opens into the middle nasal meatus. The posterior cells vary in number from two to six or more and drain into the superior nasal meatus.

Sphenoidal Sinuses

The *sphenoidal sinuses* are normally paired and occupy the body of the sphenoid bone (see Figs. 22-1 and 22-2). Anatomists state that only one sphenoidal sinus is often present; however, more than two sphenoidal sinuses are never present. The sphenoidal sinuses vary considerably in size and shape and are usually asymmetric. They lie immediately below the sellae turcica and extend between the dorsum sellae and the posterior ethmoidal air cells. The sphenoidal sinuses open into the sphenoethmoidal recess of the nasal cavity.

Summary of Pathology

Please refer to Chapter 20 for a summary of pathology for this chapter.

SUMMARY OF ANATOMY

Paranasal sinuses
maxillary sinuses
frontal sinuses
  intersinus septum
ethmoidal sinuses
  anterior ethmoidal cells
  middle ethmoidal cells
  posterior ethmoidal cells
sphenoidal sinuses

EXPOSURE TECHNIQUE CHART ESSENTIAL PROJECTIONS

PARANASAL SINUSES

Part	cm	kVp*	tm	mA	mAs	AEC	SID	IR	Dose† (mrad)
Paranasal (all) *Lateral*‡	15	70	0.04	200s	8		48″	8 × 10 in	35
Frontal and Anterior Ethmoidal *PA Axial (Caldwell)*‡	20	75		200s		○○ ●	48″	8 × 10 in	285
Maxillary *Waters*‡	24	75		200s		○○ ●	48″	8 × 10 in	280
Maxillary and Sphenoidal *Open-Mouth Waters*‡	24	75	0.14	200s	28		48″	8 × 10 in	230
Ethmoidal and Sphenoidal *SMV*‡	23	75		200s		○○ ●	48″	8 × 10 in	363

s, Small focal spot.
*kVp values are for a three-phase, 12-pulse generator.
†Relative doses for comparison use. All doses are skin entrance for average adult at cm indicated.
‡Bucky, 16:1 grid. Screen/film speed 300.

Technical Considerations

Radiographic density is probably more critical and more misleading in the sinuses than in any other region of the body (Figs. 22-3 to 22-5). Overpenetration of the sinuses diminishes or completely obliterates existing pathologic conditions, and underpenetration can simulate pathologic conditions that do not exist.

Depending on the technique employed, the milliampere-second (mAs) and kilovolt (peak) (kVp) factors should be balanced so that both soft tissue structures and bony structures are demonstrated. Although good contrast is desirable, soft tissue areas may not be visualized with high contrast.

Whenever possible, radiographs of the paranasal sinuses should be made with the patient in the *upright position.* This position is best for demonstrating the presence or absence of fluid and differentiating between fluid and other pathologic conditions. The value of the upright position in sinus examinations was pointed out by Cross[1] and Flecker.[2]

The paranasal sinuses vary not only in size and form but also in position. The cells of one group frequently encroach on and resemble those of another group. This characteristic of the sinuses, together with their proximity to the vital intracranial organs, makes accurate radiographic demonstration of their anatomic structure of prime importance. The patient's head must be carefully placed in a sufficient number of positions so that the projections of each group of cavities are as free of superimposed bony structures as possible. The radiographs must be of such quality that it is possible to distinguish the cells of several groups of sinuses and their relationship to the surrounding structures.

[1]Cross KS: Radiography of the nasal accessory sinuses, *Med J Aust* 14:569, 1927.
[2]Flecker H: Roentgenograms of the antrum, *AJR* 20:56, 1928 (letter).

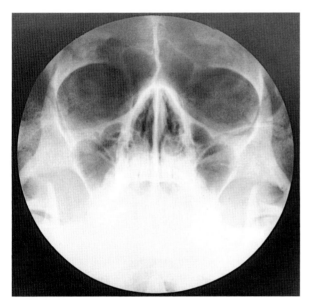

Fig. 22-3 Correctly exposed radiograph of sinuses.

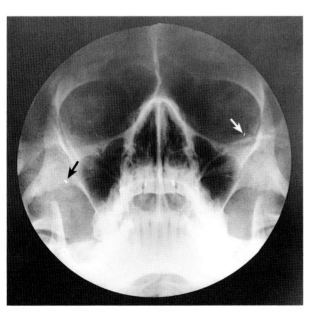

Fig. 22-4 Overexposed radiograph of sinuses demonstrating two artifacts caused by dirt on screens *(arrows).*

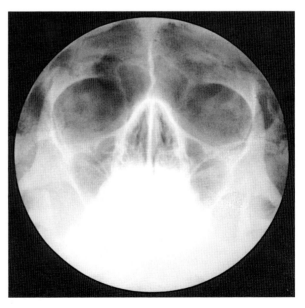

Fig. 22-5 Underexposed radiograph of sinuses.

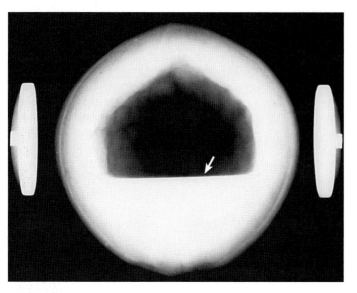

Fig. 22-6 Coconut, vertical position: horizontal central ray. Air-fluid level is demonstrated *(arrow)*.

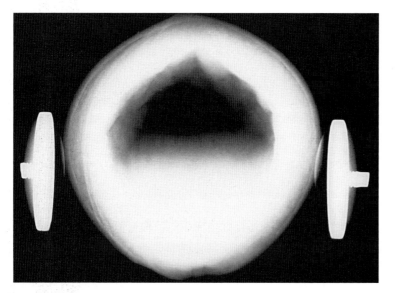

Fig. 22-7 Coconut, vertical position: central ray angled 45 degrees upward. Note that air-fluid level is not as sharp.

Unless sinus radiographs are almost perfect technically, they are of little diagnostic value. For this reason a precise technical procedure is necessary in radiography of the paranasal sinuses. The first requirements are a small focal spot and clean imaging screens that have perfect contact. The radiographic contrast must similarly distinguish the sinuses from the surrounding structures. The head must be carefully positioned and rigidly immobilized, and respiration must be suspended for the exposures.

The effect of both body position and central ray angulation is clearly demonstrated in radiographs of a coconut held in position by head clamps. Fig. 22-6 shows a sharply defined air-fluid level. This coconut was placed in the vertical position, and the central ray was directed horizontally. Fig. 22-7 was also taken with the coconut in the vertical position, but the central ray was directed upward at an angle of 45 degrees to demonstrate the gradual fading of the fluid line when the central ray is *not* horizontal. This effect is much more pronounced in actual practice because of structural irregularities. Fig. 22-8 was made with the coconut in the horizontal position and the central ray directed vertically. The resultant radiograph shows a homogeneous density throughout the cavity of the coconut, with no evidence of an air-fluid level.

Exudate contained in the sinuses is not fluid in the usual sense of the word but is commonly a heavy, semigelatinous material. The exudate, rather than flowing freely, clings to the walls of the cavity and takes several minutes, depending on its viscosity, to shift position. For this reason, when the position of a patient is changed or the patient's neck is flexed or extended to position the head for special projections, *several minutes* should be allowed for the exudate to gravitate to the desired location before the exposure is made.

Although numerous sinus projections are possible, with each serving a special purpose, many are used only when required to demonstrate a specific lesion. The consensus is that five standard projections adequately demonstrate all of the paranasal sinuses in the majority of patients. The following steps are observed in preparing for these projections:

- Use a suitable protractor to check and adjust the position of the patient's head to ensure accurate positioning.
- Have the patient remove dentures, hairpins, and ornaments such as earrings and necklaces before proceeding with the examination.
- Because the patient's face is in contact with the IR holder or the IR itself for many of the radiographs, these items should be cleaned before the patient is positioned.

Even with the most hygienic patients, the hair and face on patients are naturally oily and leave a residue. If a patient is sick, the residue is worse. During positioning of the patient's head, the hair, mouth, nose, and eyes come in direct contact with the vertical grid device, tabletop, or IR. Medical asepsis can be promoted by placing a paper towel or sheet between the imaging surface and the patient. As standard procedure, the contacted area should be cleaned with a disinfectant before and after positioning.

Radiation Protection

Protection of the patient from unnecessary radiation is a professional responsibility of the radiographer. (See Chapter 1 for specific guidelines.) In this chapter, radiation shielding of the patient is not specified or illustrated because the professional community and the federal government have reported that placing a lead shield over the patient's pelvis does not significantly reduce gonadal exposure during radiography of the paranasal sinuses. However, shielding the abdomen of pregnant women is recommended.

Infants and children, however, should be protected by radiation shielding of the thyroid and thymus glands and the gonads. The protective lead shielding used to cover the thyroid and thymus glands can also assist in immobilizing the pediatric patient.

The most effective way to protect the patient from unnecessary radiation is to restrict the radiation beam by using *proper collimation*. Taking care to ensure that the patient is properly instructed and immobilized also reduces the chance of having to repeat the procedure, thereby further limiting the radiation exposure received by the patient.

PROJECTIONS REMOVED

Advances in CT have virtually eliminated the need for many projections of the sinuses. The following projections have been eliminated from this chapter. These projections may be reviewed in their entirety in the tenth edition and other previous editions of this atlas.

Ethmoidal, sphenoidal, and maxillary sinuses
- PA projections

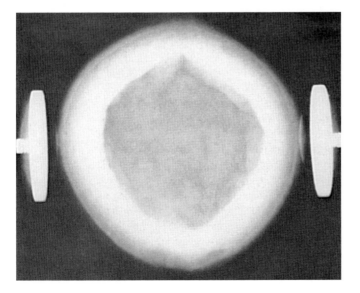

Fig. 22-8 Coconut, horizontal position: vertical central ray. Note no evidence of air-fluid level.

⚘ LATERAL PROJECTION
R or L position

Image receptor: 8 × 10 inch (18 × 24 cm)

Position of patient
- Seat the patient before a vertical grid device with the body placed in the RAO or LAO position so that the head can be adjusted in a true lateral position.

Position of part
- Rest the side of the patient's head on the vertical grid device, and adjust the head in a true lateral position. The midsagittal plane of the head is parallel with the plane of the IR, and the interpupillary line is perpendicular to the plane of the IR.
- The infraorbitomeatal line (IOML) is positioned horizontally to ensure proper extension of the head. This position places the IOML parallel with the transverse axis of the vertical grid device (Fig. 22-9).
- *Respiration:* Suspend.

Central ray
- Directed *horizontal,* entering the patient's head ½ to 1 inch (1.3 to 2.5 cm) posterior to the outer canthus
- Center the IR to the central ray.
- Immobilize the head.

Structures shown
A lateral projection shows the AP and superoinferior dimensions of the paranasal sinuses, their relationship to surrounding structures, and the thickness of the outer table of the frontal bone (Fig. 22-10).

When the lateral projection is to be used for preoperative measurements, it should be made at a 72-inch (183-cm) source–to–image-receptor distance to minimize magnification and distortion.

EVALUATION CRITERIA
The following should be clearly demonstrated:
- All four sinus groups, but the sphenoidal sinus is of primary importance
- No rotation of sella turcica
- Superimposed orbital roofs
- Superimposed mandibular rami
- Clearly visible sinuses
- Close beam restriction of sinus area
- Clearly visible air-fluid levels, if present

NOTE: If the patient is unable to assume the upright body position, a lateral projection can be obtained using the dorsal decubitus position. The horizontal beam enables fluid levels to be seen. Positioning of the part is the same, except for the IOML, which is vertical rather than horizontal.

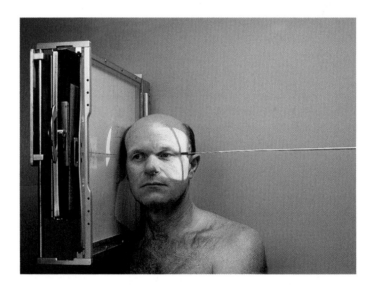

Fig. 22-9 Lateral sinuses.

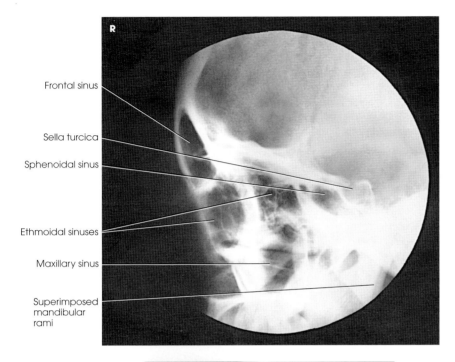

Frontal sinus

Sella turcica

Sphenoidal sinus

Ethmoidal sinuses

Maxillary sinus

Superimposed
mandibular
rami

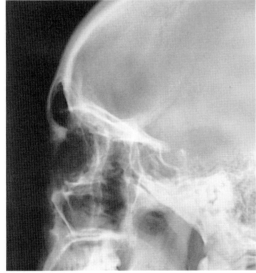

Fig. 22-10 Lateral sinuses.

♠ PA AXIAL PROJECTION

CALDWELL METHOD

Because sinus images should always be obtained with the patient in the upright body position and a *horizontal* direction of the central ray, the Caldwell method is easily modified when a head unit or other vertical grid device capable of angular adjustment is used. For the modification, all anatomic landmarks and localization planes remain unchanged.

Image receptor: 8 × 10 inch (18 × 24 cm)

Position of patient

- Seat the patient facing a vertical grid device.
- Center the midsagittal plane of the patient's body to the midline of the grid.

Position of part

Angled grid technique

- Before positioning the patient, tilt the vertical grid device down so that an angle of 15 degrees is obtained (Fig. 22-11, *A*).
- Rest the patient's nose and forehead on the vertical grid device, and center the nasion to the IR.
- Adjust the midsagittal plane and orbitomeatal line (OML) of the patient's head perpendicular to the plane of the IR.
- Note that this positioning places the OML perpendicular to the angled IR and 15 degrees from the horizontal central ray (Fig. 22-12, *A*).
- Immobilize the head.
- *Respiration:* Suspend.

Vertical grid technique

- When the vertical grid device cannot be angled, slightly extend the patient's neck, rest the tip of the nose on the grid device, and center the nasion to the IR.
- Position the patient's head so the OML forms an angle of 15 degrees with the horizontal central ray. For support, place a radiolucent sponge between the forehead and the grid device (see Figs. 22-11, *B* and 22-12, *B*).
- Adjust the midsagittal plane of the patient's head perpendicular to the plane of the IR.
- Immobilize the head.
- *Respiration:* Suspend.

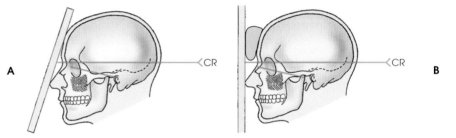

Fig. 22-11 PA axial sinuses: Caldwell method. **A,** IR tilted 15 degrees. **B,** Same projection with vertical IR.

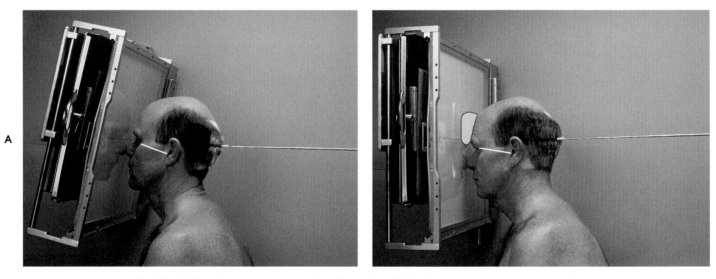

Fig. 22-12 PA axial sinuses: Caldwell method. **A,** IR tilted 15 degrees. **B,** Same projection with vertical IR.

Frontal and Anterior Ethmoidal Sinuses

Central ray

- Directed *horizontal* to exit the nasion. Note that the 15-degree relationship between the central ray and the OML remains the same for both techniques.
- Center the IR to the central ray.

NOTE: The *angled grid technique* is preferred because it brings the IR closer to the sinuses, thereby increasing resolution. Angulation of the grid device provides a natural position for placement of the patient's nose and forehead.

Structures shown

The angled grid technique and vertical grid technique demonstrate the frontal sinuses lying superior to the frontonasal suture; the anterior ethmoidal air cells lying on each side of the nasal fossae and immediately inferior to the frontal sinuses; and the sphenoidal sinuses projected through the nasal fossae just inferior to or between the ethmoidal air cells (Fig. 22-13). The dense petrous pyramids extend from the inferior third of the orbit inferiorly to obscure the superior third of the maxillary sinus. This projection is used primarily for demonstration of the frontal sinuses and anterior ethmoidal air cells.

The following should be clearly demonstrated:

- Equal distance between the lateral border of the skull and the lateral border of the orbits, indicating no rotation
- Petrous ridge symmetric on both sides
- Petrous ridge lying in the lower third of the orbit
- Frontal sinuses lying above the frontonasal suture and the anterior ethmoidal air cells lying above the petrous ridges
- Frontal and anterior ethmoidal air cells
- Clearly visible air-fluid levels, if present
- Close beam restriction of the sinus area

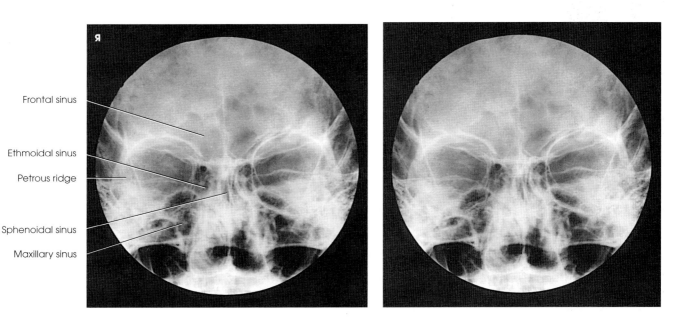

Fig. 22-13 PA axial sinuses.

Frontal sinus
Ethmoidal sinus
Petrous ridge
Sphenoidal sinus
Maxillary sinus

Frontal and anterior ethmoidal sinuses

♠ PARIETOACANTHIAL PROJECTION

WATERS METHOD

Image receptor: 8 × 10 inch (18 × 24 cm)

For the Waters method[1,2] the goal is to hyperextend the patient's neck just enough to place the dense petrosae immediately below the maxillary sinus floors (Fig. 22-14). When the neck is extended too little, the petrosae are projected over the inferior portions of the maxillary sinuses and thus obscure underlying pathologic conditions (Fig. 22-15). When the neck is extended too much, the maxillary sinuses are foreshortened and the antral floors are not demonstrated.

---

[1]Waters CA: A modification of the occipitofrontal position in the roentgen examination of the accessory nasal sinuses, *Arch Radiol Ther* 20:15, 1915.
[2]Mahoney HO: Head and sinus positions, *Xray Techn* 1:89, 1930.

Position of patient

- Place the patient seated in an upright position, facing the vertical grid device.
- Center the midsagittal plane of the patient's body to the midline of the grid device.

Position of part

- Because this position is relatively uncomfortable for the patient to hold, have the IR and equipment in position so that the examination can be performed quickly.
- Hyperextend the patient's neck to approximately the correct position, and then center the IR to the acanthion.

- Rest the patient's chin on the vertical grid device and adjust it so that the midsagittal plane is perpendicular to the plane of the IR.
- Using a protractor as a guide, adjust the head so that the OML forms an angle of 37 degrees from the plane of the IR (Figs. 22-14 and 22-16). As a positioning check for the average-shaped skull, the mentomeatal (MML) line should be approximately perpendicular to the IR plane.
- Immobilize the head.
- *Respiration:* Suspend.

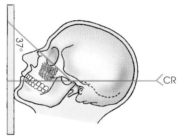

Fig. 22-14 Proper positioning. Petrous ridges are projected below maxillary sinuses.

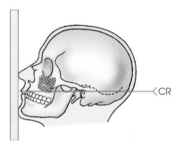

Fig. 22-15 Improper positioning. Petrous ridges are superimposed on maxillary sinuses.

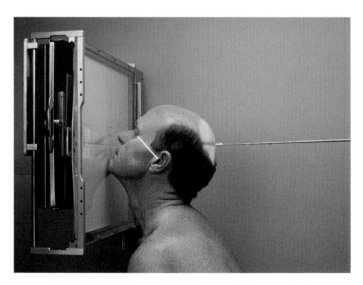

Fig. 22-16 Parietoacanthial sinuses: Waters method.

Maxillary Sinuses

Central ray
- *Horizontal* to the IR and exiting the acanthion

Structures shown
The image shows a parietoacanthial projection of the maxillary sinuses, with the petrous ridges lying inferior to the floor of the sinuses (Fig. 22-17). The frontal and ethmoidal air cells are distorted.

The Waters method is also used to demonstrate the foramen rotundum. The images of these structures are seen, one on each side, just inferior to the medial aspect of the orbital floor and superior to the roof of the maxillary sinuses.

The following should be clearly demonstrated:
- Petrous pyramids lying immediately inferior to the floor of the maxillary sinuses
- Equal distance between the lateral border of the skull and the lateral border of the orbit on both sides, indicating no rotation
- Orbits and maxillary sinuses symmetric on each side
- Maxillary sinuses
- Close beam restriction of the sinus area
- Clearly visible air-fluid levels, if present

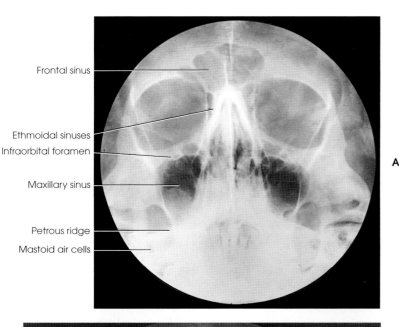

Frontal sinus

Ethmoidal sinuses
Infraorbital foramen

Maxillary sinus

Petrous ridge
Mastoid air cells

A

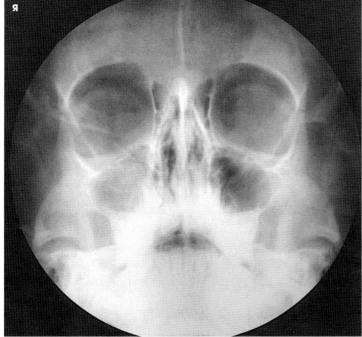

B

Fig. 22-17 A, Parietoacanthial sinuses: Waters method. **B,** Same projection. Note the clouded *(lighter)* appearance of the right maxillary sinus caused by fluid-filled sinus.

♠ PARIETOACANTHIAL PROJECTION

OPEN-MOUTH WATERS METHOD

Image receptor: 8 × 10 inch (18 × 24 cm)

This method provides an excellent demonstration of the sphenoidal sinuses projected through the open mouth. For patients who cannot be placed in position for the submentovertical (SMV) projec-tion, the *open-mouth Waters method* and lateral projections may be the only techniques for demonstrating the sphenoidal sinuses. Because the open-mouth position is relatively uncomfortable for the patient to hold, the radiographer must have the IR and equipment in position to perform the examination quickly.

Position of part

- Hyperextend the patient's neck to approximately the correct position, and then position the IR to the acanthion.

- Rest the patient's chin on the vertical grid device, and adjust it so that the midsagittal plane is perpendicular to the plane of the IR.
- Using a protractor as a guide, adjust the patient's head so that the OML forms an angle of 37 degrees from the plane of the IR. The MML will not be perpendicular (Fig. 22-18).
- Have the patient *slowly open the mouth wide open* while holding the position.
- Immobilize the head.
- *Respiration:* Suspend.

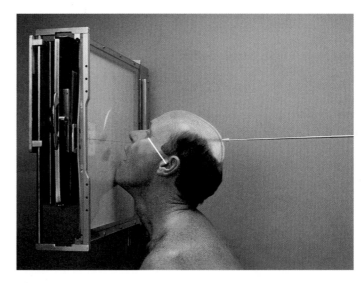

Fig. 22-18 Parietoacanthial sinuses: open-mouth Waters method.

Maxillary and Sphenoidal Sinuses

Central ray
- *Horizontal* to the IR and exiting the acanthion

Structures shown
The open-mouth Waters method demonstrates the sphenoidal sinuses projected through the open mouth along with the maxillary sinuses (Fig. 22-19).

EVALUATION CRITERIA

The following should be clearly demonstrated:
- Petrous pyramids lying immediately inferior to the floor of the maxillary sinuses
- Equal distance between the lateral border of the skull and the lateral border of the orbit on both sides, indicating no rotation
- Orbits and maxillary sinuses symmetric on each side
- Maxillary sinuses
- Close beam restriction of the sinus area
- Clearly visible air-fluid levels, if present
- Sphenoidal sinuses projected through the open mouth

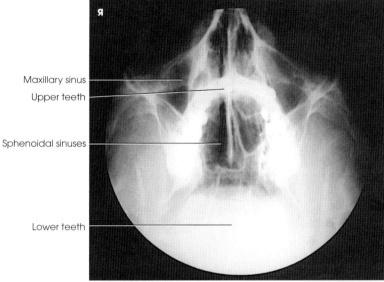

Maxillary sinus

Upper teeth

Sphenoidal sinuses

Lower teeth

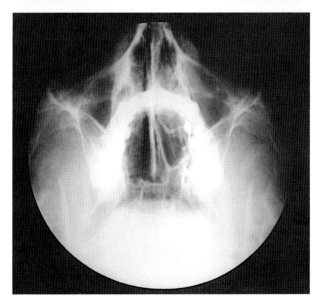

Fig. 22-19 Open-mouth Waters modification demonstrates the sphenoidal sinuses projected through the open mouth along with the maxillary sinuses.

Paranasal sinuses

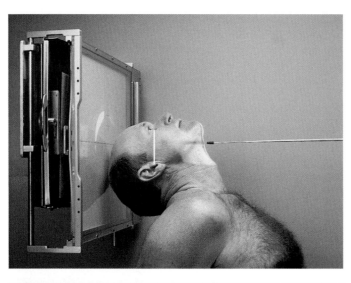

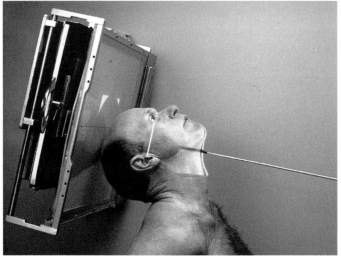

Fig. 22-20 SMV sinuses.

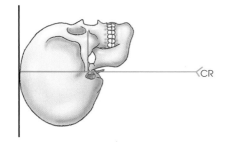

Fig. 22-21 Upright radiography, preferred position of skull.

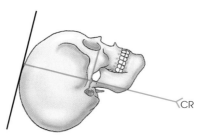

Fig. 22-22 Upright radiography.

▲ SUBMENTOVERTICAL PROJECTION

Image receptor: 8 × 10 inch (18 × 24 cm)

Position of patient

The success of the SMV projection depends on placing the IOML as nearly parallel as possible with the plane of the IR and directing the central ray perpendicular to the IOML.

The upright position is recommended for all paranasal sinus radiographs and is also more comfortable for the patient. The following steps are observed:

- Use a chair that supports the patient's back to obtain greater freedom in positioning the patient's body to place the IOML parallel with the IR.
- Seat the patient far enough away from the vertical grid device so that the head can be fully extended (Figs. 22-20, *A* and 22-21).
- If necessary to examine short-necked or hypersthenic patients, angle the vertical grid device downward to achieve a parallel relationship between the grid and the IOML (Figs. 22-20, *B* and 22-22). The disadvantage of angling the vertical grid device is that the central ray is not horizontal and air-fluid levels may not be demonstrated as easily as when the central ray is truly horizontal.

Position of part

- Hyperextend the patient's neck as far as possible, and rest the head on its vertex. If the patient's mouth opens during hyperextension, ask the patient to keep the mouth closed to move the mandibular symphysis anteriorly.
- Adjust the patient's head so that the midsagittal plane is perpendicular to the midline of the IR.
- Adjust the tube so that the central ray is perpendicular to the IOML (see Fig. 22-20).
- Immobilize the patient's head. In the absence of a head clamp, place a suitably backed strip of adhesive tape across the tip of the chin and anchor it to the sides of the radiographic unit. Do not put the adhesive surface directly on the patient's skin.
- *Respiration:* Suspend.

Central ray

- *Horizontal* and perpendicular to the IOML through the sella turcica. The central ray enters on the midsagittal plane approximately ¾ inch (1.9 cm) anterior to the level of the external acoustic meatus.

Structures shown

The SMV projection for the sinuses demonstrates a symmetric image of the anterior portion of the base of the skull. The sphenoidal sinus and ethmoidal air cells are shown (Fig. 22-23).

EVALUATION CRITERIA

The following should be clearly demonstrated:

- Equal distance from the lateral border of the skull to the mandibular condyles on both sides, indicating that the midsagittal plane is perpendicular (no tilt)
- Anterior frontal bone superimposed by mental protuberance, indicating that the IOML is parallel (full extension)
- Mandibular condyles anterior to petrous pyramids
- Clearly visible air-fluid levels, if present

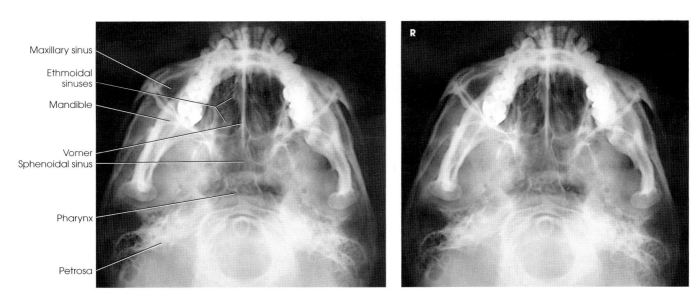

Maxillary sinus
Ethmoidal sinuses
Mandible
Vomer
Sphenoidal sinus
Pharynx
Petrosa

Fig. 22-23 SMV sinuses.

Ethmoidal and sphenoidal sinuses

23

MAMMOGRAPHY

VALERIE F. ANDOLINA

Orthogonal 90-degree mediolateral projection of the patient as in Fig. 23-70, demonstrating successful placement of the needle-wire system within the lesion (*arrow*). The lesion was found to be a 9-mm infiltrating ductal carcinoma.

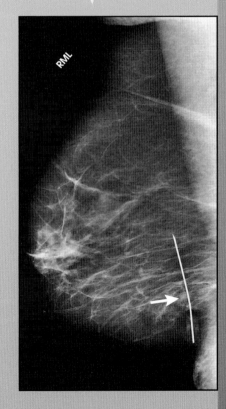

SUMMARY OF PROJECTIONS

PROJECTIONS, POSITIONS, AND METHODS

Page	Essential	Anatomy	Projection	Position	Method
422	▲	Breast	Craniocaudal		
424	▲	Breast	Mediolateral oblique		
428		Breast	Craniocaudal		IMPLANT
430		Breast	Craniocaudal		IMPLANT DISPLACED
432		Breast	Mediolateral oblique		IMPLANT
433		Breast	Mediolateral oblique		IMPLANT DISPLACED
441		Breast	Variable		MAGNIFICATION
442		Breast	Variable		SPOT COMPRESSION
444	▲	Breast	Mediolateral		
446		Breast	Lateromedial		
448	▲	Breast	Exaggerated craniocaudal		
450		Breast	Craniocaudal		CLEAVAGE
452		Breast	Craniocaudal		ROLL LATERAL
452		Breast	Craniocaudal		ROLL MEDIAL
454		Breast	Tangential		
456		Breast	Variable		COAT-HANGER
458		Breast	Caudocranial		
460		Breast	Mediolateral oblique		AXILLARY TAIL
462		Breast	Lateromedial oblique		
464		Breast	Superolateral to inferomedial oblique		

Icons in the Essential column indicate projections frequently performed in the United States and Canada. Students should be competent in these projections.

Principles of Mammography

INTRODUCTION AND HISTORICAL DEVELOPMENT

The worldwide incidence of breast cancer is increasing. In the United States, one in eight women who live to the age of 95 years will develop breast cancer sometime during her lifetime. Breast cancer is one of the most common malignancies diagnosed in women; only lung cancer kills more women overall. Research has failed to reveal the precise etiology of breast cancer, and only a few major factors, such as family history, are known to increase a woman's risk of developing the disease. Yet most women who develop breast cancer have no family history of the disease.

Despite its frequency, breast cancer is one of the most treatable cancers. Because this malignancy is most treatable when it is detected early, efforts have been directed toward developing breast cancer screening and early detection methods. Breast cancer mortality rates have declined by 2.3% per year from 1990 to 2000 in all women, with larger increases in women younger than 50 years of age. This is most likely the result of earlier detection and improved treatments.[1]

Mammography is the most important innovation in breast cancer control since the radical mastectomy was introduced by Halstead in 1898. The primary goal of mammography is to detect breast cancer before it is palpable. The combination of early detection, diagnosis, and treatment has resulted in a steady increase in survival rates. In fact, the overall mortality rate for breast cancer has finally decreased for American women.

[1]American Cancer Society: *Cancer facts and figures 2004*, Atlanta, 2004, American Cancer Society, p 9.

Before the radical mastectomy was introduced, breast cancer was considered a fatal disease. Fewer than 5% of patients survived 4 years after diagnosis, and the local recurrence rate for surgically treated breast cancer was higher than 80%. Radical mastectomy increased the 4-year survival rate to 40% and reduced the rate of local recurrence to approximately 10%. Although this was certainly a great step forward, no additional improvement in breast cancer survival rates occurred over the next 60 years. However, some of the principles of breast cancer management were developed and remain valid:

1. Patients in the early stage of the disease respond well to treatment.
2. Patients with advanced disease do poorly.
3. The earlier the diagnosis, the better the chances of survival.

Reflecting these principles, the theory of removing all palpable breast masses in hopes of finding earlier cancers was developed, and it was recognized that careful physical examination of the breast could detect some early breast cancers. However, most patients with breast cancer still were not diagnosed until their disease was advanced. This fact, coupled with the dismal breast cancer survival statistics, highlighted the need for a tool for the early detection of breast cancer. Mammography filled that need (Fig. 23-1).

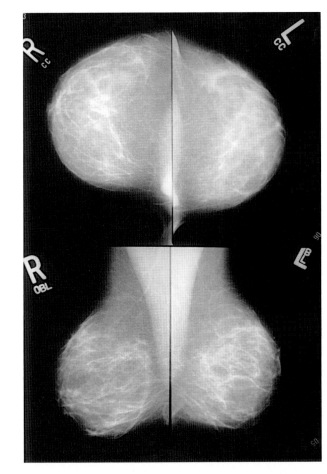

Fig. 23-1 A four-image, bilateral mammogram of a 37-year-old woman. Craniocaudal and mediolateral oblique projections demonstrate normal, symmetric breast parenchyma.

In 1913, Soloman, a German physician, reported the radiographic appearance of breast cancers. Using radiographic studies of cancerous breasts removed at surgery, he described the mechanism of how breast cancer spread. The first published radiograph of a living person's breast, made by Kleinschmidt, appeared in a 1927 German medical textbook on malignant tumors. Although publications on mammography appeared in South America, the United States, and Europe during the 1930s, the use of mammography for the diagnosis of breast cancer received little clinical interest. A few pioneers, including LeBorgne in Uruguay, Gershon-Cohen in the United States, and Gros in Germany, published excellent comparisons of mammographic and pathologic anatomy and developed some of the clinical techniques of mammography. At that time the significance of breast microcalcifications was also well understood.

By the mid-1950s, mammography was considered a reliable clinical tool because of such refinements as low-kilovoltage x-ray tubes with molybdenum targets and high-detail, industrial-grade x-ray film. During this time, Egan in the United States and Gros in Germany popularized the use of mammography for diagnosing and evaluating breast cancer. Breast xerography was introduced in the 1960s and was popularized by Wolfe and Ruzicka. Xerography substantially lowered the radiation dose received by the patient compared with the dose received using industrial-grade x-ray film (Fig. 23-2). Because many physicians found the xerographic images easier to understand and evaluate, xeromammography became widely used for evaluating breast disease. The first attempts at widespread population screening began at this time.

The combination of higher-resolution, faster-speed x-ray film and an intensifying screen was first introduced by the duPont Company. As a result, radiation exposure to the patient was reduced even more. Improved screen-film combinations were developed by both Kodak and duPont in 1975. By this time, extremely high-quality mammography images could be produced with very low patient radiation exposures. Since 1975, faster lower-dose films, magnification techniques, and grids for scatter reduction have been introduced. It is now known that high-quality mammography, careful physical examination, and monthly breast self-examination (BSE) can result in the detection of breast cancer at an early stage—when it is most curable.

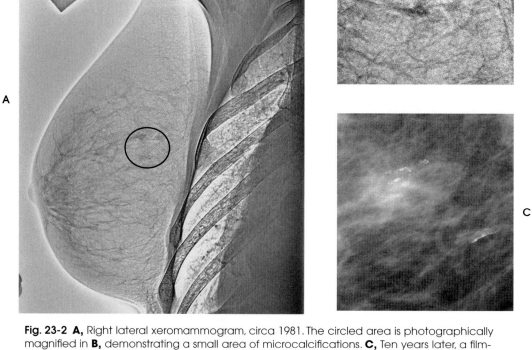

Fig. 23-2 A, Right lateral xeromammogram, circa 1981. The circled area is photographically magnified in **B,** demonstrating a small area of microcalcifications. **C,** Ten years later, a film-screen magnification study shows the same calcifications. This was proven to be ductal carcinoma in situ (DCIS) on biopsy.

The Breast Cancer Detection Demonstration Project (BCDDP) was implemented in 1973. In this project, 280,000 women underwent annual screening for breast cancer for 5 years at 29 locations throughout the United States. Organized by the American Cancer Society (ACS) and the National Cancer Institute (NCI), this project demonstrated unequivocally that screening, physical examination, mammography, and BSE could provide an early diagnosis. In the BCDDP, more than 41% of all the cancers were found using only mammography, and an even greater proportion of early breast cancers were found only with mammography. The BCDDP was not designed to demonstrate that *early* detection of breast cancer would lead to increased survival rates, but definite evidence from carefully controlled studies in The Netherlands, Sweden, and Germany showed that early diagnosis of breast cancer leads to an increase in curability. In the United States, the Health Insurance Plan study in New York City performed mammography screenings on women older than 50 years of age and demonstrated the same benefits in reduced mortality rates after early diagnosis of breast cancer.

Mammography must be performed well to be fully effective. In 1992, the Mammography Quality Standards Act (MQSA) was implemented to mandate the maintenance of high-quality breast cancer screening programs. The American College of Radiology (ACR) had been a proponent of high standards in breast imaging since 1967 and implemented an optional Mammography Accreditation Program in 1989. It was not until 1994 that mammography became the only radiographic examination to be fully regulated by the federal government. The MQSA requires formal training and continuing education for all members of the breast imaging team. In addition, imaging equipment must be inspected regularly, and all quality assurance activities must be documented. Facilities are also required to identify the individuals who are responsible for communicating mammogram results with the patient, providing follow-up, tracking patients, and monitoring outcomes. The goal of the MQSA is for high-quality mammography to be performed by those most qualified to do so and by those who are willing to accept full responsibility for providing that service with continuity of care.

RISK VS. BENEFIT

In the mid-1970s the media-influenced public perception was that radiation exposure from diagnostic x-rays would actually induce more breast cancers than would be detected. Although radiation dosage during a mammography examination has decreased dramatically since the 1970s, fear of radiation exposure still causes some women to refuse mammography, and many women who undergo the examination are concerned about exposure levels and the resultant risk of carcinogenesis. To assuage these fears, the radiographer must understand the relationship between breast irradiation and breast cancer, as well as the relative risks of mammography, in light of the natural incidence of breast cancer and the potential benefit of the examination. No direct evidence exists to suggest that the small doses of diagnostic x-rays used in mammography can induce breast cancer. It has been demonstrated, however, that large radiation doses can increase the incidence of breast cancer and that the risk is dose dependent. The evidence to support the increased risk of breast cancer from breast irradiation comes from studies of three groups of women in whom the incidence of breast cancer increased after they were exposed to large doses of radiation. These groups are as follows: (1) women exposed to the atomic bombs at Hiroshima and Nagasaki; (2) women with tuberculosis who received multiple fluoroscopic examinations of the chest; and (3) women who were treated with radiation for postpartum mastitis. However, the radiation dose received by these women (600 to 700 rads) was many times higher than the dose received from mammography.

Mean glandular dose (MGD) provides the best indicator of radiation risk to the patient. In 1997, the average MGD for a two-projection screen-film-grid mammogram for all facilities in the United States inspected under MQSA was 320 mrad.[1] Using that level as a gauge, the lifetime risk of mortality from mammography-induced radiation is 5 deaths per 1 million patients. In other terms, the risk received from having an x-ray mammogram using a screen-film combination is equivalent to smoking several cigarettes, driving 60 miles in an automobile, or being a 60-year-old man for 10 minutes.

An important observation in the previously mentioned population studies is that the breast tissue of females in their teenage years to early 20s seems to be much more sensitive to radiation than the breast tissue of women older than 30 years of age. Because breast irradiation is a concern, radiologic examinations need to be performed with only the radiation dose that is necessary for providing accurate detection.

---

[1]Haus AG: Screen-film and digital mammography image quality and radiation dose considerations, *Radiol Clin North Am* 38:871, 2000.

Principles of mammography

409

Mammography

BREAST CANCER SCREENING

The frequency with which women should undergo screening mammography depends on their age and personal risk of developing breast cancer. The current recommendations from the ACS and the ACR are that all women older than 40 years of age should undergo annual mammography and should continue yearly mammography for as long as they are in reasonably good health otherwise. A baseline examination made sometime before the onset of menopause is useful for comparison during subsequent evaluations. High-risk patients should consider beginning screening mammography at an earlier age.

The term *screening mammography* is applied to a procedure performed on an asymptomatic patient or a patient who presents without any known breast problems. For a procedure to be used as a screening method, it must meet the following criteria:
1. It must be simple.
2. It must be acceptable.
3. It must demonstrate high sensitivity.
4. It must demonstrate high specificity.
5. It must be reproducible.
6. It must be cost-effective.
7. It must have a low risk-vs.-benefit ratio.

Mammography is a relatively simple procedure that takes only about 15 minutes to complete. The acceptability of mammography, which is the only radiographic procedure used to screen cancer, has been confirmed in numerous studies. However, mammography cannot detect all cancerous lesions. Therefore an annual clinical breast examination is recommended by the ACS. Many physicians also recommend that women perform monthly BSEs. Even when mammography is performed properly, approximately 10% of cancers remain radiographically occult, particularly in the dense breast and the augmented breast. Even so, mammography has greater sensitivity and specificity for detecting breast tumors than any other currently available noninvasive diagnostic technique. When compared with magnetic resonance imaging (MRI), sonography, and digital techniques, mammography is more cost effective and more reproducible when quality control standards are maintained. Yet mammography must be performed properly to maintain these characteristics. As with other imaging modalities, high-quality mammography requires an extremely dedicated staff with the appropriate training and expertise.

Breast cancer screening studies have shown that early detection is essential to reducing mortality and that the most effective approach is to combine clinical breast examination with mammography at directed intervals. Although massive screening efforts initially could appear cost prohibitive, the actual cost of screening is, in the long term, much less than the expenses involved in caring for patients with advanced breast disease.

The preceding discussion describes the screening of patients who do not have significant breast symptoms. All patients with clinical evidence of significant or potentially significant breast disease should undergo a *diagnostic mammogram* and subsequent workup as necessary. Diagnostic mammograms are problem-solving examinations in which specific projections are obtained to rule out cancer or to demonstrate a suspicious area seen on the routine screening projections. They are also indicated if a woman presents with a palpable mass or other symptom. The area of interest may be better demonstrated using image enhancement methods such as focal spot compression and a magnification technique. Further workup may be necessary if mammography does not demonstrate a correlative mass. Alternative imaging modalities such as sonography are often used to complete a successful workup. The radiologist and radiographer direct and conduct the diagnostic mammogram to facilitate an accurate interpretation.

Although most diagnostic mammograms conclude with probable benign findings, some women are asked to return for subsequent mammograms in 3 or 6 months to assess for interval changes. Other women must consult with a specialist or surgeon about possible options such as fine-needle aspiration biopsy (FNAB), core biopsy, or excisional biopsy.

Although it is an excellent tool for detecting breast cancer, mammography does *not* diagnose breast cancer. Some lesions may appear consistent with malignant disease but turn out to be completely benign conditions. Therefore breast cancer can be diagnosed only by a pathologist through the evaluation of tissue extracted from the lesion. After interpreting the diagnostic workup, the radiologist must carefully determine whether surgical intervention is warranted.

RISK FACTORS

Assessing a woman's risk for developing breast cancer is a complicated process. An accurate patient history must be elicited to identify the potential individual risk factors. The radiologist considers these known risks after interpreting the mammogram. Except for gender, factors that are known to influence the development of breast cancer include age, hormonal history, and family history.

Age

The incidence of breast cancer increases with age.

Hormonal history

Hormones influence the glandular tissue of the breast during breast development, pregnancy, and lactation; however, hormone levels decline at the onset of menopause. As a result, the glandular breast tissue is more sensitive to carcinogens during menarche. High-risk women include those with early menses (beginning before the age of 12 years), late menopause (occurring after 52 years of age), first birth after age 30 years, and nulliparity.

Family history

A woman whose daughter, sister, or mother previously developed breast cancer, especially at an early age, is at higher risk of developing the disease. However, studies have shown that only 13.6% of known breast cancers are found in women with a family history of the disease. Furthermore, a true genetic disorder has been identified in only 5% to 10% of women with breast cancer.[1] In 1994, researchers isolated two breast cancer genes—BRCA1 and BRCA2. Subsequently, commercial screening tests were developed. However, the accuracy of these tests has not yet been clinically accepted. In addition, widespread genetic testing raises ethical concerns associated with identifying appropriate candidates for genetic screening and determining what is done with the information derived from the testing.

---

[1]National Cancer Institute: www.cancer.gov. Accessed August 16, 2006.

Breast

The terms *breast* and *mammary gland* are often used synonymously. Anatomy textbooks tend to use the term *mammary gland,* whereas radiography textbooks tend to use the term *breast.* The breasts (mammary glands) are lobulated glandular structures located within the *superficial fascia* of the anterolateral surface of the thorax of both males and females. The mammary glands divide the superficial fascia into anterior and posterior components. Therefore the mammary tissue is completely surrounded by fascia and is enveloped between the anterior and posterior layers of the superficial fascia. In females, the breasts are secondary sex characteristics and function as accessory glands to the reproductive system by producing and secreting milk during lactation. In males, the breasts are rudimentary and without function. Male breasts are only rarely subject to abnormalities, such as neoplasms, that require radiologic evaluation.

Female breasts vary considerably in size and shape, depending on the amount of fat and glandular tissue and the condition of the suspensory ligaments. Each breast is usually cone-shaped, with the base or posterior surface of the breast overlying the *pectoralis major* and *serratus anterior* muscles. These muscles extend from the second or third rib inferiorly to the sixth or seventh rib and from near the lateral margin of the sternum laterally toward the anterior axillary plane. An additional portion of breast tissue, the *axillary prolongation* or *axillary tail* (AT), extends from the upper lateral base of the breasts into the *axillary fossa* (Fig. 23-3).

The breast tapers anteriorly from the base, ending in the *nipple* that is surrounded by a circular area of pigmented skin called the *areola.* The breasts are supported by *Cooper's ligaments,* suspensory ligaments that extend from the posterior layers of the superficial fascia through the anterior fascia into the subcutaneous tissue and skin. It is the condition of these ligaments, and not the relative fat content, that gives the breasts their firmness or lack of firmness.

The adult female breast consists of 15 to 20 *lobes,* which are distributed such that more lobes are superior and lateral than inferior and medial. Each lobe is divided into many *lobules,* which are the basic structural units of the breast. The lobules contain the glandular elements, or *acini.* Each lobule consists of several acini, a number of draining ducts, and the interlobular stroma or connective tissue. These elements are part of the breast parenchyma and participate in hormonal changes. By the late teenage years to early 20s, each breast contains several hundred lobules. The lobules tend to decrease in size with increasing age and particularly after pregnancy—a normal process called *involution.*

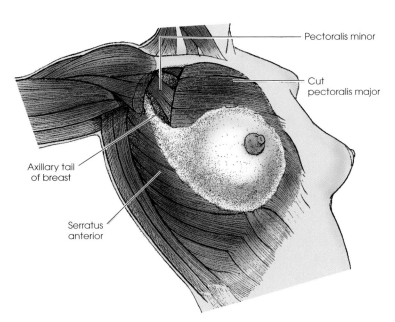

Fig. 23-3 Relationship of the breast to the chest wall. Note the extension of breast tissue posteriorly into the axilla.

The openings of each *acinus* join to form *lactiferous ductules* that drain the lobules, which in turn join to form 15 to 20 lactiferous ducts, one for each lobe. Several lactiferous ducts may combine before emptying directly into the nipple. As a result, there are usually fewer duct openings on the nipple than there are breast ducts and lobes. The individual lobes are incompletely separated from each other by the Cooper's ligaments. The space between the lobes also contains fatty tissue and additional connective tissue. A layer of fatty tissue surrounds the gland, except in the area immediately under the areola and nipple (Fig. 23-4).

The lymphatic vessels of the breast drain laterally into the *axillary lymph nodes* and medially into the chain of *internal mammary lymph nodes* (see Fig. 25-6). Approximately 75% of the lymph drainage is toward the axilla, and 25% of the drainage is toward the internal mammary chain. The number of axillary nodes varies from 12 to 30 (sometimes more). The axilla is occasionally radiographed during breast examinations to evaluate the axillary nodes. The internal mammary nodes are situated behind the sternum and manubrium and, if enlarged, are occasionally visible on a lateral chest radiograph.

The radiographer should take into account breast anatomy and patient body habitus to successfully image as much breast tissue as possible. Cassette size must be appropriate for the breast being imaged. Larger breasts will not be entirely demonstrated on small image receptors (IRs). Conversely, smaller breasts should not be imaged on larger cassettes because (1) other body structures may interfere with the compression device and thus produce an unacceptable image and (2) the pectoral muscle and the skin are likely to become taut from upward stretching of the arm, preventing the breast tissue from being completely pulled onto the film.

The natural mobility of the breast is also an important consideration. The lateral and inferior aspects of the breast are mobile, whereas the medial and superior aspects are fixed. The breast should always be positioned by moving the mobile aspects toward the fixed tissues. Likewise, the radiographer should avoid moving the compression paddle against fixed tissues because this will cause less breast tissue to be imaged.

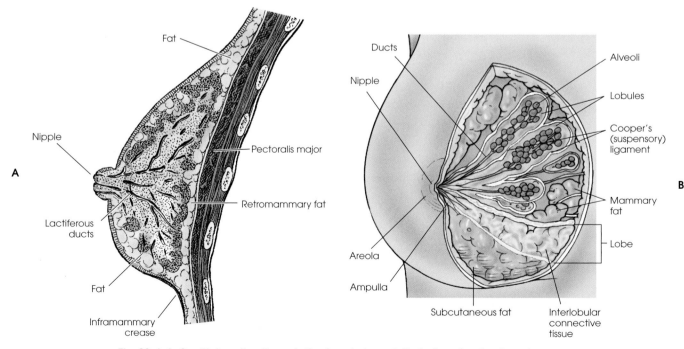

Fig. 23-4 A, Sagittal section through the female breast, illustrating structural anatomy. **B,** Breast: anterior view.

Tissue Variations

The *glandular* and *connective tissues* of the breasts are soft tissue–density structures. The ability to demonstrate radiographic detail within the breast depends on the fat within and between the breast lobules and the fat surrounding the breasts. The postpubertal adolescent breast contains primarily dense connective tissue and casts a relatively homogeneous radiographic image with little tissue differentiation (Fig. 23-5). The development of glandular tissue decreases radiographic contrast. During pregnancy, significant hypertrophy of glands and ducts occurs within the breasts. This change causes the breasts to become extremely dense and opaque. After the end of lactation, considerable involution of glandular and parenchymal tissues usually occurs and these tissues are replaced with increased amounts of *fatty tissue*. Fat accumulation varies markedly among individuals. This normal fat accumulation significantly increases the natural radiographic contrast within the breasts (Fig. 23-6). The breasts of patients with fibrocystic parenchymal conditions may not undergo this involution (Fig. 23-7).

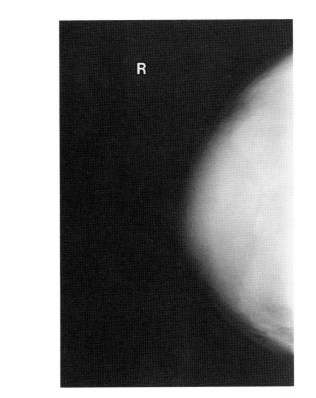

Fig. 23-5 Craniocaudal projection of normal breast in a 19-year-old woman who has never been pregnant. Note the dense glandular tissues with small amounts of fat. In women who do not become pregnant, the breasts may remain dense for many years.

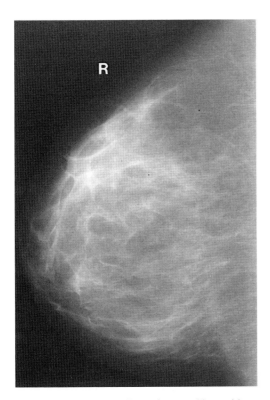

Fig. 23-6 Mediolateral projection of normal breast in a 24-year-old woman who has had two pregnancies. Note decreased volume of glandular tissue and increased amount of fat.

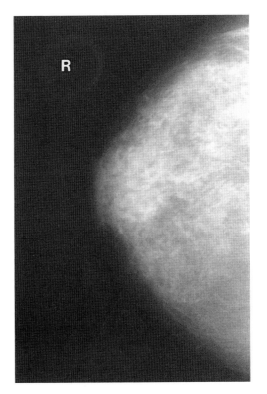

Fig. 23-7 Craniocaudal projection of breast of a 42-year-old woman with fibrocystic condition, illustrating prominent dilated ducts.

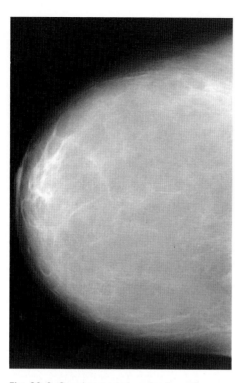

Fig. 23-8 Craniocaudal projection of normal breasts of a 68-year-old woman. Most of the glandular tissue is atrophic. Some glandular tissue remains in the lateral breast posteriorly and in the retroareolar area.

The glandular and connective tissue elements of the breast can regenerate as needed for subsequent pregnancies. After menopause, the glandular and stromal elements undergo gradual atrophy (Fig. 23-8). External factors such as surgical menopause and ingestion of hormones may inhibit this normal process. From puberty through menopause, mammotrophic hormones influence cyclic changes in the breasts. Thus the glandular and connective tissues are in a state of constant change (Fig. 23-9).

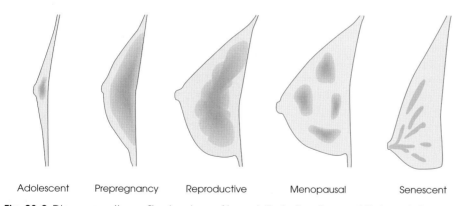

Adolescent   Prepregnancy   Reproductive   Menopausal   Senescent

Fig. 23-9 Diagrammatic profile drawings of breast, illustrating the most likely variation and distribution of radiographic density *(shaded areas)* related to the normal life cycle from adolescence to senescence. This normal sequence may be altered by external factors such as pregnancy, hormone medications, surgical menopause, and fibrocystic breast condition.

EXPOSURE TECHNIQUE CHART ESSENTIAL PROJECTIONS

MAMMOGRAPHY

Part	cm	kVp*	tm	mA†	mAs	AEC	SID	IR	Dose‡ (mrad)
Mammogram:									
CC§	5	25		100		●	60 cm	18 × 24 cm	910
MLO§	5	25		100		●	60 cm	18 × 24 cm	1030
ML§	5	25		100		●	60 cm	18 × 24 cm	1030
XCCL§	5	25		100		●	60 cm	18 × 24 cm	910

CC, Craniocaudal; *MLO*, mediolateral oblique; *ML*, mediolateral; *XCCL*, exaggerated craniocaudal.
*kVp values are for a one-phase, high frequency generator.
†Used with the 0.3-mm focal spot.
‡Relative doses for comparison use. All doses are skin entrance for average adult at cm indicated.
§Bucky, 4:1 grid. Screen/film speed 180.

SUMMARY OF ANATOMY

Mammary gland (breast)	axillary fossa	axillary lymph nodes
superficial facia	nipple	internal mammary
pectoralis major muscle	areola	lymph nodes
serratus anterior muscle	Cooper's ligaments	glandular tissue
axillary prolongation (axillary tail)	lobes	connective tissue
	acini	fatty tissue
	lactiferous ductules	

SUMMARY OF PATHOLOGY

Condition	Definition
Breast Carcinoma	Malignant new growth composed of epithelial cells
Calcification	Deposit of calcium salt in tissue; characteristics may suggest either benign or malignant processes
Cyst	Closed epithelial sac containing fluid or a semisolid substance
Epithelial Hyperplasia	Proliferation of the epithelium of the breast
Fibrosis	Formation of fibrous tissue in the breast
Tumor	New tissue growth where cell proliferation is uncontrolled
Fibroadenoma	Benign tumor of the breast containing fibrous elements
Intraductal Papilloma	A benign, neoplastic papillary growth in a duct

Tissue variations

415

Breast Imaging

EVOLUTION OF MAMMOGRAPHY SYSTEMS

Because the breast is composed of tissues with very similar densities and effective atomic numbers, little difference in attenuation is noticed when conventional x-ray equipment and technique are used. Therefore manufacturers have developed imaging systems that optimally and consistently produce images with high contrast and resolution.

Diligent research and development began in the 1960s, and the first dedicated mammography unit was introduced in 1967 by CGR (France) (Fig. 23-10). In the 1970s, increased awareness of the elevated radiation doses prevalent in mammography served as the catalyst for the rapid progression of imaging systems. In the 1970s and early 1980s, xeromammography, named for the Xerox Corporation that developed it, was widely used (see Fig. 23-2). This method used much less radiation than the direct-exposure silver-based films that were available. Eventually, film manufacturers introduced several generations of mammography film-screen systems that used even less exposure and improved tissue visualization. Each subsequent new system showed improvement in contrast and resolution while minimizing patient dose.

In the 1980s, the ACR accreditation program established quality standards for breast imaging to optimize mammographic equipment, processors, and screen-film systems to ensure the production of high-quality images. This program was expanded in the 1990s to include quality control and personnel qualifications and training. The voluntary ACR program has become the model from which MQSA operates, and the ACR has been instrumental in designing the clinical practice guidelines for quality mammography in the United States. The evolution of mammography has resulted in the implementation of radiographic systems designed specifically for breast imaging.

MAMMOGRAPHY EQUIPMENT

In recent years, equipment manufacturers have produced dedicated mammography units that have high-frequency generators, a variety of tube and filter materials, focal spot sizes that allow tissue magnification, and specialized grids to help improve image quality, as well as streamlined designs and ergonomic patient positioning aids.

The high-frequency generators offer more precise control of kilovolt (peak) (kVp), milliamperes (mA), and exposure time. The linearity and reproducibility of the radiographic exposures using high-frequency generators is uniformly excellent. The greatest benefit of these generators, however, may be the efficient waveform output that produces a higher effective energy x-ray beam per set kVp and mA. High-frequency generators are not as bulky, and they can be installed within the single-standing mammography unit operating on single-phase incoming line power, thus facilitating easy installation and creating a less intimidating appearance (Fig. 23-11).

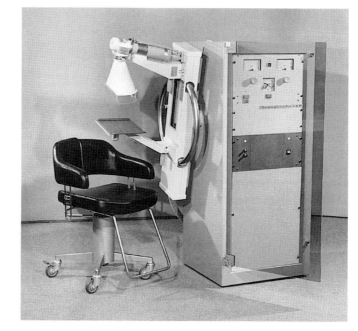

Fig. 23-10 First dedicated mammography system: Senographe by CGR (France).

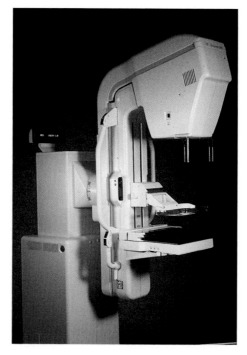

Fig. 23-11 Senographe DMR by General Electric (Milwaukee, Wis).

Specialized grids were developed for mammography during the 1980s to reduce scatter radiation and increase the image contrast in mammography. Most units employ moving linear focused grids, but some manufacturers have developed very specialized grids. For example, the Hologic (Lorad) High Transmission Cellular (HTC) Grid employs a honeycomb-pattern, multidirectional design. All dedicated mammography units today, with the exception of slit-scan digital units, still employ grids.

As manufacturers of dedicated mammography equipment sought to improve image quality, they have tried many different combinations of tube and filter materials. The most widely accepted combinations used at this time are Molybdenum target with Molybdenum filter (Mo/Mo), Molybdenum target with Rhodium filter (Mo/Rh), or Rhodium target with Rhodium filter (Rh/Rh). Mo/Mo is used most often, but Mo/Rh and Rh/Rh are used for better penetration of more dense, thick-tissued breasts.

As manufacturers sought to improve image quality, they knew that technologists and physicians were also interested in the comfort of their patients. They worked to make the examination more tolerable for patients, more ergonomically acceptable, and more efficient for the technologist performing the examination, while developing positioning aids to increase visualization of the tissue. Some of these include the obvious: the more rounded corners on Bucky devices and compression paddles, the automatic release of compression after exposure, and the foot pedal controls.

METHOD OF EXAMINATION

It is advisable to dress patients in open-front gowns because the breast must be bared for the examination. Due to the sensitivity of the radiographic films and techniques used for mammography, the image will reveal even the slightest wrinkle in any cloth covering. Patients should remove any deodorant and powder from the axilla region and breast because these substances can resemble calcifications on the resultant image. Before the breast is radiographed, a complete history is taken, and a careful physical assessment is performed, noting all biopsy scars, palpable masses, suspicious thickenings, skin abnormalities, and nipple alterations (Fig. 23-12).

NAME

Department of Diagnostic Imaging

M.R.#

MAMMOGRAPHY QUESTIONNAIRE

Please answer the following questions:

Today's date: _____

1. Your current age: _____

Age at menopause: _____

2. Have you ever had a mammogram? ☐ Yes ☐ No   Last mammogram was in _____ (year)
   Where? _____

   Your signature will allow the release of prior mammograms should they be needed.

   Signature: _____

3. Family history of breast cancer: (please √) ☐ Mother ☐ Sister ☐ Grandmother ☐ Aunt ☐ Daughter
   Was breast cancer found: ☐ Before menopause? ☐ After menopause?

4. Are you taking birth control pills or other female hormones? ☐ Yes ☐ No   Since: _____

5. Have you had your breasts examined by a physician or nurse in the past year? ☐ Yes ☐ No

6. Do you have breast implants? ☐ Yes ☐ No

7. PROBLEMS:
   A. Have you had prior breast surgery/biopsy?..... ☐ Yes ☐ No — ☐ Right ☐ Left
      If yes, when? _____
      Was your biopsy positive for cancer?.............. ☐ Yes ☐ No — ☐ Right ☐ Left
      Have you had radiation therapy?................... ☐ Yes ☐ No — ☐ Right ☐ Left

   B. Do you have breast lumps?.............................. ☐ Yes ☐ No — ☐ Right ☐ Left

   C. Is there pain in the breast?............................... ☐ Yes ☐ No — ☐ Right ☐ Left

   D. Do you have any skin or nipple discharge?..... ☐ Yes ☐ No — ☐ Right ☐ Left

   E. If you answered "yes" to any of the above, please localize area on the diagram below.
      (The technologist can assist you with this.)

Lump = "O"
Surgery/scar = "–"
Skin change = "#"
Mole = " • "

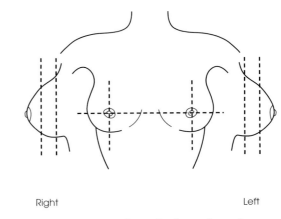

Right   Left

Fig. 23-12 Sample mammography patient questionnaire.

(Courtesy The Permanente Medical Group, Inc., Richmond, Calif.)

Both breasts are routinely radiographed obtaining craniocaudal (CC) and mediolateral oblique (MLO) projections. Image enhancement methods such as spot compression and magnification technique are often useful. It is sometimes necessary to enhance images or vary the projections in order to better characterize lesions and calcifications. In symptomatic patients, the examination should not be limited to the symptomatic breast. Both breasts should be examined for comparison purposes and because significant radiographic findings may be demonstrated in a clinically normal breast.

EXAMINATION PROCEDURES

This section describes procedures for conducting mammographic examinations using dedicated systems. The following steps should be observed:

- If possible, examine previous mammographic studies of patients who are undergoing subsequent mammography screening. These images should be evaluated for positioning, compression, and exposure factors to determine whether any improvement in image quality is required for the current study. Then position the breast consistently so that any lesion can be accurately localized and a valid comparison can be made with prior studies.
- Determine the correct film size for the patient, and use the smallest possible size to fully image all of the breast tissue. Positioning the breast on a film that is too large will cause the skin and muscles to overextend, reducing the amount of posterior tissue imaged.
- Explain the procedure simply and completely to the patient before beginning the examination. It should never be assumed that the patient is fully aware of what the mammographer is about to do, even if the patient has had prior examinations.
- In many cases, the routine projections will not sufficiently demonstrate all of the breast tissue and additional projections may be necessary. To allay patient concerns, the mammographer should explain to the patient *before* beginning the procedure why additional projections are sometimes needed and that they do not necessarily indicate a potential problem.
- Before positioning the patient's breast and applying compression, consider the natural mobility of the breast so that patient discomfort can be minimized. The inferior and lateral portions of the breast are mobile, whereas the superior and medial portions are fixed. Whenever possible, the mobile tissues should be moved toward the fixed tissues.
- For each of the two basic breast projections, ensure that the breast is firmly supported and adjusted so that the nipple is directed forward.
- Profile the nipple, if possible. Obtaining an image of the posterior breast tissue should be the primary consideration, and positioning of the nipple in profile is not always possible. An additional projection to profile the nipple can be obtained if necessary. Alternatively, a marker may be used to clearly locate the nipple that is not in profile, in which case an additional image may not be needed.
- Apply proper compression to the breast. Compression is an important factor in achieving a high-quality mammogram. The primary objective of compression is to produce uniform breast thickness from the nipple to the most posterior

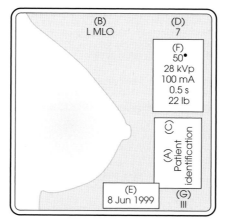

Fig. 23-13 Correct labeling of mammography image: MLO projection.

TABLE 23-1

Labeling codes for mammographic positioning

Projection/method	Labeling code	Purpose
Craniocaudal	CC	Routine
Mediolateral oblique	MLO	Routine
Implant displaced	ID	Augmented breast
Spot compression		Define
Magnification technique	M (used as prefix)	Define
Mediolateral	ML	Localize; define
Lateromedial	LM	Localize; define
Exaggerated craniocaudal	XCCL	Localize
CC for cleavage	CV	Define
CC with roll	RL (rolled lateral) and RM (rolled medial) (both used as suffix)	Localize; define Localize; define
Tangential	TAN	Localize; define
Caudocranial	FB	Define
MLO for axillary tail	AT	Localize; define
Lateromedial oblique	LMO	
Superolateral to inferomedial oblique	SIO	Define

From Bassett L et al, editors: *Quality determinants of mammography,* AHCPR Pub No 95-0632, Rockville, Md, 1994, U.S. Department of Health and Human Services.

aspect of the breast. Properly applied compression spreads the breast so that the tissue thickness is more evenly distributed over the image and better separation of the glandular elements is achieved. A rigid, radiolucent mammography compression paddle facilitates breast compression. Generally, compression is applied initially using a hands-free control, and then applied manually during the final phase of compression. The compression should be taut but not painful. The skin of the properly compressed breast should feel tight when lightly tapped with the fingertips. When evaluating images, compare the degree of compression with that in previous mammograms and note any variations. If a patient is unable to tolerate an adequate amount of compression, document this information on the patient history form for the radiologist.

- Place identification markers (Fig. 23-13) according to the following standard convention:
  A. Before processing, photographically expose a permanent identification label that includes the facility's name and address, the date of the examination, and the patient's name, age, date of birth, and medical number on the image. Include the initials of the person performing the examination on the identification label (C).
  B. On the cassette near the patient's axilla, place a radiopaque marker indicating both the side examined and the projection used (Table 23-1).
  C. Label the mammography cassette with an identification number (Arabic numeral is suggested by the ACR).

- Mammography film labeling may also include the following:
  D. A separate date sticker or perforation
  E. A label indicating the technical factors used: kVp, milliampere-seconds, target material, degree of obliquity, density setting, exposure time, compression thickness, etc. This is often included on the automatic identification labeling system that most manufacturers now offer with their units.
  F. Facilities with more than one unit must identify the mammographic unit used (Roman numerals are suggested by the ACR).

- For patients with palpable masses, a radiopaque (BB or X-spot) marker may be used to identify the location of the mass. A different type of radiopaque marker may be used to identify skin lesions, scars, or moles. This is determined by the policy of the facility.

- When using automatic exposure control (AEC), position the variable-position detector at the chest wall, the mid-breast, or the anterior breast, depending on breast composition and size. The appropriate location of the AEC detector must be determined for each individual patient. If possible, the detector should be placed under the most glandular portion of the breast, usually just posterior to the nipple.

- When reviewing images, assess contrast and density for optimal differentiation of breast tissues. Anatomic markers should be visible. The projections of one breast should be compared with the same projections of the contralateral breast to evaluate symmetry and consistency of positioning. All images should be absent of motion blur, artifacts, and skin folds. Images must be evaluated for potentially suspicious lesions and calcifications that may require image enhancement methods.

- To evaluate whether sufficient breast tissue is demonstrated, the radiographer should measure the depth of the breast from the nipple to the chest wall on both the CC and MLO projections. The posterior nipple line (PNL) is an imaginary line that is "drawn" obliquely from the nipple to the pectoralis muscle, or edge of the image, whichever comes first on the MLO projection. On the CC projection, the PNL is "drawn" from the nipple to the chest wall, or to the edge of the image, whichever comes first. The PNL on the CC should be within 1 cm of depth of the PNL on the MLO projection (Fig. 23-14).

- Between examinations, use a disinfectant to clean the cassette tray surface, compression paddle, patient handle grips, and face guard.

- If practical, a heating pad may be used to warm the cassette tray surface to enhance patient comfort.

- Remember that mammography is a team effort involving both the patient and the mammographer. Therefore acknowledge the individual needs of each patient to facilitate the cooperation and trust necessary to successfully complete the procedure. The nature of the interaction between the radiographer and the patient will more than likely determine whether the patient chooses to have subsequent mammograms.

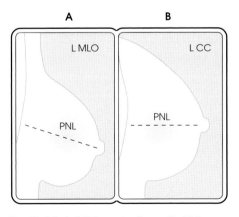

Fig. 23-14 A, MLO projection with PNL drawn. **B,** CC projection with PNL drawn. The PNL of the CC projection should be within 1 cm of the PNL of the MLO projection.

Summary of Mammography Projections

Before beginning to learn mammography projections, the student of radiography should carefully study the illustrative summary of mammography projections shown in the box. Familiarity with the different projection names and abbreviations will enhance the student's understanding of the detailed discussions of the projections presented in this chapter.

DESCRIPTIVE TERMINOLOGY

For the referring physician, the technologist and the radiologist to all communicate efficiently regarding an area of concern within a breast, descriptive terminology has been developed. When describing an area of concern, the laterality (right or left) must accompany the description (Fig. 23-15).

The breast is divided into four quadrants: the upper-outer (UOQ), lower-outer (LOQ), upper-inner (UIQ), and lower-inner (LIQ). Clock-time is also used to describe the location of a specific area of concern within the breast. Note that 2:00 in the right breast is in the UIQ, whereas 2:00 in the left breast is in the UOQ. This opposite labeling applies to all clock-times; therefore it is important to identify the correct breast, clock-time, and quadrant. Also note the distance of the abnormality from the nipple, which is the only fixed point of reference in the breast. The terms *subareolar* and *peri-areolar* describe the area directly beneath the nipple, and near (or around) the nipple area respectively.

Routine Projections of the Breast

Mammography is routinely performed using the CC and MLO projections.

ILLUSTRATIVE SUMMARY OF MAMMOGRAPHY PROJECTIONS

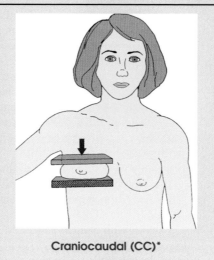

Craniocaudal (CC)*

Mediolateral oblique (MLO)*

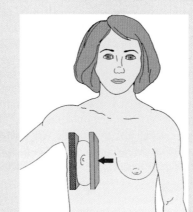

Mediolateral (ML)*

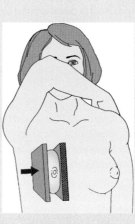

Lateromedial (LM)

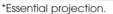

*Essential projection.

ILLUSTRATIVE SUMMARY OF MAMMOGRAPHY PROJECTIONS—cont'd

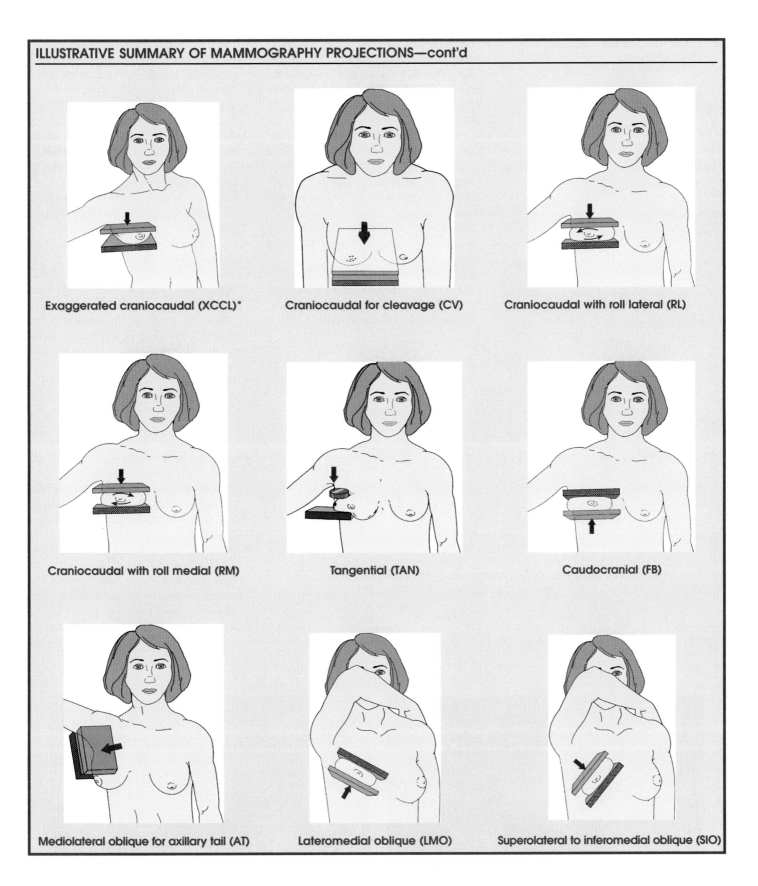

Exaggerated craniocaudal (XCCL)*

Craniocaudal for cleavage (CV)

Craniocaudal with roll lateral (RL)

Craniocaudal with roll medial (RM)

Tangential (TAN)

Caudocranial (FB)

Mediolateral oblique for axillary tail (AT)

Lateromedial oblique (LMO)

Superolateral to inferomedial oblique (SIO)

♠ CRANIOCAUDAL (CC) PROJECTION

Image receptor: 18 × 24 cm or 24 × 30 cm

Position of patient

- Have the patient stand facing the cassette holder, or seat the patient on an adjustable stool facing the holder.

Position of part

- While standing on the medial side of the breast to be imaged, elevate the inframammary fold to its maximum height.
- Adjust the height of the cassette to the level of the inferior surface of the patient's breast.

- Use both hands to gently pull the breast onto the cassette holder while instructing the patient to press the thorax against the cassette holder. Have the patient lean slightly forward from the waist.
- Keep the breast perpendicular to the chest wall. The technologist should use his or her fingertips to gently pull the posterior tissue forward onto the IR.
- Center the breast over the AEC detector, with the nipple in profile if possible.
- Immobilize the breast with one hand, being careful not to remove this hand until compression begins.
- Use the other hand to drape the opposite breast over the corner of the cassette. This maneuver improves demonstration of the medial tissue.

- Have the patient hold onto the grab bar with the contralateral hand. This helps steady the patient as you continue positioning.
- Placing your arm against the patient's back with your hand on the shoulder of the affected side, make certain her shoulder is relaxed and in external rotation.
- Rotate the patient's head away from the affected side.
- Lean the patient toward the machine, and rest the patient's head against the face guard.
- Make certain no other objects obstruct the path of the beam.
- With the hand on the patient's shoulder, gently slide the skin up over the clavicle.
- Using the hand that is anchoring the patient's breast, pull the lateral tissue on the cassette holder without sacrificing medial tissue.
- Inform the patient that compression of the breast will be used. Bring the compression paddle into contact with the breast while sliding the hand toward the nipple.
- Slowly apply compression until the breast feels taut.
- Check the medial and lateral aspects of the breast for adequate compression.
- Instruct the patient to indicate whether the compression becomes uncomfortable.
- After full compression is achieved and checked, move the AEC detector to the appropriate position, and instruct the patient to stop breathing (Fig. 23-16).
- Make the exposure.
- Release breast compression immediately.

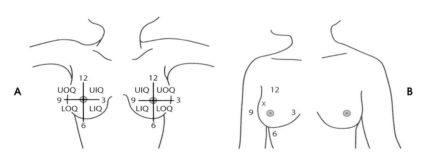

Fig. 23-15 A, Each breast is viewed as a clock and divided into four quadrants to describe the location of a lesion: the UOQ, UIQ, LOQ, or LIQ. Always describe an abnormality in a consistent manner. For example, the location of the abnormality denoted by the "x" in **B** would be described as "right breast UOQ at approximately the 10:30 position."

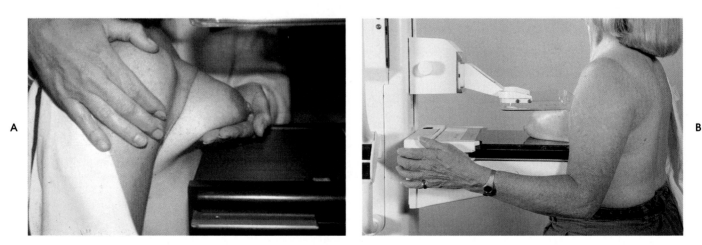

Fig. 23-16 A, Lift the breast to adjust the level of the cassette to the elevated inframammary fold. **B,** CC projection.

Central ray

- Perpendicular to the base of the breast

Structures shown

The CC projection demonstrates the central, subareolar, and medial fibroglandular breast tissue. The pectoral muscle is demonstrated in approximately 30% of all CC images.[1]

---

[1]Bassett L, Heinlein R: Good positioning key to imaging of breast, *Diagn Imaging* 9:69, 1993.

The following should be clearly demonstrated:

- The PNL extending posteriorly to the edge of the image and measuring within 1 cm of the depth of PNL on MLO projection (Fig. 23-17)
- All medial tissue, as shown by the visualization of medial retroglandular fat and the absence of fibroglandular tissue extending to posteromedial edge of image
- Nipple in profile (if possible) and at midline, indicating no exaggeration of positioning
- For emphasis of medial tissue, exclusion of some lateral tissue
- Pectoral muscle seen posterior to medial retroglandular fat in about 30% of properly positioned CC images
- Slight medial skin reflection at the cleavage, ensuring adequate inclusion of posterior medial tissue
- Uniform tissue exposure if compression is adequate

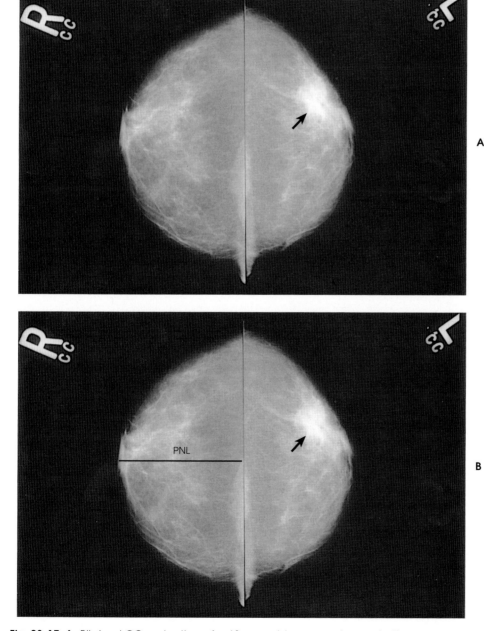

Fig. 23-17 A, Bilateral CC projection of a 63-year-old woman, demonstrating proper positioning. The CC projection should include maximum medial breast tissue with the nipples centered. Breast cancer *(arrow)* is visible on the left *(L)* breast. **B,** CC projections with the PNL demonstrated.

♠ MEDIOLATERAL OBLIQUE (MLO) PROJECTION

Image receptor: 18 × 24 cm or 24 × 30 cm

Position of patient
- Have the patient stand facing the cassette holder, or seat the patient on an adjustable stool facing the holder.

Position of part
- Determine the degree of obliquity of the C-arm apparatus by rotating the tube until the long edge of the cassette is parallel to the upper third of the pectoral muscle of the affected side. The degree of obliquity should be between 30 and 60 degrees, depending on the patient's body habitus.
- Adjust the height of the cassette so that the superior border is level with the axilla.
- Instruct the patient to elevate the arm of the affected side over the corner of the cassette holder and to rest the hand on the handgrip adjacent to the cassette. The patient's elbow should be flexed.
- Place the upper corner of the cassette as high as possible into the patient's axilla between the pectoral and latissimus dorsi muscles so that the cassette is behind the pectoral fold.

- Be certain that the patient's affected shoulder is relaxed and leaning slightly anterior. Then placing the flat surface of the hand along the lateral aspect of the breast, gently pull the patient's breast and pectoral muscle anteriorly and medially.
- Holding the breast between the thumb and fingers, gently lift it up, out, and away from the chest wall.
- Rotate the patient's body toward the cassette while asking the patient to bend slightly at the waist.
- Center the breast with the nipple in profile if possible, and hold the breast in position.
- Hold the breast up and out by rotating the hand so that the base of the thumb and the heel of the hand support the breast (fingers are pointing away from breast).
- Inform the patient that compression of the breast will be used. Continue to hold the breast up and out while sliding the hand toward the nipple as the compression paddle is brought into contact with the breast.

- Slowly apply compression until the breast feels taut. The corner of the compression paddle should be inferior to the clavicle.
- Check the superior and inferior aspects of the breast for adequate compression.
- Instruct the patient to indicate whether the compression becomes uncomfortable.
- Pull down on the patient's abdominal tissue to open the inframammary fold.
- Instruct the patient to hold the opposite breast away from the path of the beam.
- After full compression is achieved, move the AEC detector to the appropriate position, and instruct the patient to stop breathing (Fig. 23-18).
- Make the exposure.
- Release breast compression immediately.

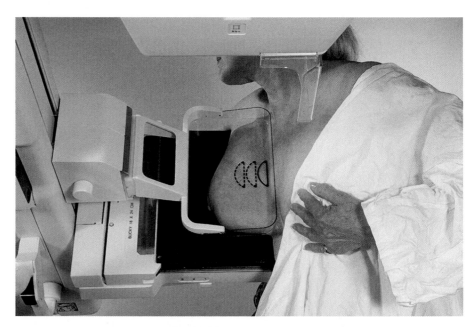

Fig. 23-18 MLO projection.

Central ray

- Perpendicular to the base of the breast
- The C-arm apparatus is positioned at an angle determined by the slope of the patient's pectoral muscle (30 to 60 degrees). The actual angle is determined by the patient's body habitus: tall, thin patients require steep angulation, whereas short, stout patients require shallow angulation.

Structures shown

The MLO projection usually demonstrates most of the breast tissue, with emphasis on the lateral aspect and AT.

EVALUATION CRITERIA

The following should be clearly demonstrated:

- PNL measuring within 1 cm of the depth of PNL on CC projection[1] (While drawing the imaginary PNL obliquely following the orientation of breast tissue toward the pectoral muscle, use the fingers to measure its depth from nipple to pectoral muscle or to the edge of the image, whichever comes first [Fig. 23-19].)
- Inferior aspect of the pectoral muscle extending to the PNL or below it if possible

---

[1]Bassett L: Clinical image evaluation, *Radiol Clin North Am* 33:1027, 1995.

- Pectoral muscle showing anterior convexity to ensure a relaxed shoulder and axilla
- Nipple in profile if possible
- Open inframammary fold
- Deep and superficial breast tissues well separated when the breast is adequately maneuvered up and out from the chest wall
- Retroglandular fat well visualized to ensure inclusion of deep fibroglandular breast tissue
- Uniform tissue exposure if compression is adequate

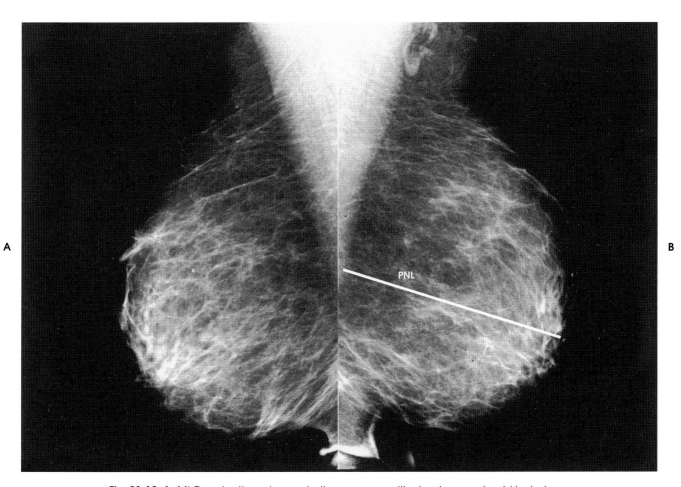

Fig. 23-19 A, MLO projections demonstrating proper positioning. Images should include pectoral muscle to the level of the nipple, posterior breast tissue, and junction of inframammary fold and abdominal skin. **B,** The PNL is demonstrated.

Routine Projections of the Augmented Breast

Mammography is clearly the preferred and most reliable technique for breast cancer screening. This technique has an 80% to 90% true-positive rate for detecting cancer in breasts that do not contain implants. However, millions of women in the United States have undergone augmentation mammoplasty for cosmetic or reconstructive purposes. The true-positive (pathologic-mammographic) breast cancer detection rate decreases to approximately 60% in patients with augmented breasts because implants can obscure up to 85% of breast structures, potentially hiding a small cancer that could normally be detected with mammography at an early and curable stage.

Successful radiography of the augmented breast requires a highly skilled mammographer. During the examination, precautions must be taken to avoid rupture of the augmentation device.

Mammography of the augmented breast presents a challenge that cannot be met with the standard two-image examination of each breast. An eight-radiograph examination is preferred whenever possible. The posterior and superior aspects of the augmented breast can be satisfactorily evaluated using the CC and MLO projections. However, these four images do not adequately demonstrate the surrounding breast parenchyma.

The initial two projections may be combined with the Eklund, or implant displaced (ID), technique. For the Eklund method, the implant is pushed posteriorly against the chest wall so that it is excluded from the image, and the breast tissue surrounding the implant is pulled anteriorly and compressed. This positioning improves both compression of breast tissue and visualization of breast structures. The CC and MLO projections are often performed using the ID technique.

Complications frequently associated with breast augmentation include fibrosis, increased fibrous tissue surrounding the implant, shrinking, hardening, leakage, and pain. Because mammography alone cannot fully demonstrate all complications, both sonography and MRI are also used for breast examinations in symptomatic patients. Whether sonography or MRI is used as the adjunct imaging for following mammography for patients with suspected implant rupture varies from practice to practice.

Sonography of the breast has proved useful in identifying implant leakage when implant rupture is suggested by mammographic findings and clinical examination and occasionally when leakage is not suspected. It has also successfully identified leakage that has migrated to the axillary lymph nodes. Although sonography is not yet recommended as a screening modality for implant leakage, it has enhanced the mammographic examination.

MRI is currently the most commonly used modality for the diagnostic evaluation of the augmented breast. Although MRI offers several diagnostic advantages, the cost and time-consuming nature of the procedure inhibits its use as a screening modality. MRI has proved useful, however, as a preoperative tool in locating the position of an implant, identifying the contour of the deformity, and confirming rupture and leakage migration patterns. The sensitivity and specificity of MRI have been as high as 94% and 97%, respectively.[1]

---

[1]Orel SG: MR imaging of the breast, *Radiol Clin North Am* 38:899, 2000.

CRANIOCAUDAL PROJECTION WITH FULL IMPLANT

Image receptor: 18 × 24 cm or 24 × 30 cm

Position of patient

- Have the patient stand facing the cassette holder, or seat the patient on an adjustable stool facing the holder.

Position of part

- Turn the AEC *off,* and preselect a *manual* technique.
- Follow the same positioning sequence as for the standard CC projection.
- Inform the patient that compression of the breast will be used. Bring the compression paddle into contact with the breast, and slowly apply enough compression to immobilize the breast only. Compression should be *minimal.* The anterior breast tissue should still feel soft.
- Select the appropriate exposure factors, and instruct the patient to stop breathing.
- Make the exposure.
- Release compression immediately.

Central ray

• Perpendicular to the base of the breast

Structures shown

The image should show the entire implant and surrounding posterior breast tissue with suboptimal compression of the anterior fibroglandular breast tissue (Fig. 23-20).

The following should be clearly demonstrated:

■ Implant projected over fibroglandular tissue, extending to posterior edge of image

■ Posterior breast tissue on medial and lateral aspects extending to chest wall

■ Nipple in profile, if possible, and at midline, indicating no exaggeration of positioning

■ Nonuniform compression of anterior breast tissue

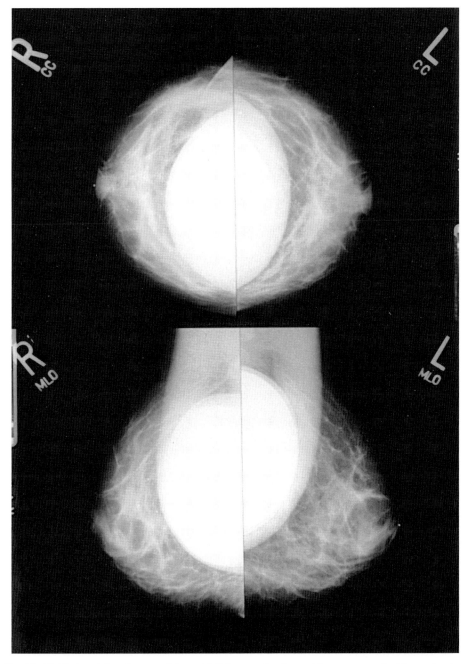

Fig. 23-20 Bilateral, four-image CC and MLO examination of the augmented breasts of a 37-year-old woman. Implants have been surgically placed behind the pectoral muscle. Additional radiographs should be obtained using the Eklund (ID) technique to complete the eight-radiograph study (see Fig. 23-22).

CRANIOCAUDAL PROJECTION WITH IMPLANT DISPLACED (CC ID)

Image receptor: 8 × 24 cm or 24 × 30 cm

Position of patient

- Have the patient stand facing the cassette holder, or seat the patient on an adjustable stool facing the holder.

Position of part

- While standing on the medial side of the breast to be imaged, elevate the inframammary fold to its maximum height.
- Adjust the height of the cassette to the level of the inferior surface of the breast.
- Standing behind the patient, place both arms around the patient and locate the anterior border of the implant by walking the fingers back from the nipple toward the chest wall.

- Once the anterior border of the implant has been located, gently pull the anterior breast tissue forward onto the cassette holder (Fig. 23-21). Use the hands and the edge of the cassette to keep the implant displaced posteriorly.
- Center the breast over the AEC detector with the nipple in profile if possible.
- Hold the implant back against the chest wall. Slowly apply compression to the anterior skin surface, being careful not to allow the implant to slip under the compression paddle. As compression continues, the implant should be seen bulging behind the compression paddle.
- Apply compression until the anterior breast tissue is taut. Compared with the full-implant projection, an additional 2 to 5 cm of compression should be achieved with the implant displaced.
- Instruct the patient to indicate whether the compression becomes uncomfortable.
- When full compression is achieved, move the AEC detector to the appropriate position and instruct the patient to stop breathing.
- Make the exposure.
- Release breast compression immediately.

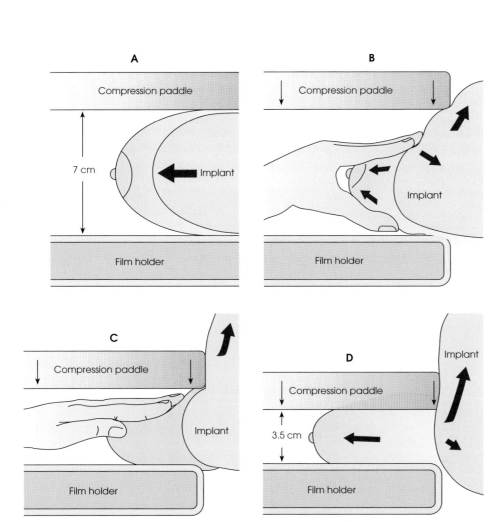

Fig. 23-21 A, Breast with implant and normal positioning techniques. **B** to **D,** Eklund technique of pushing the implant posteriorly against the chest wall, pulling the breast anteriorly, and compressing the tissue.

(From Eklund GW et al: Improved imaging of the augmented breast, *AJR* 151:469, 1988.)

Central ray

• Perpendicular to the base of the breast

Structures shown

This projection demonstrates the implant displaced posteriorly. The anterior and central breast tissue is seen projected free of superimposition with uniform compression and improved tissue differentiation (Fig. 23-22).

The following should be clearly demonstrated:

■ Breast tissue superior and inferior to the implant pulled forward with the anterior breast tissue projected free of the implant

■ PNL extending posteriorly to edge of implant, measuring within 1 cm of depth of PNL on MLO projection with implant displaced

■ Implant along posterior edge of image, flattened against chest wall

■ Image sharpness enhanced by increased compression and reduced scatter

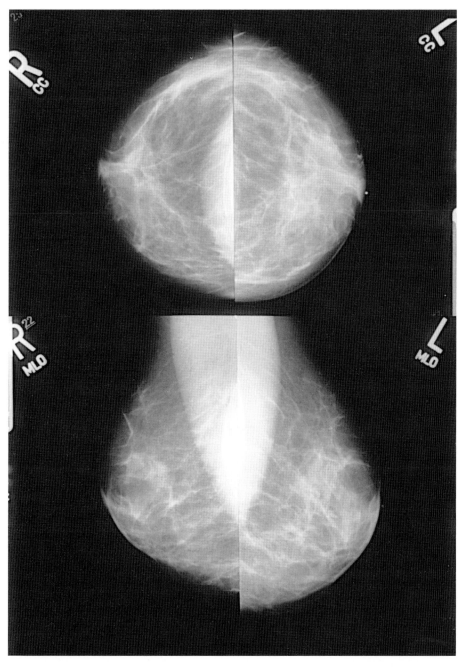

Fig. 23-22 Bilateral, four-image with ID examination of the same patient as in Fig. 23-20, using the Eklund, or ID, technique. The implants are pushed back for better visualization of surrounding breast tissue.

MEDIOLATERAL OBLIQUE (MLO) PROJECTION WITH FULL IMPLANT

Image receptor: 18 × 24 cm or 24 × 30 cm

Position of patient
- Have the patient stand facing the cassette holder, or seat the patient on an adjustable stool facing the holder.

Position of part
- Turn the AEC *off* and preselect a *manual* technique.
- Follow the same positioning sequence as for the standard MLO projection.
- Inform the patient that compression of the breast will be used. Continue to hold the breast up and out while sliding the hand toward the nipple as the compression paddle is brought into contact with the breast.

- Slowly apply enough compression to immobilize the breast only. Compression should be minimal, and the anterior breast tissue should still feel soft.
- Pull down on the patient's abdominal tissue to open the inframammary fold.
- Select the appropriate exposure factors, and instruct the patient to stop breathing.
- Make the exposure.
- Release breast compression immediately.

Central ray
- Perpendicular to the cassette
- The C-arm apparatus is positioned at an angle determined by the slope of the patient's pectoral muscle (30 to 60 degrees). The actual angle is determined by the patient's body habitus: tall, thin patients require steep angulation, whereas short, stout patients require shallow angulation.

Structures shown
The image shows the entire implant and surrounding posterior breast tissue with suboptimal compression of the anterior fibroglandular breast tissue (see Fig. 23-20).

EVALUATION CRITERIA

The following should be clearly demonstrated:
- Implant projected over fibroglandular tissue, extending to posterior edge of image
- Posterior breast tissue on the inferior aspect, extending to chest wall
- Nipple in profile if possible
- Open inframammary fold
- Breast adequately maneuvered up and out from chest wall
- Nonuniform compression of anterior breast tissue

Mammography

MEDIOLATERAL OBLIQUE PROJECTION WITH IMPLANT DISPLACED (MLO ID)

Image receptor: 18 × 24 cm or 24 × 30 cm

Position of patient
- Have the patient stand facing the cassette holder, or seat the patient on an adjustable stool facing the holder.

Position of part
- Determine the degree of obliquity of the C-arm apparatus by rotating the tube until the long edge of the cassette is parallel to the upper third of the pectoral muscle of the affected side. The degree of obliquity should be between 30 and 60 degrees, depending on the patient's body habitus.
- Adjust the height of the cassette so that the superior border is level with the axilla.
- Instruct the patient to elevate the arm of the affected side over the corner of the cassette holder and to rest the hand on the handgrip adjacent to the cassette. The patient's elbow should be flexed.
- Standing in front of the patient, locate the anterior border of the implant by walking the fingers back from the patient's nipple toward the chest wall.
- After locating the anterior border of the implant, gently pull the anterior breast tissue forward onto the cassette holder. Use the edge of the cassette and the hands to keep the implant displaced posteriorly.
- Center the breast over the AEC detector with the nipple in profile if possible.

- Hold the anterior breast tissue up and out so that the base of the thumb and the heel of the hand support the breast (fingers are pointing away from breast).
- Hold the implant back against the chest wall. Slowly apply compression to the anterior skin surface, being careful not to allow the implant to slip under the compression paddle. As compression continues, the implant should be seen bulging behind the compression paddle.
- Apply compression until the anterior breast tissue is taut. Compared with the full-implant projection, an additional 2 to 5 cm of compression should be achieved with the implant displaced.
- Instruct the patient to indicate whether the compression becomes uncomfortable.
- Pull down on the patient's abdominal tissue to open the inframammary fold.
- Instruct the patient to hold the opposite breast away from the path of the beam.
- When full compression is achieved, move the AEC detector to the appropriate position and instruct the patient to stop breathing.
- Make the exposure.
- Release breast compression immediately.

Central ray
- Perpendicular to the cassette
- The C-arm apparatus is positioned at an angle determined by the slope of the patient's pectoral muscle (30 to 60 degrees). The actual angle is determined by the patient's body habitus: tall, thin patients require steep angulation, whereas short, stout patients require shallow angulation.

Structures shown
This image shows the implant displaced posteriorly. The anterior and central breast tissue is seen projected free of superimposition with uniform compression and improved tissue differentiation (see Fig. 23-22).

EVALUATION CRITERIA
The following should be clearly demonstrated:
- Breast tissue superomedial and inferolateral to the implant with anterior breast tissue projected free of the implant
- PNL extending obliquely to edge of implant, measuring within 1 cm of depth of PNL on CC projection with implant displaced
- Implant projected over fibroglandular tissue, extending to posterior edge of image
- Posterior breast tissue on inferior aspect of breast, extending to chest wall
- Nipple in profile if possible
- Open inframammary fold
- Breast adequately maneuvered up and out from chest wall
- Image sharpness enhanced by increased compression and reduced scatter

Routine Projections of the Male Breast

EPIDEMIOLOGY OF MALE BREAST DISEASE

In the United States, approximately 1300 men develop breast cancer every year, and one third of those men die of the disease. Although most men who develop breast cancer are 60 years of age and older, juvenile cases have been reported. Based on the medical literature, very few studies are being conducted to ascertain the relevance of breast cancer incidence in men. Nearly all male breast cancers are primary tumors. Because men have significantly less breast tissue, smaller breast lesions are palpable and diagnosed at early stages. Other symptoms of breast cancer in men include nipple retraction, crusting, discharge, and ulceration.

Gynecomastia, a benign excessive development of the male mammary gland, can make malignant breast lesions more elusive to palpation. Gynecomastia occurs in up to 40% of male breast cancer patients. However, a histologic relationship between gynecomastia and male breast cancer has not been definitely established. Because gynecomastia is caused by a hormonal imbalance, it is believed that abnormal hormonal function may increase the risk of male breast cancer. Other associated risk factors for male breast cancer include increasing age, positive family history, and Klinefelter's syndrome.[1]

Breast cancer treatment options are limited among male patients. Because men have less breast tissue, lumpectomy is not considered practical. A modified radical mastectomy is usually the preferred surgical procedure. Radiation and systemic therapy is considered when the tumor is located near the chest wall or if indicated by lymph node analysis. Like female breast cancer, the prognosis for male breast cancer is directly related to the stage of the disease at diagnosis. An early diagnosis indicates a better chance of survival. Survival rates among male patients with localized breast carcinomas are positive: 97% survive for 5 years.

[1]Appelbaum A et al: Mammographic appearance of male breast disease, *Radiographics* 19:559, 2001.

MALE MAMMOGRAPHY

Male breast anatomy varies significantly from female breast anatomy in that the pectoral muscle is highly developed in men. The radiographer must take this variance into consideration. The standard CC and MLO projections may be applied with success in many male patients (Figs. 23-23 through 23-26). However, for men (or women) with large pectoral muscles, the radiographer may perform the caudocranial (FB) projection instead of the standard CC because it may be easier to compress the inferior portion of the breast. In addition, the lateromedial oblique (LMO) projection may replace the standard MLO (see pp. 458-459 and 462-463).

These supplemental projections allow the radiographer to successfully accommodate the patient with prominent pectoral muscles. Some facilities also use narrower compression paddles (8 cm in width) for compressing the male breast or the small female breast.[1] The smaller paddle permits the radiographer to hold the breast in position while applying final compression. A wooden spoon or spatula can also be used to hold the breast in place.

[1]Eklund GW, Cardenosa G: The art of mammographic positioning, *Radiol Clin North Am* 30:21, 1992.

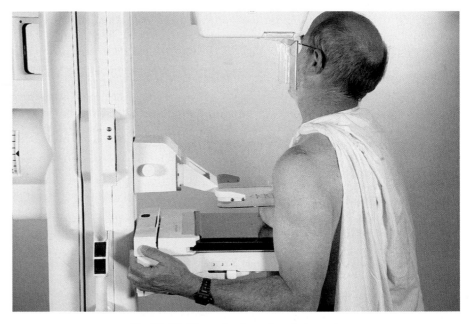

Fig. 23-23 CC projection of male breast.

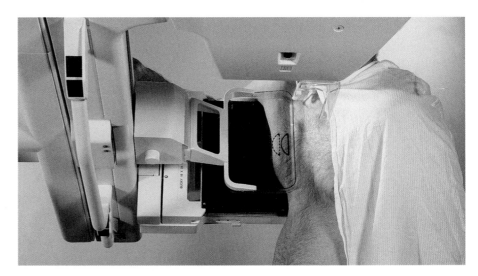

Fig. 23-24 MLO projections of male breast.

Because most men who undergo mammography present with outward symptoms, mammography of the male breast is considered a *diagnostic* examination. The radiographer should work closely with the radiologist to achieve a thorough demonstration of the potential abnormality. In the male breast, most tumors are located in the subareolar region. Careful attention should be given to positioning the nipple in profile and to adequate compression of this area to allow the best visualization of this tissue.

Calcifications are rare in male breast cancer cases. When present, they are usually larger, rounder, and more scattered than the calcifications associated with female breast cancer. Spot compression and magnification technique are common image enhancement methods for demonstrating the morphology of calcifications (see pp. 440-443).

Techniques other than mammography are used to diagnose male breast cancer.

FNAB and excisional biopsy of palpable lesions are standard methods of diagnosis. Histologically, most breast cancers in men are ductal, with most being infiltrating ductal carcinoma.

Because breast cancer is traditionally considered a "woman's disease," the radiographer should remain sensitive to the feelings of the male patient by providing not only physical comfort but also psychologic support.

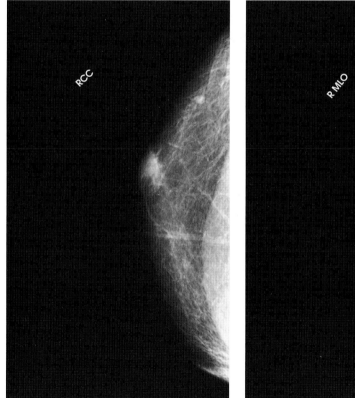

Fig. 23-25 CC projection of a 62-year-old male.

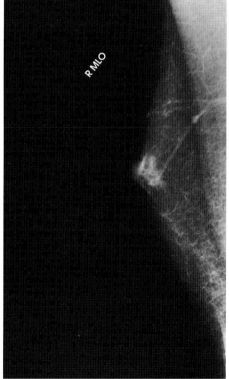

Fig. 23-26 MLO projection of the patient in Fig. 23-25.

TABLE 23-2

Supplemental projections/methods and their suggested applications

Projection/method	Application(s)
Spot compression	Defines lesion or area through focal compression; separates overlying parenchyma
Magnification (M)	Combines with spot compression to demonstrate margins of lesion; delineates microcalcifications
Mediolateral (ML)	Localization; demonstrates air-fluid-fat levels; defines lesion located in lateral aspect of breast; complements mediolateral oblique (MLO) projection
Lateromedial (LM)	Localization; demonstrates air-fluid-fat levels; defines lesion located in medial aspect of breast
Exaggerated cranio-caudal (XCCL)	Visualizes lesions in deep outer aspect of breast that are not seen on standard CC
CC for cleavage (CV)	Visualizes deep medial breast tissue; demonstrates medial lesion in true transverse/axial plane
CC with roll (RL, RM)	Triangulates lesion seen only on CC projection; defines location of lesion as in either superior or inferior aspect of breast
Tangential (TAN)	Confirms dermal vs. breast calcifications; demonstrates obscure palpable lump over subcutaneous fat
Coat-hanger	Demonstrates a palpable lump in posterior tissue that is difficult to immobilize with conventional techniques
Caudocranial (FB)	Visualizes superior breast tissue; defines lesion located in superior aspect of breast; replaces standard CC for patients with kyphosis or prominent pectoral muscles
MLO for axillary tail (AT)	Focal compression projection of AT
Lateromedial oblique (LMO)	Demonstrates medial breast tissue; replaces standard MLO for patients with pectus excavatum, prominent pacemakers, prominent pectoral muscles, Hickman catheters, and postoperative open heart surgery
Superolateral to infero-medial oblique (SIO)	Visualizes upper-inner quadrant and lower-outer quadrant, which are normally superimposed on MLO and LMO projections

Significant Mammographic Findings

The routine projections are not always adequate in completely demonstrating a patient's breast tissue, or a specific area may require clearer delineation. Supplemental projections complement the routine projections and have distinct applications (Table 23-2). The mammographer should fully understand the value of each projection and its ability to demonstrate significant findings in the breast. This section provides a brief overview of significant mammographic findings in their most common radiographic presentation and provides suggested correlative supplemental projections. The language related to mammographic findings must be appreciated for the mammographer and the radiologist to work collaboratively toward a successful diagnostic examination.

The *mass* is the most common presentation of a potential abnormality in the breast. It is identified on two projections of the affected breast. A mass has a convex shape or an outward contour to its margins. If a suspected mass is only identified on one projection, the mammographer must strive to position the breast so that the area in question is demonstrated on at least two projections. For example, if the suspected mass is only seen on the MLO projection in the deep medial aspect of the breast, a CC projection for cleavage may complement the standard CC projection. Conversely, if the mass is seen in the extreme lateral aspect, an exaggerated craniocaudal (XCCL) projection laterally would be the projection of choice. In a sense the radiographer is collecting evidence to prove whether the mass is real or merely a summation shadow of superimposed breast parenchyma. Once a mass has been successfully identified on two projections, the radiologist describes the mass according to the following characteristics:

- *Shape* is a good predictor of the malignant or benign nature of the mass. Round, oval, or lobular masses are probably benign. Irregularly shaped masses are suspicious.
- *Margin* characteristics help predict whether a mass is malignant or benign. Well-defined circumscribed masses are probably benign. Microlobulated masses have a 50% chance of being malignant. Masses with obscured, ill-defined, indistinct margins are suspicious. Spiculated margins may indicate malignancy. Postbiopsy scarring may appear as a spiculated mass, and an accurate patient history revealing previous breast biopsies can prevent an unnecessary workup (Fig. 23-27).
- The tissue *density* of the mass can predict whether it is malignant or benign. Masses consisting of mostly fat are usually benign, whereas masses consisting of variable fibroglandular tissue could be malignant.
- Although *size* cannot predict whether a lesion is malignant or benign, clinical management is the same regardless of size. The radiologist may request spot compression images to confirm mass characteristics. Magnification projections may be warranted if calcifications or spiculations are present within the mass. Sonography may be appropriate to determine whether the mass is a simple cyst (Fig. 23-28).
- The malignant or benign nature of a mass cannot be determined based on *location*. Most cancers are detected in the UOQ of the breast; however, most breast lesions—malignant or benign—are found in that quadrant. Cancer can occur in any region of the breast with a certain degree of probability. It is important to determine the location of a lesion for additional diagnostic procedures such as core biopsy or open surgical biopsy.

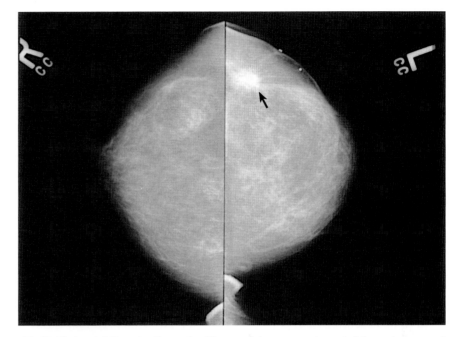

Fig. 23-27 Bilateral CC projections of a 55-year-old woman whose left breast was surgically altered as a result of previous breast cancer. Lumpectomy scar is visible on left breast *(arrow)*. Surgical scars can mimic characteristics of breast cancer.

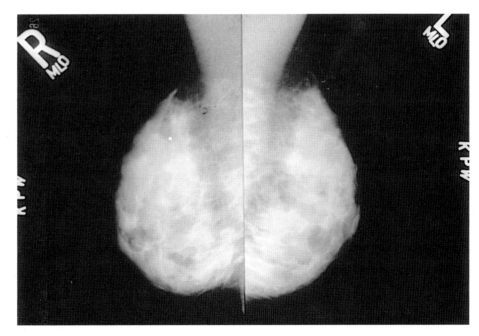

Fig. 23-28 Bilateral MLO projections of a 27-year-old woman who stopped breastfeeding 2 months before having this mammogram. Dense parenchyma with multinodularity throughout all quadrants is demonstrated bilaterally. A lead marker in the upper quadrant of the right breast marks a palpable mass; sonographic examination proved the mass to be solid.

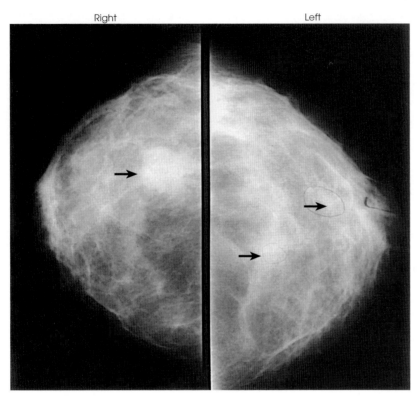

Fig. 23-29 CC projections of right and left breasts in a 28-year-old woman who is 4 months postpartum and not breastfeeding. The right breast contains a large mass *(arrow)* palpable on physical examination. The left breast contains two smaller nonpalpable masses *(arrows)* with microcalcifications. All three lesions were breast cancers.

- *Interval change* may increase the suspicion of malignancy. The radiologist carefully compares current images with previous ones and notes whether the mass is newly apparent, an interval enlargement is present, the borders have become nodular and/or ill defined, a mass has increased in density, or calcifications have appeared (Fig. 23-29).
- Almost all (98%) of the axillary lymph nodes are located in the UOQ. The nodes are well circumscribed, may have a central or peripheral area of fat, and can be kidney bean shaped. If the lymph nodes appear normal, they are rarely mentioned in the context of an identifiable mass on the radiology report.
- Examples of benign stellate lesions include radial scar, fat necrosis, breast abscess, and sclerosing adenosis. Examples of benign circumscribed masses include fibroadenoma (Fig. 23-30), cyst, intramammary lymph node, hematoma, and galactocele.
- A *density* is seen on only one projection, is not confirmed three-dimensionally, may represent superimposed structures, and may have scalloped edges and/or concave borders. The radiologist may request spot compression projections, rolled projections, or angled projections to confirm or deny the presence of a real density. A suspicious density seen on only one projection within the breast is usually a summation shadow of superimposed breast parenchyma and will disappear when the breast tissue is spread apart.

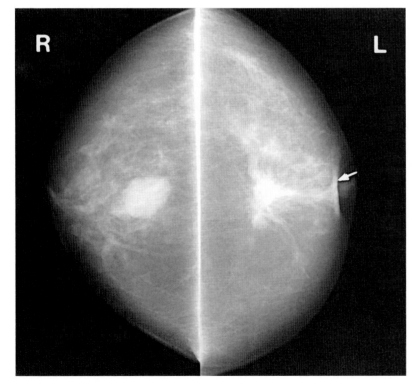

Fig. 23-30 CC projections of bilateral breast masses. Left breast *(L)* contains an irregular carcinoma that is producing considerable spiculation, nipple retraction *(arrow)*, and skin thickening. Right breast *(R)* contains fibroadenoma.

Mammography

- *Calcifications* are often normal metabolic occurrences within the breast and are usually benign (Fig. 23-31). However, approximately 15% to 25% of microcalcifications found in asymptomatic women are associated with cancer. These calcifications can have definitive characteristics. Yet because of size, some microcalcifications are more difficult to interpret. The most valuable tool for defining microcalcifications is the properly performed magnification projection. Using this image, the radiologist can ascertain whether the calcifications are suspicious and warrant any further workup.
- Benign calcifications may have one or more of the following attributes: moderate size, scattered location, round shape, and, usually, bilateral occurrence. In addition, they may be eggshell (lucent center), arterial (parallel tracks), crescent, or sedimented ("teacup" milk of calcium). Calcifications may also represent a fibroadenoma ("popcorn") and postsurgical scarring (sheets or large strands of calcium). The projection suggested for better defining sedimented milk of calcium is the 90-degree lateral projection—lateromedial (LM) or mediolateral (ML). If possible, the mammographer should select the lateral projection that places the suspected area closest to the IR. The 90-degree lateral is also used as a triangulation projection before needle localization and for the demonstration of air-fluid-fat levels.

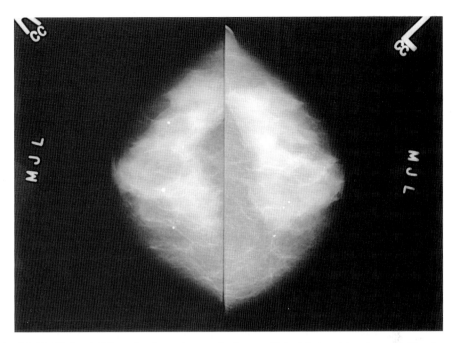

Fig. 23-31 Bilateral CC projections demonstrating multiple, bilateral, benign calcifications.

Significant mammographic findings

- Suspicious calcifications are small (occurring in groups of five or more), located within the breast parenchyma (vs. dermal), localized in distribution, and branching and linear in shape (Fig. 23-32). Dermal or skin calcifications can mimic suspicious microcalcifications within the breast parenchyma. The tangential (TAN) projection is best suited for resolving this discrepancy.
- Other supplemental projections are intended to offer alternative methods for tailoring the mammographic procedure to the specific abilities of the patient and the requirements of the interpreting physician. Often, however, the need for additional projections is only determined after careful examination of the standard projections. Therefore throughout mammographic procedures, the radiographer should consistently evaluate the images, keeping foremost in mind the optimal demonstration of possible findings. The mammographer may develop the expertise to predict and perform supplemental projections that demonstrate or rule out suspected breast abnormalities. As with all radiographic procedures, image evaluation is a critical component of high-quality imaging systems. In doing so, the mammographer becomes an integral member of the breast imaging team, actively participating in the workup of a symptomatic patient.

Image Enhancement Methods

The spot compression technique and the magnification technique are designed to enhance the image of the area under investigation.

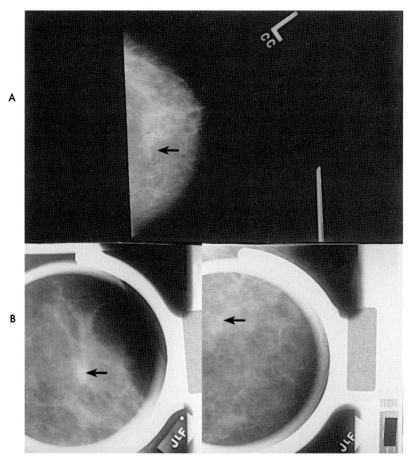

Fig. 23-32 Microcalcifications are an early sign of breast cancer. **A,** A mass with calcifications *(arrow).* **B,** This type of mass is best visualized with two right-angle projections *(arrows).*

MAGNIFICATION TECHNIQUE (M USED AS PREFIX)

Image receptor: 18 × 24 cm

Position of patient

- Have the patient stand facing the cassette holder, or seat the patient on an adjustable stool facing the holder.

Position of part

- Attach the firm, radiolucent magnification platform designed by the equipment manufacturer to the unit. The patient's breast will be positioned on the platform between the compression device and a nongrid IR.
- Select the smallest focal spot target size (0.1 mm or less is preferred). Most units will only allow magnification images to be exposed using the correct focal spot size.

- Select the appropriate compression paddle (regular or spot compression). Collimate according to the size of the compression paddle.
- Reposition the patient's breast to obtain the projection that best demonstrates the area of interest. The angle of the C-arm can be adjusted to accommodate any projection normally performed using a traditional grid technique.
- When full compression is achieved, move the AEC detector to the appropriate position and instruct the patient to stop breathing (Fig. 23-33).
- Make the exposure.
- Release breast compression immediately.

Central ray

- Perpendicular to the area of interest

Structures shown

This technique magnifies the area of interest with improved detail, facilitating the determination of the characteristics of microcalcifications (Fig. 23-34) and the margins (or lack of definitive margins) of suspected lesions (Fig. 23-35).

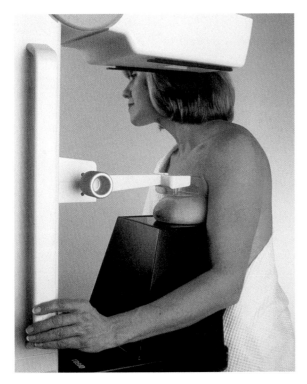

Fig. 23-33 Radiolucent platform placed between breast and film holder causes the breast image to be enlarged.

(Courtesy Lorad Corp.)

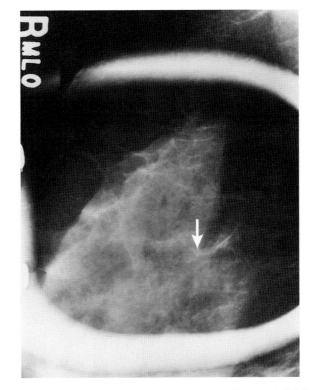

Fig. 23-34 Spot compression used with magnification in MLO projection, demonstrating microcalcifications *(arrow).*

EVALUATION CRITERIA

The following should be clearly demonstrated:

- Area of interest within collimated and compressed margins
- Improved delineation of number, distribution, and morphology of microcalcifications
- Enhanced architectural characteristics of focal density or mass
- Uniform tissue exposure if compression is adequate

SPOT COMPRESSION TECHNIQUE

Image receptor: 18×24 cm

Position of patient

- Have the patient standing facing the cassette holder, or seat the patient on an adjustable stool facing the holder.
- This technique is often performed in conjunction with the magnification technique.

Position of part

In conjunction with magnification technique

- Place a firm, radiolucent magnification platform designed for use with the dedicated mammography equipment on the unit, between the patient's breast and a nongrid cassette device (see p. 441).
- Select the smallest focal spot target size (0.1 mm or less is preferred).

For palpable masses

A TAN projection combined with spot compression and the magnification technique is most often used to image a palpable mass; however, the spot compression technique in a previously imaged projection is also requested by many radiologists.

- Select the appropriate focal compression device.
- Reposition the patient's breast to obtain the projection that best demonstrates the suspected abnormality.
- Mark the location of the palpable mass with a felt-tip pen.
- Center the area of interest under the compression device.
- Inform the patient that compression of the breast will be used. Bring the compression paddle into contact with the breast, and slowly apply compression until the breast feels taut.

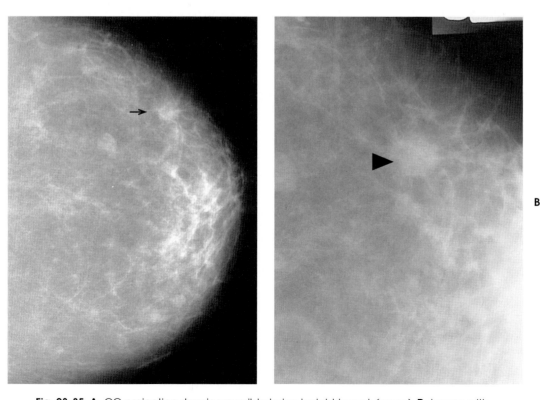

Fig. 23-35 A, CC projection showing possible lesion in right breast *(arrow)*. **B,** Image with 2× magnification in the same patient, convincingly demonstrating a lesion with irregular margin *(arrowhead)*.

- Instruct the patient to indicate whether the compression becomes uncomfortable.
- When full compression is achieved, move the AEC detector to the appropriate position and instruct the patient to stop breathing (Fig. 23-36).
- Make the exposure.
- Release breast compression immediately.

For nonpalpable masses

- While viewing the routine mammogram, measure the location of the area of interest from a reference point (the nipple), using either a tape measure or the fingertips.
- Select the appropriate focal compression device.
- Reposition the patient's breast to obtain the projection from which the measurements were taken.
- Using the same reference point, transfer the measurements taken from the mammogram onto the patient.
- Mark the area of interest with a felt-tip pen.
- Center the area of interest under the compression device.
- Inform the patient that compression of the breast will be used. Bring the compression paddle into contact with the breast, and slowly apply compression until the breast feels taut.
- Instruct the patient to indicate whether the compression becomes uncomfortable.

- When full compression is achieved, move the AEC detector to the appropriate position, and instruct the patient to stop breathing.
- Make the exposure.
- Release breast compression immediately.

Central ray

- Perpendicular to the area of interest

Structures shown

The spot compression technique resolves superimposed structures seen on only one projection, better visualizes small lesions located in the extreme posterior breast, separates superimposed ductal structures in the subareolar region, and improves visualization in areas of dense tissue through localized compression (Fig. 23-37).

EVALUATION CRITERIA

The following should be clearly demonstrated:

- Area of interest clearly seen within compressed margins
- Close collimation to the area of interest unless contraindicated by radiologist

- Improved recorded detail through the use of close collimation and magnification technique employing a microfocal spot
- Uniform tissue exposure if compression is adequate

NOTE: Densities caused by the superimposition of normal breast parenchyma disappear on spot compression images.

Supplemental Projections

Supplemental projections described in the following section include the 90-degree ML projection, the CC projection for cleavage, and others. These projections are designed to delineate areas not visualized or not clearly seen on the routine projections.

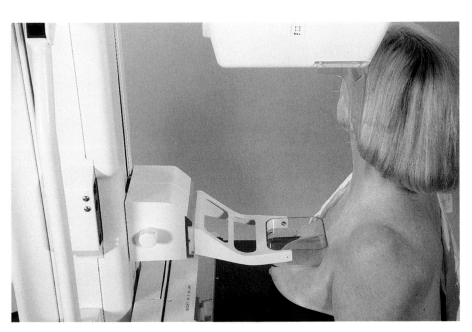

Fig. 23-36 Spot compression used with CC projection.

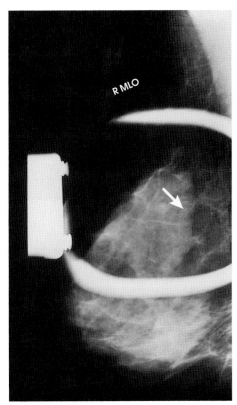

Fig. 23-37 Spot compression of suspicious area containing microcalcifications (*arrow*). The lesion was later biopsied and was found to be ductal carcinoma in situ, an early stage of cancer.

♠ 90-DEGREE MEDIOLATERAL (ML) PROJECTION

Image receptor: 18 × 24 cm or 24 × 30 cm

Position of patient
- Have the patient stand facing the cassette holder, or seat the patient on an adjustable stool facing the holder.

Position of part
- Rotate the C-arm assembly 90 degrees, with the x-ray tube placed on the medial side of the patient's breast.
- Have the patient bend slightly forward. Position the superior corner of the cassette high into the axilla, with the patient's elbow flexed and the affected arm resting behind the cassette.

- Ask the patient to relax the affected shoulder.
- Pull the breast tissue and pectoral muscle superiorly and anteriorly, ensuring that the lateral rib margin is pressed firmly against the edge of the cassette.
- Rotate the patient slightly laterally to help bring the medial tissue forward.
- Gently pull the medial breast tissue forward from the sternum, and position the nipple in profile.
- Hold the patient's breast up and out by rotating the hand so that the base of the thumb and the heel of the hand support the breast.
- Inform the patient that compression of the breast will be used. Continue to hold the patient's breast up and out while sliding the hand toward the nipple as the compression paddle is brought into contact with the breast. Do not allow the breast to droop (Fig. 23-38).
- Slowly apply compression until the breast feels taut.
- Instruct the patient to indicate whether compression becomes uncomfortable.
- Ask the patient to hold the opposite breast away from the path of the beam.
- When full compression is achieved, move the AEC detector to the appropriate position, and instruct the patient to stop breathing (Fig. 23-39).
- Make the exposure.
- Release breast compression immediately.

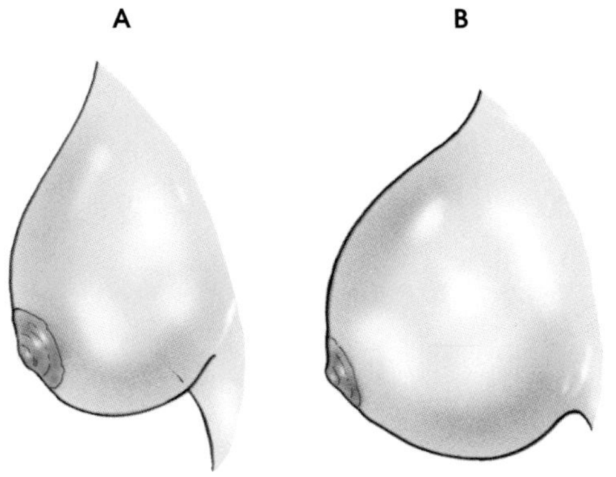

Fig. 23-38 A, Lateral profile of breast demonstrating inadequate compression and a drooping breast. **B,** Lateral profile of properly compressed breast. Note how compression has overcome the effect of gravity and how the breast is spread out over a greater area.

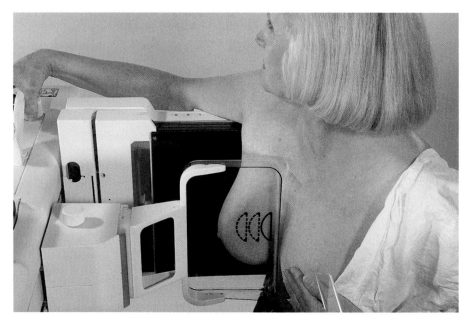

Fig. 23-39 ML projection.

Central ray

- Perpendicular to the base of the breast

Structures shown

This projection demonstrates lesions on the lateral aspect of the breast in the superior or inferior aspects. It resolves superimposed structures seen on the MLO projection, localizes a lesion seen on one (or both) of the initial projection(s), and demonstrates air-fluid and fat-fluid levels in breast structures (i.e., milk of calcium, galactoceles) and in pneumocystography.

Breast

EVALUATION CRITERIA

The following should be clearly demonstrated:

- Nipple in profile
- Open inframammary fold
- Deep and superficial breast tissues well separated when breast is adequately maneuvered up and out from chest wall (Figs. 23-40 and 23-41)
- Retroglandular fat well visualized to ensure inclusion of deep fibroglandular breast tissue
- Uniform tissue exposure if compression is adequate

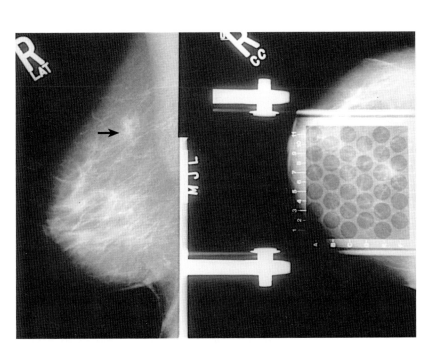

Fig. 23-40 ML projection is often used as a preliminary projection in a breast localization procedure. The arrow denotes the lesion.

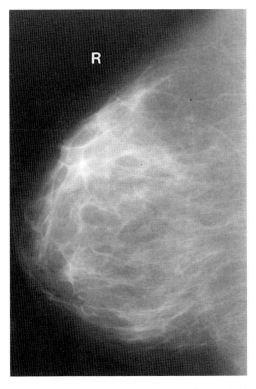

Fig. 23-41 ML projection of a normal breast of a 24-year-old woman.

90-DEGREE LATEROMEDIAL (LM) PROJECTION

Image receptor: 18 × 24 cm or 24 × 30 cm

Position of patient

- Have the patient stand facing the cassette holder, or seat the patient on an adjustable stool facing the holder.

Position of part

- Rotate the C-arm assembly 90 degrees, with the x-ray tube placed on the lateral side of the patient's breast.
- Position the superior corner of the cassette at the level of the jugular notch.
- Have the patient flex the neck slightly forward.
- Have the patient relax the affected shoulder, flex the elbow, and rest the affected arm over the top of the cassette.
- Pull the breast tissue and pectoral muscle superiorly and anteriorly, ensuring that the patient's sternum is pressed firmly against the edge of the cassette.
- Rotate the patient slightly medially to help bring the lateral tissue forward.

- Have the patient rest her chin on the top edge of the cassette holder to help loosen the skin in the medial aspect of the breast.
- Position the nipple in profile.
- Hold the patient's breast up and out. Do not let it droop.
- Inform the patient that compression of the breast will be used. Bring the compression paddle past the latissimus dorsi muscle and into contact with the breast. Then slowly apply compression while sliding the hand out toward the nipple until the patient's breast feels taut.
- Instruct the patient to indicate whether the compression becomes uncomfortable.
- When full compression is achieved, move the AEC detector to the appropriate position, and instruct the patient to stop breathing (Fig. 23-42).
- Make the exposure.
- Release breast compression immediately.

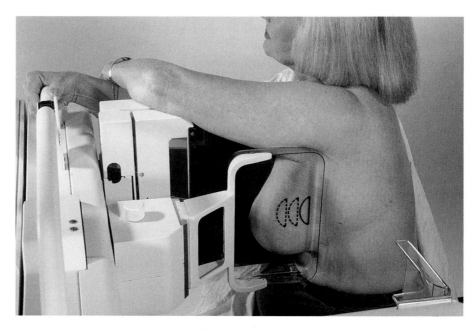

Fig. 23-42 LM projection.

Central ray

• Perpendicular to the base of the breast

Structures shown

This projection demonstrates lesions on the medial aspect of the breast in the superior or inferior aspects (Fig. 23-43). It resolves superimposed structures seen on the MLO projection, localizes a lesion seen on one (or both) of the initial projection(s), and demonstrates air-fluid and fat-fluid levels in breast structures (i.e., milk of calcium, galactoceles) and in pneumocystography.

The following should be clearly demonstrated:
■ Nipple in profile
■ Open inframammary fold
■ Deep and superficial breast tissues well separated when breast is adequately maneuvered up and out from chest wall
■ Retroglandular fat well visualized to ensure inclusion of deep fibroglandular breast tissue
■ Uniform tissue exposure if compression is adequate

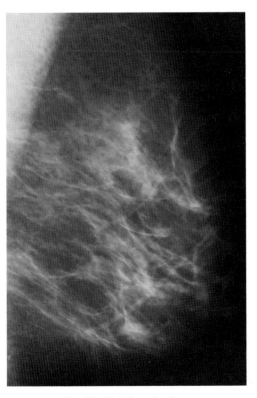

Fig. 23-43 LM projection.

⚘ EXAGGERATED CRANIOCAUDAL (XCCL) PROJECTION

Image receptor: 18 × 24 cm or 24 × 30 cm

Position of patient

- Have the patient stand facing the cassette holder, or seat the patient on an adjustable stool facing the holder.

Position of part

- Elevate the inframammary fold to its maximum height.
- Adjust the height of the cassette accordingly.
- Use both hands to gently pull the breast onto the cassette holder while instructing the patient to press the thorax against the cassette tray.
- Slightly rotate the patient medially to place the lateral aspect of the breast on the cassette.

- Place an arm against the patient's back with the hand on the shoulder of the affected side, making certain that the shoulder is relaxed in external rotation.
- Slightly rotate the patient's head away from the affected side.
- Have the patient lean toward the machine and rest the head against the face guard.
- Rotate the C-arm assembly mediolaterally 5 degrees to eliminate overlapping of the humeral head.
- Inform the patient that compression of the breast will be used. Smoothen and flatten the breast tissue toward the nipple while bringing the compression paddle into contact with the breast.
- Slowly apply compression until the breast feels taut.
- Instruct the patient to indicate whether the compression becomes uncomfortable.
- When full compression is achieved, move the AEC detector to the appropriate position, and instruct the patient to stop breathing (Figs. 23-44 and 23-45).
- Make the exposure.
- Release breast compression immediately.

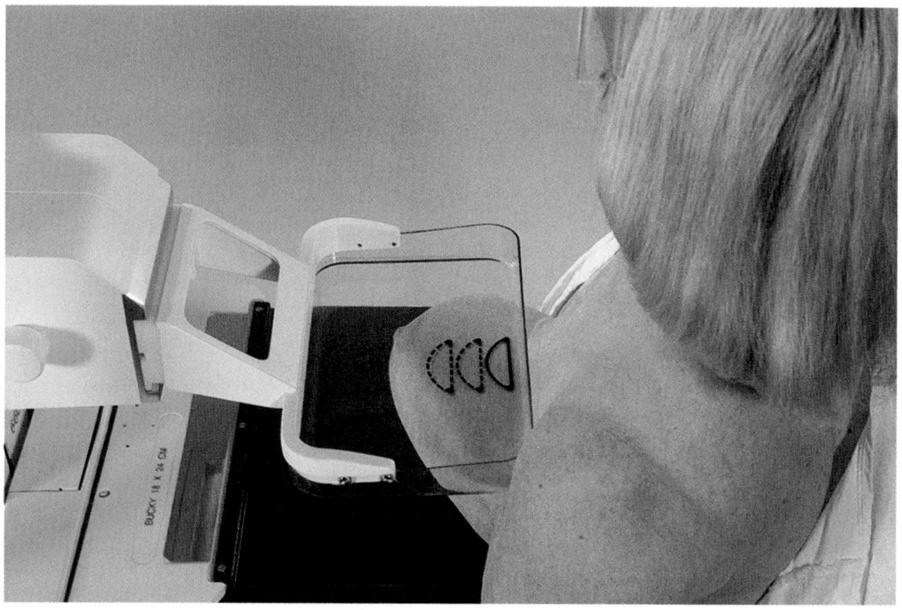

Fig. 23-44 XCCL projection.

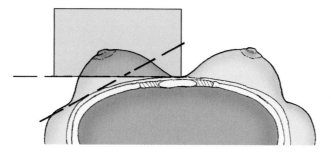

Fig. 23-45 Superior profile illustrating how placement of the flat edge of the cassette against the curved chest wall excludes a portion of the breast tissue *(shaded area)*. Dashed line indicates placement of cassette for exaggerated position.

Central ray

- Angled 5 degrees mediolaterally to the base of the breast

Structures shown

This projection demonstrates a superoinferior projection of the lateral fibroglandular breast tissue and posterior aspect of the pectoral muscle. It also demonstrates a sagittal orientation of a lateral lesion located in the AT of the breast.

The following should be clearly demonstrated:

- Retroglandular fat well visualized to ensure inclusion of deep fibroglandular breast tissue on lateral aspect of breast and lower axillary region
- Pectoral muscle visualized over lateral chest wall (Fig. 23-46)
- Humeral head projected clear of image with use of a 5-degree ML angle
- Uniform tissue exposure if compression is adequate

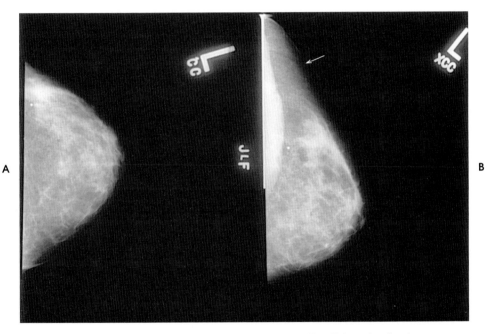

A   **B**

Fig. 23-46 A, CC projection of left breast. **B,** XCCL projection. This projection is exaggerated laterally to demonstrate AT *(arrow)*. Note also visualization of the pectoral muscle.

CRANIOCAUDAL PROJECTION FOR CLEAVAGE (CV)

Image receptor: 18 × 24 cm or 24 × 30 cm

Position of patient

- Have the patient stand facing the cassette holder, or seat the patient on an adjustable stool facing the holder.

Position of part

- Turn the AEC *off*, and preselect a *manual* technique. The radiographer may use AEC only if enough breast tissue is positioned over the AEC detector. The cleavage may be intentionally offset for this purpose.
- Determine the proper height of the cassette by elevating the inframammary fold to its maximum height.
- Adjust the height of the cassette accordingly.
- Standing behind the patient, use both hands to gently lift and pull both breasts forward onto the cassette holder while instructing the patient to press the thorax against the cassette tray.

- Pull as much medial breast tissue as possible onto the cassette holder.
- Slightly rotate the patient's head away from the affected side.
- Have the patient lean toward the machine and rest the head against the face guard.
- Ask the patient to hold the grip bar with both hands to keep in position on the cassette.
- Place one hand at the level of the patient's jugular notch, and then slide the hand down the patient's chest while pulling down as much deep medial tissue as possible.
- Inform the patient that compression of the breast will be used. Bring the compression paddle into contact with the breasts, and slowly apply compression until the breast feels taut. Using a quadrant compression paddle will allow better compression of the cleavage area and will also allow more of the area of interest to be pulled into the imaging area. If a quadrant paddle is used, collimate to the area of compression to better visualize the detail of the tissue.
- Instruct the patient to indicate when the compression becomes uncomfortable.
- When full compression is achieved, move the AEC detector to the appropriate position if AEC is used, and instruct the patient to hold the breath (Fig. 23-47).
- Make the exposure.
- Release breast compression immediately.

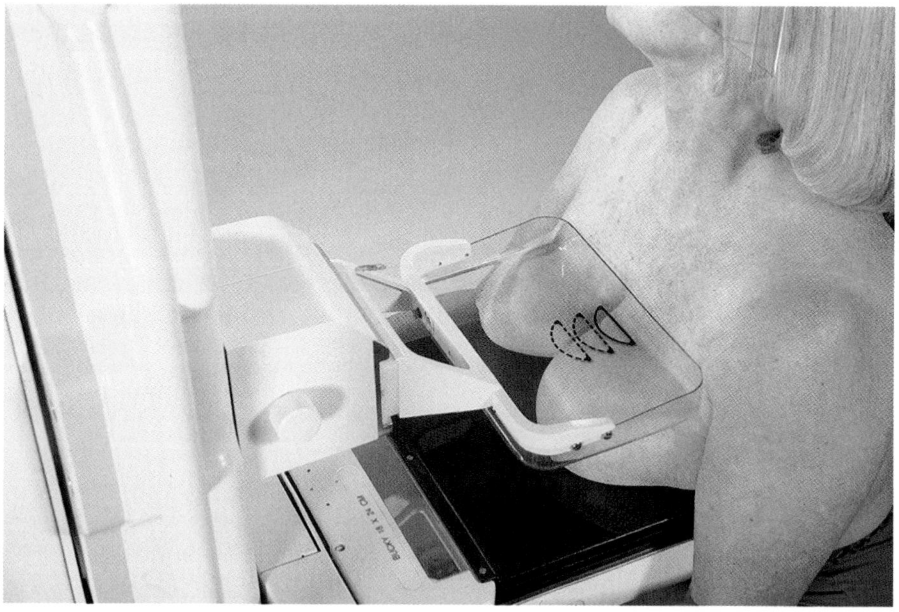

Fig. 23-47 Craniocaudal projection for cleavage. Note that cleavage is slightly off-center so that AEC is under breast tissue.

Central ray

• Perpendicular to either the area of interest or the centered cleavage

Structures shown

This projection demonstrates lesions located in the deep posteromedial aspect of the breast.

The following should be clearly demonstrated:

■ Area of interest over the central portion of the cassette (over the AEC detector if possible) with cleavage slightly off-centered or with cleavage centered to the cassette and manual technique selected (Fig. 23-48)

■ Deep medial tissue of affected breast

■ All medial tissue included, as shown by the visualization of medial retro-glandular fat and the absence of any fibroglandular tissue extending to posteromedial edge of imaged breasts

■ Uniform tissue exposure if compression is adequate (Retroareolar regions may not be adequately compressed because of emphasis on the deep medial tissue. It is not necessary to image all of the breast tissue on this projection.)

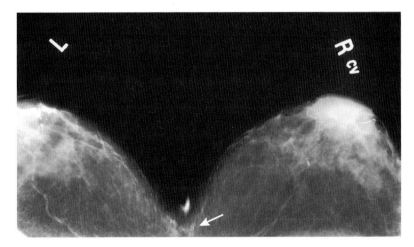

Fig. 23-48 CV demonstrating benign calcifications located in deep medial tissue *(arrow)*. With a centered cleavage, the manual technique should be selected.

CRANIOCAUDAL PROJECTION WITH ROLL LATERAL OR ROLL MEDIAL (RL OR RM USED AS SUFFIX)

Image receptor: 18 × 24 cm or 24 × 30 cm

Position of patient

- Have the patient stand facing the cassette holder, or seat the patient on an adjustable stool facing the holder.

Position of part

- Reposition the patient's breast in the projection that best demonstrates the suspected superimposition (usually the CC projection).
- Place the hands on opposite surfaces of the patient's breast (superior/inferior), and roll the surfaces in opposite directions. The direction of the roll is not important as long as the mammographer rolls the superior surface in one direction and the inferior surface in the other direction. In a sense the mammographer is very gently rotating the breast approximately 10 to 15 degrees (Fig. 23-49).

- Place the patient's breast onto the cassette surface with the lower hand while holding the rolled position with the upper hand.
- Note the direction of the superior surface roll (lateral or medial), and label the image accordingly. For example, if the superior aspect of the breast is rolled medially, the image should be labeled RM.
- Inform the patient that compression of the breast will be used. Bring the compression paddle into contact with the breast, and slide the hand out while rolling the breast tissue.
- Slowly apply compression until the breast feels taut.
- Instruct the patient to indicate whether the compression becomes uncomfortable.
- When full compression is achieved, move the AEC detector to the appropriate position and instruct the patient to hold the breath (Fig. 23-50).
- Make the exposure.
- Release breast compression immediately.

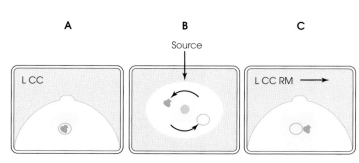

Fig. 23-49 A, CC projection demonstrating a lesion that may represent superimposition of two structures. If spot compression fails to resolve these structures, a CC projection with the roll position may be performed. **B,** Anterior view of CC projection, with arrows indicating rolling of superior and inferior breast surfaces in opposite directions to separate superimposed structures. **C,** CC projection with RM, demonstrating resolution of two lesions. The arrow indicates the direction of the roll of the superior surface of the breast.

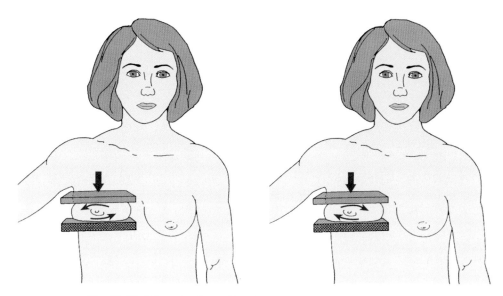

Fig. 23-50 CC projection with lateral and medial roll, respectively.

Mammography

Central ray

- Perpendicular to the base of the breast
- Alternatively, the standard CC projection may be performed with the C-arm assembly rotated 10 to 15 degrees either mediolaterally or lateromedially to eliminate superimposition of breast tissue. This is often the preferred method because it allows easier duplication of the projection during subsequent examinations.

Structures shown

This position demonstrates separation of superimposed breast tissues (also known as *summation shadow*), particularly those seen only on the CC projection. The position also helps determine whether a lesion is located in the superior or inferior aspect of the breast (Fig. 23-51).

The following should be clearly demonstrated:

- Suspected superimposition adequately resolved
- Suspected lesion in either superior or inferior aspect of breast
- PNL extending posteriorly to edge of image, measuring within 1 cm of the depth of PNL on MLO projection
- All medial tissue included, as shown by the visualization of medial retroglandular fat and the absence of fibroglandular tissue extending to posteromedial edge of image
- Nipple in profile and at midline, indicating no exaggeration of positioning. The nipple is used as a point of reference to distinguish the location of the suspected lesion, if it exists.
- Some lateral tissue possibly excluded to emphasize medial tissue visualized
- Slight medial skin reflection at cleavage, ensuring that posterior medial tissue is adequately included
- Uniform tissue exposure if compression is adequate

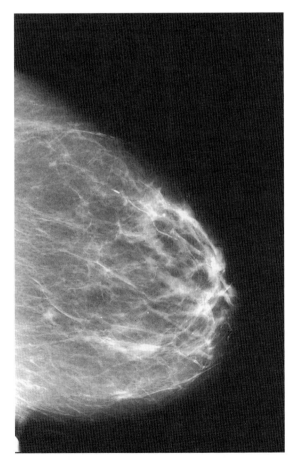

Fig. 23-51 CC projection with RL.

TANGENTIAL (TAN) PROJECTION

Image receptor: 18 × 24 cm

Position of patient
- Have the patient stand facing the cassette holder, or seat the patient on an adjustable stool facing the holder.

Position of part

For a palpable mass
The TAN projection is most often performed with use of the magnification technique.
- Select either a standard, quadrant, or spot compression paddle.
- Locate the area of interest by palpating the patient's breast.
- Place a radiopaque marker or BB on the mass.
- Using the imaginary line between the nipple and the BB as the angle reference (Fig. 23-52), rotate the C-arm apparatus until the central ray is directed tangential to the breast at the point identified by the BB marker (the "shadow" of the BB will be projected onto the cassette surface).
- Using the appropriate compression paddle (regular or spot compression), compress the breast and skin area while ensuring that enough breast tissue covers the AEC detector area.
- Slowly apply compression until the breast feels taut.
- Instruct the patient to indicate whether the compression becomes uncomfortable.
- When full compression is achieved, move the AEC detector to the appropriate position, and instruct the patient to stop breathing (Figs. 23-53 and 23-54).
- Make the exposure.
- Release breast compression immediately.

For skin localization or nonpalpable dermal calcifications, two projections are necessary: (1) a localization projection (which depends on the area of interest) and (2) a TAN projection.

Localization projection
- From the routine CC and MLO projections, determine the quadrant in which the area of interest is located.
- Determine which projection will best localize the area of interest—the CC or 90-degree lateral projection.
- Turn off the automatic compression release, and inform the patient that compression will be continued while the first image is processed.
- Using a localization compression paddle, position the C-arm and breast so that the paddle opening is positioned over the quadrant of interest.
- Slowly apply compression until the breast feels taut.
- Instruct the patient to indicate whether the compression becomes uncomfortable.
- When full compression is achieved, move the AEC detector to the appropriate position, and instruct the patient to stop breathing.
- Make the exposure.
- *Do not release compression.* Keep the breast compressed while the initial image is processed.

Tangential projection
- Check the initial image, and locate the area of interest using the alphanumeric identifiers.
- With the patient's breast still under compression, locate the corresponding area on the breast and place a radiopaque marker or BB over the area.
- Release breast compression, and replace the localization compression paddle with a regular or spot compression paddle.
- Rotate the C-arm apparatus until the central ray is directed tangential to the breast at the point identified by the BB marker (the "shadow" of the BB will be projected onto the cassette surface).
- Compress the area while ensuring that enough breast tissue covers the AEC detector area.

- Slowly apply compression until the breast feels taut.
- Instruct the patient to indicate whether the compression becomes uncomfortable.
- When full compression is achieved, move the AEC detector to the appropriate position, and instruct the patient to stop breathing.
- Make the exposure.
- Release breast compression immediately.

Central ray
- Perpendicular to the area of interest

Structures shown
This projection demonstrates superficial lesions close to the skin surface with minimal parenchymal overlapping. It also shows skin calcifications or palpable lesions projected over subcutaneous fat (Fig. 23-55).

The following should be clearly demonstrated:
- Palpable lesion visualized over subcutaneous fat
- Tangential radiopaque marker or BB marker accurately correlated with palpable lesion
- Minimal overlapping of adjacent parenchyma
- Calcification in parenchyma or skin
- Uniform tissue exposure if compression is adequate

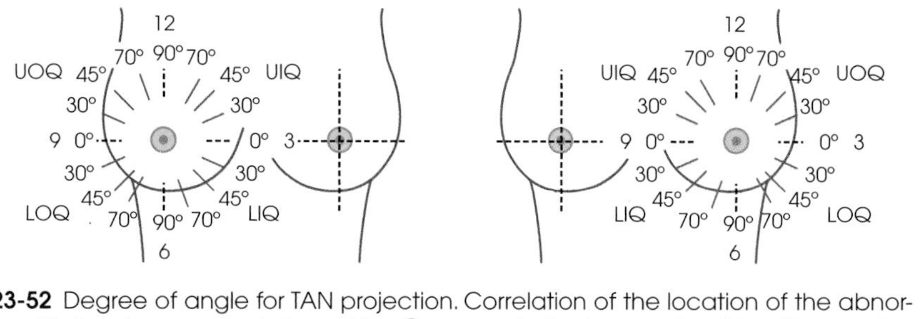

Fig. 23-52 Degree of angle for TAN projection. Correlation of the location of the abnormality with the degree of rotation of the C-arm; note that an angle of the C-arm will demonstrate both an upper quadrant and a lower quadrant abnormality tangentially.

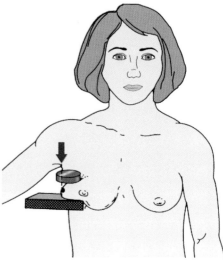

Fig. 23-53 TAN projection.

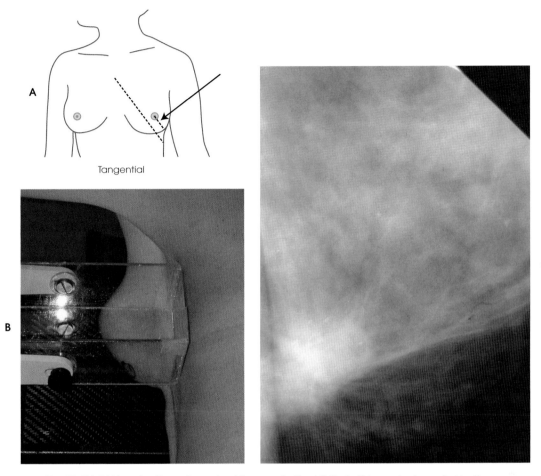

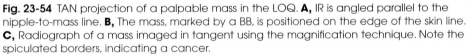

Fig. 23-54 TAN projection of a palpable mass in the LOQ. **A,** IR is angled parallel to the nipple-to-mass line. **B,** The mass, marked by a BB, is positioned on the edge of the skin line. **C,** Radiograph of a mass imaged in tangent using the magnification technique. Note the spiculated borders, indicating a cancer.

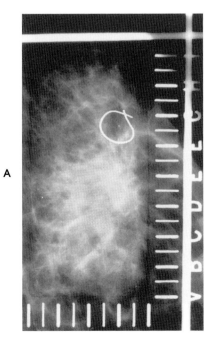

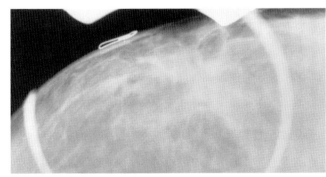

Fig. 23-55 A, A 90-degree ML projection performed with a localization compression paddle to determine the location of suspicious microcalcifications. Note that the mammographer placed a wire on the surface of the breast, encircling the area in question. **B,** TAN projection with spot compression of the localized area demonstrating benign dermal calcifications.

(From Wentz G: *Mammography for radiologic technologists,* ed 2, New York, 1997, McGraw-Hill.)

"COAT-HANGER" PROJECTION

This specialized positioning is seldom used, but is very useful when imaging a palpable lesion located in the extreme posterior breast tissue. Sometimes lesions in this area tether themselves to the chest wall and resist being pulled forward to be visualized on a routine projection. This procedure is a variation of the TAN projection and should be labeled as such. It is generally performed using magnification and tight collimation. The coat-hanger projection captures and isolates the palpable lump for imaging (Fig. 23-56).

Image receptor: 18 × 24 cm

Position of patient
- Have the patient stand facing the cassette holder, or seat the patient on an adjustable stool facing the holder.

Position of part
- Place the magnification platform designed for use with the dedicated mammography unit on the equipment. If using a coat-hanger for positioning, remove the compression paddle. Otherwise, insert the spot compression paddle upside down. The chest wall edge of the compression device will be used to hold the mass in place.
- Place a lead BB over the palpable mass.
- Using your hands, determine the projection most likely to image the lump with no superimposition of other tissue. Place the area of clinical concern at the edge of the breast in a tangent plane to the film.

- The palpable area of clinical concern is captured with a corner of a wire coat-hanger or an inverted spot compression device. No additional compression is needed.
- It may be necessary to use a manual technique if the amount of tissue captured within the coat-hanger or inverted compression device does not cover the AED detector.

Central ray
- Perpendicular to the film

Structures shown
The area of clinical concern is positively identified and visualized with the advantages of magnification mammography.

EVALUATION CRITERIA
The following should be clearly demonstrated:
- Area of interest within collimated and self-compressed margins

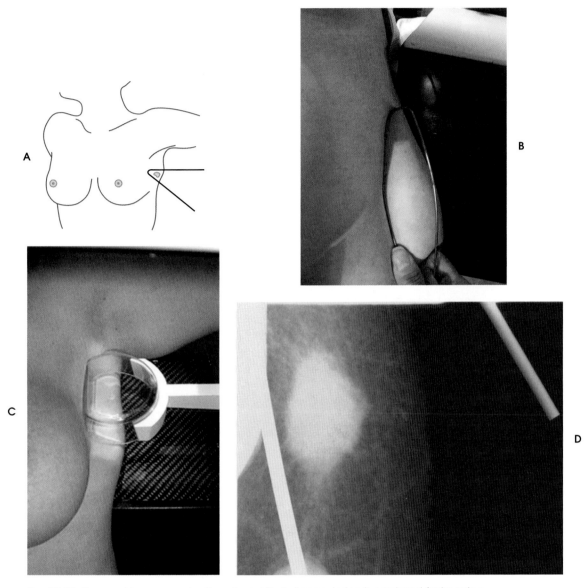

Fig. 23-56 The coat-hanger projection. **A** and **B,** A slippery lesion is captured for imaging by the angle of a wire coat-hanger. **C,** An inverted spot compression device can sometimes achieve the same results. **D,** Radiograph of lesion imaged using the coat-hanger projection. This lesion was not able to be viewed on the routine projections because of its position within the breast and the elastic nature of the lesion.

CAUDOCRANIAL (FB) PROJECTION

Image receptor: 18 × 24 cm or 24 × 30 cm

Position of patient
- Have the patient stand facing the cassette holder.

Position of part
- Rotate the C-arm apparatus 180 degrees from the rotation used for a routine CC projection.
- Standing on the medial side of the breast to be imaged, elevate the inframammary fold to its maximum height.

- Adjust the height of the cassette so that it is in contact with the superior breast tissue.
- Lean the patient slightly forward while gently pulling the elevated breast out and perpendicular to the chest wall. Hold the breast in position.
- Have the patient rest the affected arm over the top of the cassette holder.
- Inform the patient that compression of the breast will be used. Bring the compression paddle from below into contact with the patient's breast while sliding the hand toward the nipple.
- Slowly apply compression until the breast feels taut.

- Instruct the patient to indicate whether the compression becomes uncomfortable.
- To ensure that the patient's abdomen is not superimposed over the path of the beam, have the patient pull in the abdomen or move the hips back slightly.
- When full compression is achieved, move the AEC detector to the appropriate position, and instruct the patient to stop breathing (Fig. 23-57).
- Make the exposure.
- Release breast compression immediately.

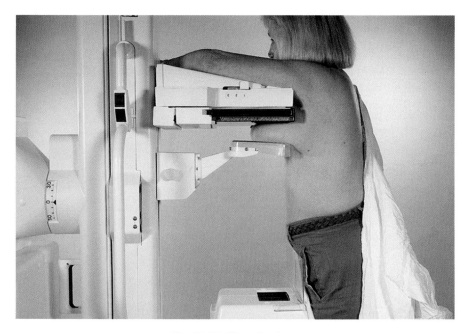

Fig. 23-57 FB projection.

Central ray

• Perpendicular to the base of the breast

Structures shown

This projection shows an inferosuperior projection of the breast for the improved visualization of lesions located in the superior aspect as a result of reduced object–to–image-receptor distance. The FB projection may also facilitate a shorter route for needle-wire insertion to localize an inferior lesion (Figs. 23-58 and 23-59). The projection is also used as a replacement for the standard CC in patients with prominent pectoral muscles or kyphosis.

The following should be clearly demonstrated:

■ Superior breast tissue/lesions clearly visualized
■ For needle localization images, inferior lesion visualized within specialized fenestrated compression plate
■ Patient's abdomen projected clear of image
■ Inclusion of fixed posterior tissue of superior aspect of breast
■ PNL extending posteriorly to edge of image, measuring within 1 cm of depth of PNL on MLO projection

■ All medial tissue included as shown by visualization of medial retroglandular fat and absence of fibroglandular tissue extending to posteromedial edge of image
■ Nipple in profile, if possible, and at midline, indicating no exaggeration of positioning
■ Some lateral tissue possibly excluded to emphasize medial tissue
■ Slight medial skin reflection at cleavage, ensuring that posterior medial tissue is adequately included
■ Uniform tissue exposure if compression is adequate

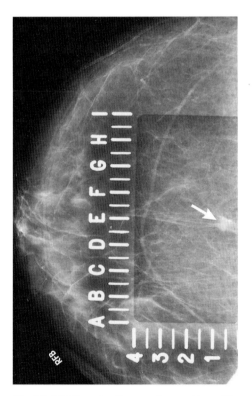

Fig. 23-58 FB projection performed in a 57-year-old woman to facilitate the shortest route for localizing a lesion identified in the inferior aspect of the breast *(arrow).*

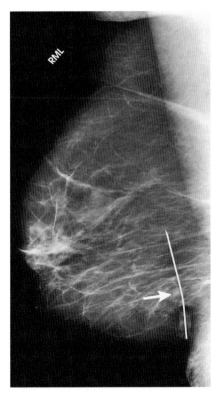

Fig. 23-59 Orthogonal 90-degree ML projection of the patient in Fig. 23-58, demonstrating successful placement of the needle-wire system within the lesion *(arrow).* The lesion was found to be a 9-mm infiltrating ductal carcinoma.

MEDIOLATERAL OBLIQUE PROJECTION FOR AXILLARY TAIL (AT)

Image receptor: 18 × 24 cm or 24 × 30 cm

Position of patient

• Have the patient stand facing the cassette holder, or seat the patient on an adjustable stool facing the holder.

Position of part

• Determine the degree of obliquity of the C-arm apparatus by rotating the tube until the long edge of the cassette is parallel with the AT of the affected side. The degree of obliquity varies between 10 and 45 degrees.
• Adjust the height of the cassette so that the superior border is just under the axilla.

• Instruct the patient to elevate the arm of the affected side over the corner of the cassette and to rest the hand on the handgrip adjacent to the cassette holder. The patient's elbow should be flexed.
• Have the patient relax the affected shoulder and lean it slightly anterior. Using the flat surface of the hand, gently pull the tail of the breast anteriorly and medially onto the cassette holder, keeping the skin and tissue smooth and free of wrinkles.
• Ask the patient to turn her head away from the side being examined and to rest her head against the face guard.
• Inform the patient that compression of the breast will be used. Continue to hold the breast in position while sliding the hand toward the nipple as the compression paddle is brought into contact with the AT (Fig. 23-60).

• Slowly apply compression until the breast feels taut. The corner of the compression paddle should be inferior to the clavicle. To avoid patient discomfort caused by the corner of the paddle and to facilitate even compression, remind the patient to keep her shoulder relaxed.
• Instruct the patient to indicate whether the compression becomes uncomfortable.
• When full compression is achieved, move the AEC detector to the appropriate position, and instruct the patient to stop breathing. It may be necessary to increase exposure factors if compression is not as taut as in the routine projections.
• Make the exposure.
• Release breast compression immediately.

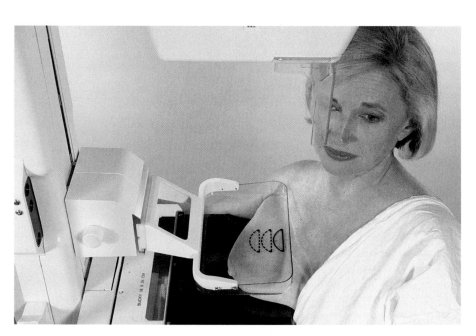

Fig. 23-60 MLO projection for AT.

Central ray

- Perpendicular to the cassette
- The angle of the C-arm apparatus is determined by the slope of the patient's AT.

Structures shown

This projection demonstrates the AT of the breast, with emphasis on its lateral aspect.

The following should be clearly demonstrated:

- ■ AT with inclusion of axillary lymph nodes under focal compression (Fig. 23-61)
- ■ Uniform tissue exposure if compression is adequate
- ■ Slight skin reflection of affected arm on superior border of image

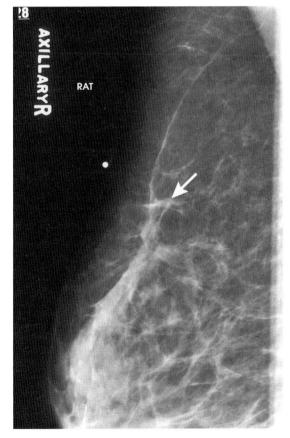

Fig. 23-61 MLO projection for AT of a 68-year-old woman, demonstrating ill-defined stellate mass measuring 8 mm *(arrow)*. Biopsy confirmed the lesion to be an infiltrating ductal carcinoma.

LATEROMEDIAL OBLIQUE (LMO) PROJECTION

Image receptor: 18 × 24 cm or 24 × 30 cm

Position of patient
- Have the patient stand facing the cassette holder, or seat the patient on an adjustable stool facing the holder.

Position of part
- Determine the degree of obliquity of the C-arm apparatus by rotating the assembly until the long edge of the cassette is parallel with the upper third of the pectoral muscle of the affected side. The central ray enters the inferior aspect of the breast from the lateral side. The degree of obliquity should be between 30 and 60 degrees, depending on the body habitus of the patient.

- Adjust the height of the cassette so that its superior border is level with the jugular notch.
- Ask the patient to place the opposite hand on the C-arm. The patient's elbow should be flexed.
- Lean the patient toward the C-arm apparatus, and press the sternum against the edge of the cassette, which will be slightly off center toward the opposite breast.
- Have the patient relax the affected shoulder and lean it slightly anterior. Gently pull the patient's breast and pectoral muscle anteriorly and medially with the flat surface of the hand positioned along the lateral aspect of the breast.
- Scoop breast tissue up with the hand, gently grasping the breast between fingers and thumb.
- Center the breast with the nipple in profile, if possible, and hold the breast in position.

- Inform the patient that compression of the breast will be used. Continue to hold the patient's breast up and out while sliding the hand toward the nipple as the compression paddle is brought into contact with the LOQ of the breast.
- Slowly apply compression until the breast feels taut.
- Instruct the patient to indicate whether the compression becomes uncomfortable.
- Pull down on the patient's abdominal tissue to open the inframammary fold.
- Ask the patient to rest the affected elbow on the top edge of the cassette.
- When full compression is achieved, move the AEC detector to the appropriate position, and instruct the patient to stop breathing (Fig. 23-62).
- Make the exposure.
- Release breast compression immediately.

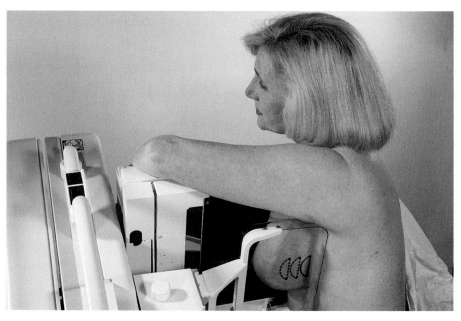

Fig. 23-62 LMO projection.

Mammography

Central ray
- Perpendicular to the cassette
- The C-arm apparatus is positioned at an angle determined by the slope of the patient's pectoral muscle (30 to 60 degrees). The actual angle is determined by the patient's body habitus: tall, thin patients require steep angulation, whereas short, stout patients require shallow angulation.

Structures shown

This projection demonstrates a true reverse projection of the routine MLO projection and is typically performed to better demonstrate the medial breast tissue. It is also performed if the routine MLO cannot be completed because of one or more of the following conditions: pectus excavatum, post open-heart surgery, prominent pacemaker, males or females with prominent pectoralis muscles, or Port-A-Cath (Hickman catheters).

The following should be clearly demonstrated:
- Medial breast tissue clearly visualized (Fig. 23-63)
- PNL measuring within 1 cm of the depth of the PNL on the CC projection (While drawing the PNL obliquely, following the orientation of the breast tissue toward the pectoral muscle, measure its depth from nipple to pectoral muscle or to the edge of the image, whichever comes first.)
- Inferior aspect of the pectoral muscle extending to nipple line or below it if possible
- Pectoral muscle with anterior convexity to ensure a relaxed shoulder and axilla
- Nipple in profile if possible
- Open inframammary fold
- Deep and superficial breast tissues well separated when breast is adequately maneuvered up and out from chest wall
- Retroglandular fat well visualized to ensure inclusion of deep fibroglandular breast tissue
- Uniform tissue exposure if compression is adequate

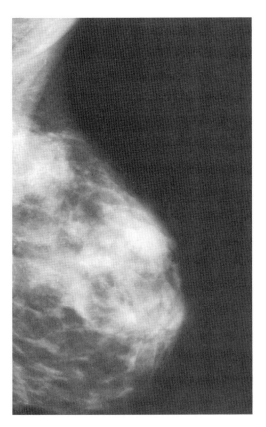

Fig. 23-63 LMO projection.

(From Svane G: *Screening mammography,* St Louis, 1993, Mosby.)

SUPEROLATERAL TO INFEROMEDIAL OBLIQUE (SIO) PROJECTION

Image receptor: 18 × 24 cm or 24 × 30 cm

Position of patient

- Have the patient stand facing the cassette holder, or seat the patient on an adjustable stool facing the holder.

Position of part

- Rotate the C-arm apparatus so that the central ray is directed at an angle to enter the superior and lateral aspect of the affected breast. The LIQ will be adjacent to the cassette.
- Adjust the degree of C-arm obliquity according to the body habitus of the patient, or, when the SIO projection is being used as an additional projection to more clearly image an area of the tissue without superimposition of surrounding tissue, adjust the C-arm to the degree of angulation required by the radiologist, generally a 20- to 30-degree angle.

- Adjust the height of the cassette to position the patient's breast over the center of the cassette.
- Instruct the patient to rest the hand of the affected side on the handgrip adjacent to the cassette holder. The patient's elbow should be flexed. For shallow-angled SIO projections, the arm on the affected side should lie straight against the patient's side. The handgrip is held by the hand on the contralateral side.
- Place the upper corner of the cassette along the sternal edge adjacent to the upper inner aspect of the patient's breast.
- With the patient leaning slightly forward, gently pull as much medial tissue as possible away from the sternal edge while holding the breast up and out. The breast should not droop. Be sure that the patient's back remains straight during positioning and that she does not lean to the side or toward the film holder.
- Inform the patient that compression of the breast will be used. Continue to hold the breast up and out.
- Bring the compression paddle under the affected arm and into contact with the patient's breast while sliding the hand toward the patient's nipple. For the shallow-angled SIO, the affected arm at the patient's side should be bent at the elbow to avoid superimposition of the humeral head over the breast tissue.
- Slowly apply compression until the breast feels taut. The upper corner of the compression paddle should be in the axilla for the standard SIO projection.
- Instruct the patient to indicate whether the compression becomes uncomfortable.
- When full compression is achieved on the standard SIO, help the patient bring the arm up and over with the flexed elbow resting on top of the cassette.
- Gently pull down on the patient's abdominal tissue to smooth out any skin folds.
- Move the AEC detector to the appropriate position, and instruct the patient to stop breathing (Fig. 23-64).
- Make the exposure.
- Release breast compression immediately.

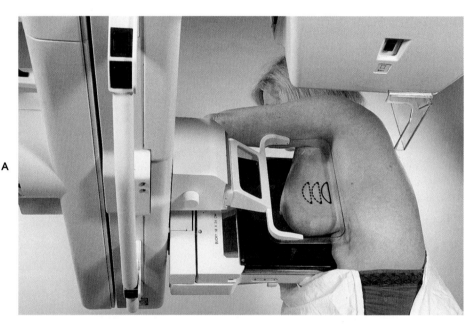

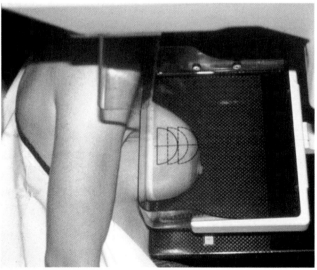

Fig. 23-64 A, SIO projection. **B,** Shallow-angled SIO with the arm down.

Central ray

- Perpendicular to the cassette
- The C-arm apparatus is positioned at an angle determined by the patient's body habitus or tissue composition.

Structures shown

This projection demonstrates the UIQ and LOQ of the breast free of superimposition. In addition, lesions located in the lower inner aspect of the breast are shown with better recorded detail. This projection may also be used to replace the MLO ID projection in patients with encapsulated implants (Fig. 23-65).

The following should be clearly demonstrated:

- UIQ and LOQ free of superimposition (These quadrants are superimposed on both the MLO and the LMO projections.)
- Lower inner aspect of breast visualized with greater detail
- Nipple in profile if possible
- Deep and superficial breast tissues well separated when breast is adequately maneuvered up and out from chest wall
- Retroglandular fat well visualized to ensure inclusion of deep fibroglandular breast tissue
- Uniform tissue exposure if compression is adequate.

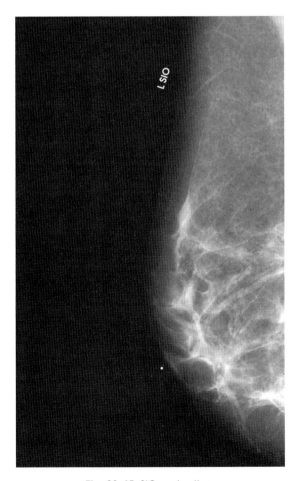

Fig. 23-65 SIO projection.

Localization of Nonpalpable Lesions

When mammography identifies a non-palpable lesion that warrants biopsy, the abnormality must be accurately located so that the smallest amount of breast tissue is removed for microscopic evaluation, thereby minimizing trauma to the breast. This technique conserves the maximum amount of normal breast tissue unless extensive surgery is indicated.

Nonpalpable breast lesions can be localized using three techniques: (1) needle-wire localization for open surgical biopsy, (2) fine-needle aspiration biopsy (FNAB), and (3) large-core needle biopsy (LCNB). Needle-wire localization uses a needle that contains a hooked guide wire to lead the surgeon directly to the suspicious tissue.

FNAB uses a hollow small-gauge needle to extract tissue cells from a suspicious lesion. FNAB can potentially decrease the need for surgical excisional biopsy by identifying benign lesions and by diagnosing malignant lesions that will require extensive surgery rather than excisional biopsy.

LCNB obtains small samples of breast tissue by means of a 9-, 11-, or 14-gauge needle with a trough adjacent to the tip of the needle. Because larger tissue samples are obtained with LCNB, clinical support exists for using this technique instead of surgical excisional biopsy. LCNB may be used with sonographic guidance. In this case, a linear array transducer of 7.5 MHz or higher should be used. Free-hand positioning of the needle is usually preferred with this modality. LCNB is also used in conjunction with stereotactic localization guidance systems (discussed later in this chapter). The method used depends on the preference of the radiologist and the surgeon and is typically determined by the degree of experience and success with each respective method. With all three methods, images are used to triangulate the location of the lesion to be biopsied.

The Advanced Breast Biopsy Instrumentation (ABBI) device is another type of tissue acquisition device that can be mounted to a stereotactic biopsy table. This method removes tissue by insertion of an oscillating cannula with diameters measuring up to 2 cm, making it possible to remove a lesion as a single, intact specimen, along with a large core of surrounding tissue. The clinical value and efficacy of this method is still being explored.[1]

---

[1]Liberman L: Clinical management issues in percutaneous core breast biopsy, *Radiol Clin North Am* 38:791, 2000.

Needle-wire localization is a predominant method for localizing nonpalpable lesions for open surgical biopsy. The four most common needle-wire localization systems are the Kopans, Homer (18-gauge), Frank (21-gauge), and Hawkins (20-gauge) biopsy guides. With each system, a long needle containing a hooked wire is inserted into the breast so that the tip approximates the lesion. A small incision (1 to 2 mm) at the entry site may be necessary to facilitate insertion of a larger-gauge needle. Once the wire is in place, the needle is withdrawn over the wire (Fig. 23-66). The hook on the end of the wire anchors the wire within the breast tissue. The surgeon cuts along the guidewire and removes the breast tissue around the wire's hooked end. Alternatively, the surgeon may choose an incision site that intercepts the anchored wire distant from the point of wire entry. Some radiologists also inject a small of amount of methylene blue dye to visually label the proper biopsy site. After needle-wire localization, the patient is properly bandaged and taken to the surgical area for excisional biopsy (Fig. 23-67). Ideally, the radiologist and surgeon should review the localization images together before the excisional biopsy.

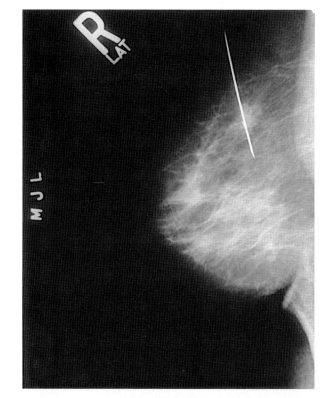

Fig. 23-66 ML projection demonstrating needle-wire localization system within a lesion.

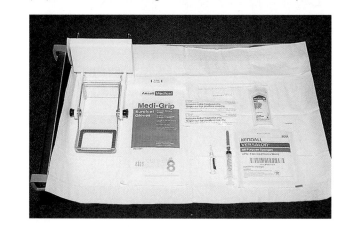

Fig. 23-67 Material for breast localization using specialized compression plate: alphanumeric localization compression plate, sterile gloves, topical antiseptic, alcohol wipe, local anesthetic, 5-mL syringe, 25-gauge needle, scalpel blade, sterile gauze, tape, and needle-wire localization system.

BREAST LESION LOCALIZATION WITH A SPECIALIZED COMPRESSION PLATE

Many mammography units have a specialized compression plate with an opening that can be positioned over a breast lesion. Through this opening a localizing needle-wire can be introduced into the breast. The initial mammogram and a 90-degree lateral projection are usually reviewed together to determine the shortest distance from the skin to the breast lesion. For example, a lesion in the inferior aspect of the breast may be best approached from the medial, lateral, or inferior surface of the breast but not from the superior surface.

The opening in the specialized fenestrated compression plate may consist of a rectangular cutout with radiopaque alphanumeric grid markings along at least two adjacent sides. Alternatively, the plate may contain several rows of holes, each large enough to accommodate the insertion of a localization needle (Fig. 23-68).

Needle-localization procedures vary from radiologist to radiologist. As a result, no standardized procedure exists. However, the following steps are typically observed:

- Perform preliminary routine full-breast projections to confirm the existence of the lesion (Figs. 23-69 and 23-70). Note that the MLO projection may be replaced by a 90-degree lateral projection.

- Obtain an informed consent after discussing the following subjects with the patient:
  1. Full explanation of the procedure
  2. Full description of potential problems: vasovagal reaction, excessive bleeding, allergic reaction to lidocaine, and possible failure of the procedure (failure rate of 1% to 10%)
  3. Answers to patient's preliminary questions

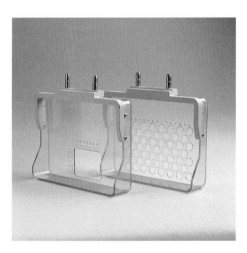

Fig. 23-68 Compression plates specifically designed for breast localization procedure.

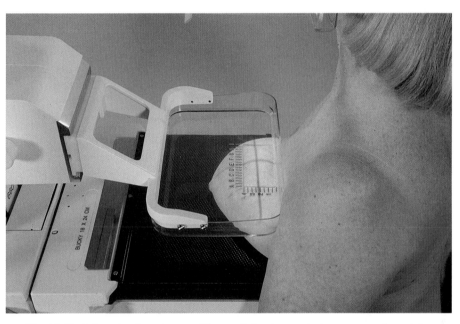

Fig. 23-69 CC projection shown with specialized open-hole compression plate.

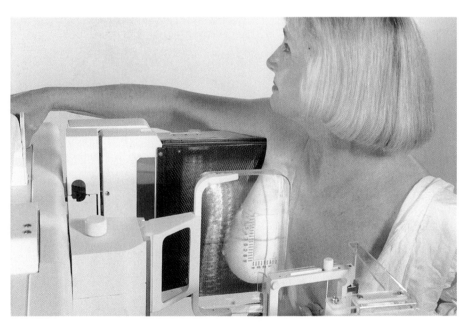

Fig. 23-70 ML projection shown with specialized open-hole compression plate.

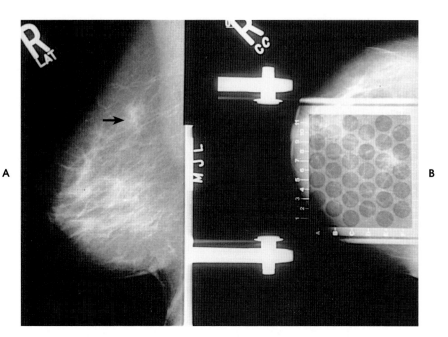

Fig. 23-71 Preliminary projections for breast localization procedure. **A,** Lateral projection is obtained to determine depth of lesion *(arrow).* **B,** Compression plate immobilizes breast for needle-wire insertion on the CC projection. Note that the alphanumeric grid demonstrates that the lesion is located nearest to E7 junction. The needle-wire will be inserted through the posterior aspect of hole E7.

- Position the patient so that the compression plate is against the skin surface closest to the lesion as determined from the preliminary images.
- Tell the patient that compression will not be released until the needle has been successfully placed and that the patient is to hold as still as possible.
- Make a preliminary exposure using compression. Ink marks placed at the corners of the paddle window determine whether the patient moves during the procedure.
- Process the image without removing compression. The resultant image shows where the lesion lies in relation to the compression plate opening (Fig. 23-71).
- Clean the skin of the breast over the entry site with a topical antiseptic.
- Apply a topical anesthetic if necessary.
- Insert the localizing needle and guide-wire into the breast perpendicular to the compression plate and parallel to the chest wall, moving the needle directly toward the underlying lesion. Advance the needle to the estimated depth of the lesion. Because the breast is compressed in the direction of the needle's insertion, it is better to pass beyond the lesion than to be short of the lesion.
- With the needle in position, make an exposure (Fig. 23-72). Then slowly release the compression plate, leaving the needle-wire system in place. Obtain an additional projection after the C-arm apparatus has been shifted 90 degrees (Fig. 23-73). These two radiographs are used to determine the position of the end of the needle-wire relative to the lesion.

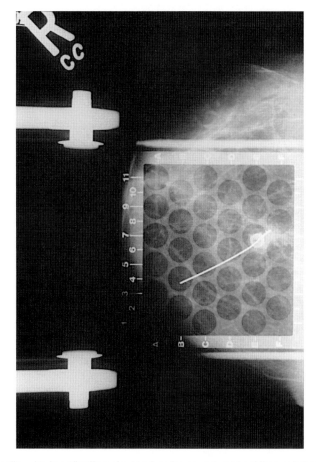

Fig. 23-72 Needle-wire localization device has been advanced through hole in compression plate to approximate location of lesion in CC projection.

- Reposition the needle-wire, and repeat the exposures if necessary.
- When the needle is accurately placed within the lesion, withdraw the needle but leave the hooked guidewire in place.
- Place a gauze bandage over the breast.
- Transport the patient to surgery along with the final localization images.

BREAST LESION LOCALIZATION WITHOUT A SPECIALIZED COMPRESSION PLATE

If a specialized fenestrated compression plate is not available or preferred, the following procedure is observed:

- Obtain preliminary routine full-breast projections to confirm the existence of the lesion. The MLO projection may be replaced by a 90-degree lateral projection.
- Obtain an informed consent after discussing the following subjects with the patient:
  1. Full explanation of the procedure
  2. Full description of potential problems: vasovagal reaction, excessive bleeding, allergic reaction to lidocaine, and possible failure of the procedure (failure rate of 1% to 10%)
  3. Answers to patient's preliminary questions

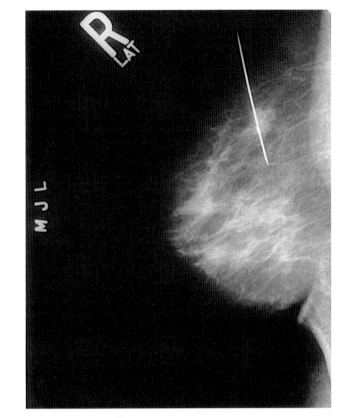

Fig. 23-73 Second projection is obtained after x-ray tube is rotated 90 degrees. This projection allows depth of needle-wire localization system to be determined. Fenestrated compression plate is replaced with standard compression plate.

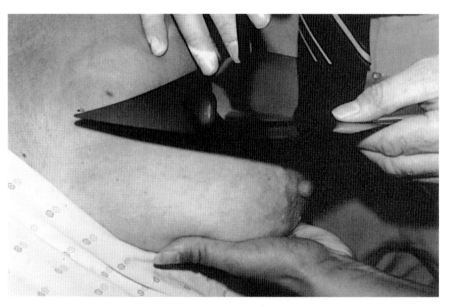

Fig. 23-74 Mammographer supports breast while physician superimposes CC projection mammogram over breast. This technique is used to locate breast lesion in reference to skin surface.

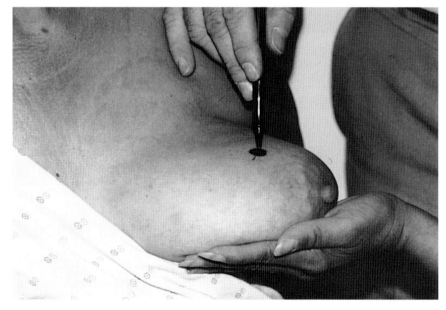

Fig. 23-75 Ink mark is placed on breast surface directly over breast lesion, locating lesion in CC projection. This technique is also used to place a mark over the lesion to locate the lesion in an ML projection.

- Using the preliminary images, place an ink mark on the breast surface indicating the position of the lesion on each image. Taping alphanumeric radiopaque markers to the breast for the preliminary images can help define the position of the lesion relative to the breast surface in each projection. Because the breast is compressed for the exposures, it must resemble the compressed position to accurately place the markers. Using the hands, the mammographer reproduces this compression while the physician marks the surface of the breast at the appropriate sites (Figs. 23-74 and 23-75). Triangulation of the two surface marks fixes the three-dimensional (3D) location of the lesion.
- Clean the skin of the breast over the entry site with a topical antiseptic.
- Apply a topical anesthetic if necessary.
- Insert the needle, preferably parallel to the chest wall, toward the lesion for the predetermined distance (Fig. 23-76).
- Image the breast in the CC and 90-degree lateral projections with the needle-wire in place so that the exact location of the wire relative to the lesion can be determined.
- Reposition the needle-wire, and repeat the exposures if necessary.
- When the needle is accurately placed within the lesion, withdraw the needle and leave the hooked guidewire in place (Figs. 23-77 and 23-78).
- Place a gauze bandage over the breast.
- Transport the patient to surgery along with the final localization images.

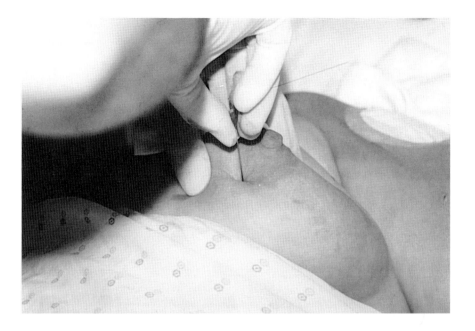

Fig. 23-76 Frank biopsy needle and guidewire is inserted into breast perpendicular to chest wall at site directly anterior to lesion. Site and depth of insertion are selected by triangulation using external skin marks.

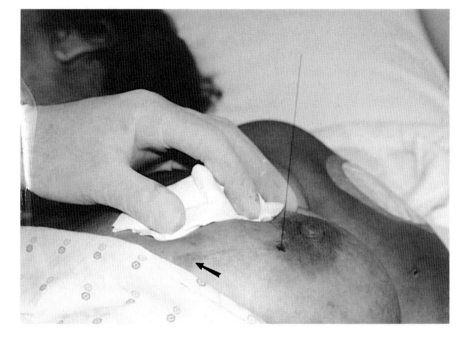

Fig. 23-77 After inserting needle and guidewire to depth of lesion, needle is removed, leaving guidewire in place. Lateral skin mark used for selecting needle insertion site is seen *(arrow)*.

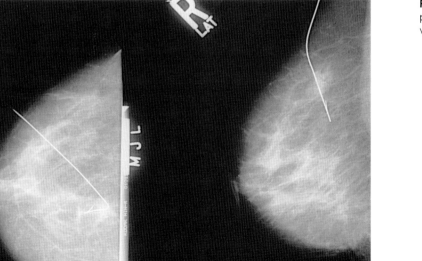

Fig. 23-78 CC and true lateral right-angle projections demonstrate relationship of wire to lesion. Needle has been removed.

STEREOTACTIC PROCEDURES

Approximately 80% of nonpalpable lesions identified by mammography are not malignant. Nonetheless, a breast lesion cannot be definitely judged benign until it has been microscopically evaluated. Stereotactic intervention, or *stereotaxis,* is a minor surgical procedure used to determine the benign or malignant nature of suspicious breast lesions. Stereotaxis guided by mammographic or ultrasound imaging is the preferred method for obtaining biopsy specimens of nonpalpable or equivocally symptomatic breast lesions. Most women with a mammographic and/or clinical breast abnormality are candidates for stereotactic core needle biopsy. The only exceptions are patients who cannot cooperate for the procedure, patients who have mammographic findings at the limits of perception, and patients with lesions of potentially ambiguous histology.

Stereotaxis is used to differentiate between benign and malignant breast lesions. The benefits of stereotaxis over conventional surgical biopsy are less pain, less scarring, shorter recovery time, less patient anxiety, and lower cost.

Because stereotaxis can expedite pathology results, potential surgical decisions such as those regarding lumpectomy or mastectomy can be made with minimal delay. When operating on the basis of a core biopsy diagnosis of cancer, surgeons are more likely to obtain clean (negative) lumpectomy margins with the first excision. Axillary lymph nodes, which are evaluated to ascertain metastases, are also sampled at the time of the initial surgery. Thus the woman with a known diagnosis of breast cancer may avoid a second operation.

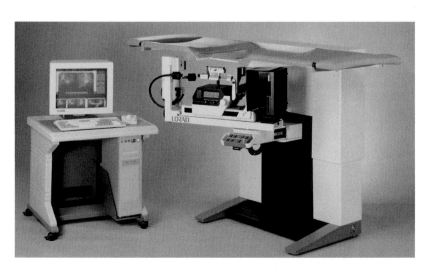

Fig. 23-80 Prone stereotactic biopsy system with digital imaging.

(Courtesy Delta Medical Systems, Inc., Milwaukee, Wis.)

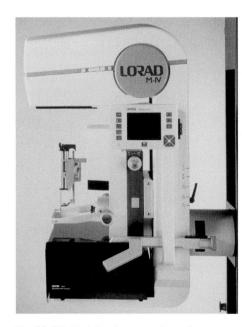

Fig. 23-79 Upright stereotactic system attached to a dedicated mammography unit.

(Courtesy Trex Medical Corp., LORAD Division, Danbury, Conn.)

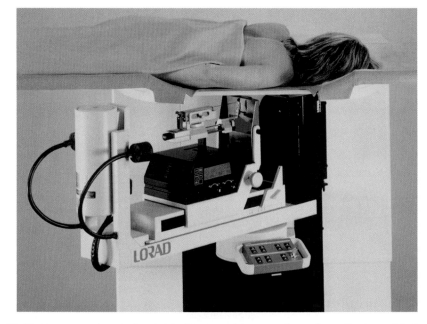

Fig. 23-81 Open aperture in the table for prone biopsy system allows the breast to be positioned beneath the table.

(Courtesy Trex Medical Corp., LORAD Division, Danbury, Conn.)

Stereotactic breast biopsy requires a team approach involving a radiologist, a mammographer, a pathologist, and a specially trained nurse or technologist. Stereotactic prone biopsy tables and upright add-on devices used for biopsy intervention are both commercially available. The disadvantages of the upright add-on system include a limited working space, an increased potential for patient motion, and a greater potential for vasovagal reactions (Fig. 23-79). The dedicated prone system is more expensive than the add-on system. It also requires a larger space and should not be used for conventional mammography (Figs. 23-80 and 23-81). However, the success or failure of core needle breast biopsy depends more on the experience and interest of the diagnostic team than on the particulars of the system that is used.

In stereotactic breast biopsy, 3D triangulation is used to identify the exact location of a breast lesion. A digitizer calculates X, Y, and Z coordinates (Figs. 23-82 and 23-83). The X coordinate identifies transverse location (right to left), the Y coordinate designates depth (front to back), and the Z coordinate identifies the height of the lesion (top to bottom). It is important to note that different stereotactic systems will have different methods for calculating a "Z" value, depending on the center of rotation of the localization device. The operator should be familiar with the system in use so that accurate adjustments of the localization device can be made. Two exposures of a single position are taken at a difference of 30 degrees—one exposure at +15 degrees

and the other at −15 degrees from the perpendicular. Precision of these angles is important. Also, with certain systems, the sequence of these images is significant in providing a correct value of lesion depth. The resultant image localizes the lesion in three dimensions. The resultant images are referred to as the *stereo image* (Fig. 23-84). The physician can use the stereo image to determine the appropriate approach for reaching the breast lesion. Imaging with stereotactic units is available as either conventional screen-film or small-field (5 × 5 cm) digital imaging. Although conventional screen-film systems are considerably less expensive, digital imaging is preferred due to its shorter acquisition time.

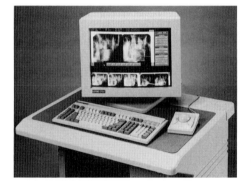

Fig. 23-82 Digitizer calculates and transmits X, Y, and Z coordinates to stage, or "brain," of biopsy system, where biopsy gun is attached. This information is used to determine placement of biopsy needle.

(Courtesy Trex Medical Corp., LORAD Division, Danbury, Conn.)

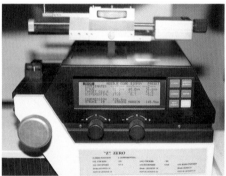

Fig. 23-83 Stage of biopsy system supports biopsy gun. The X, Y, and Z coordinates are displayed.

(Courtesy Delta Medical Systems, Inc., Milwaukee, Wis.)

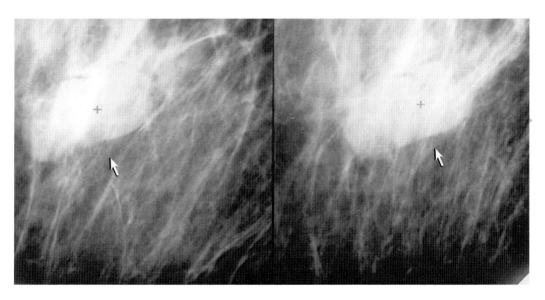

Fig. 23-84 Stereo images demonstrating 3D visualization of breast lesion before intervention *(arrows).*

Before beginning the procedure, the physician reviews the initial mammographic images to determine the shortest distance from the surface of the skin to the breast lesion. If the exact lesion location is identified, the biopsy needle can be inserted through the least amount of breast with only minimal trauma to the breast. For example, a lesion located in the lateral aspect of the UOQ is approached from the lateral aspect, whereas a lesion located in the medial and superior portion of the breast is approached from above. After the best approach to the lesion has been determined, the affected breast is positioned and compressed for a scout image to localize the breast lesion. Once the breast lesion has been localized, stereo images are taken to triangulate the lesion so that proper coordinates can be calculated and dialed into the biopsy table stage. The breast is aseptically cleansed to minimize infection. Pain associated with the procedure can be effectively managed using a local anesthetic to numb the skin at the area where the biopsy needle enters.

Three general methods can be used to localize a breast lesion. The physician's preference generally determines the procedure that is performed. With needle-wire localization, the surgeon uses the hooked guidewire to find the biopsy site. In FNAB, cells are extracted from a suspicious lesion with a thin needle. LCNB obtains core samples of tissue by means of a larger needle with a groove adjacent to its tip. All three procedures can be performed using prone or upright stereotactic breast biopsy systems. However, because LCNB with stereotactic guidance is becoming the preferred localization method, it is discussed in depth in this chapter.

The physician decides where the first and subsequent passes (biopsy needle travels through the breast tissue to reach the breast lesion) are to be made. After the skin is anesthetized, a small incision is made with a scalpel to facilitate entry of the needle into the breast. A spring-loaded biopsy device is then used to power the needle back and forth through the target. A set of stereo images is obtained to confirm correct direction of the needle (Fig. 23-85). The first pass is made by placing the biopsy needle within the lesion and obtaining a "postfire" image to confirm the correct needle placement. This image determines the course of subsequent passes. Redigitization (use of a digitizer to repeat the steps needed to calculate the new triangulation coordinates) can be performed to obtain additional samples. Alternatively, the physician can estimate where to move the biopsy needle based on the initial needle location within the breast. It is important to remember that LCNB tissue samples are obtained using a needle with a trough adjacent to the needle tip. With the needle located inside the lesion, a sheath or needle cover slides over the trough of the needle. The sheath cuts the tissue sample within the trough and holds the sample in place while the needle is withdrawn. When the needle is outside the breast, the sheath is pulled back, exposing the tissue sample. The sample is then transferred to a specimen container for transportation to the laboratory. A minimum of 5 and as many as 20 tissue samples are obtained to ensure accurate sampling of the abnormality. The time required to perform a stereotactic procedure is approximately 40 to 50 minutes.

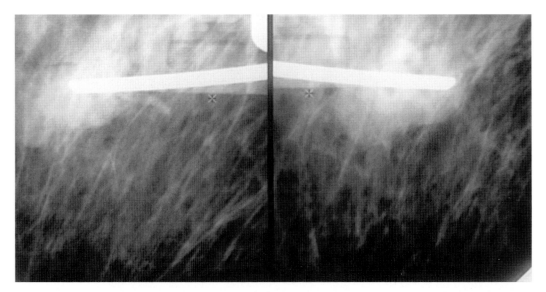

Fig. 23-85 Postfire stereo images demonstrating placement of biopsy needle inside lesion.

An alternative technique known as vacuum-assisted core biopsy uses a 14-, 11-, or 9-gauge probe that is inserted under stereotactic or sonographic guidance to align the probe's aperture within the lesion. Tissue is gently vacuum aspirated into the probe's aperture. A rotating cutter is advanced to cut and capture the tissue sample. The cutter is then withdrawn without removing the probe from the lesion, and the specimen is transported in the cutter to a tissue collection chamber. Multiple samples may be obtained by rotating the probe in vivo without multiple insertions. Once the biopsy is complete, a radiopaque clip can be deployed through the probe and into the biopsy site to mark the area for future reference. The larger amount of tissue sampled with this technique is reported to improve accuracy in diagnosing atypical ductal hyperplasia and ductal carcinoma in situ lesions.[1]

After the LCNB procedure is completed, the breast is cleansed and bandaged using sterile technique. Compression to the biopsy site is necessary to prevent excessive bleeding, and a cold compress is applied to minimize discomfort and swelling of the related tissues.

The patient may be asked to return within 24 to 48 hours so that the breast can be examined to ensure that no bleeding or infection has occurred. The physician who performed the biopsy discusses the biopsy results and subsequent treatment options, if applicable, with the patient.

[1]Dershaw DD: Equipment, technique, quality assurance, and accreditation for image-guided breast biopsy procedures, *Radiol Clin North Am* 38:773, 2000.

Breast Specimen Radiography

When open surgical biopsy is performed, the suspected lesion must be contained in its entirety in the tissue removed during the biopsy. Very small lesions that are characterized by tissue irregularity or microcalcifications on a mammographic image and that are nonpalpable in the excised specimen may not be detectable on visual inspection; therefore a radiographic image of the biopsied tissue may be necessary to determine that the entire lesion has been removed. Compression of the specimen is necessary to identify lesions, especially lesions that do not contain calcifications. Magnification imaging is used to help to better visualize microcalcifications. Specimen radiography is often performed in an immediate post-excision procedure while the patient is still under anesthesia. Speed is therefore imperative. The film type, technical factors, and procedure for handling the specimen must be established before the procedure is started. Cooperation among the radiologist, mammographer, surgeon, and pathologist is a necessity. Together, a system of identifying the orientation of the tissue sample to the patient's breast (anterior, posterior, medial, or lateral aspect of the sample) can be applied to aid in determining that the lesion has been completely removed. Extremely fine-grain, nonscreen film may be used because patient exposure is no longer a factor. The exposure factors depend on the thickness of the specimen and the film that is used (Fig. 23-86).

It may be helpful to obtain one image of the breast specimen for the radiologist and another for the pathologist. The pathologist often uses the specimen radiograph to precisely locate the area of concern. The next step is to match the actual specimen to the specimen radiograph before the specimen is dissected. Marking the area of concern by placing a radiopaque object, such as a 1- or 2-inch needle, directly at the area of concern helps the pathologist locate the abnormality more accurately.

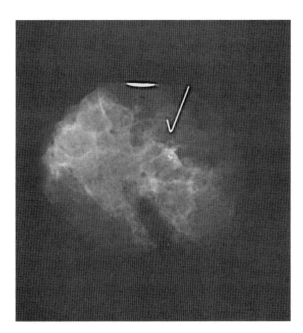

Fig. 23-86 Radiograph of surgical specimen containing suspicious microcalcifications.

Ductography (Examination of Milk Ducts)

When a nipple discharge is localized in one of the multiple duct openings on the nipple, the milk duct can be studied using an opaque contrast medium. The purpose of the examination is to rule out an intraductal cancer or to determine whether a benign mass such as a papilloma is the cause of the discharge. The equipment and supplies for the examination include the following: a sterile hypodermic syringe (usually 1 to 3 mL); a 30-gauge ductography cannula with a smooth, round tip; a skin cleansing agent; sterile gauze sponges or cotton balls; paper tape; a waste basin; and an organic, water-soluble, iodinated contrast medium.

After the nipple is cleansed, a small amount of discharge is expressed to identify the correct ductal opening. The cannula is inserted into the orifice of the duct, and undiluted iothalamate meglumine or iopamidol is gently injected. So that the patient does not experience unnecessary discomfort and extravasation does not occur, the injection is terminated as soon as the patient experiences a sense of fullness, pressure, or pain. The cannula is taped in place before positioning the patient for the radiographs. If cannulation is unsuccessful, a sterile local anesthetic gel or warm compress may be applied to the nipple and areola and the procedure is reattempted. If ductography is unsuccess-ful after several attempts, the procedure may be rescheduled in 7 to 14 days. Upon successful injection, the following guidelines are observed:

- Immediately obtain radiographs with the patient positioned for the CC and lateral projections of the subareolar region using magnification technique (Fig. 23-87). If needed, MLO or rolled CC and rolled MLO magnification projections may be obtained to resolve superimposed ducts.
- Employ the exposure techniques used in general mammography.
- Leave the cannula in the duct to minimize leakage of contrast material during compression and to facilitate reinjection of the contrast medium without the need for recannulation.
- If the cannula is removed for the images, do not apply vigorous compression because it would cause the contrast medium to be expelled.

Computer-Aided Detection and Computer-Aided Diagnosis

When performing mammographic interpretation, the radiologist must locate any suspicious lesions (sensitivity) and then determine the probability that the lesion is malignant or benign (specificity). Even with high-quality, screen-film mammography, some breast cancers are missed on initial interpretation. Double-reading of screening mammograms by a second radiologist can improve detection rates by approximately 10%.[1] Recently, efforts have been made to develop and apply a computer-aided detection system to achieve the same result as double-reading. It has also been found that double-reading plus the use of CAD can increase detection rates by an additional 8%.[2]

Computer-aided detection and computer-aided diagnosis (CAD) are methods by which a radiologist can use computer analysis of digitally acquired images as a "second opinion" before making a final interpretation. CAD works much like a spell-check on a computer; an area is pointed out for the radiologist to check, but it is up to the radiologist to decide whether the area is suspicious enough to warrant any additional procedures. CAD requires that the mammographic image exist in a digital format to facilitate computer input. This is more commonly accomplished with use of an optical scanner; however, the use of images directly acquired with full-field digital techniques is emerging as a preferred method. The computer may detect lesions that are missed by the radiologist, thereby minimizing the possibility of false-negative readings (Fig. 23-88). Once a lesion is detected, the computer can be programmed with basic

[1]Kopans DB: Double-reading, *Radiol Clin North Am* 38:719, 2000.
[2]Destounis SV et al: Can computer-aided detection with double reading of screening mammograms help decrease the false-negative rate? Initial experience, *Radiology* 232:578, 2004.

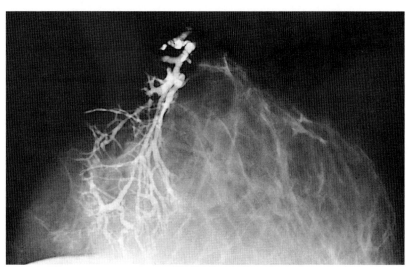

Fig. 23-87 CC projection of opacified milk ducts.

algorithms to estimate the likelihood of malignancy, thereby increasing true-positive rates. Ultimately, the objective of this technology is to improve early detection rates and minimize the number of unnecessary breast biopsies. Another advantage of CAD is that computers are not subject to the bias, fatigue, or distractions to which a radiologist may be subject.

Multicenter studies are being conducted to determine the sensitivity of computer detection programs. The sensitivity of CAD for detecting clusters of microcalcifications has been shown to approach 90%.[1] In another study, one algorithm has been shown to identify more than 80% of missed lesions that proved conspicuous in retrospect. These results have led the U.S. Food and Drug Administration to approve a commercial computer-aided detection system for clinical use.[2] The sensitivity of CAD for correctly identifying microcalcifications is remarkable (98% accuracy). In the identification of masses, CAD demonstrated a 74.7% accuracy. Furthermore, during clinical application, CAD has not shown a significant increase in false-positive mammograms.

CAD has demonstrated meaningful clinical application not only in screening mammography but also in the analysis of basic chest radiography and computed tomography of the lung. The successful clinical application of CAD in these areas will certainly result in its complete integration with full-field digital imaging systems in the future.

[1]Vyborny CJ et al: Computer-aided detection and diagnosis of breast cancer, *Radiol Clin North Am* 38:725, 2000.
[2]Roehrig J et al: Clinical results with R2 image checker system. In Karssemeijer N et al, editors: *Digital imaging '98,* Dordrecht, The Netherlands, 1998, Kluwer Academic.

Full-Field Digital Mammography

Mammography has been the last area in the field of radiography to take advantage of digital technology. In addition to the many technical issues with full-field digital mammography (FFDM), the prohibitive cost of the equipment and its maintenance do not make digital mammography practical for all facilities.

FFDM units allow radiologists to electronically manipulate the digital images, potentially saving patients from undergoing additional projections and therefore additional radiation. The ability to manipulate the digital images improves the sensitivity of mammography, especially in women with dense breast tissue. The results of the ACRIN DMIST study, a multi-facility, multi-unit study comparing film/screen mammography to digital mammography, was published in September of 2005.[1] The authors of this study concluded that FFDM would benefit some patients, specifically women under the age of 50, premenopausal and perimenopausal women, and women of any age with dense breast tissue. Because there are patients who will benefit from digital mammography, it is destined to become more dominant in the future. In the meantime, if FFDM is unavailable to

[1]Pisano E et al: Diagnostic performance of digital versus film mammography for breast cancer screening, *N Engl J Med* 353:1773, 2005.

women who fall within these benefit guidelines, they should continue having film-screen mammography studies, as it has successfully been used as a screening tool for breast cancer for more than 35 years.

Digital breast imaging requires a much finer resolution than other body imaging. FFDM images are extremely large files that require a great deal of archival space in the picture archiving and communication system (PACS). Due to regulations safeguarding the image quality of mammography, the images cannot be interpreted on a traditional PACS workstation; they can be interpreted only on special five-megapixel monitors. Innovative solutions and approaches to FFDM continue to be developed. A promising offshoot of FFDM is breast tomosynthesis, a 3D imaging technology that involves acquiring images of a stationary, compressed breast at multiple angles during a short scan. These images are then reconstructed into thin, high-resolution slices that can be displayed individually or in a dynamic cine mode.

The ultimate goal of these pursuits should not be lost in the technology itself or in the formidable economic climate of health care today. The purpose of breast cancer screening is to save lives, regardless of the method or medium. The efficacy of mammography has been proved. The continued improvement of mammographic image quality by using digitally based image manipulation is a certainty.

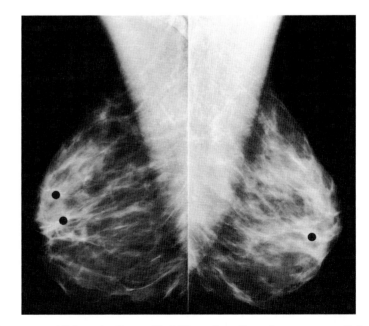

Fig. 23-88 Bilateral MLO projections with CAD markers. These images were digitally acquired by an optical scanner and analyzed by a computer. Areas indicated by markers were benign.

(Courtesy R2 Technology, Inc., Los Altos, Calif.)

Breast MRI

Breast MRI has proven to be most useful in patients with proven breast cancer to assess for multifocal/multicentric disease, chest wall involvement, chemotherapy response, or tumor recurrence or to identify the primary site in patients with occult breast disease.

INDICATIONS

Extent of disease/assessment of residual disease

MRI can be helpful for patients who have had a lumpectomy and have positive margins and no evidence of residual disease on conventional imaging (mammography, ultrasound). Postoperative mammography can help detect residual calcifications but is limited for residual mass. MRI is very sensitive for detection of residual mass and identifies other potential suspicious sites seen on MRI only.

Assessing tumor recurrence

Assessment of tumor recurrance can be very complicated on MRI because scars can enhance for 1 to 2 years after surgery. Suggestion of recurrence can be made by MRI, yet the cost of the procedure should be weighed against a less-expensive needle biopsy of the area.

Occult primary breast cancer

Patients with axillary metastases suspicious for primary breast cancer with a negative physical exam, mammogram, and ultrasound are good candidates for MRI because of its high sensitivity for invasive cancers. MRI has been shown to detect 90% to 100% of cancers if tumor is present in the breast. If the primary site is detected, the patient may be spared a mastectomy and MRI can influence patient surgical management.

Neoadjuvant chemotherapy response

In patients with advanced breast cancer, MRI may be able to predict earlier which patients are responding to chemotherapy. Mammography and physical exam can sometimes be limited by fibrosis. Studies suggest that MRI may be better at assessing patients' response to treatment.[1]

---

[1]Yeh E et al: Prospective comparison of mammography, sonography, and MRI in patients undergoing neoadjuvant chemotherapy for palpable breast cancer, *AJR* 184:868, 2005.

High-risk screening

MRI holds promise in BRCA1 or 2 carriers, who have up to an 85% risk of developing breast cancer in their lifetime. The risk of bilateral and premenopausal breast cancer is much higher in these women. A recent study published in the *New England Journal of Medicine* concluded that MRI is "more sensitive than mammography in detecting tumors in women with an inherited susceptibility of breast cancer."[1] Currently not all insurance companies cover breast MRI in these high-risk women.

Women who are found to have foci on MRI suspicious of cancer need to have these verified by biopsy. Often these areas are reexamined with directed ultrasound for potential biopsy. If these lesions are not found by conventional imaging, confirmation with an MRI-guided biopsy would be necessary before committing the patient to potential lumpectomy and/or mastectomy.

---

[1]Kriege M et al: Efficacy of MRI and mammography for breast cancer screening in women with a familial or genetic predisposition, *N Engl J Med* 351:427, 2004.

Thermography and Diaphanography

Beginning in the 1950s, thermography and diaphanography were actively investigated in the hope that breast cancer and other abnormalities could be diagnosed using nonionizing forms of radiation. These two diagnostic tools are seldom used today.

Thermography is the photographic recording of the infrared radiation emanating from a patient's body surface. The resulting thermogram demonstrates areas of increased temperature, with a temperature increase often suggesting increased metabolism. (More complete information on this technique is provided in the fourth through eighth editions of this atlas.)

Diaphanography is an examination in which a body part is transilluminated using selected light wavelengths and special imaging equipment. With this technique the interior of the breast is inspected using light directed through its exterior wall. The light exiting the patient's body is then recorded and interpreted. The rapid advances in mammography have essentially eliminated the use of this technique for evaluating breast disease. (More complete information on diaphanography is given in this chapter in the fourth through eighth editions of this atlas.)

Conclusion

Radiographic examination of the breast is a technically demanding procedure. Success depends in large part on the skills of the mammographer—more so than in most other areas of radiology. In addition to skill, the mammographer must have a strong desire to perform high-quality mammography and must be willing to work with the patient to allay qualms and to obtain cooperation. In the course of taking the patient's history and physically assessing and radiographing the breasts, the mammographer may be asked questions about breast disease, BSE, screening guidelines, and breast radiography that the patient has been reluctant to ask other health care professionals. The knowledge, skill, and attitude of the mammographer may be lifesaving for the patient. Although most patients do not have significant breast disease when first examined, statistics show that approximately 12% of patients develop breast cancer at some time during their lifetime. An early positive mammography encounter may make the patient more willing to undergo mammography in the future. When properly performed, breast radiography is safe, and it presently is the best hope for significantly reducing the mortality of breast cancer.

Suggested reading

Adler D, Wahl R: New methods for imaging the breast: techniques, findings and potential, *AJR* 164:19, 1995.

American Cancer Society: Breast cancer facts and figures 1999/2000 (website): www.cancer.org. Accessed April 2001.

Andolina V, Lille S, Willison K: *Mammographic imaging: a practical guide*, ed 2, Philadelphia, 2001, Lippincott Williams & Wilkins.

Appelbaum A et al: Mammographic appearance of male breast disease, *Radiographics* 19:559, 2001.

Bassett L: Clinical image evaluation, *Radiol Clin North Am* 33:1027, 1995.

Bassett L: Imaging of breast masses, *Radiol Clin North Am* 38:669, 2000.

Bassett L, Heinlein R: Good positioning key to imaging of breast, *Diagn Imaging* 9:69, 1993.

Bassett L et al, editors: *Quality determinants of mammography*, AHCPR Pub No 95-0632, Rockville, Md, 1994, U.S. Department of Health and Human Services.

Burbank F: Stereotactic breast biopsy of atypical hyperplasia and ductal carcinoma in situ lesions: improved accuracy with directional, vacuum-assisted biopsy, *Radiology* 202:843, 1997.

Burbank F, Parker SH, Fogarty TJ: Stereotactic breast biopsy: improved tissue harvesting with Mammotome, *Am Surg* 62:738, 1996.

Carr J et al: Stereotactic localization of breast lesions: how it works and methods to improve accuracy, *Radiographics* 21:463, 2001.

Dershaw DD: Equipment, technique, quality assurance, and accreditation for image-guided breast biopsy procedures, *Radiol Clin North Am* 38:773, 2000.

Dershaw DD et al: Mammographic findings in men with breast cancer, *AJR* 160:267, 1993.

Donegan WL: Cancer of the male breast. In Donegan WL, Spratt JS, editors: *Cancer of the breast*, ed 4, Philadelphia, 1995, Saunders.

Eklund GW, Cardenosa G: The art of mammographic positioning, *Radiol Clin North Am* 30:21, 1992.

Eklund GW et al: Improved imaging of the augmented breast, *AJR* 151:469, 1988.

F-D-C Reports, Inc: *ImageChecker unanimously endorsed by radiology panel. Medical devices, diagnostics, and instrumentation: "the gray sheet,"* 24:20, 1998.

Feig S: Breast masses. Mammographic and sonographic evaluation, *Radiol Clin North Am* 30:67, 1992.

Fundamentals of mammography: the quest for quality positioning: guidebook for radiologic technologists, Albuquerque, 1993, American Society of Radiologic Technologists.

Haus A, Yaffe M: Screen-film and digital mammography image quality and radiation dose considerations, *Radiol Clin North Am* 38:871, 2000.

Healy B: BRCA genes: bookmarking, fortunetelling, and medical care, *N Engl J Med* 336:1448, 1997 (editorial).

Henderson IC: Breast cancer. In Murphy GP, Lawrence WL, Lenhard RE, editors: *Clinical oncology,* Atlanta, 1997, American Cancer Society.

Homer M, Smith T, Safaii H: Prebiopsy needle localization. Methods, problems, and expected results, *Radiol Clin North Am* 30:139, 1992.

Jackson V: The status of mammographically guided fine needle aspiration biopsy of nonpalpable breast lesions, *Radiol Clin North Am* 30:155, 1992.

Kimme-Smith C: New and future developments in screen-film mammography equipment and techniques, *Radiol Clin North Am* 30:55, 1992.

Kopans DB: Double reading, *Radiol Clin North Am* 38:719, 2000.

Krainer M et al: Differential contributions of BRCA1 and BRCA2 to early-onset breast cancer, *N Engl J Med* 336:1416, 1997.

Liberman L: Clinical management issues in percutaneous core breast biopsy, *Radiol Clin North Am* 38:791, 2000.

Logan-Young W, Hoffman N: *Breast cancer: a practical guide to diagnosis,* Rochester, NY, 1994, Mt. Hope Publishing.

Logan-Young W et al: The cost effectiveness of fine-needle aspiration cytology and 14-gauge core needle biopsy compared with open surgical biopsy in the diagnosis of breast cancer; *Cancer* 82:1867, 1998.

Love S: *Dr. Susan Love's breast book,* ed 2, Reading, Mass, 1995, Perseus.

Mammography quality control manual, rev. ed, Chicago, 1999, American College of Radiology.

National Cancer Institute CancerNet: www.cancernet.nci.nih.gov. Accessed April 2001.

Nishikawa R et al: Computerized detection of clustered microcalcifications: evaluation of performance on mammograms from multiple centers, *Radiographics* 15:443, 1995.

Orel SG: MR imaging of the breast, *Radiol Clinc North Am* 38:899, 2000.

Parker SL, Burbank F: A practical approach to minimally invasive breast biopsy, *Radiology* 200:11, 1996.

Parker SL et al: Percutaneous large-core breast biopsy: a multi-institutional study, *Radiology* 193:359, 1994.

Parker SL et al: Cancer statistics, 1997, *CA Cancer J Clin* 47:5, 1997.

Prechtel K, Pretchel V: Breast carcinoma in the man. Current results from the viewpoint of clinic and pathology, *Pathologe* 18:45, 1997.

Roehrig J et al: Clinical results with R2 image checker system. In Karssemeijer N et al, editors: *Digital imaging '98,* Dordrecht, The Netherlands, 1998, Kluwer Academic.

Rozenberg S et al: Principal cancers among women: breast, lung, and colorectal, *Int J Fertil* 41:166, 1996.

Schmidt R, Wolverton D, Vyborny C: Computer-aided diagnosis in mammography. In: *RSNA categorical course in breast imaging* [syllabus], Oak Park, Ill, 1995, RSNA.

Skolnick AA: Ultrasound may help detect breast implant leaks, *JAMA* 267:786, 1992.

Slawson SH et al: Ductography: how to and what if? *Radiographics* 21:133, 2001.

Vyborny CJ: Computer-aided detection and computer-aided diagnosis of breast cancer, *Radiol Clin North Am* 38:725, 2000.

Wentz G: *Mammography for radiologic technologists,* ed 2, New York, 1997, McGraw-Hill.

ADDENDUM B: SUMMARY OF ABBREVIATIONS, VOLUME TWO

AAA	Abdominal aortic aneurysm
ACR	American College of Radiology
AML	Acanthiomeatal line
AP	Anteroposterior
ASRT	American Society of Radiologic Technologists
BE	Barium enema
BPH	Benign prostatic hyperplasia
BUN	Blood urea nitrogen
CDC	Centers for Disease Control and Prevention
CPR	Cardiopulmonary resuscitation
CR	Central ray
CT	Computed tomography
CTC	CT colonography
CVA	Cerebrovascular accident
EAM	External acoustic meatus
ED	Emergency department
ERCP	Endoscopic retrograde cholangiopancreatography
GML	Glabellomeatal line
GSW	Gunshot wound
HSG	Hysterosalpingography
IAM	Internal acoustic meatus
IOML	Infraorbitomeatal line
IPL	Interpupillary line
IR	Image receptor
IUD	Intrauterine device
IV	Intravenous
IVP	Intravenous pyelogram
IVU	Intravenous urography
KUB	Kidneys, ureters, and bladder
M-A	Miller-Abbott
MML	Mentomeatal line
MPR	Multiplanar reconstruction
MRI	Magnetic resonance imaging
MVA	Motor vehicle accident
NPO	nil per os (nothing by mouth)
OID	Object–to–image-receptor distance
OML	Orbitomeatal line
PA	Posteroanterior
PTC	Percutaneous transhepatic cholangiography
RUQ	Right upper quadrant
SID	Source–to–image-receptor distance
SMV	Submentovertical
TEA	Top of ear attachment
TMJ	Temporomandibular joint
UGI	Upper gastrointestinal
VC	Virtual colonoscopy
VCUG	Voiding cystourethrogram

INDEX

Page numbers followed by *f* indicate figures; *t,* tables;
b, boxes.

I-1

Index

Index

Index

Index

Index

Index

Index

Index

Index

Index

Index

Index

Index

Index

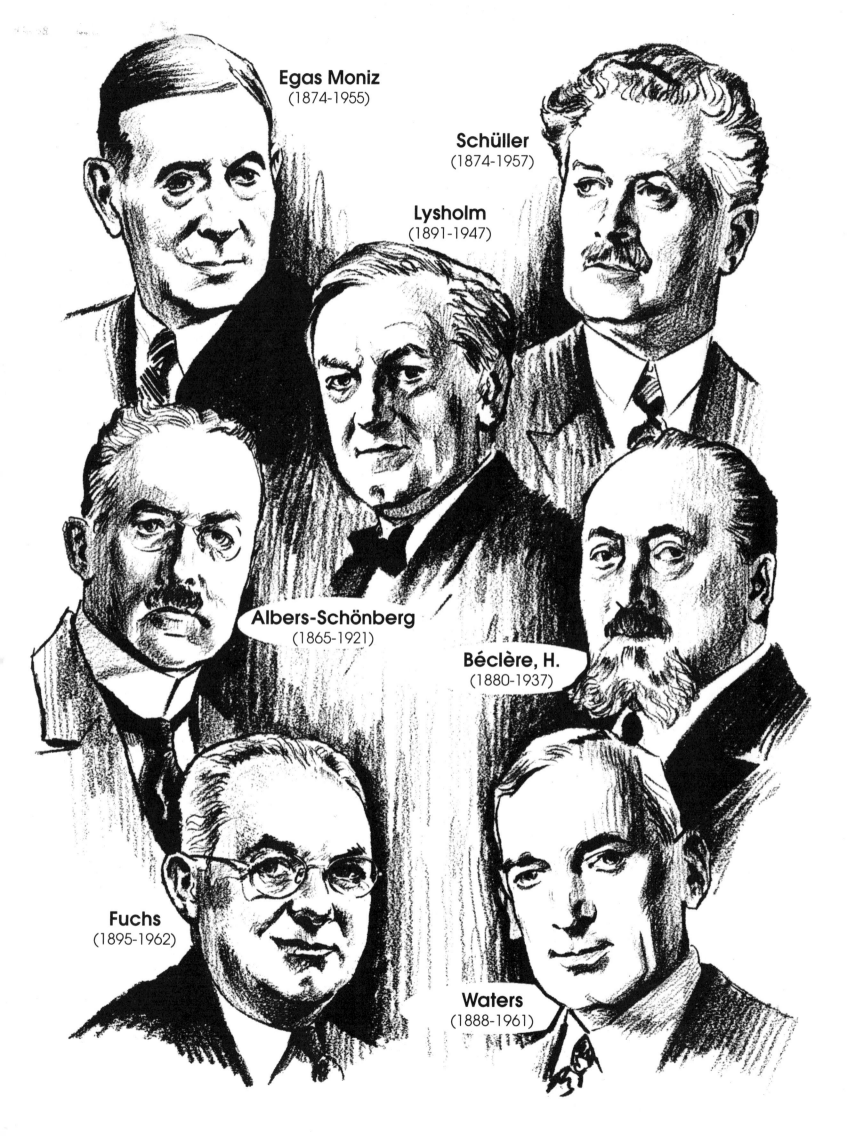

Egas Moniz
(1874-1955)

Schüller
(1874-1957)

Lysholm
(1891-1947)

Albers-Schönberg
(1865-1921)

Béclère, H.
(1880-1937)

Fuchs
(1895-1962)

Waters
(1888-1961)